Food, diet and obesity

Related titles from Woodhead's food science, technology and nutrition list:

Functional foods, ageing and degenerative disease
(ISBN-13: 978-1-85573-725-9; ISBN-10: 1-85573-725-6)
This important collection reviews the role of functional foods in helping to prevent a number of degenerative conditions, from osteoporosis and obesity to immune system disorders and cancer. Introductory chapters discuss the regulation of functional foods in the EU and the role of diet generally in preventing degenerative disease. Part I examines bone and oral health, the use of diet to control osteoporosis, the use of functional ingredients to improve bone strength, and ways of maintaining dental health. Part II discusses how obesity can be controlled, whilst Part III looks at gut health and maintaining the immune function using functional ingredients. The book concludes by reviewing research on functional foods and cancer.

Functional foods, cardiovascular disease and diabetes
(ISBN-13: 978-1-85573-735-8; ISBN-10: 1-85573-735-3)
Cardiovascular disease and diabetes pose a serious and growing risk to the health of the population in the developed world. Edited by a leading authority, this important collection reviews the role of functional foods in helping to prevent these chronic diseases. Part I examines the importance of diet in the prevention of cardiovascular disease and diabetes, with chapters on fat soluble nutrients, antioxidants and iron intake. Part II focuses on the role of phytochemicals in preventing cardiovascular disease, including chapters on isoflavones and plant sterols. Part III addresses the control of dietary fat, including the use of polyunsaturated fatty acids and fat replacers. The final part of the book reviews the use of starch and other functional ingredients in controlling cardiovascular disease.

The nutrition handbook for food processors
(ISBN-13: 978-1-85573-464-7; ISBN-10: 1-85573-464-8)
Over the past decade there has been a dramatic increase in research on the relationship between nutrition and health. Given the current interest of consumers in more nutritious food, food processors are increasingly concerned with understanding the nature of nutrient loss during food processing. This book brings together an international team of experts to summarise key findings on diet and nutrient intake, the impact of nutrients on health, and how food processing operations affect the nutritional quality of foods.

Details of these books and a complete list of Woodhead's food science, technology and nutrition titles can be obtained by:

- visiting our web site at www.woodheadpublishing.com
- contacting Customer Services (e-mail: sales@woodhead-publishing.com; fax: +44 (0) 1223 893694; tel.: +44 (0) 1223 891358 ext.30; address: Woodhead Publishing Ltd, Abington Hall, Abington, Cambridge CB1 6AH, England)

If you would like to receive information on forthcoming titles, please send your address details to: Francis Dodds (address, tel. and fax as above; e-mail: francisd@woodhead-publishing.com). Please confirm which subject areas you are interested in.

Food, diet and obesity

Edited by
David J. Mela

1871535
LIBRARY
ACC. No. 36035031
DEPT.
CLASS No.
UNIVERSITY OF CHESTER

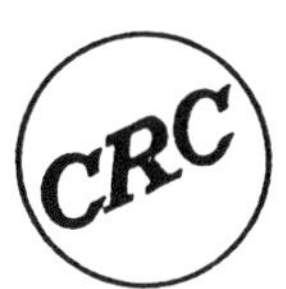

CRC Press
Boca Raton Boston New York Washington, DC

WOODHEAD PUBLISHING LIMITED
Cambridge England

Published by Woodhead Publishing Limited, Abington Hall, Abington
Cambridge CB1 6AH, England
www.woodheadpublishing.com

Published in North America by CRC Press LLC, 6000 Broken Sound Parkway, NW, Suite 300, Boca Raton FL 33487, USA

First published 2005, Woodhead Publishing Limited and CRC Press LLC
© 2005, Woodhead Publishing Limited
The authors have asserted their moral rights.

This book contains information obtained from authentic and highly regarded sources. Reprinted material is quoted with permission, and sources are indicated. Reasonable efforts have been made to publish reliable data and information, but the authors and the publishers cannot assume responsibility for the validity of all materials. Neither the authors nor the publishers, nor anyone else associated with this publication, shall be liable for any loss, damage or liability directly or indirectly caused or alleged to be caused by this book.

Neither this book nor any part may be reproduced or transmitted in any form or by any means, electronic or mechanical, including photocopying, microfilming and recording, or by any information storage or retrieval system, without permission in writing from Woodhead Publishing Limited.

The consent of Woodhead Publishing Limited does not extend to copying for general distribution, for promotion, for creating new works, or for resale. Specific permission must be obtained in writing from Woodhead Publishing Limited for such copying.

Trademark notice: Product or corporate names may be trademarks or registered trademarks, and are used only for identification and explanation, without intent to infringe.

British Library Cataloguing in Publication Data
A catalogue record for this book is available from the British Library.

Library of Congress Cataloging in Publication Data
A catalog record for this book is available from the Library of Congress.

Woodhead Publishing ISBN-13: 978-1-85573-958-1 (book)
Woodhead Publishing ISBN-10: 1-85573-958-5 (book)
Woodhead Publishing ISBN-13: 978-1-84569-054-0 (e-book)
Woodhead Publishing ISBN-10: 1-84569-054-0 (e-book)
CRC Press ISBN-10: 0-8493-3440-3
CRC Press order number: WP3440

The publishers' policy is to use permanent paper from mills that operate a sustainable forestry policy, and which has been manufactured from pulp which is processed using acid-free and elementary chlorine-free practices. Furthermore, the publishers ensure that the text paper and cover board used have met acceptable environmental accreditation standards.

Typeset by SNP Best-set Typesetter Ltd., Hong Kong
Printed by TJ International Limited, Padstow, Cornwall, England.

Contents

Contributor contact details

(* indicates main point of contact)

Chapter 1

Professor B. M. Popkin
School of Public Health
University of North Carolina at Chapel Hill
CB 8120
123 W. Franklin Street
Chapel Hill, NC
27516-3997
USA

E-mail: popkin@unc.edu

Chapter 2

Dr Camilla Verdich
Institute of Preventative Medicine
Copenhagen University Hospital
Kommunehospitalet, Entrance 23A
DK 1399, Copenhagen K
Denmark

E-mail: CV@ipm.hosp.dk

Dr Karine Clément
INSERM 'Avenir'
EA 3502
Paris VI University Nutrition Department
Hôtel-Dieu

Place du Parvis Notre-Dame
75004 Paris, France

E-mail: karine.clement@htd.ap-hop-paris.fr

Thorkild I. A. Sorensen, Professor, Dr Med Sci
Danish Epidemiology Science Centre
Institute of Preventative Medicine
Copenhagen University Hospital
Entrance 23A
DK 1399 Copenhagen K
Denmark

E-mail: tias@ipm.hosp.dk

Chapter 3

Professor Arne Astrup
Department of Human Nutrition
Centre for Advanced Food Studies
The Royal Veterinary and Agricultural University
Rolighedsvej 30
DK-1958
Frederiksberg C
Denmark

E-mail: ast@kvl.dk

Chapter 4

Professor Klaas R. Westerterp
Department of Human Biology
Maastricht University
PO Box 616
6200 MD Maastricht
The Netherlands

E-mail: K.Westerterp@HB.Unimaas.NL

Chapter 5

Dr M. I. Goran
Room 208-D
Department of Preventive Medicine
University of Southern California
1540 Alcazar Street
Los Angeles, CA
90033
USA

E-mail: goran@usc.edu

Chapter 6

Professor C. P. Herman
Department of Psychology
University of Toronto
Toronto, Ontario
M5S 3G3
Canada

E-mail: herman@psych.utoronto.ca

Chapter 7

Dr C. de Graaf
Division of Human Nutrition
Wageningen University
PO Box 8129
6700 EV Wageningen
The Netherlands

E-mail: kees.deGraaf@wur.nl

Chapter 8

Professor B. J. Rolls
Department of Nutritional Sciences
The Pennsylvania State University
226 Henderson Building
University Park, PA
16802-6501
USA

E-mail: bjr4@psu.edu

Chapter 9

Dr S. Whybrow
The Rowett Research Institute
Greenburn Road
Bucksburn
Aberdeen
AB21 9SB

E-mail: S. Whybrow@Rowett.ac.uk

Chapter 10

Dr Manny Noakes
CSIRO Health Sciences and Nutrition

PO Box 10041
Adelaide BC
SA 5000
Australia

E-mail: manny.noakes@csiro.au

Chapter 11

Dr Karen Teff
Division of Diabetes, Endocrinology and Metabolism
National Institute of Diabetes, Digestive and Kidney Disease
6707 Democracy Boulevard
Bethesda, MD
20892-5460
USA

E-mail: teffk@niddk.nih.gov

Chapter 12

Dr P. Clifton
CSIRO Health Sciences and Nutrition
PO Box 10041
Adelaide BC
SA 5000
Australia

E-mail: peter.clifton@csiro.au

Chapter 13

Professor R. D. Mattes
Department of Food and Nutrition
Purdue University
700 W State Street
West Lafayette, IN
47907-2059
USA

E-mail: mattes@purdue.edu

Chapter 14

Professor Julie Miller Jones
Department of Nutrition and Food Science
College of St Catherine
4030 Valentine Ct
Arden Hills, MN

55112
USA

E-mail: juliemjones@comcast.net

Chapter 15

Professor G. Harvey Anderson
Department of Nutritional Sciences
University of Toronto
FitzGerald Building
150 College Street
Toronto
Ontario
M5S 3E2
Canada

E-mail: Harvey.anderson@utoronto.ca

Chapter 16

Dr Kjeld Rahbek Ryttig
Farmaservice
Solhøj 13
DK-2990 Nivå
Denmark

E-mail: kjeld@ryttig.dk

Chapter 17

Professor Hans C. M. van Trijp
Marketing and Consumer Behaviour Group
Wageningen University
PO Box 8129
6700 EV Wageningen
The Netherlands

E-mail: Hans.vanTrijp@wur.nl

Chapter 18

Dr Monika Leonhardt
Institute of Animal Sciences
Swiss Federal Institute of Technology
Schorenstr 16
CH-8603 Schwerzenbach
Switzerland

E-mail: monika.leonhardt@inw.agrl.ethz.ch

Chapter 19

Dr James W. Anderson*
Metabolic Research Group
University of Kentucky
1030 South Broadway, Suite 5
Lexington, KY
40504
USA

E-mail: janders@uky.edu

Elizabeth C. Konz, RD, PhD
Graduate Center for Nutritional Sciences
Metabolic Research Group
University of Kentucky
1030 South Broadway Suite 5
Lexington, KY
40504
USA

Phone: 859-257-4058 ext. 81249
Fax: 859-257-8410
E-mail: eckonz0@email.uky.edu

Chapter 20

Hollie Raynor, PhD, RD
Brown Medical School
The Miriam Hospital
Weight Control and Diabetes Research Center
196 Richmond Street
Providence, RI
02903
USA

E-mail: hraynor@lifespan.org

Professor R. R. Wing
Brown Medical School
The Miriam Hospital
Weight Control and Diabetes Research Center
196 Richmond Street
Providence, RI
02903
USA

E-mail: rwing@lifespan.org

Chapter 21

Professor S. I. Barr
Department of Food, Nutrition and Health
Faculty of Land and Food Systems
University of British Columbia
2205 East Mall
Vancouver
British Columbia
V6T 1Z4
Canada

E-mail: sibarr@interchange.ubc.ca

Chapter 22

Dr C. Bell
School of Exercise and Nutritional Sciences
Deakin University
Geelong Waterfront Campus
Gheringhap Street
Geelong
Victoria 3217
Australia

E-mail: cbell@deakin.edu.au

Chapter 23

Dr M. S. Westerterp-Plantenga
Department of Human Biology
Maastricht University
PO Box 616
6200 MD Maastricht
The Netherlands

E-mail: M.Westerterp@HB.unimaas.nl

Chapter 24

Dr David J. Mela
Unilever Food & Health Research Institute
PO Box 114
3130 AC Vlaardingen
The Netherlands

E-mail: david.mela@unilever.com

Preface

The global epidemic of obesity raises important questions for health professionals, food companies and consumers, regarding the potential role of diet in the cause, prevention and treatment of excessive weight gain.

Scientifically, the solution can appear deceptively simple. The positive energy balance which leads to obesity can be readily corrected by just eating less or being more physically active. On the other hand, the environmental conditions of developing and developed economies have increasingly tended to facilitate excessive energy intake whilst minimising the need or opportunities to be physically active. Furthermore, obesity reflects an unusual interplay of these environmental conditions with a general underlying biological predisposition, plus individual variations in lifestyle and behaviour, which make weight control a constant challenge for many consumers. Thus, while the proximate causes and solutions are indeed 'simple' and certainly amenable to individual action, changes in the food and lifestyle environment will be critical to realistically addressing current trends at a population level.

The health implications and consumer desires related to obesity create both obligations and opportunities for nutrition professionals in the food industry. Key challenges are to apply current understanding to make everyday food products more 'weight-friendly', to identify and prove the efficacy of 'functional' foods, and to communicate responsibly and effectively around products and services for weight control.

Actions by industrial and health professionals to implement change and innovation need to be based on the best scientific evidence, and have support from independent experts. A major goal of this book was, therefore, to assemble current expert views on the relationships amongst food, energy balance and obesity. The intention is to provide an overview of current understanding and implications to support evidence-based action and innovation, with a particular emphasis on commercial products and services. The book is broadly organized around the themes of: 1) contributing factors, including physiology, lifestyle and behaviour; 2) macronutrients, including fibre and reduced-energy ingredients; and 3) public health and commercial strategies, including weight loss products and potential 'functional' ingredients.

As editor, I was gratified that so many top international experts responded enthusiastically to my invitation to contribute to this book, providing thoughtful and authoritative chapters that comprehensively address the key issues. They have provided a wealth of food for thought, which can be used to understand and evaluate many different avenues for further action and application. I thank the contributors for their willingness to share their knowledge and experience, and hope that readers will find ways to apply these in developing and delivering effective and sustainable weight control benefits for consumers.

Dave Mela

1

Global trends in obesity

B. M. Popkin, University of North Carolina, USA

1.1 Introduction

This chapter explores shifts in nutrition transition from the period termed the receding famine pattern to one dominated by nutrition-related non-communicable diseases (NR-NCDs). It examines the shifts in obesity and the speed of these changes, summarizes dietary and physical activity changes and provides some sense of the health effects and economic costs. The focus is on the world but special emphasis is given to the less understood shifts occurring in the lower- and middle-income countries of Asia, Africa, the Middle East and Latin America. This chapter shows that changes are occurring at great speed and at earlier stages of countries' economic and social development. The burden of disease from NR-NCDs is shifting towards the poor and the costs are also becoming greater than those for undernutrition. Elsewhere, we cover in detail the stages of the nutrition transition and underlying conceptual framework (Popkin, 2003).

The major themes covered in this chapter are:

- The shift in the stages of the nutrition transition are occurring rapidly and this is seen in the speed of change in obesity around the world.
- The prevalence rates and dynamic shifts in obesity in the developing world match if not exceed those in the higher income countries.
- Dietary shifts are occurring that are fairly comparable across the developing world but different from those found in the USA and in other developed countries.
- Physical activity patterns, while much less studied, appear to be changing equally dramatically.

- The burden of obesity is shifting rapidly toward the poor and lower socio-economic status groupings.
- Income growth, long-term declines in food prices, urbanization and rapid dissemination of mass media are key determinants.
- The future trends appear to be as fast if not faster than current ones.
- The requirement for large-scale programme and policy action is great.

1.2 Trends in obesity

In a series of papers published in a recent issue of *Public Health Nutrition* (available as pdf files in the Bellagio papers section of *www.nutrans.org*), the current levels of overweight in countries as diverse as Mexico, Egypt and South Africa are shown to be equal or greater than those in the United States. Moreover, the rate of change in obesity in lower- and middle-income countries is shown to be much greater than in higher-income countries (see Popkin, 2002, for the overview). Figure 1.1(a) presents the level of obesity and overweight in several illustrative countries. Most interesting is the fact that many of these countries with quite high overweight levels are very low-income. Moreover, it probably surprises many people that the levels of obesity of several countries – all with much lower income levels than the USA – are so high.

Figure 1.1(b) shows how quickly overweight and obesity status has emerged as a major public health problem in some of these countries. Compared with the USA and European countries, where the annual increase in the prevalence of overweight and obesity is about 0.25 for each, the rates of change are very high in Asia, North Africa, and Latin America – two to five times greater than in the USA.

The burden is shifting towards the poor! We show that a large number of low- and moderate-income countries already have a greater likelihood that adults residing in lower-income or lower educated households are overweight and obese relative to adults in higher income or education households (Monteiro *et al.*, 2004). This study, based on multi-level analysis of 37 nationally representative data sets, shows that countries with a GNP per capita over about $2500 are likely to have a burden of obesity greater among the poor. It also provides some idea of the set of risk factors causing obesity and other NCDs that are changing rapidly, including poor diets, inactivity, smoking and drinking.

These changes are occurring in both urban and rural areas. In one recent paper in which we examined overweight and obesity in nationally representative cross-sectional surveys on women aged 20–49 (n = 148 579) conducted from 1992 to 2000 in 36 developing countries from all regions and stages of economic development (Mendez *et al.*, 2005). We examined associations between the nutritional status of urban and rural women with national socioeconomic development indicators – gross national income

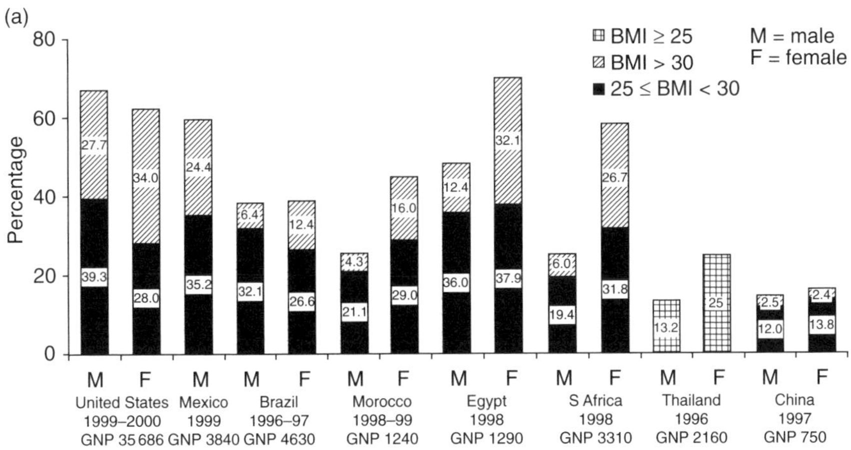

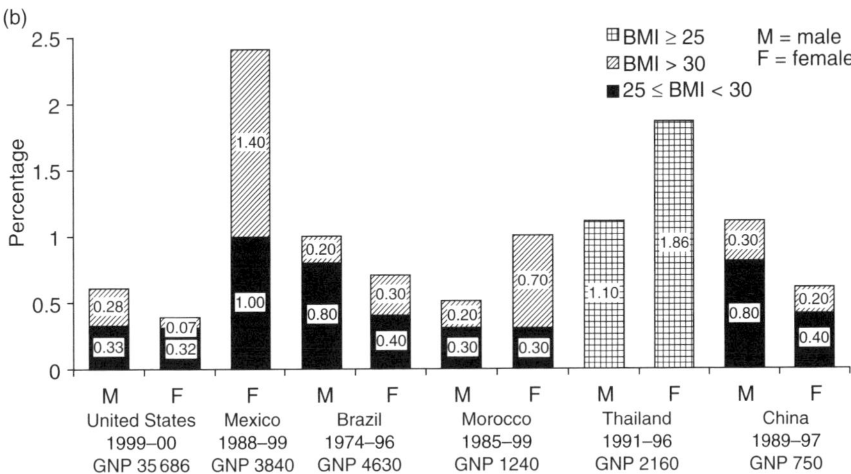

Fig. 1.1 (a) Obesity patterns and trends across the developing world; (b) obesity trends among adults in selected developing countries (the annual percentage point increases in prevalence) (*Source*: Popkin (2002) *Pub Health Nutr* 5: 93–103).

(GNI) and urbanization. Many countries had high levels of overweight in both urban and rural women. Overweight exceeded underweight in the great majority of countries: the median ratio of over- to underweight was 5.8 in urban and 2.1 in rural areas. Countries with high GNI and urbanization levels had not only high absolute levels of overweight, but small urban–rural differences in overweight and very high ratios of over- to underweight. However, even many of the poorest countries also had fairly high levels of rural overweight, and ratios of over- to underweight ≥1.0.

1.3 Dietary shifts: more fat, more added caloric sweeteners, more animal source foods

The diets of the developing world are shifting rapidly, particularly with respect to fat, caloric sweeteners and animal source foods (Popkin, 2003; Popkin and Du, 2004).

1.3.1 Edible oil

In the popular mind, the Westernization of the global diet continues to be associated with increased consumption of animal fats. Yet the nutrition transition in developing countries typically begins with major increases in the domestic production and imports of oilseeds and vegetable oils, rather than meat and milk (see Drewnowski and Popkin, 1997 for details). Fat intake increases with income, but there have also been dramatic changes in the aggregate income–fat relationship (Du *et al.*, 2004). Most significantly, even poor nations had access to a relatively high-fat diet by 1990, when a diet deriving 20% of energy (kcal) from fat was associated with countries having a GNP of only $750 per capita. In 1962, the same energy diet (20% from fat) was associated with countries having a GNP of $1475 (both GNP values in 1993 dollars).

This dramatic change arose principally from a major increase in the consumption of vegetable fats. In 1990, these accounted for a greater proportion of dietary energy than animal fats for countries in the lowest 75% of countries (all of which have incomes below $5800 per capita) of the per capita income distribution. The change in edible vegetable fat prices, supply, and consumption is unique because it affected rich and poor countries equally, but the net impact is relatively much greater on low-income countries.

1.3.2 Caloric sweeteners

Sugar is the world's predominant sweetener; however, we use the term caloric sweetener instead of added sugar, as there is such a range of non-sugar products used today. High fructose corn syrup is a prime example as it is the sweetener used in all US soft drinks. The overall trends show a large increase in caloric sweetener consumed (see Popkin and Nielsen, 2003). In 2000, 306 kcals were consumed per person per day, about a third more than in 1962; caloric sweeteners also accounted for a larger share of both total energy and total carbohydrates consumed. All measures of caloric sweetener increase significantly as GNP per capita of the country and urbanization increase. However, the interaction between income growth and urbanization is important.

1.3.3 Animal source foods

The revolution in animal source foods (ASF) refers to the increase in demand and production of meat, fish, and milk in low-income developing countries. The International Food Policy Research Institute's Christopher Delgado has studied this issue extensively in a number of seminal reports and papers (summarized in Delgado, 2003; Delgado *et al.*, 1999). Most of the world's growth in production and consumption of these foods comes from the developing countries. Thus, developing countries will produce 63% of meat and 50% of milk in 2020. It is a global food activity, transforming the grain markets for animal feed. It also leads to resource degradation, rapid increases in feed grain imports, rapid concentration of production and consumption and social change.

1.4 Physical activity changes at work, leisure, home, and travel

There are several linked changes in physical activity occurring jointly. One is a shift away from the high energy expenditure activities such as farming, mining and forestry towards the service sector. Elsewhere, we have shown this large effect (Popkin, 1999). Reduced energy expenditures in the same occupation are a second change. Other major changes relate to mode of transportation, home production and activity patterns during leisure hours. There is a marked shift away from walking to mass transportation and motorcycle use in the developing world and toward car use in the developed world. Mechanization of home production, ranging from the purchase of more processed food products to washing machines, fuel-powered stoves, microwaves and refrigerators are some of the myriad of technological changes that have reduced activity during home production (e.g. Lanningham-Foster *et al.*, 2003).

China provides interesting illustrations. Using a nationwide survey in China, Table 1.1 shows that the proportion of urban adults (male and female) working in occupations where they participate in vigorous activity patterns has decreased. In rural areas, however, there has been a shift for some towards increased physical activity linked to holding multiple jobs and more intensive effort. For rural women, there is a shift towards a larger proportion engaged in more energy-intensive work, but there are also sections where light effort is increasing. In contrast, for rural men there is a small decrease in the proportion engaged in light work effort.

In China, 14% of households acquired a motorized vehicle between 1989 and 1997. In one study we showed that the odds of being obese were 80% higher ($P < 0.05$) for men and women in households that owned a motorized vehicle compared to those which did not own a vehicle (Bell *et al.*, 2002).

Table 1.1 Labor force distribution amongst adults, aged 20 to 45, by level of activity

		Light		Vigorous	
		1989	1997	1989	1997
Urban	Male	32.7	38.2	27.1	22.4
	Female	36.3	54.1	24.8	20.8
Rural	Male	19.0	18.7	52.5	59.9
	Female	19.3	25.5	47.4	60.0

Source: China Health and Nutrition Survey, 1989–1997.

Television ownership has sky-rocketed in China, leading to greater inactivity during leisure time (see Du *et al.*, 2002).

1.5 Some key causes of change

How do we understand the causes of the changes that have occurred? First, economic theory would clearly predict the changes in diet and activity that we see. Obtaining a more varied and tasteful diet and a less burdensome work pattern is an important choice desired by most individuals. The choices being made are rational. Preferences for dietary sugars and fats are regarded by many as an innate human trait. Sweetness, in particular, serves as the major cue for food energy in infancy and childhood, and preferences for sweet taste are observed in all societies around the globe (Drewnowski, 1987). An argument has been made that preferences for dietary fats are also either innate or learned in infancy or childhood (Drewnowski, 1989). References to the desirable qualities of milk and honey (i.e. fat and sugar), cream, butter and animal fats are found throughout recorded history.

Second, an important factor is the interaction between income and consumption preferences. As we have shown in several studies, not only is income increasing, but the structure of consumption is shifting, and additional higher-fat foods are being purchased with additional income (Du *et al.*, 2004; Guo *et al.*, 2000). The China example illustrates the point: for the same extra dollar of income, an average Chinese person is purchasing higher calorie food today than s/he would have done for the same extra yuan a decade ago.

A third element is lower food prices. Delgado (2003) documents the large long-term reduction in the real costs of basic commodities in the developing world over the past several decades. He has shown that inflation-adjusted prices of livestock and feed commodities fell sharply from the early 1970s to the early 1990s, stabilized in the mid-1990s in most cases and fell again thereafter (Delgado *et al.*, 1999). Others have shown how important cost constraints might be (Guo *et al.*, 1999; Darmon *et al.*, 2002).

Fourth, we might point to the centralization of the mass media and the generation of major pushes to promote selected dietary patterns directly and indirectly via these media. There is as yet little in the way of rigorous analysis to link shifts in mass media coverage to the consumption or work patterns in the developing world, but there is an emerging literature on increased television ownership and viewing (for example, Du *et al.*, 2002; Tudor-Locke *et al.*, 2003). There is a profound cultural side not only to the globalization of mass media, but also to the related penetration of Western-style fast food outlets into the developing world. There is some evidence that these changes affect the entire culture of food production and consumption (Jin, 2000).

Fifth, an added push has come from technological factors that affect work and leisure, productivity and effort. Most of the changes affecting home production, from piped water to electricity to microwave ovens and lower-cost gas and butane ovens, reduce domestic effort. Similarly, the onset of mass transportation, the availability of cheap motor scooters and cycles and buses reduce energy expenditure in transportation. Similar profound changes affect all types of work. The computer revolution, the availability of small gas-powered systems for ploughing and many others affect the work of farmers and other workers. Importantly, the reduction in the cost of producing and distributing food, and of work-related technology, is affected by urbanization. More dense residential development cuts the costs for marketing, distribution and even production in many cases.

Finally, there are other changes in household purchasing, preparation and eating behavior that matter greatly. These include location of the purchase, consumption of food, and the processing of the foods purchased, *inter alia*. Elsewhere we have discussed the rapid shifts in sources of calories away from at-home preparation and consumption to away-from-home purchase and consumption (e.g. Nielsen *et al.*, 2002; Bisgrove and Popkin, 1996; McGuire and Popkin, 1989). There are few systematic studies of location of preparation and consumption in the developing world; however, it is clear that many important changes are occurring in both the level of processed food consumed at home and the proportion of meals consumed away from home. As the food system changes and as incomes rise, these changes are expected to intensify. Reardon and Berdegué's work on supermarkets in Latin America represents one example of a major shift in the marketing of food in the developing world (Reardon and Berdegué, 2002).

1.6 Future trends

It is always difficult to predict the future with any certainty. This is certainly the case for such a dynamic situation as relates to obesity or energy imbalance. Data presented on dietary trends give some sense that the rate of change of poor energy dense diets might be accelerating (see also Popkin, 2002). At the same time we have limited data on physical activity and energy expenditure trends so it is very hard to understand how changes will occur in this component. The data most available – information on the annual prevalence rate of change in overweight and obesity (see Fig. 1.1(a)) – are available for a small sample of countries.

The available data do suggest a rate of change in obesity in the 1–2% of the population per year for adults but there is inadequate trend data to extend this change to children aged 2–18 (see one of the limited studies, Wang *et al.*, 2002). The little data for youth would lead us to assume the rate of change in the prevalence point of overweight for youth would be only 0.5 to 0.75 vs. 1.0 to 1.5 for adults.

1.7 Implications and recommendations

The nutrition transition is most rapid, particularly in moderate income countries such as China, Mexico and Brazil. The populations involved are large. Therefore, policies and programmes must be designed to understand fully what is happening and why, and to address these issues in all their dimensions. Developing countries have paid little attention to the colossal transitions summarized in this review, and to their current and future impacts. There have been few projects and policies that have addressed diet-related chronic diseases. The evidence reviewed here indicates some elements of programmes that have been successful in limited ways. There is, however, still little experience in the field. It is important to establish a series of small, community-based projects as well as to review, evaluate and initiate national policies.

First and foremost, at national level, is the need for coordinated food and agricultural policies that consider diet-related chronic diseases. Second is pricing policy. Third are the large-scale activities that promote important, healthful components of traditional eating patterns, as in the Republic of Korea (e.g. Kim *et al.*, 2000; Lee *et al.*, 2002). Fourth are efforts, such as those in Brazil, to begin to build public awareness of the elements of the food-based dietary guidelines and physical activity patterns (Coitinho *et al.*, 2002). Finally, at community and institution levels, the main example is the school nutrition and fitness programme of Singapore. There are few examples of other community-based efforts that appear relevant at this time. Clearly, reducing child obesity and inactivity are major aspects of any programme. In most developing countries the emerging environment is highly conducive to increased obesity. Environmental assessments and changes are needed. Schools and preschools are the places to begin. From current research, many other components of programmes and policies can be identified, but there has been little large-scale implementation and evaluation.

In the promotion of physical activity and reduction of inactivity, current thinking seems to be focused on a combination of a more supportive environment: including programmes and facilities at schools, worksites, and in neighborhoods etc., and changes in educational and behavioral activities. Figure 1.2 summarizes some of the options that are being considered for improving physical activity in higher income countries. Without more research and focus on these issues at a national level, it will not be possible to set priorities or to consider programme options, especially for disadvantaged groups.

For school-based programmes, the essential set of potential strategies needed to make the food environment more health-enhancing include promoting meaningful ways of increasing consumption of lower-energy, denser, more healthful foods (e.g. fruit, vegetables and whole grains) and discouraging the consumption of foods high in fat and sodium. Similarly, attention to making healthy changes in physical activity is essential. There are a myriad of examples of what is needed, but only the most systematic efforts, such as those found in Singapore, tend to work. Operations research is needed here. Many of the programme elements needed to create successful school nutrition or other national or local efforts require piloting and evaluation. In the nutrition sector, most developing countries still focus on addressing the problems of undernutrition, even when the costs of diet-related NCDs are becoming greater than those of undernutrition. Operations research and capacity building are needed to break through this problem. The sharing and comparison of examples of successful operations research in this field could assist for the development of country-specific programmes and policies.

Many elements of a national plan must be country specific. For example, in China, the promotion of consumption of key foods, in particular soybean foods, are seen as important. This has required a major shift in agricultural policy, whereby soybean has been classified as a cash crop and not a staple, and its pricing has become more flexible. The Ministry of Agriculture now has more latitude to increase consumption of soybean products; for example, the promotion of more soybean-based foods. The qualitative 1999 Dietary Guidelines for Chinese Residents for the PRC reflect the multidimensionality of diets as well as the nutritional epidemiological transition. They aim to: reduce extremes of poverty and excess; promote good health; enhance immunity; reduce risks of stunting and rickets; and prevent CVD, hypertension, osteoporosis, and some cancers. The PRC is also considering ways to prevent further obesity, but no programmes and policies have emerged yet. Indeed, there is a general lack of proven programmes and policies to address the nutrition transition, as this review shows.

Asian countries and Pacific Small Island Developing States (SIDS) are not yet ready for the urgently needed, large-scale programme and policy initiatives to combat diet-related NCDs. Moreover, the development of food and nutrition policies and health policies represents a new and

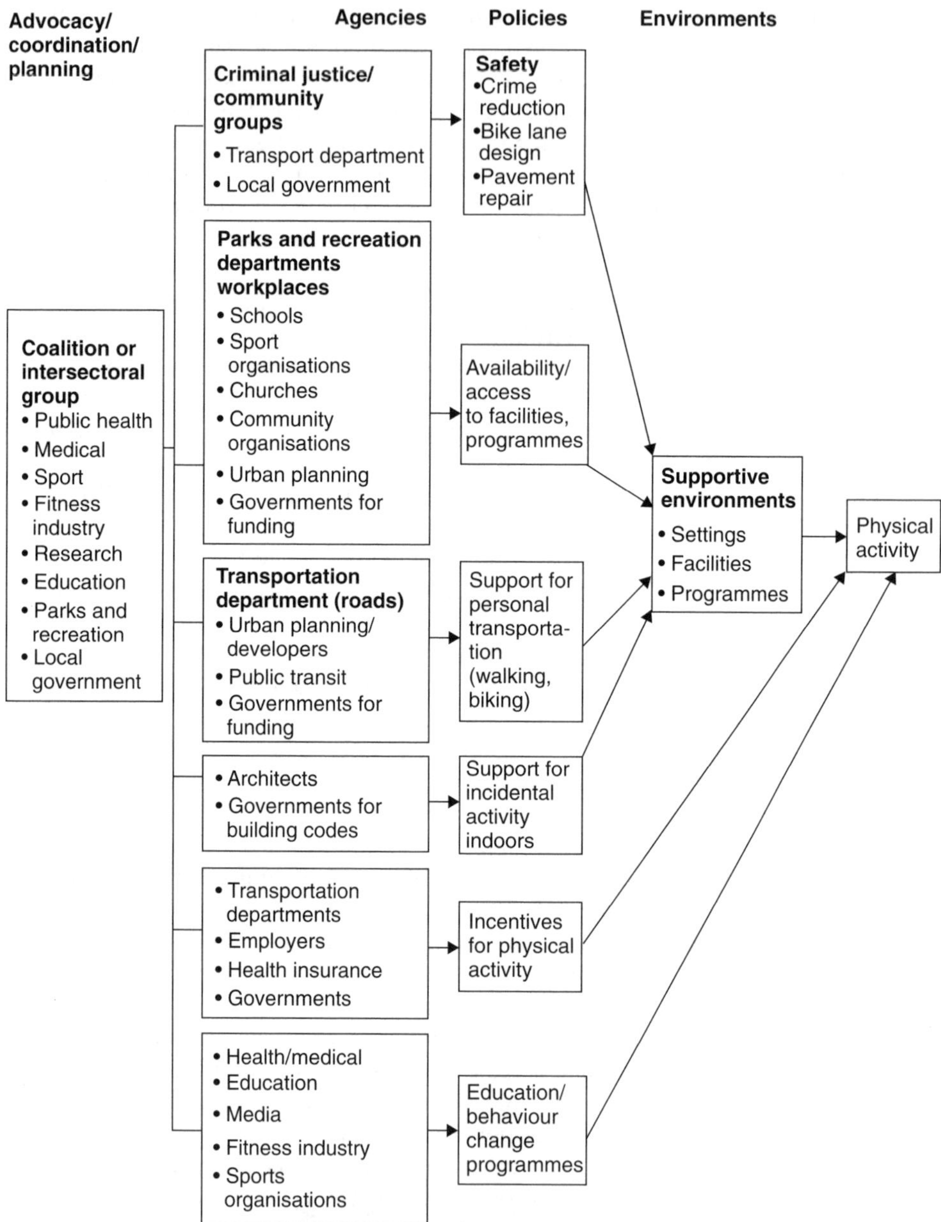

Fig. 1.2 The development of policy and environmental interventions to promote physical activity (*Source*: Jim Sallis, San Diego State University, USA).

pressing agenda for countries where problems of dietary excess and deficit exist side by side. In such countries, the prevailing policies to address deficits in the agricultural and health sectors are quite different from those needed to address problems of excess. Dietary guidelines, like the example cited above for the PRC, will be most successful if combined with systematic promotion of healthful diets. Additional elements might emerge from the examples discussed above and from future programmes, as these are evaluated for effectiveness and cost-effectiveness. Therefore, it is still premature to think of developing national investment plans. The funding and evaluation of pilot studies are, however, needed as a key step forward. The need for action is most urgent in the middle and high income countries that are further along in the nutrition transition, and in which undernutrition is becoming an issue of the past. However, even the lower low income countries have to think about the problems that are emerging from this transition in urban areas; for example, the impending diabetes epidemic in urban South Asia. The nutrition transition and diet-related chronic diseases in developing countries appear more concentrated in urban areas, where the following are greater than in rural areas: inactivity; consumption of a more energy dense diet; obesity; and many other environmental factors that promote NCDs. It would be most useful to include, as a major component of an urban nutrition strategy, NCD prevention focused on dietary, activity and body composition changes.

Capacity building is also a key need. As has been shown here, most developing countries have yet to invest significantly in prevention of diet-related NCDs. Most of these countries lack institutions that can assist macroeconomic development planners to incorporate food and nutrition issues, related to both under- and overnutrition. Some, such as the PRC, wish to develop this capability. Similarly, it is crucial to develop trained personnel and institutions for the creation of a new array of monitoring, screening and programmes and policies related to the nutrition components of NCDs. The following elements merit emphasis: school health; trade and food production; licensing and pricing policies; national, particularly urban, monitoring; mass media; and the establishment of guidelines to promote healthful elements of traditional diets and to discourage unhealthful elements of new diets.

Little is still known about patterns and trends in diets and physical activity and the causes of these trends. Large forces of global trade, technological changes in work and leisure, mass media and urbanization are linked with these massive shifts in diets and in activity. The challenge is to seek greater understanding of underlying causes of these changes, so as to address their negative effects.

There is not enough experience in most developing countries as yet to move to full-scale programmes. What is emerging is a clear need for a life cycle strategy for urban nutrition. There are also unique and important capacity building components that could be initiated immediately. Implementation and evaluation of pilot studies will be necessary. Finally, it is important to continue research on the underlying causes of the nutrition transition.

1.8 Sources of further information and advice

There are few major texts on this topic to date. There are two excellent sources for further exploration of the nutrition transition around the world and its implications. Both focus on the developing world. One is the book by Caballero and Popkin (2002), *The Nutrition Transition: Diet and Disease in the Developing World* (see Reference section). This text provides a broad overview of the critical elements of the transition, including agricultural, demographic, dietary and physical activity dimensions. Its chapter authors are eminent and include one Nobel laureate. It also has indepth case studies from Brazil and China.

The second is a publication composed of papers presented at the Bellagio conference on the nutrition transition in the developing world. The meeting was organized to allow us to assess current low and moderate income industrializing countries experience related to the nutrition transition and provide ideas for pushing forth a broader public health agenda in this area. Many of the papers were country studies which capture the key trends in dietary, physical activity, body composition and NR-NCDs that could be measured on a large-scale basis. Data are very scarce in many countries, in particular for diet and physical activity, so the main common denominator is data on overweight and obesity. Overall, we know that four-fifths of the world's burden of NR-NCDs comes from the low and moderate income countries. These papers provide some insights into ways that the key nutritional risk factors have changed.

A second set of papers explored a series of questions. These were: Is the speed of change greater today? Is there anything about the great rapidity of change in diet, activity and body composition that matters? Is the biology different? How do we interpret the high levels of both under-nutrition and overweight in the same household and are there important programmematic issues related to this topic and that of managing under nutrition during this rapid transition?

A second component relates to the issue of food and nutrition programme design. How do we get policy makers to focus on prevention of poor dietary and activity patterns and accelerated obesity? How do the politics of hunger interact with these new concerns? Are there unique points about the cardiovascular disease epidemic to consider?

A third set of papers focused on the early efforts in low and moderate income countries to prevent many of the most adverse dimensions of the rapid shift to the NR-NCD pattern. The general message is that a combination of national and local efforts focused on changes not only in the economic and physical environment but also use of mass media and various settings (work, school, community) are needed to create the wide-scale changes needed.

This full set of papers is in the February 2002 supplementary issue of *Public Health Nutrition*. The papers can all be obtained from the internet. Interested parties can go to the public website: *www.nutrans.org/*. Click on the Bellagio conference to access the papers.

1.9 References

BELL, A., COLIN, K., GE, K. and POPKIN, B. M. (2002), 'The road to obesity or the path to prevention. Motorized Transportation and obesity in China', *Obes. Res.*, **10**, 277–83.

BISGROVE, E. and POPKIN, B. M. (1996), 'Does women's work improve their nutrition? Evidence from the Urban Philippines', *Soc. Sci. Med.*, **43**, 1475–88.

CABALLERO, B. and POPKIN, B. M. (2002), *The Nutrition Transition: Diet and Disease in the Developing World*, London: Academic Press, 261.

COITINHO, D., MONTEIRO, C. A. and POPKIN, B. M. (2002), 'What Brazil is doing to promote healthy diets and active lifestyles?' *Public Health Nutr.*, **5** (1A), 263–7.

DARMON, N., FERGUSON, E. L. and BRIEND, A. (2002), 'A cost constraint alone has adverse effects on food selection and nutrient density: an analysis of human diets by linear programming', *J. Nutr.*, **132**, 3764–71.

DELGADO, C. L. (2003), 'Rising consumption of meat and milk in developing countries has created a new food revolution', *J. Nutr.*, **133**, 3907S–10S.

DELGADO, C. L., ROSEGRANT, M. W., STEINFELD, H., EHUI, S. K. and COURBOIS, C. (1999), 'Livestock to 2020: the next food revolution', Washington, DC: International Food Policy Research Institute.

DREWNOWSKI, A. (1987), 'Sweetness and obesity', in Dobbing J, *Sweetness*, London: Springer-Verlag.

DREWNOWSKI, A. (1989), 'Sensory preferences for fat and sugar in adolescence and in adult life', in Murphy C. W., Cain S. and Hegsted D. M., *Nutrition and the Chemical Senses in Aging*, New York: Academy of Sciences.

DREWNOWSKI, A. and POPKIN, B. M. (1997), 'The nutrition transition: new trends in the global diet', *Nutr. Rev.*, **55**, 31–43.

DU, S., LU, B., ZHAI, F. and POPKIN, B. M. (2002), 'The nutrition transition in China: a new stage of the Chinese diet', in Caballero B. and Popkin B. M., *The Nutrition Transition: Diet and Disease in the Developing World*, London: Academic Press.

DU, S., MROZ, T. A., ZHAI, F. and POPKIN, B. M. (2004), Rapid income growth adversely affects diet quality in China – particularly for the poor!' *Soc. Sci. Med.*, **59**, 1505–15.

GUO, X., POPKIN, B. M., MROZ, T. A. and ZHAI, F. (1999), 'Food price policy can favorably alter macronutrient intake in China', *J. Nutr.*, **129**, 994–1001.

GUO, X., MROZ, T. A., POPKIN, B. M. and ZHAI, F. (2000), 'Structural changes in the impact of income on food consumption in China, 1989–93', *Econ. Dev. Cult. Change*, **48**, 737–60.

JIN, J. (2000), *Feeding China's Little Emperors: Food, Children, and Social Change*. Palo Alto, CA: Stanford University Press.

KIM, S., MOON, S. and POPKIN, B. M. (2000), 'The nutrition transition in South Korea.' *Am. J. Clin. Nutr.*, **71**, 44–53.

LANNINGHAM-FOSTER, L., NYSSE, L. J. and LEVINE, J. A. (2003), 'Labor saved, calories lost: the energetic impact of domestic labor-saving devices', *Obes. Res.*, **11**, 1178–81.

LEE, M.-J., POPKIN, B. M. and KIM, S. (2002), 'The unique aspects of the nutrition transition in South Korea: the retention of healthful elements in their traditional diet', *Public Health Nutr.*, **5** (1A), 197–203.

MENDEZ, M. A., MONTEIRO, C. A. and POPKIN, B. M. (2005), 'Overweight now exceeds underweight among women in most developing countries!', *Am. J. Clin. Nutr.*, **81**, 714–21.

MCGUIRE, J. and POPKIN, B. M. (1989), 'Beating the zero sumgame: women and nutrition in the third world', *Food Nutr. Bull.*, **11** (4), 38–63; Part II **12** (1), 3–11.

MONTEIRO, C. A., CONDE, W. L., LU, B. and POPKIN, B. M. (2004), 'Obesity and inequities in health in the developing world', *Int. J. Obes.*, **28**, 1181–6.

NIELSEN, S. J., SIEGA-RIZ, A. M. and POPKIN, B. M. (2002), 'Trends in energy intake in the US between 1977 and 1996: similar shifts seen across age groups', *Obes. Res.*, **10**, 370–8.

POPKIN, B. M. (1999), Urbanization, lifestyle changes and the nutrition transition. *World Dev.*, **27**, 1905–16.

POPKIN, B. M. (2002), 'The shift in stages of the nutrition transition in the developing world differs from past experiences!', *Public Health Nutr.*, **5** (1A), 205–14.

POPKIN, B. M. (2003), 'The nutrition transition in the developing world', *Dev. Policy Rev.*, **21** (5), 581–97.

POPKIN, B. M. and DU, S. (2003), 'Dynamics of the nutrition transition toward the animal foods sector in China and its implications: a worried perspective', *J. Nutr.*, **133**, 3898S–906S.

POPKIN, B. M. and NIELSEN, S. J. (2003), 'The sweetening of the world's diet', *Obes. Res.*, **11**, 1325–32.

TUDOR-LOCKE, C., AINSWORTH, B. A., ADAIR, L. S. and POPKIN, B. M. (2003), 'Physical activity in Filipino youth: the Cebu Longitudinal Health and Nutrition Survey', *Int. J. Obes.*, **27**, 181–90.

REARDON, T. and BERDEGUÉ, J. A. (2002), 'The rapid rise of supermarkets in Latin America: challenges and opportunities for development', *Dev. Policy Rev.*, **20** (4), 371–88.

WANG, Y., MONTEIRO, C. A. and POPKIN, B. M. (2002), 'Trends of overweight and underweight in children and adolescents in the United States, Brazil, China, and Russia', *Am. J. Clin. Nutr.*, **75**, 971–7.

Part I

Contributing factors

2

Nutrient–gene interactions contributing to the development of obesity

C. Verdich, Danish Epidemiology Science Centre, K. Clément, INSERM, France and T. Sorensen, Copenhagen University Hospital, Denmark

2.1 Introduction

By the year 2000, being overweight or obese was more common than being normal weight among the adult population in many European countries and in the United States. Also among children and adolescents, the prevalence of obesity is increasing (Strauss and Pollack, 2001; Reilly and Dorosty, 1999; Thomsen *et al.*, 1999; Sorensen *et al.*, 1997). The World Health Organization has classified this as a global epidemic of obesity, and emphasised that it is not restricted to the industrialised countries (World Health Organization, 1997).

The epidemic of obesity has major costs on the individual level. The costs encompass excess mortality and morbidity from cardiovascular diseases, type 2 diabetes, and certain forms of cancers, osteoarthritis and sleep apnoea. Moreover, obese subjects tend to suffer from various forms of social stigmatisation and discrimination contributing to low quality of life.

The medical-care costs burden of obesity is considerable, and increasing along with the epidemic. Obesity and its related co-morbidities are estimated to account for 5.5–7% of the total health care expenditure in the United States, and 2.0–3.5% in other Western countries (Thompson and Wolf, 2001). Obesity causes a considerable increase in sick leave, and risk of early retirement (Seidell, 1998). Unfortunately, current strategies for prevention and treatment of obesity have failed to reverse the epidemic of obesity, and therefore a continued search for modifiable causes is mandatory.

The development of obesity is determined by both genetic and environmental factors. A considerable proportion of the between-subject variation in body weight is determined by genetic differences, but part of the variation must also be attributed to differences in environment. Whereas changes in the environment must be responsible for the increasing prevalence of obesity, genetic factors together with environmental factors are expected to determine who will become obese, and to which degree obesity will develop. Thus, genetic factors influence the distribution of obesity in a given environment, in a given population, at a given time.

It is generally assumed that the genes and the environment interact in some way, but there is a considerable uncertainty about how this interaction takes place. There must be a tight interaction between the genes and the environment, fully integrated in the biological system that constitutes the organism of any species. This type of interaction does not in itself contribute to the inter-individual differences, and particularly not to the explanation of why some become and stay obese and others do not. If gene–environment interaction contributes to this kind of difference, there must be between-subject variations that cannot be attributed to the genetic differences and/or the environmental differences as such. Thus, this type of gene–environment interaction implies that the response to a certain environmental exposure depends on the particular genotype, and vice versa, that the effect of a particular genotype depends on the environmental exposures.

The aim of the present chapter is to present an overview of the topics related to studying the role of genetic and environmental factors, and especially the role of nutrient–gene interaction, in the control of obesity. The strategies for identifying 'nutrient-sensitive genes' and the current knowledge on nutrient–gene interactions with a putative role in obesity will be presented.

2.2 Genetic influences on obesity

2.1 Role of genetic factors in obesity

Estimating the role of genetic factors in obesity

The estimated quantitative role of genetic factors varies dependent of study type. In family studies, the heritability has been estimated to 20–40% (Maes *et al.*, 1997). The correlations between full siblings are higher than between parents and their offspring, which suggest non-additive genetic influences, possibly due to intra- and inter-locus gene–gene interactions, or higher degree of shared environment between siblings than between parents and their offspring.

However, family studies do not allow separation of genetic effects and effects of shared family environment, which may be achieved in studies of adopted children and their biological and adoptive families and by twin studies. In adoption studies, the resemblance between the adoptee and the biological family members, i.e. parents, full and half-siblings can be ascribed

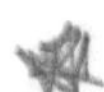

solely to genetic factors. This approach has suggested that genetic factors account for 20–40% of between-subject differences in obesity and associated phenotypes (Maes *et al.*, 1997; Stunkard *et al.*, 1986; Sorensen *et al.*, 1989).

Studies of monozygotic and dizygotic twins have revealed a much greater resemblance in the degree of obesity between monozygotic twins than between dizygotic twins, indicating that the resemblance is related to their similar genetic background rather than to their shared environment. These types of studies indicate a higher heritability, indicating that up to 60–80% of the between-subject differences can be ascribed to genetic factors. It might be argued that monozygotic twins may tend to share more environmental factors than dizygotic twins, which would lead to an overestimation of the heritability. However, twins raised apart show the same resemblance in body weight as twins raised together (Stunkard *et al.*, 1990).

Also, adoption and twin studies suggest that there are non-additive genetic influences, but generally they are difficult to disentangle from shared environmental influences, which naturally make studies of gene–environment interactions in this setting difficult. Both twin studies and adoption studies have indicated that the childhood family environment plays a minor – if any – role in adult obesity and associated phenotypes, whereas the rearing environment may have some influence while the child lives in the parents' home (Sorensen, 1996). This indicates that the within family resemblance in BMI in adults can be ascribed almost exclusively to genetic background (Sorensen *et al.*, 1992; Vogler *et al.*, 1995).

Selecting the optimal obesity phenotype for genetic research

Obesity represents merely the extreme in continuously distributed phenotypes. Although standardised categorisation of subjects as normal-weight and obese may be relevant in relation to treatment and prevention of obesity, arbitrary classification may hamper the identification of genetic and environmental factors contributing to the between-subject variation in obesity and related traits. Studies aiming to elucidate the role of genetic components and nutrient–gene interactions in obesity should ideally involve detailed characteristics of the obesity state, including a broad range of obesity-related and intermediate phenotypes (Comuzzie and Allison, 1998). Specification such as body fat percentage, or body fat distribution, and the use of intermediate phenotypes such as energy expenditure, fat oxidation and plasma levels of hormones expected to be involved in the regulation of energy balance, has several advantages. Firstly, assessment of body composition gives a more refined measure of the degree of fat accumulation, as compared to body weight and BMI. Secondly, assessment of parameters related to adipose tissue metabolism, energy expenditure and appetite regulation offers the possibility of studying genetic factors involved in the regulation of energy balance, and exploring the mechanisms of action. Thirdly, it is conceivable that intermediate phenotypes, such as energy expenditure or fat oxidation, may be less influenced by environmental factors than BMI *per se*. Indeed, when addressing the role of specific candidate genes, the phenotypic profile should include intermediate phenotypes presumed to be closely linked to the function of the candidate genes. Finally, recognising obesity as a complex heterogeneous phenotype it is of importance to address the common traits, i.e. the high body weight, as well as the heterogeneity with regard to, for example, abdominal fat accumulation, insulin sensitivity, lipid metabolism, etc. Studying the changes in the phenotype in response to environmental manipulation, e.g. changes in body weight, body composition, or abdominal obesity induced by changes in energy balance, is another potentially profitable approach to study the effect of different genotypes, and it may be particularly suitable to the study of gene–environment interaction.

2.2.2 Candidate genes and the mechanism behind their role of genetic factors

A major aim in obesity research is to identify single gene variants involved in the development of obesity and to explore and clarify the interaction between specific gene variants and specific environmental factors, with the prospect of transforming this knowledge directly into techniques for identification of individuals at risk for developing obesity, and developing strategies for specific prevention and treatment.

However, as judged from the phenotypic segregation pattern in the families, the general between-subject variations in body weight and other obesity-related phenotypes undoubtedly involve a complex oligo- or polygenic non-Mendelian pattern of inheritance.

Challenges in identifying obesity genes

There are two strategic approaches for identifying potential candidate genes. The first is to study the association between obesity or obesity-related phenotypes and already identified candidate genes selected on the basis of their known or presumed biological function, and the second one is to search for regions in the genome which appear to be linked to the obese phenotypes (Clement *et al.*, 2002a).

A great number of research groups have contributed to this field by studying candidate genes of interest in cohorts of obese patients. For this purpose they have constituted banks of clinical data and DNA in large cohorts of obese patients and controls. Group of patients and their families have been characterised with regard to clinical and biological parameters related to obesity.

In association studies, the frequency of DNA variations between groups of subjects (i.e. obese vs. non-obese) is compared, or a measurable phenotype (body mass index, fat mass, skin folds, waist/hip ratio) in subjects carrying or not carrying the given polymorphism is compared. Such association studies have been conducted in many populations collected in Europe and in North America. They have provided a huge number of putative susceptibility genes, but with small or uncertain effects (Snyder *et al.*, 2004; Swarbrick and Vaisse, 2003). This strategy has been used for both adults (Clement *et al.*, 2002a) and children (Clement and Ferre, 2003).

For the candidate genes that have shown association to the obese phenotype in one population, the general situation is lack of replication in independent populations. Association studies encounter many pitfalls, including doubtful links between the physiological roles of the candidate genes and body weight regulation. Selecting candidate genes based on rodent models of monogenic forms of obesity have been considered for genetic studies of human obesity. Although previous studies have led mainly to the discovery of rare forms of obesity in humans, it is likely that key regulatory genes discovered in animal forms of monogenic obesity may reveal genetic factors involved in the common forms of obesity in humans.

There are also difficulties related to statistical aspects including too small sample sizes of obese and controls, non-representative control groups, biased population stratification, false-positive results due to multiple testing and suppression of negative results. This state of affairs has led to development of recommendations that should secure more robust results: sufficient sample size, necessity of replication in independent groups, statistical correction for multiple testing and functional assessment of the gene variant (Cardon and Bell, 2001; Tabor *et al.*, 2002). However, only few published studies have met these criteria, such as the study on the recently described new obesity candidate gene, GAD2 (Boutin *et al.*, 2003).

Whereas the candidate gene approach may be successful in addressing the genetic factors influencing mono- or oligogenic traits, this approach seems destined to fail when studying polygenic inheritance where many different genes contribute to the phenotype in interaction with environmental factors and other genes (Comuzzie *et al.*, 2001; Comuzzie and Allison, 1998; Sorensen and Echwald, 2001). One set of problems is related to the identification of importance only in co-existence with other obesity genes, which are present in the selected populations. Another set of problems is related to the study size of relevant candidate genes as described. Further, genes identified as major obesity genes in family-based linkage studies may turn out to be of major importance only in co-existence with other obesity genes which are present in the selected populations, and have only minor influence on the common forms of obesity.

Another set of problems is related to the study size and statistical power, which in these settings is even more demanding. In very large studies it may be possible to study the gene–gene interactions, whereas collection of detailed information regarding the environment, e.g. the habitual lifestyle and thorough phenotypic profile including the response to dietary interventions is feasible only in smaller studies. Moreover, the success of addressing the gene–gene and gene–environment interaction may depend highly on the inclusion of genes and environmental factors with major effects in the model, since even relatively large effects of 'minor' genes will only become evident after adjustment for major effect (Williams, 1984). Thus, the 'major-effect' factors will need to be clarified before the 'minor-effect' factors can be addressed.

The other approach for identifying obesity genes does not involve any *a priori* hypothesis about the genes and their function. Linkage analyses in families offer the possibility of studying the co-segregation of chromosomal markers with obesity or related phenotypes. The technique of genome-wide scan offers a new way of identifying candidate genes, which can then be examined further using the candidate gene approach.

Genome-wide scans have been performed in populations originating from Europe (France, Germany, Finland, Denmark), United States and Canada (Snyder *et al.*, 2004; Swarbrick and Vaisse, 2003; Clement *et al.*, 2002a). The genome-wide scan has been performed mostly in adult populations where the severity of obesity varied (Bell *et al.*, 2004; Adeyemo *et al.*, 2003; Newman *et al.*, 2003; Suviolahti *et al.*, 2003; van Tilburg *et al.*, 2003), but also more recently in families where children sib pairs were collected (Meyre *et al.*, 2004).

In North America, the genome-wide scan has been performed either in Caucasian families, or in selected populations with less admixture such as Pima Indians, Amish, Mexican, Indian or African Americans. Usually, families in which obesity-related traits segregate are analysed using 400 to 600 polymorphic markers regularly spanning the genome, with the goal of finding the genes and pathways underlying these complex traits. The genome-wide scan approach has provided more than 30 genome-wide scans for obesity and related phenotypes.

In general, the validity of chromosomal loci identified in genetic linkage is increased if the association between the loci and the phenotype has been replicated in other studies. Twenty-five regions of the human genome harbour quantitative trait loci (QTL) replicated in two to five studies with high lod score (Snyder *et al.*, 2004; Suviolahti *et al.*, 2003; van Tilburg *et al.*, 2003). Some of the QTLs could explain a significant part of the variance of obesity-related phenotypes. Polymorphisms of candidate genes situated in the regions of linkage to obesity have been identified (Boutin *et al.*, 2003; Durand *et al.*, 2004). Some haplotypes are associated with a higher risk of obesity or diabetes. Genetic maps record annually the genes and polymorphisms implicated in the various European and American populations. Despite the power of current analyses, it has been difficult to draw conclusions concerning the role of these tested candidate genes in fully explaining links observed on the genome, which include thousands of bases. The risks associated with the development of obesity or diabetes, in subjects with these variants, are generally moderate and should be placed in the context of other, lifestyle-related, risk factors.

In mice, hundreds of QTLs have been linked to body weight or body fat (Snyder *et al.*, 2004). Among them at least six different chromosomal loci (DO1-6) have been identified by genetic mapping studies after crosses of mice strain differentially sensitive to diet-induced obesity (e.g. the AKR/J being the most sensitive strain and the SWR/J, the less sensitive strain to high fat diet) (West and York, 1998). However, the corresponding genes explaining the linkage have not been found in mice or in humans, even in chromosomal regions showing high and replicated statistical linkage.

The multi-factorial nature of obesity with a polygenic, non-Mendelian inheritance is probably responsible for the lack of success of gene identification. Several years will probably be needed to clone the genes located in the regions of linkage but the time needed for gene identification will possibly be reduced considerably thanks to the use of strategies combining analysis of genome scans and gene expression (see below).

Monogenic forms of human obesity

Although studying the role of single gene variants may not solve the enigma of obesity, this approach has led to the discovery and classification of a series of rare monogenic types of obesity, which might contribute to the understanding of the molecular basis of a number of well-known rare syndromes in which obesity is a main feature, such as the Bardet–Biedl syndrome, Prader–Willi syndrome, Alstrom and Cohen syndromes. For several of the identified genes, it remains unclear what the role of these genes are in the complex pathogenesis of the disease.

The discovery and characterisation of these rare monogenic forms of obesity provide valuable insight into the complex physiological pathways involved in the control of fat tissue size and energy balance. Such discoveries may pave the way for developing new pharmacological aids for treating obesity, irrespective of the cause. During the last decade, several rare monogenic forms of obesity have been described, involving the genes encoding for the fat cell hormone leptin (LEP) and its receptor (LEPR), pro-opiomelanocortine (POMC) and its converting enzyme, pro-hormone convertase 1, and finally the melanocortin 4 receptor (MC4R) (Clement *et al.*, 2002a). The examples below describe monogenic forms of obesity, in which the discovery of the underlying genetic cause has led to new insight into the pathways involved in the regulation of body weight.

In 1994, the product of the ob-gene, the 16 kd peptide hormone, referred to as 'leptin', was described for the first time (Zhang *et al.*, 1994) followed by the description of the rodent leptin receptor (Lee *et al.*, 1996). Mice lacking either functional leptin (ob/ob mice) or leptin receptor (db/db mice) are severely obese. Rare homozygous loss-of-function mutations in the human leptin and leptin receptor genes have been shown to lead to symptoms similar to those seen in ob/ob and db/db animals, including early onset of severe obesity, abnormal eating behaviour, and hypogonadotropic hypogonadism (Clement *et al.*, 1998; Montague *et al.*, 1997; Ozata *et al.*, 1999). Several studies have suggested a possible association between more common polymorphisms in the human leptin and leptin receptor gene and obesity, but it has not been possible to confirm these associations (Cancello *et al.*, 2004).

The role of genetic variants of the Melanocortin 4 receptor (MC4R), the receptor for alpha-melanocyte-stimulating hormone (αMSH), in the regulation of body weight and obesity in humans has been addressed in several studies (Sina *et al.*, 1999; Vaisse *et al.*, 1998, 2000). The frequency of rare heterozygous MC4-R missense and frameshift mutations has been found to be 4% in a population of morbidly obese subjects (Vaisse *et al.*, 2000) but low in normal weight subjects. Altogether, these findings suggest a dominant pattern of inheritance with variable penetrance and reduced expressivity (Vaisse *et al.*, 2000), although also recessive, and dominant negative pattern inheritance have been described (Biebermann *et al.*, 2003; Farooqi *et al.*, 2000). The molecular mechanisms for the effect of these mutations on body weight regulation are multiple including impaired trafficking of the receptor to the cell surface, impaired binding of αMSH, and impaired ability to generate cAMP (Lubrano-Berthelier *et al.*, 2003; Yeo *et al.*, 2003; Nijenhuis *et al.*, 2003). Among obese subjects, phenotypic characteristics have been shown not to differ between carriers and non-carriers of the mutations, but carriers tended to have a higher prevalence of childhood obesity (Vaisse *et al.*, 2000). Binge eating has been suggested as a major phenotypic trait in obese carriers of MC4R mutations (Branson *et al.*, 2003), but these findings are controversial, and have for instance not been confirmed in a more recent study (Hebebrand *et al.*, 2004).

Where other known forms of monogenetic obesity are recessive, and associated with other endocrine abnormalities, functional polymorphisms of the MC4-R gene have been suggested to be associated with a dominant non-syndromic form of obesity, and it is the most frequent genetic cause of obesity described to date (Sina *et al.*, 1999; Vaisse *et al.*, 2000). Others have, however, identified features of a distinct syndrome, including increased linear growth, hyperphagia and elevated insulin levels (Farooqi *et al.*, 2003). These clinical traits have, however, not been retrieved in all the tested populations.

Different types of obesity mutations

Until recently, mutations in the coding regions have been the major focus in the research addressing obesity genes. Localising the coding region of a gene is far less complicated than localising all of the regulatory elements. In addition, knowing the structure and the function of the gene product, it is possible to predict the potential effect of changes in a specific area of the coding region. However, mutations in the non-coding region have gained increasing attention. Addressing the regulatory regions of putative obesity genes may lead to discovery of gene variants involved in obesity. In addition, combining genotyping with studies of the gene expression in specific tissues and in response to specific exposures, such as changes in fat intake or calorie restriction, will improve the understanding of the specific mechanisms of gene regulation and the mechanism for regulatory gene variants.

During the last years, mutations and polymorphisms in the promoters of several putative obesity genes including 5HT receptor, CART, UCP2, UCP3, TNFalpha, resistin, leptin and more recently adiponectin have been suggested to be associated with obesity-related phenotypes (Cancello *et al.*, 2004; Engert *et al.*, 2002; Esterbauer *et al.*, 2001; Halsall *et al.*, 2001; Hoffstedt *et al.*, 2000; Mammes *et al.*, 2000; Rosmond *et al.*, 2000; Yamada *et al.*, 2002). However, several of these observations are challenged by negative findings, and still need to be replicated in additional studies.

Physiological mechanisms behind the genetic effects in obesity
Development of obesity is very slow, ongoing for several years, and is typically considered to be a result of inappropriate adaptation of the systems involved in control of energy balance to either a primarily increased energy intake or reduced energy expenditure, leading to a passive accumulation of surplus energy as body fat.

Studies addressing the heritability of intermediate phenotypes have suggested that 30–50% of between-subject differences in metabolic variables, and 25–50% of between-subject variation in energy intake can be ascribed to genetic factors (Bouchard *et al.*, 1989; de Castro, 1993). These findings suggest that the search for specific genetic effects should encompass both components of the energy balance.

However, the paradigm of obesity as a passive storage of the surplus of energy may be insufficient. Active accumulation of fat in the adipose tissue, due to dys-regulations of the adipose tissue balance between release of fat and fat accumulation, followed by a subsequent corresponding regulatory adjustment of the energy balance should be considered (Sorensen, 2003b).

Table 2.1 illustrates the pathways in which genetic polymorphisms may affect the physiological pathways involved in the regulation of energy balance, hereby increasing the susceptibility to developing obesity in a given environmental setting. Examples of putative candidate genes are given for each pathway.

2.2.3 The epidemic of obesity, the role of environment and the interaction between genes and lifestyle

As mentioned, there is no doubt that obesity is strongly influenced by environmental factors and that changes in the environment with which our genetic background interacts, must be the direct cause of the rapid increase in the prevalence of obesity worldwide. This implies that prevention of obesity may be achieved through modification of the environmental factors. However, knowing the basis for the gene–environment interactions in obesity may pave the way for more targeted prevention strategies, and hereby a better success in the prevention of obesity. Given that genetic factors mediated the susceptibility to obesity in a given environmental setting and that different genes provide susceptibility to different types of

Table 2.1 The different mechanisms by which genetics are expected to play a role in the development of obesity. Examples of putative candidate genes are given for each category. The genes are annotated with the approved gene symbol (Human Genome Nomenclature Database)

Level	Physiological mechanism	Candidate genes
Adipose tissue		
Auto regulation	Adipocyte differentiation, fat accumulation	FOXC2, PPARA, PPARD, PPARG, RXRA, RXRB
Metabolic function	Balance between fat release and fat accumulation	VLDLR, LIPE, LPL, SCD, UCP2, ADRB1, ADREB2, ADRB3, ADRA2A, ADRA2B, INSR
Endocrine function	Signals from adipose tissue to central regulation of energy balance	LEP, LEPR, NPPA, SPARC, TNF, IL6, AMP1
Energy intake		
Central	Hypothalamic neurotransmitters or receptors	NPY, NPYR, POMC, MC4R, LEPR, CART, 5HT2C, CCKAR, AGRP, GHSR, POMC
Peripheral	Hormones or other signalling compounds involved in appetite regulation	CCK, APOA4, GHRL, PPY, GCG
Food preferences	Preference for sweet, fat, aversion to certain fruits and vegetables due to high sensitivity to bitter taste	TAS1R, TAS2R
Energy expenditure		
Central	Hypothalamic neurotransmitters or receptors	MC4R, MC3R
Mediator	Symphatoadrenergic system	ADRB1, ADREB2, ADRB3, ADRA2A, ADRA2B
Effector	EE as such, Fat oxidation	UCP1, UCP2, UCP3

environmental influences, the context of environment will be a critical factor in determining which genes will be identified (Barsh *et al.*, 2000; Leibel, 1997).

In a restrictive environment characterised by low food resources and high demand for physical activity, obesity may be a rare phenomenon. Since the restrictive environment may have been prevailing throughout the development of mankind, it can be speculated that the physiological defence against weight loss and under-nutrition are stronger than the defence mechanisms protecting against weight gain. As hypothesised by Neel in the 1960s, gene variants now associated with type 2 diabetes and obesity have helped our early ancestors survive in a restrictive environment (Neel, 1999). This theory, commonly referred to as 'the thrifty gene hypothesis', states that what is now seen as a susceptibility to obesity and diabetes may indeed be a conserved mechanism of economical management of body energy resources.

Basically, weight gain will only occur when energy intake exceeds energy expenditure, and it may therefore be stated that the reason why more and more people are becoming obese is that they either eat too much or have too low level of physical activity. This highly simplified statement may capture the essence of the mechanism by which our environment and our behaviour promotes obesity, although there is no convincing evidence available to support the contention. Thus, there is no evidence precluding the alternative hypothesis that the epidemic is due to an increased primary accumulation of fat in the adipose tissue that subsequently leads to a corresponding adjustment of the energy intake relative to the energy expenditure. Further, the prevailing opinion does not hold any other keys to prevention than telling the public to eat less and increase their physical activity, which has not succeeded in reducing the prevalence of obesity. Obviously, a more refined strategy for prevention is needed, and one of the major challenges in obesity research is to identify the environmental factors responsible for the increasing prevalence and reveal the interaction between environmental and genetic factors.

Macronutrient composition of the diet and obesity

Although fat intake is one of the potential obesity promoting factors that has gained most attention in obesity research, the role of fat intake in development of obesity is still controversial, and the findings are not consistent. In animal models, changing from a low-fat diet to a high-fat diet leads to an increase in body fatness and an increase in the inter-individual and interstrain variation in body fatness, suggesting a genetic susceptibility to become obese on a high fat diet (West *et al.*, 1995; Salmon and Flatt, 1985). Epidemiological studies have not so far led to any clear conclusions on the role of fat intake and obesity in humans (Lissner and Heitmann, 1995). In general, cross-sectional studies have indicated positive associations between dietary fat energy percentage and body weight, but such studies cannot distinguish between possible effects of obesity on the fat intake, vice versa or common effects on both obesity and fat intake of an underlying third factor.

There are some paradoxical observations regarding the relationship between reported fat intake and obesity that raise the suspicion that there is no simple relation between the two. In the USA and in many European countries, fat intake has decreased during the last decade, whereas the prevalence of obesity has increased. This may be interpreted as an indication that reducing dietary fat may not lead to a concomitant reduction in obesity. However, increased under-reporting of fat intake may bias these observations (Heitmann *et al.*, 2000), and subgroups of the population may have increased their fat intake and become obese, whereas others may have reduced their fat intake. In line with the findings from animal models, a high habitual fat energy percentage has been shown to be associated with a higher mean BMI, as compared to low fat consumers (Macdiarmid *et al.*, 1996). Another common feature between animal and human studies is that between-subject variation is higher in high fat consumers, and that some individuals appear to be protected from developing obesity even when consuming a high fat diet (Macdiarmid *et al.*, 1996).

Results from prospective observational studies do not support that high fat intake lead to later obesity. However, also these studies are inconsistent, and may be confounded by people modifying food intake in order to prevent changes in body weight or that for other reasons the baseline food recording does not reflect food habits during the follow-up period (Lissner and Heitmann, 1995).

Intervention studies generally support the hypothesis about a relationship between fat intake, energy intake and eventual weight change. *Ad libitum* intake of a low fat diet has been shown to induce a mean weight loss of 1–4 kg over a period of 1–12 months, and has further shown a dose–response relationship between the reduction in fat intake and weight loss (Astrup *et al.*, 2000a,b). Although a weight loss of 0.5–1 kg per month may occur during the first month of such an intervention, weight loss will in many cases tend to level off, which may be due either to adaptation to the diet or to cessation of compliance. If the dietary effect holds over longer periods of time, then reduction of fat intake may be effective in prevention of further development of obesity.

Fat content and energy density of the diet are highly correlated, and only a few studies have targeted the effect of energy density and fat content separately. These studies have indicated that energy density rather than fat content *per se* may favour increase in energy intake. However, it might be hypothesised that, in subjects with a genetic predisposition to low fat oxidation and high fat accumulation in adipose tissue, fat intake *per se* could be expected to promote obesity. Further, genetic factors may influence the satiety effect of fat and the preference for fat and may cause some people to markedly increase their food intake in response to a high fat diet.

Taken together, both animal studies, epidemiological observational studies, and intervention studies offer substantial support to the hypothesis that high fat energy percentage or high energy density may play a role in the development of obesity. Increase in dietary carbohydrate and protein energy percentage will cause a reduction in dietary fat energy percentage, and vice versa. Epidemiological studies have suggested a positive association between fat–sugar ratio in the diet and BMI (Bolton-Smith and Woodward, 1994). Recent intervention studies have, however, shown similar weight losses in groups of obese subjects following an energy restricted diet with either low or medium fat content (Pelkman *et al.*, 2004; Petersen *et al.*, 2003). With respect to the type of carbohydrates, intervention studies have indicated no differences in weight loss during intake of a low-fat diet rich in either simple or complex carbohydrates (Saris *et al.*, 2000). However, there is evidence that high intake of simple carbohydrates in liquid form (soft drinks) may predispose to weight gain (DiMeglio and Mattes, 2000; Ludwig *et al.*, 2001; Raben *et al.*, 2002), and that reducing the intake of carbonated drinks sweetened with sugar can limit the development of obesity in school children (James *et al.*, 2004). Animal studies have indicated inverse relationships between dietary protein content and energy intake with between-strain differences in response, which suggest a nutrient–gene interaction (West *et al.*, 1995). Intervention studies have suggested that a low-fat high-protein diet may lead to a larger weight reduction compared with a low-fat high-carbohydrate diet (Baba *et al.*, 1999; Skov *et al.*, 1999). Recent intervention studies suggest that low carbohydrate diet with a high protein and fat content (the so-called Atkins diet) may be superior to the low-fat–high-carbohydrate diet in terms of weight reduction (Foster *et al.*, 2003; Samaha *et al.*, 2003). However, large-scale intervention studies are required to determine long-term safety and efficacy of these dietary strategies for both prevention and treatment.

Other dietary factors

During later years, several lines of studies have indicated a relationship between dairy calcium and regulation of body weight (Zemel, 2004). Observational studies have shown a lower prevalence of obesity and rate of weight gain for subjects reporting a high calcium intake (Heaney, 2003; Teegarden, 2003). In addition, intervention studies have indicated that high intake of dairy calcium may aid intentional weight loss and prevent weight gain (Davies *et al.*, 2000).

2.3 Nutrient-sensitive genes

2.3.1 Definition of nutrient-sensitive genes

Naturally, numerous genes are involved through their gene products in the entire biological system regulating and responding to food intake and processing and metabolisation of nutrients. In the present context, the nutrient-sensitive genes are defined as genes of which the transcriptional activity is influenced – enhanced or reduced or even turned on or off by – reduced or increased energy intake (calorie restriction and overfeeding, respectively) or by specific nutrients. Thus, this is a general biological phenomenon common to individuals of a species, and it should be distinguished from nutrient–gene interaction, which refers to inter-individual differences between members of a species.

2.3.2 Nutrient-sensitive candidate genes

The study of expression of specific candidate genes during changes in the nutritional environment, e.g. during fasting or intake of food enriched in fat, is an alternative approach in finding genetically defined pathways. Several candidate genes have been tested to decipher whether or not their level of expression in key tissues involved in body weight regulation (in humans, mostly adipose tissue and muscle) is modulated by change of environmental conditions.

Most of the human studies have aimed at analysing the changes of expression after drastic caloric restriction in obese subjects (very low calorie diet, VLCD). Most of the genes studied encode proteins involved in three different functional groups: (i) metabolic enzymes and related signalling proteins or receptors such as the hormone-sensitive lipase (HSL), the lipoprotein lipase (LPL) involved in triglyceride hydrolysis and synthesis, respectively, adrenoreceptor genes and uncoupling proteins; (ii) factors involved in adipogenic process such as the transcription factors C/EBP, PPAR and SREBP1c; (iii) proteins secreted by adipose tissue such as leptin, TNFα and inflammation-related proteins such as interleukin 8. As expected, severe caloric restriction leading to increased lipolysis and decreased lipid synthesis and improvement of insulin sensitivity in adipose tissue was associated with increased expression of HSL (Kolehmainen *et al.*, 2002; Richelsen *et al.*, 2000) and alpha-2-adrenergic receptor (Stich *et al.*, 1997, 2002), and in some but not all studies of adiponectin (Garaulet *et al.*, 2004; Liu *et al.*, 2003), as well as decreased expression of the LPL (Richelsen *et al.*, 2000), leptin, and TNFα genes (Bastard *et al.*, 1999). The adipose tissue transcription factors are also mobilised in this situation (Bastard *et al.*, 1999; Kolehmainen *et al.*, 2002; Redonnet *et al.*, 2002). The change in expression of new adipose tissue genes was also observed, although the exact role of these factors in the physiology of adipocyte is not known. Adiponutrin is an example of such a situation. This newly identified non-secreted adipocyte protein was shown to be regulated by changes in energy balance in rodents. Human studies indicated that adiponutrin gene expression is highly regulated by changes in energy balance either in the very short term or longer term (Baulande *et al.*, 2001; Liu *et al.*, 2004).

Some of the changes in gene expression induced by weight loss have not been consistently reproduced, and the discrepancies may be attributed to the time of adipose tissue sampling over the course of weight loss. In some studies, tissue biopsies were obtained during active weight loss, whereas in others the biopsies were performed after weight stabilisation, which probably is associated with a new metabolic status.

2.3.3 Expression profiling of nutrient-sensitive genes

The possibilities of studying multiple gene expression patterns in response to various nutritional conditions opened a new era for seeking pathways involved in the response to nutritional changes. The key issue is to dissect and characterise the regulatory pathways and networks involved in energy balance and to define the resulting signalling patterns in gene expression. This approach will facilitate a more integrative picture of the complex biologic process.

The technology for the study of many RNA at the same time, i.e. micro-array, is now available (Copland *et al*., 2003). Micro-array technology is based on the simple concept of dot blot and northern blot analysis, where the hybridisation is reversed, as the probes are put on a filter and the bulk RNA is labelled. One can study very large numbers (~100 000) of cDNA sequences or synthetic DNA oligomers on a glass slide (or other substrate like filters) in known locations on a grid. The target RNA sample is labelled and hybridised. The measured amount of RNA bound to each square in the grid reflects the level of expression of the gene.

While initially used for simple organisms (e.g. yeast), this approach now indexes thousands of known and newly discovered genes into various large groups defined by expression similarities in terms of physiological pathways, for example respiration, cell division, and response to chemical or thermal stress. Micro-array DNA screening is now applied to the understanding of complex diseases including cancer and ageing. This technique can be applied to many other both basic and clinical research problems, including the consequence of nutritional changes on the modification of gene transcripts.

In humans, these techniques have been used to define molecular signatures of the physiology of insulin and thyroid hormone action. Variations in gene expression in muscle of healthy men treated with triiodothyronine (T3) has been investigated using cDNA micro-arrays representing 24 000 human genes (Clement *et al*., 2002b). It showed up-regulated genes encoding for proteins involved in a wide range of cellular functions including transcriptional control, mRNA maturation, protein turnover, signal transduction, cellular trafficking and energy metabolism. A lot of these genes were new targets of T3 action (Clement *et al*., 2002; Viguerie and Langin, 2003). Similar findings were made regarding the transcription consequences of insulin action in muscle. By analysing the global changes in mRNA levels after a hyper-insulinemic euglycemic clamp in healthy subjects, it was observed that a large number of transcripts were significantly modified. Most of the genes with known function are novel targets of insulin, and may define a transcriptional signature of insulin action in human skeletal muscle (Rome *et al*., 2003). Studies in diabetics of different origin have also showed differential modulation of key genes involved in different cellular processes such as cell respiration or transcriptional control of gene involved in glucose and lipid metabolism (Permana *et al*., 2004). Other studies are, however, necessary to prove the primary roles of these genes and their importance in determining insulin resistance and development of diabetes.

Increasing data suggest that adipose tissue produces inflammation and immunity molecules suspected to be involved in obesity and related complications. However, the pattern of expression and the nutritional regulation of these molecules are not well understood in humans. By analysing gene expression profiles of subcutaneous white adipose tissue from obese subjects during low calorie diet (VLCD) using cDNA microarray, it was described that calorie restriction-induced weight loss leads to the regulation of a wide variety of genes and in particular inflammation-related molecules in human adipose tissue. Weight loss decreases the expression of inflammatory markers in white adipose tissue of obese subjects and leads to the concomitant increased expression of molecules with anti-inflammatory properties. The vast majority of the gene transcripts were expressed in cells from the stroma vascular fraction of adipose tissue. This type of study also paves the way to future clinical and cellular studies aimed at determining the impact of these molecular adaptations on the development of insulin resistance (Clement *et al.*, 2004).

Although information and resources are growing, it should be kept in mind that there are difficulties and pitfalls in the interpretation of microarray data, and progress still has to be made. One aspect is the tremendous source of variability at many levels. Thus, mRNA measurements are inherently highly variable (biological variability). The variability also depends on the level of expression of the gene (low vs. highly expressed genes). The methods by themselves induce variability: mRNA extraction, hybridisation (variability due to temperature, time, mixing), probe labelling (the chemistry of the fluorescent label is different), image analysis and scanning (laser and detector). In addition, measurement of thousands of values can result in the observation of large differences that are only attributable to the random normal distribution of the data, and adequate procedures for multiple testing have to be applied.

The goal of future projects in this field should aim at characterising clusters of genes that are recruited or modified by the given nutritional conditions, their links in biological families, their co-regulation in different tissues, gene markers specific for some nutrients, differences/similarities in different models, and eventually the patterns of tissue expression in individuals with different genetic polymorphisms in these genes. Another challenge will be to relate the groups of genes mobilised by environmental changes and the regions of linkage with obesity, so as to identify tissue targets which might be located in these regions. The integration of all information coming from expression patterns observed in the various models of energy restriction or abundance in human is among the objectives.

2.4 Interactions between genetic background and diets

Nutrient–gene interaction deals with the differential functional and eventual phenotypic effects of different doses – ranging from zero to excessive amounts – of total energy intake or specific nutrients, in combination with different gene variants. Nutrient–gene interaction addresses inter-individual differences within a species, for example, the biological basis for development of obesity in some but not in other individuals. Genetic differences that induce different risks and degrees of obesity without modifying the response to differences in the diet, e.g. its fat content, may not be considered to contribute to nutrient–gene interactions. Similarly, dietary differences that induce different risks and degrees of obesity, without modification of the effects of genetic differences, do not contribute to nutrient–gene interactions. The nutrient–gene interaction can, of course, operate at the level of modifications of the transcriptional activity of nutrient-sensitive genes, but not necessarily so. The nutrient–gene interaction may as well take place at any downstream post-transcriptional step in the function of nutrient-sensitive genes and of other genes of which the transcriptional activity is not nutrient-sensitive. On the other hand, the search for polymorphisms in genes involved in nutrient–gene interaction may become very profitable, and the technology now makes this feasible on a genome-wide basis.

The classical example and model of nutrient–gene interaction is phenylketonuria (Følling's disease), which leads to severe mental retardation in the carriers of a mutation in the gene for the enzyme phenylalanine hydroxylase if the subjects are fed a diet containing the amino acid phenylalanine while the brain is growing. If the individuals with this mutation avoid phenylalanine in the diet during this period, then the brain develops normally, and they may return to a normal diet, containing phenylalanine, when they are grown up (women with the mutation who get pregnant should, however, return to the restricted diet in order to protect the brain development of their unborn child).

2.4.1 Strategies for analysing the interaction between genetic background and diet

There are several strategies for addressing the possible interaction between genetic background and diet composition in the development of obesity. Both animal models and human studies allow for the study of the interaction between genotype and diet and between diet and gene expression. Animal studies can be designed to address the effect of a specific genetic modification on susceptibility to the obesity promoting effect of a high-fat diet, and the effect of diet on gene expression in various tissues and organs. However, only human studies will reveal the complex interaction between genetic and environmental factors responsible for human obesity and hence for the current epidemic of obesity. Human studies addressing the nutrient–gene interaction in obesity can be divided into epidemiological observational studies and intervention studies, addressing the interaction of various environmental factors with either overall genetic predisposition for development of obesity or with specific gene variants.

Epidemiological observational studies

Interaction between overall change in environment and genetic background may be revealed in studies of subjects of different ethnic origin who have been exposed to a so-called Westernised environment. One example is the increase in the prevalence of obesity in Japanese migrating to Hawaii or the USA (Curb and Marcus, 1991). In some ethnic groups, such as the Pima Indians living in Arizona, and the population in the Western Samoa, adoption of a Western lifestyle has led to a prevalence of obesity exceeding that in the USA and other Western countries (Knowler *et al.*, 1991; Krosnick, 2000; Hodge *et al.*, 1994). Finally, the recent dramatic increase in the prevalence of obesity in Mauritius, has been shown to be more pronounced among Creole than in Indian, and less pronounced in Chinese Mauritians (Hodge *et al.*, 1996). Although cultural differences may still play a role, such findings suggest an interaction between a 'thrifty genotype' prevailing in some ethnic groups and the Western lifestyle (Hodge *et al.*, 1996). The apparently specific genetic predisposition for obesity of the Pima Indians in Arizona has been studied thoroughly, but so far the specific genetic background has not been identified.

Prospective studies can address the association between habitual diet and weight changes over time for subjects with different degrees of genetic predisposition. Using this approach, Heitmann and colleagues investigated the interaction between genetic predisposition to obesity and fat intake in the Prospective Study of Women in Gothenburg, Sweden (Heitmann *et al.*, 1995). Baseline fat intake adjusted for total energy intake was found to be positively related to subsequent 6-year weight gain only in women who were already overweight, who had at least one obese parent, and whose fat intake at baseline exceeded 40% of the total energy. This observation suggests the existence of a genetic predisposition for gaining weight on a high fat diet, but confirmation in other studies is needed. The finding is in accordance with clinical studies showing a reduced fat oxidation rate following a high-fat test meal in post-obese subjects, with a genetic predisposition to obesity, compared with never obese subjects (Astrup *et al.*, 1994; Raben *et al.*, 1994).

A few epidemiological observational studies have addressed the interaction between lifestyle factors and specific gene variants in relation to obesity and related phenotypes.

The EPIC–Heidelberg study is a large European prospective investigation study of the potential interaction between dietary fatty acid intake, assessed by food frequency questionnaire, and common allelic variants of candidate genes on the obesity phenotypes (Nieters *et al.*, 2002). They found that the Pro12Ala variant of one of the nuclear receptor peroxisome proliferator-activated receptor genes, the PPARγ2 gene, as well as common polymorphisms in the leptin, and tumor necrosis factor (TNFα) gene, may interact with the intake of linoleic acid and arachidonic acid (Nieters *et al.*, 2002). Subjects carrying the Ala allele of the PPARγ 2 gene had a higher odds ratio for obesity with high intake of arachidonic acid compared with subjects homozygous for the Pro allele. The analysis initially showed that total fat intake as well as intake of *n*-6 polyunsaturated fatty acids were significant predictors of obesity, but when linoleic and arachidonic acid were included in the analysis the effect of total fat intake was not longer significant. Thus, this study suggests a specific nutrient–gene interaction between common polymorphisms in candidate genes and dietary intake of *n*-6 fatty acids in obesity.

Prospective population-based cohort studies have suggested gene–nutrient interaction involving the PPARγ2 gene and fat intake. Based on a study including about 600 non-diabetic subjects, Luan and colleagues have shown an interaction between the ratio of polyunsaturated fat to saturated fat (P:S ratio) and the Pro12Ala polymorphism on both BMI and fasting insulin. With a low P:S ratio the Ala carriers had a higher BMI than subjects homozygote for the Pro allele, whereas the opposite was seen in subjects with a high P:S ratio (Luan *et al.*, 2001). Data from the Québec Family Study have suggested that carriers of the Ala allele in general have a higher BMI, and larger fat depots, but that total fat intake and intake of SFA is associated with features of the metabolic syndrome and degree of obesity only in subjects homozygous for the Pro allele (Robitaille *et al.*, 2003). These findings are supported by data from the Nurses' Health Study, recently indicating an interaction between total fat intake, and fat composition, and the Pro12Ala gene variant in determining both BMI and HDL cholesterol (Memisoglu *et al.*, 2003). A positive association between total fat intake and body weight was seen in women homozygous for the Pro allele, with no association between fat intake and body weight in carriers of the Ala allele. Further an inverse association was seen between MUFA intake and body weight in Ala carriers only (Memisoglu *et al.*, 2003).

In addition to the studies focusing on the PPARγ gene variant, Martinez and colleagues have recently shown an interaction between the Gln27Glu variant in the beta adrenergic receptor and habitual carbohydrate intake, indicating that women carrying Glu27 and having a carbohydrate intake above the median are more prone to obesity (Martinez *et al.*, 2003). Further the possible role of the PPARα L162V variant in the metabolic syndrome has recently been investigated, finding no difference in the frequency of the V allele in cases as compared to controls, although the V allele was associated with a higher plasma level of apolipoprotein B and triglycerides (Robitaille *et al.*, 2004). No differences in BMI or waist circumference were observed between carriers of the V allele and subjects homozygous for the L allele. However, in subjects homozygous for the L allele, habitual intake of total fat and saturated fat was positively associated with waist circumference, whereas such association was not seen in carriers of the V allele (Robitaille *et al.*, 2004).

These studies emphasise the interaction of this gene with interindividual differences in nutritional habits, but the studies may also provide explanations of the discrepancies found in usual association studies that neglect the role of the environment.

On the other hand, the methodological issues pertaining to the search for candidate genes are even more problematic in the study of nutrient–gene interaction. In both of the above-mentioned studies on fatty acids, habitual dietary intake was estimated by food frequency questionnaires, which implies a considerable uncertainty. As stated by Luan and colleagues, the absence of an interaction between total fat intake or fat energy percentage may be due to the difficulties in assessment of absolute intakes of fat and total energy intake by this technique (Luan *et al.*, 2001). Indeed, dealing with large populations, in which the environment is well controlled, is generally very difficult.

Intervention studies

Studies on controlled overfeeding and calorie restriction in monozygotic twins have been taken to suggest a relatively strong genetic component in the effect of change in energy intake, i.e. a nutrient-gene interaction (Bouchard *et al.*, 1990; Bouchard and Tremblay, 1997; Hainer *et al.*, 2000).

In the overfeeding study, 12 pairs of monozygotic lean male twins were fed a 4.2 MJ per day energy surplus in 6 out of 7-week days during a 100-day period (Bouchard *et al.*, 1990). Both BMI as well as the degree of visceral obesity increased in most twins, but there was a considerable inter-individual variation. However, the intra-pair resemblance was much greater than the between-pair resemblance. This phenotypic correlation may suggest that the genetic identity of the twin pairs also make them more similar in the response to the enforced dietary changes, whereas the genetic differences between the twin pairs are responsible for the greater differences in response to the same dietary challenge. This seems plausible, but, on the other hand, the similarity within the twin pairs can also be due to preceding shared environment that influences the response to the dietary change. The distinction between the genetic and the environmental interpretation of the phenotypic correlation among monozygotic twins requires, as in the classical twin study design, a corresponding investigation of dizygotic twins under the assumption that the shared environmental influences are the same for mono- and dizygotic twins. The fact that the phenotypic correlation among these monozygotic twin pairs is less than 1.0, unambiguously demonstrates (assuming negligible measurement errors) the role of the environmental influences – preceding or during the experiment – that are not identical within the twin pairs. Similar considerations apply to the study of the effects of caloric restriction on weight loss among monozygotic twins pairs (Hainer *et al.*, 2000). Further, the study of lean subjects not necessarily predisposed to develop obesity and of already obese subjects may limit the applicability of the results to the process of development of obesity.

The twin overfeeding study has been used as platform for the investigation of the effects of several common polymorphisms in genes assumed to play a role in regulation of body weight. Ukkola and colleagues have published several studies showing that gene variants in genes coding for the uncoupling proteins UCP1, UCP2, and UCP3, the IGF2, the IGF binding protein 1, the beta2 adrenergic receptor, the glucocorticoid receptor, the Na^+–K^+ ATPase alpha2, adipsin and resistin are associated with the initial change in body weight, body composition, and metabolic parameters in response to overfeeding, and to recovery from the weight gain induced by overfeeding (summarised in Ukkola and Bouchard, 2004). However, these analyses may have some limitations that must be taken into account. The 24 subjects included in the study represented 12 pairs of monozygotic twins, but was handled in one set of analyses as if they were unrelated persons, and by using only the phenotypic means of the 12 pairs in another set of analyses.

Several other studies have addressed the effect of candidate gene variants on response to weight loss intervention in humans. Carriers of the C allele of the Ser(T) 343 Ser(C) polymorphism of the leptin receptor gene have been shown to experience a greater weight loss during calorie restriction than subjects homozygous for the T allele (Mammes *et al.*, 2001). In a study including 163 overweight and obese subjects, Fumeron and colleagues addressed the possible effect of the Bcl 1 restriction polymorphism of the UCP gene on weight loss achieved during 4 months of calorie restriction (Fumeron *et al.*, 1996). Carriers of the UCP polymorphism lost more weight than non-carriers. Further, subjects homozygous for the polymorphism had the greatest weight loss, indicating a dose-response effect of this gene variant on weight loss (Fumeron *et al.*, 1996).

A recent study addressing the effects of the Trp64Arg polymorphism of the beta 3 adrenergic receptor, and the –55C to T mutation of the promoter of the UCP3 gene reports that subjects carrying the mutation in both genes show the lowest reduction in abdominal adipose tissue, and no change in fasting glucose and FFA level, as well as postprandial responses of insulin and glucose following a glucose load in response to energy restriction (Kim *et al.*, 2004). The weight loss was not dependent on genotype, but the beneficial effect on abdominal fat mass and blood markers was most pronounced in the subjects homozygous for the wild-type alleles of both genes and hereafter in the subjects carrying only the UCP3 mutation (Kim *et al.*, 2004). Other studies have indicated that the Arg allele is associated with an impaired response to weight reduction in Japanese subjects (Sakane *et al.*, 1997; Shiwaku *et al.*, 2003; Xinli *et al.*, 2001). A German study has indicated that subjects carrying the Arg allele of Trp64Arg, and the Arg allele of the Gly972Arg polymorphism in the insulin receptor substrate 1 (IRS-1) gene, experience low weight reduction in response to calorie restriction (Benecke *et al.*, 2000). Several studies have failed to identify any association between the Trp64Arg polymorphism of the beta 3 adrenergic receptor and weight loss success (Fumeron *et al.*, 1996; Rawson *et al.*, 2002). Taken together, the role of the Trp64Arg polymorphism in determining weight loss may be highly dependent on interaction with other specific genes or overall genetic background.

Several studies have addressed the possible effect of the Pro12Ala variant of the PPARγ 2 gene in intervention trials. Nicklas and colleagues have addressed its possible effect on weight loss, metabolic response to the weight loss and weight regain following a six-month dietary intervention in women (Nicklas *et al.*, 2001). Weight loss did not differ between women carrying the Ala allele and women homozygous for the Pro allele. However fat oxidation was significantly decreased following the weight loss intervention only in Ala carriers. In addition, carriers of the Ala allele presented a larger reduction in insulin response to an oral glucose tolerance test compared with women homozygous for the Pro allele. Finally, 12-month weight regain was greater in Ala carriers.

Lindi and colleagues have studied the effect of the Pro12Ala PPARγ polymorphism on long-term weight change in response to energy and fat restriction and increased physical activity. The weight loss in the subjects homozygous for the Ala allele was significantly greater than in subjects homozygous for the Pro allele, and the weight loss for subjects with the Pro/Ala genotype was close to that of the Pro/Pro subjects (Lindi *et al.*, 2002). Further, Lindi and colleagues have reported that carriers of the Ala allele have a greater reduction in serum triacylglycerol in response to long-term fish oil supplementation as compared to subjects with the Pro12Pro genotype (Lindi *et al.*, 2003).

A French group recently carried out an intervention study (called RIVAGE) to investigate the interactions between diets (Mediterranean or low-fat types vs. standard Western type), risk factors for cardiovascular disease and gene polymorphisms in about 300 patients who were randomised into two groups over periods of 3 and 12 months. They studied several genes encoding for proteins that are known to be modulated in response to diet. In a first analysis performed in a subgroup of 100 subjects, they found, for example, that several common SNPs located in the Apolipoprotein E, ApoA VI, micosomal transfer protein (MTP), intestinal fatty acid protein (FABP2) might be associated with the metabolic response to diet (Vincent *et al.*, 2002). The study has not yet provided results pertaining to obesity or weight change. In addition, a recent systematic review has indicated that genetic variations in several of the apolipoproteins may contribute to the heterogeneity in the lipid response to dietary intervention (Masson *et al.*, 2003).

Combining genome wide scanning for gene polymorphisms and expression

The advances in biotechnology now allow for combining the search for gene polymorphisms, possibly generating a basis for nutrient–gene interaction, and the gene expression profiling on a genome-wide basis. Thus, the overlap between gene profiling studies, the whole genome scan and the candidate gene map available in humans and rodents will constitute important steps.

The development of data mining tools is essential to develop and fully exploit these new opportunities.

A proof-of-concept of this new approach was recently provided by a study in which gene expression studies and genome wide scan was combined in standard inbred mice strains (C57BL/6J and DBA/2J) (Schadt *et al.*, 2003). The strains were crossed together and the F2 generation yielded by these crosses was fed a high-fat diet for 4 months. All animals were carefully phenotyped with regard to obesity-related traits and metabolic parameters. Subcutaneous fat pad mass was measured and animals were categorised as either lean or obese if they were below or above the first or last quartile of fat amount, respectively. In the first step, using micro-arrays, the authors compared the differential gene expression levels in the liver of obese and lean animals. The gene profiling study showed that 30% of the genes differentially mobilised in the animals could represent molecular signatures of the thin and the obese status, respectively. Among the 300 highly-ranked genes with a differential expression in thin and obese animals, two different profiles of gene expression were observed in the liver of the obese animals, thus separating these animals in different obese categories based on their gene expression levels in the liver. The second step aimed at identifying genes or regions that contributed to the increased fat mass. Genome-wide scans were utilized to detect chromosomal regions showing linkage with obesity-related phenotypes in these animals. The variation of liver gene expression in the animal strains was also used as a quantitative trait (eQTL). The linkage study not only identified chromosomal regions involved in the control of adiposity, but also in the control of the liver gene expression. Specific chromosomal regions discriminated the two types of obese mice with different patterns of liver expression. Some genes or chromosomal regions that may be involved both in the regulation of genes expressed in the liver (with a different pattern of expression in lean and obese) and in adiposity will probably be identified. The future will tell us if they are good targets for intervention (Schadt *et al.*, 2003).

Current large-scale international studies

Large multi-centre studies are currently addressing the nutrient–gene interaction in obesity. One of these is the NUGENOB study 'Nutrient Gene Interaction in Human Obesity – Implications for Dietary Guidelines' which was funded by a European Commission grant under the Fifth Framework Programme. Approximately 750 obese subjects and 115 normal weight reference subjects were included in the study. All subjects completed a 3-day food diary to assess habitual diet, and completed questionnaires addressing dietary habits and lifestyle, and family history of obesity and related diseases. All subjects completed a 1-day clinical investigation programme including assessment of metabolic responses to a high-fat test meal. Obese subjects were then randomised to a hypocaloric dietary intervention with either moderate or low fat content. Novel candidate genes possibly involved

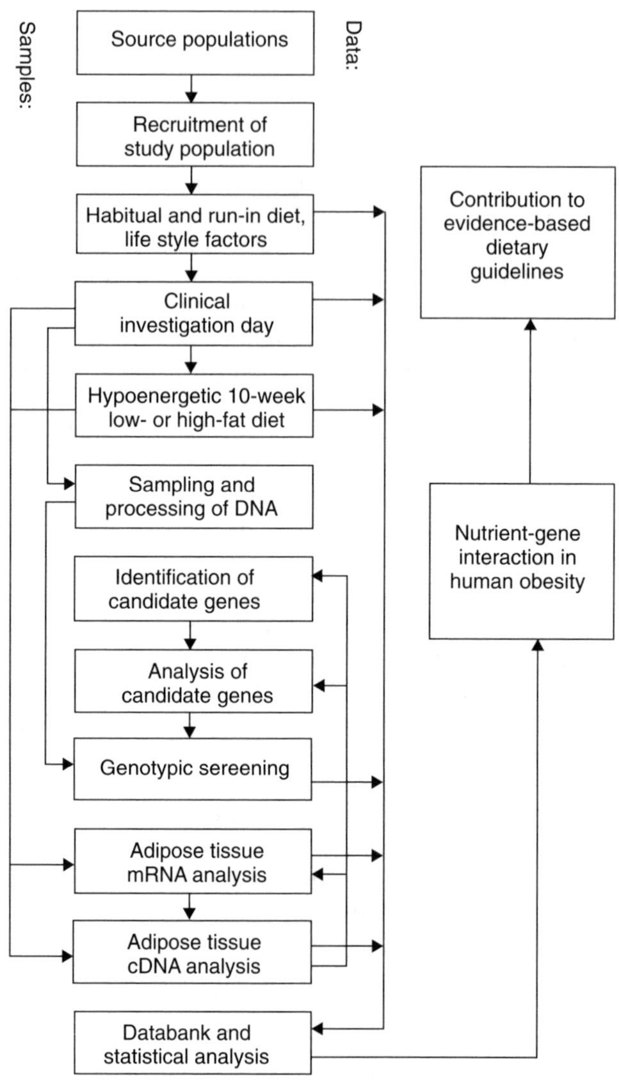

Fig. 2.1 Outline of the NUGENOB project (EU grant QLK1-CT-2000-00618).

in pathogenesis of obesity were identified based on linkage results obtained in data outside the project (Boutin *et al.*, 2003; Meyre *et al.*, 2004), as well as bioinformatics. Candidate gene variants were identified through scanning of candidate genes and bioinformatics (Boutin *et al.*, 2003; Dalgaard *et al.*, 2003; Draper *et al.*, 2002; Yanagisawa *et al.*, 2003). All subjects have now been genotyped for a large number of gene polymorphisms with a putative role in the regulation of body fat accumulation. Quantitative gene expression analyses on selected genes, and microarray based gene expression profiling have been conducted on adipose tissue samples taken in obese subjects before and after the dietary intervention (Dahlman *et al.*, 2005; Viguerie *et al.*, 2005b). The outline of the NUGENOB project is illustrated in Fig. 2.1. The study specifically aims at addresses the nutrient–gene interactions by investigating the effect of genotype on the metabolic response to a high-fat test meal, the effect of genotype on weight loss, including the interaction between genotype and diet, and finally the changes in adipose tissue gene expression in response to energy restriction, and changes in dietary fat content. In addition to improving the understanding of nutrient–gene interaction, the project aims to improve the understanding of the specific mechanisms underlying the well-documented genetic predisposition to obesity, and the specific pathways involved in the regulation of adipose tissue fat accumulation and metabolism.

Another multi-centre project is the 'Diet and Obesity' project, which is also funded by the European Commission within the Fifth Framework Programme. This project addresses the causes of weight gain with particular focus on an energy-dense, high fat diet, including the mechanisms of susceptibility to weight gain and diet preferences, using both animal models and human epidemiological and interventional models (Mercer, 2001). The project aims at addressing the mechanism and defining the factors that predispose some individual to prefer a high-fat diet and to gain weight on this type of diet. Nutrient–gene interaction will be addressed by attempting to identify the genes and the gene variants responsible for the differences in susceptibility to the obesity-promoting effect of a high-fat diet. The project will aim at defining diagnostic biomarkers of susceptibility or resistance to excess weight gain on a high-fat diet, and to identify the mechanistic basis of post-dieting weight gain, addressing both the central and the peripheral regulatory systems.

2.5 Managing obesity: dietary and other strategies

There are several strategies for inducing weight loss in overweight and obese subjects. However, in most cases the long-term success is limited as the majority of subjects regain all lost weight within 3–5 years. Obesity is a chronic condition, and it therefore seems evident that some form of lifelong intervention may be needed in order to maintain weight loss in obese subjects. On the other hand, the long-term benefit of this strategy is not as obvious as it might look. Thus, there is an ongoing debate regarding the evidence suggesting that weight reduction, although having beneficial effects on risk factors for cardiovascular diseases and type 2 diabetes, may be associated with increased long-term mortality (Sorensen, 2003a; Yang *et al.*, 2003). Evidently, improved primary prevention of weight gain in obesity

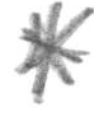

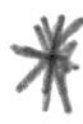

prone subjects, combined with improved strategies for management of obesity are the main tasks for the future.

2.5.1 Current strategies for the management of obesity

Even a weight reduction of 5–10% of the initial weight can markedly improve insulin sensitivity and other features of the metabolic syndrome (Bosello *et al.*, 1997; Pasanisi *et al.*, 2001; Van Gaal *et al.*, 1997). The US National Institute of Health accordingly recommends an initial weight loss of approximately 10% in obese subjects (National Institutes of Health, 1998).

It has become evident that abdominal obesity is associated with greater health risk compared to increased fat accumulation on the hips and legs (Bigaard *et al.*, 2003; Larsson *et al.*, 1984). Therefore, subjects with abdominal obesity may need more intensive treatment, especially if they also suffer from obesity-related co-morbidities. Surgical treatments of obesity as well as some of the pharmacological treatments are restricted to subjects who are massively obese. The different strategies for the treatment are all related to the severity of the obesity and not to the pathophysiological nature of the obesity.

Surgical treatment is recommended only for morbidly obese subjects, or for severely obese subjects with co-morbidities or physical conditions conferring a high risk. Several surgical techniques are available. One is gastroplasty or gastric banding, which reduces the volume of the stomach, thereby increasing post-meal satiety and inhibits intake of large meals. Another technique is intestinal bypass surgery, which reduces the intestinal absorption, but which often is associated with complications or severe side effects that require the bypass to reversed, which is then followed by rapid weight regain. In general, both the initial and the long-term weight loss are large after these treatments compared with other regimens (Colquitt *et al.*, 2003).

Most pharmacological treatments are only approved for short-term usage in obesity treatment, but the newer drugs, sibutramine and olistate, may be used for long-term treatment including prevention of weight regain. Sibutramine inhibits the central re-uptake of noradrenaline and serotonine, which reduces hunger and produces a minor increase in energy expenditure (Leung *et al.*, 2003; Luque and Rey, 2002). Orlistat inhibits pancreatic lipase, which reduces intestinal fat absorption (Leung *et al.*, 2003). This treatment also invites the patients to reduce fat intake in order to avoid steatorrhea. Both treatments should be combined with dietary intervention to achieve the optimal results. Most other pharmacological agents available reduce food intake, via modulation of the central regulatory centres in the hypothalamus, combined with a varying degree of thermogenic effect. None of the currently available drugs directly target the adipose tissue fat metabolism, but the PPARs expressed in this tissue may be a potential target (Ram, 2003).

The cornerstone of any dietary treatment of obesity is reduction of energy intake, and sustainment of a lower energy intake to prevent weight regain. The US National Institute of Health recommends an initial weight loss of approximately 10%, achieved over a 6-month period with a daily energy deficit of 300–1000 kcal, depending on the initial weight (National Institutes of Health, 1998). The dietary approach may be combined with increased physical activity, which may aid both weight loss and subsequent maintenance of the weight loss. When a great weight loss is aimed at, an initial treatment with a VLCD, providing 2.4–4.2 MJ per day may be useful. VLCD should always be followed by a more lifestyle-oriented approach, providing the patient with new eating habits that will prevent regain. Although the initial weight loss rate is high for VLCDs, the maintained weight loss after 1 year is not different between subjects who initially followed a VLCD and subjects who followed a conventional energy-restricted diet (Wadden *et al.*, 1994).

More moderate reductions in energy intake can either be obtained directly by limiting the energy intake to a certain amount of calories per day (energy restriction), or by introducing a low-fat, low-energy density diet, which indirectly will reduce energy intake (low fat *ad libitum* diet). Previous studies have indicated that the two procedures may produce similar weight loss, but that the *ad libitum* approach may in general be perceived as more pleasant (Jeffery *et al.*, 1995; Shah *et al.*, 1994). However, other studies indicate that the passive underconsumption on the *ad libitum* diet may be a temporary phenomenon (Kendall *et al.*, 1991; Stubbs *et al.*, 1998), and that continued weight reduction over a longer time period may only be achieved by some degree of deliberate energy restriction (Astrup *et al.*, 2000b). In controlled dietary intervention studies, medium- and low-fat diets may produce similar degree of weight reduction, as long as they are subjected to the same degree of energy restriction (Pelkman *et al.*, 2004; Peters *et al.*, 2003; Powell *et al.*, 1994). However, the patients ability and motivation to actively control calorie intake may be more important on a medium-fat diet than on a low-fat diet. Although there is little knowledge about interaction between dietary fat and genetic factors involved in the regulation of weight loss, it is plausible that some individuals are more susceptible than others to a high-fat diet, and hence that nutrient–gene interactions may play an important role in weight reduction.

Lifestyle modification has become one of the most commonly used strategies for prevention and treatment of obesity. The overall aim of the lifestyle modification is to induce a behavioural modification of eating and exercise patterns. The intervention will usually focus on reduction of intake of high-fat or other energy-dense foods and reduction of portion size, on reinforcement of the awareness to internal clues of hunger and satiety, on reduction of eating in response to external clues, and finally, on increase of physical activity. However, such lifestyle changes have not proven to be as effective as might be expected. There are several possible reasons for the failure. Advising at risk individuals to change their lifestyle will not have the same effect as changing the environment that promotes the maintenance of the inappropriate habits. Most people are probably aware of the healthy choices, but these choices are often not the easy choices in terms of costs, social norms, etc. Little is known about the between-subject differences in response to different types of lifestyle changes. Finally, it is still unknown if generally recommended low-fat, low-energy density diets will reduce the risk of weight gain in the population. Even if this is the case, other prevention strategies may be more effective in subgroups of obesity-prone subjects.

2.5.2 Integrating the knowledge on the genetics of obesity and nutrient–gene interaction in treatment and prevention of obesity

It seems likely that a polygenic, multifactorial disease such as obesity may be more effectively managed by individual tailoring of the treatment and prevention strategies. Other fields of nutritional science have provided insight into genetic mechanisms determining between-subject differences in nutrient requirements. One example is the above-mentioned phenylketonuria. It is now known that genetic variations in apolipoproteins, in the vitamin D receptor, and in the thermo-labile variant of the 5,10-methylenetetrahydrofolate reductase (MTHER), may induce reduced sensitivity to dietary cholesterol and increased requirement for calcium and folate, respectively, (for review see Simopoulos, 1999). Similar findings on genes or pathways involved in regulation of body fat accumulation, in sensitivity to physical inactivity and high-fat diet, and in response to anti-obesity drugs and other forms of treatment or prevention of obesity may pave the way for development of a new obesity taxonomy defining different subtypes of obesity according to sub-phenotypes as well as genetic aspects. Transforming this knowledge into new diagnostics and tailored treatment and prevention regimes may hold the key to combating the epidemic of obesity.

Research on the genetics of obesity has mainly led to the discovery of rare monogenic forms of obesity, rather than to improvement of our understanding of the genetic mechanisms behind the well-known genetic predisposition for development of common obesity. The discovery of leptin offered an effective strategy for treating the rare cases of obesity caused by lack of leptin production (Farooqi *et al.*, 1999). Current knowledge about nutrient–gene interaction in human obesity is very preliminary. However, studies have indicated that the long-term effect of dietary weight loss intervention may differ in subjects with different PPARγ genotypes (Lindi *et al.*, 2002; Nicklas *et al.*, 2001), and an interaction between dietary fat composition and PPARγ genotypes has been suggested (Luan *et al.*, 2001; Nieters *et al.*, 2002). Moreover, in obese subjects treated by gastric banding surgery, those carrying different types of mutation in the MC4 receptor may have more complications and less weight loss (Potoczna *et al.*, 2003).

In the field of pharmacogenetics, addressing the role of specific genetic variation in determining the well known between-subject differences in drug-efficacy, a recent study has indicated an association between the G-148A variant in the phenylethanolamine *N*-methyltransferase gene and 3-month weight loss in response to sibutramine treatment combined with lifestyle modification (Peters *et al.*, 2003). In addition Hauner and colleagues have shown that obese subjects with the CC genotype for the C825T polymorphism in the G-protein β3 subunit gene presents low weight loss on an energy-restriction only regimen, as compared subjects with the to TT/TC genotype, and that combining the intervention with sibutramine administration improves weight loss mainly in subjects with the CC genotype (Hauner *et al.*, 2003). Future pharmacogenetic studies are expected to pave the way for more 'personalised' treatment regimens, where both the type of medication and the dose are guided by the subjects' genotype.

Current and future large-scale research projects are aiming at identifying predictors of weight gain and weight loss, and susceptibility to environmental obesity promoting factors. Within the next decades it may therefore be possible to identify at risk individuals before they develop obesity, and to prevent the development of obesity using tailored intervention strategies. Further, tailoring the treatment and secondary prevention for obese subjects may increase the success in initial weight loss and in prevention of the subsequent regain.

Prevention and treatment of obesity clearly demand testing changes in the environmental factors to which the individual is exposed (Hill and Peters, 1998). In addition to more refined and targeted regimes for dietary intervention, advanced insight into the biological mechanisms regulating adipose tissue fat accumulation, energy expenditure and appetite regulation will offer new drug targets for the treatment of obesity. Also in pharmacological treatment of obesity, a sub-classification of the obese phenotype based on the affected genes or pathways may lead to specifically targeted treatment regimes, hopefully implying improved treatment effect and reduced side effects.

2.6 Future trends

During the last few years, the research in the field of nutrient-sensitive genes and nutrient–gene interaction with implications on body weight regulation has developed rapidly, from a research strategy focusing on the overall role of genetic factors in determining the between-subject variation in response to habitual diet or dietary interventions such as overfeeding and calorie restriction, to research protocols aimed at addressing the specific interaction between genetic factors and components of the diet.

LIBRARY, UNIVERSITY OF CHESTER

Studies have addressed the effect of calorie restriction on adipose tissue gene expression in humans (Viguerie *et al.*, 2005a). Future studies addressing the association between change in adipose tissue gene expression in response to dieting and the subsequent weight loss, the effect of diet composition on change in gene expression, and the interaction between gene polymorphisms and change in gene expression in response to dietary intervention are under way. They are expected to increase our understanding of the systems biology of adipose tissue in response to weight loss, as well as the between-subject differences in response to dietary weight loss interventions. An improved understanding of the interaction between diet composition and specific gene variants, or pathways involved in the regulation of body fat accumulation, may pave the way for a new obesity taxonomy, and for more targeted strategies for treatment.

Future large scaled multi-disciplinary projects should aim at optimising the use of new research methods in combination with already existing research methods. Metabolomics and proteomics, combined with gene expression profiling and genotype screening may provide new important insight into the system biology of obesity. This may further allow for the identification of candidate pathways involved in the development of obesity, and hence the identification of candidate drug targets for treatment and prevention of obesity, as well as biomarkers indicating the efficiency of the pathways on individual subject level. It may be speculated that, although a large number of genes and a complex interplay of environmental and genetic factors determine body fat accumulation, the number of pathways mediating the effect of these factors on body fat accumulation may be limited. Identifying the pathways could serve as a platform for a new classification, diagnostic and treatment of the common complex forms of obesity. Further, identifying biomarkers reflecting susceptibility to particular nutrients in pre-obese subjects would be a crucial step in the primary prevention of obesity.

2.7 Sources of further information and advice

2.7.1 Further reading

On Section 2.2

(Maes *et al.*, 1997) Review of the literature on the genetic and environmental factors in human obesity. This review includes family studies, twin studies, adoption studies, and advantages and disadvantages of the study designs are discussed.

(Stunkard *et al.*, 1986) An adoption study of the genetic and familial environmental effects on adult obesity. The study was based on 540 thin, medium weight, overweight and obese adoptees, their biological and adoptive parents, and their biological full and half siblings. The adoptees were selected among 3580 Danish adoptees who had reported their height and weight. The average BMI of the relatives of the selected adoptees was analysed and supported a genetic influence and no sustained influence of the rearing family environment.

(Sorensen *et al.*, 1989) An adoption study of genetic effects on obesity in adulthood. The study is based on 341 thin, medium weight, overweight and obese adoptees selected from among 4000 adoptees from the region of Copenhagen, Denmark. The association between BMI of the adoptees and their biological full and half siblings was examined.

(Comuzzie *et al.*, 2001; Comuzzie and Allison 1998) Review papers addressing the strategies for identifying candidate genes for obesity. The papers discuss the strategies for identifying candidate genes involved in the pathogenesis of complex phenotypes, expected to be determined by the action and interaction of multiple genes and environmental factors.

(Clement *et ai.*, 2002a) Review of genetics in obesity. The review presents examples of monogenetic forms of obesity, and the insight gained from these rare cases of obesity in terms of understanding the complex pathways involved in the regulation of food intake and identifying targets for future drug development. The candidate gene and the genome-wide scan approach are presented and discussed as strategies for identifying genes involved in the common forms of obesity. Updated results from genome-wide scan studies are presented. Finally, the strategies for medical application of this knowledge in terms of drug development and optimal integration of the knowledge about the genetic mechanisms in the pharmacotherapy of obesity is discussed.

(Snyder *et al.*, 2004) The tenth update of the human obesity gene map, incorporating published results through October 2003. Evidence from single-gene mutation obesity cases, Mendelian disorders exhibiting obesity as a clinical feature, quantitative trait loci (QTLs) from human genome-wide scans and various animal cross-breeding experiments, and association and linkage studies with candidate genes and other markers are reviewed. In addition, transgenic and knockout murine models exhibiting obesity as a phenotype are incorporated.

(Barsh *et al.*, 2000) Review addressing the search for human obesity genes, rodents as a model system for human obesity, and gene–environment interaction.

(West *et al.*, 1995) Study addressing the effect of varying dietary macronutrient content on the body composition and the possible interaction between genetic background and macronutrient content of the diet on body composition of different strains of mice.

(Lissner and Heitmann 1995) Review paper addressing the role of dietary fat in human obesity. The evidence for a role of dietary fat in human obesity is addressed based on the epidemiological evidence from various epidemiological methods and the consistency of these findings with experimental data is discussed.

On Section 2.3

(Copland *et al.*, 2003) Review paper describing the gene array technology. This technology is expected to pave the way for identifying candidate genes and pathways for specific diseases, a way of subclassifying diseases according to patterns of gene expression in various tissues, and a mean of identifying new molecular targets for the development of drug therapeutics.

(Clement *et al.*, 2002; Rome *et al.*, 2003) Studies applying the microarray technology addressing the effects of thyroid hormone and insulin on gene expression in human skeletal muscle. The studies also address the interpretation of microarray data.

On Section 2.4

(Lindi *et al.*, 2002, 2003; Luan *et al.*, 2001; Nicklas *et al.*, 2001; Nieters *et al.*, 2002) Studies addressing nutrient–gene interaction between fat intake or calorie restriction and the Pro12Ala variant of the PPAR gamma gene.

(Masson *et al.*, 2003) Review addressing the effect of genetic variation on the lipid response to dietary intervention.

(Schadt *et al.*, 2003) Study combining gene expression studies and genome wide scan in standard inbred mice strains. The study describes comprehensive genetic screens of mouse, plant and human transcriptomes by considering gene expression values as quantitative traits. The study identified a gene expression pattern strongly associated with obesity in a murine cross, and observed two distinct obesity subtypes, which appeared to be under the control of different loci.

On Section 2.5

(Simopoulos 1999) Review paper addressing the concept of nutrient–gene interaction and implications for dietary recommendations.

2.7.2 Useful websites

www.nugenob.org The website for the NUGENOB project, funded by the European Commission within the Fifth Framework Programme

http://www.adipositas-online.com The website for the Diet and Obesity project, funded by the European Commission within the Fifth Framework Programme

http://www.nugo.org/everyone/ The website for the European NutriGenomics Organisation. A Network of Excellence on Nutrition and Genomics funded by the European Commission within the Sixth Framework Programme http://www.flair-flow.com/ FLAIR-FLOW EUROPE disseminates information from food R&D and nutrition projects funded by the European Union

http://obesitygene.pbrc.edu/ Electronic version of the Human Obesity Gene Map (Snyder *et al.*, 2004). Claude Bouchard, Pennington Biomedical

2.8 References

ADEYEMO, A., LUKE, A., COOPER, R. *et al.* (2003), 'A genome-wide scan for body mass index among Nigerian families,' *Obes. Res.*, **11** (2), 266–73.

ASTRUP, A., GRUNWALD, G. K., MELANSON, E. L., SARIS, W. H. and HILL, J. O. (2000a), 'The role of low-fat diets in body weight control: a meta-analysis of *ad libitum* dietary intervention studies', *Int. J. Obes. Relat. Metab. Disord.*, **24** (12), 1545–52.

ASTRUP, A., RYAN, L., GRUNWALD, G. K. *et al.* (2000b), 'The role of dietary fat in body fatness: evidence from a preliminary meta-analysis of *ad libitum* low-fat dietary intervention studies', *Br. J. Nutr.*, **83** Suppl 1, S25–32.

ASTRUP, A., BUEMANN, B., CHRISTENSEN, N. J. and TOUBRO, S. (1994), 'Failure to increase lipid oxidation in response to increasing dietary fat content in formerly obese women', *Am. J. Physiol.*, **266** (4) (Pt 1), E592–9.

BABA, N. H., SAWAYA, S., TORBAY, N., HABBAL, Z., AZAR, S. and HASHIM, S. A. (1999), 'High protein vs. high carbohydrate hypoenergetic diet for the treatment of obese hyperinsulinemic subjects,' *Int. J. Obes. Relat. Metab. Disord.*, **23** (11), 1202–6.

BARSH, G. S., FAROOQI, I. S. and O'RAHILLY, S. (2000), 'Genetics of body-weight regulation', *Nature*, **404** (6778), 644–51.

BASTARD, J. P., HAINQUE, B., DUSSERRE, E. *et al.* (1999), 'Peroxisome proliferator activated receptor-gamma, leptin and tumor necrosis factor-alpha mRNA expression during very low calorie diet in subcutaneous adipose tissue in obese women', *Diabetes Metab. Res. Rev.*, **15** (2), 92–8.

BAULANDE, S., LASNIER, F., LUCAS, M. and PAIRAULT, J. (2001), 'Adiponutrin, a transmembrane protein corresponding to a novel dietary- and obesity-linked mRNA specifically expressed in the adipose lineage', *J. Biol. Chem.*, **276** (36), 33336–44.

BELL, C. G., BENZINOU, M., SIDDIQ, A. *et al.* (2004), 'Genome-wide linkage analysis for severe obesity in French Caucasians finds significant susceptibility locus on chromosome 19q', *Diabetes*, **53** (7), 1857–65.

BENECKE, H., TOPAK, H., VON ZUR, M. A. and SCHUPPERT, F. (2000), 'A study on the genetics of obesity: influence of polymorphisms of the beta-3-adrenergic receptor and insulin receptor substrate 1 in relation to weight loss, waist to hip ratio and frequencies of common cardiovascular risk factors', *Exp. Clin. Endocrinol. Diabetes*, **108** (2), 86–92.

BIEBERMANN, H., KRUDE, H., ELSNER, A., CHUBANOV, V., GUDERMANN, T. and GRUTERS, A. (2003), 'Autosomal-dominant mode of inheritance of a melanocortin-4 receptor mutation in a patient with severe early-onset obesity is due to a dominant-negative effect caused by receptor dimerization', *Diabetes*, **52** (12), 2984–8.

BIGAARD, J., TJONNELAND, A., THOMSEN, B. L., OVERVAD, K., HEITMANN, B. L. and SORENSEN, T. I. (2003), 'Waist circumference, BMI, smoking, and mortality in middle-aged men and women', *Obes. Res.*, **11** (7), 895–903.

BOLTON-SMITH, C. and WOODWARD, M. (1994), 'Dietary composition and fat to sugar ratios in relation to obesity', *Int. J. Obes. Relat. Metab. Disord.*, **18** (12), 820–8.

BOSELLO, O., ARMELLINI, F., ZAMBONI, M. and FITCHET, M. (1997), 'The benefits of modest weight loss in type II diabetes', *Int. J. Obes. Relat. Metab. Disord.*, **21** Suppl 1, S10–13.

BOUCHARD, C. and TREMBLAY, A. (1997), 'Genetic influences on the response of body fat and fat distribution to positive and negative energy balances in human identical twins', *J. Nutr.*, **127** (5) Suppl, 943S–7S.

BOUCHARD, C., TREMBLAY, A., NADEAU, A. *et al.* (1989), 'Genetic effect in resting and exercise metabolic rates', *Metabolism*, **38** (4), 364–70.

BOUCHARD, C., TREMBLAY, A., DESPRES, J. P. *et al.* (1990), 'The response to long-term overfeeding in identical twins', *N. Engl. J. Med.*, **322** (21), 1477–82.

BOUTIN, P., DINA, C., VASSEUR, F. *et al.* (2003), 'GAD2 on chromosome 10p12 is a candidate gene for human obesity', *PLoS. Biol.*, **1** (3), E68.

BRANSON, R., POTOCZNA, N., KRAL, J. G., LENTES, K. U., HOEHE, M. R. and HORBER, F. F. (2003), 'Binge eating as a major phenotype of melanocortin 4 receptor gene mutations', *N. Engl. J. Med.*, **348** (12), 1096–103.

CANCELLO, R., TOUNIAN, A., POITOU, C. and CLEMENT, K. (2004), 'Adiposity signals, genetic and body weight regulation in humans', *Diabetes Metab.*, **30** (3), 215–27.

CARDON, L. R. and BELL, J. I. (2001), 'Association study designs for complex diseases', *Nat. Rev. Genet.*, **2** (2), 91–9.

CLEMENT, K. and FERRE, P. (2003), 'Genetics and the pathophysiology of obesity', *Pediatr. Res.*, **53** (5), 721–5.

CLEMENT, K., VAISSE, C., LAHLOU, N. *et al.* (1998), 'A mutation in the human leptin receptor gene causes obesity and pituitary dysfunction, *Nature*, **392** (6674), 398–401.

CLEMENT, K., BOUTIN, P. and FROGUEL, P. (2002a), 'Genetics of obesity', *Am. J. Pharmacogenomics*, **2** (3), 177–87.

CLEMENT, K., VIGUERIE, N., DIEHN, M. *et al.* (2002b), 'In vivo regulation of human skeletal muscle gene expression by thyroid hormone', *Genome Res.*, **12** (2), 281–91.

CLEMENT, K., VIGUERIE, N., POITOU, C. *et al.* (2004), 'Weight loss regulates inflammation-related genes in white adipose tissue of obese subjects'. *Faseb. J.*, **18** (14), 1657–9.

COLQUITT, J., CLEGG, A., SIDHU, M. and ROYLE, P. (2003), 'Surgery for morbid obesity', *Cochrane Database. Syst. Rev.* no. 2, p. CD003641.

COMUZZIE, A. G. and ALLISON, D. B. (1998), 'The search for human obesity genes', *Science*, **280** (5368), 1374–7.

COMUZZIE, A. G., WILLIAMS, J. T., MARTIN, L. J. and BLANGERO, J. (2001), 'Searching for genes underlying normal variation in human adiposity', *J. Mol. Med.*, **79** (1), 57–70.

COPLAND, J. A., DAVIES, P. J., SHIPLEY, G. L., WOOD, C. G., LUXON, B. A. and URBAN, R. J. (2003), 'The use of DNA microarrays to assess clinical samples: the transition from bedside to bench to bedside', *Rec. Prog. Horm. Res.*, **58**, 25–53.

CURB, J. D. and MARCUS, E. B. (1991), 'Body fat and obesity in Japanese Americans', *Am. J. Clin. Nutr.*, **53** (6) Suppl, 1552S–5S.

DAHLMAN, I., LINDER, K., ARVIDSSON, N. E., ANDERSSON, I., LIDEN, J., VERDICH, C., SORENSEN, T. I., and ARNER, P. (2005), 'Changes in adipose tissue gene expression with energy-restricted diets in obese women', *Am. J. Clin. Nutr.*, **81** (6), 1275–85.

DALGAARD, L. T., ANDERSEN, G., LARSEN, L. H. *et al.* (2003), 'Mutational analysis of the UCP2 core promoter and relationships of variants with obesity', *Obes. Res.*, **11** (11), 1420–7.

DAVIES, K. M., HEANEY, R. P., RECKER, R. R. *et al.* (2000), 'Calcium intake and body weight', *J. Clin. Endocrinol. Metab.*, **85** (12), 4635–8.

DE CASTRO, J. M. (1993), 'Independence of genetic influences on body size, daily intake, and meal patterns of humans, *Physiol. Behav.*, **54** (4), 633–9.

DIMEGLIO, D. P. and MATTES, R. D. (2000), 'Liquid versus solid carbohydrate: effects on food intake and body weight', *Int. J. Obes. Relat. Metab. Disord.*, **24** (6), 794–800.

DRAPER, N., ECHWALD, S. M., LAVERY, G. G. *et al.* (2002), 'Association studies between microsatellite markers within the gene encoding human 11beta-hydroxysteroid dehydrogenase type 1 and body mass index, waist to hip ratio, and glucocorticoid metabolism', *J. Clin. Endocrinol. Metab.*, **87** (11), 4984–90.

DURAND, E., BOUTIN, P., MEYRE, D. *et al.* (2004), 'Polymorphisms in the amino acid transporter solute carrier family 6 (neurotransmitter transporter) member 14 gene contribute to polygenic obesity in French Caucasians', *Diabetes*, **53** (9), 2483–6.

ENGERT, J. C., VOHL, M. C., WILLIAMS, S. M. *et al.* (2002), '5′ flanking variants of resistin are associated with obesity', *Diabetes*, **51** (5), 1629–34.

ESTERBAUER, H., SCHNEITLER, C., OBERKOFLER, H. *et al.* (2001), 'A common polymorphism in the promoter of UCP2 is associated with decreased risk of obesity in middle-aged humans', *Nat. Genet.*, **28** (2), 178–83.

FAROOQI, I. S., JEBB, S. A., LANGMACK, G. *et al.* (1999), 'Effects of recombinant leptin therapy in a child with congenital leptin deficiency', *N. Engl. J. Med.*, **341** (12), 879–84.

FAROOQI, I. S., YEO, G. S., KEOGH, J. M. *et al.* (2000), 'Dominant and recessive inheritance of morbid obesity associated with melanocortin 4 receptor deficiency', *J. Clin. Invest.*, **106** (2), 271–9.

FAROOQI, I. S., KEOGH, J. M., YEO, G. S., LANK, E. J., CHEETHAM, T. and O'RAHILLY, S. (2003), 'Clinical spectrum of obesity and mutations in the melanocortin 4 receptor gene', *N. Engl. J. Med.*, **348** (12), 1085–95.

FOSTER, G. D., WYATT, H. R., HILL, J. O. *et al.* (2003), 'A randomized trial of a low-carbohydrate diet for obesity', *N. Engl. J. Med.*, **348** (21), 2082–90.

FUMERON, F., DURACK-BOWN, I., BETOULLE, D. *et al.* (1996), 'Polymorphisms of uncoupling protein (UCP) and beta 3 adrenoreceptor genes in obese people submitted to a low calorie diet', *Int. J. Obes. Relat. Metab. Disord.*, **20** (12), 1051–4.

GARAULET, M., VIGUERIE, N., PORUBSKY, S. *et al.* (2004), 'Adiponectin gene expression and plasma values in obese women during very-low-calorie diet. Relationship with cardiovascular risk factors and insulin resistance', *J. Clin. Endocrinol. Metab.*, **89** (2), 756–60.

HAINER, V., STUNKARD, A. J., KUNESOVA, M., PARIZKOVA, J., STICH, V. and ALLISON, D. B. (2000), 'Intrapair resemblance in very low calorie diet-induced weight loss in female obese identical twins', *Int. J. Obes. Relat. Metab. Disord.*, **24** (8), 1051–7.

HALSALL, D. J., LUAN, J., SAKER, P. *et al.* (2001), 'Uncoupling protein 3 genetic variants in human obesity: the c-55t promoter polymorphism is negatively correlated with body mass index in a UK Caucasian population', *Int. J. Obes. Relat. Metab. Disord.*, **25** (4), 472–7.

HAUNER, H., MEIER, M., JOCKEL, K. H., FREY, U. H. and SIFFERT, W. (2003), 'Prediction of successful weight reduction under sibutramine therapy through genotyping of the G-protein beta3 subunit gene (GNB3) C825T polymorphism', *Pharmacogenetics*, **13** (8), 453–9.

HEANEY, R. P. (2003), 'Normalizing calcium intake: projected population effects for body weight', *J. Nutr.*, **133** (1), 268S–70S.

HEBEBRAND, J., GELLER, F., DEMPFLE, A. *et al.* (2004), 'Binge-eating episodes are not characteristic of carriers of melanocortin-4 receptor gene mutations', *Mol. Psychiatry*, **9** (8), 796–800.

HEITMANN, B. L., LISSNER, L., SORENSEN, T. I. and BENGTSSON, C. (1995), 'Dietary fat intake and weight gain in women genetically predisposed for obesity', *Am. J. Clin. Nutr.*, **61** (6), 1213–17.

HEITMANN, B. L., LISSNER, L. and OSLER, M. (2000), 'Do we eat less fat, or just report so?', *Int. J. Obes. Relat. Metab. Disord.*, **24** (4), 435–42.

HILL, J. O. and PETERS, J. C. (1998), 'Environmental contributions to the obesity epidemic', *Science*, **280** (5368), 1371–4.

HODGE, A. M., DOWSE, G. K., GAREEBOO, H., TUOMILEHTO, J., ALBERTI, K. G. and ZIMMET, P. Z. (1996), 'Incidence, increasing prevalence, and predictors of change in obesity and fat distribution over 5 years in the rapidly developing population of Mauritius', *Int. J. Obes. Relat. Metab. Disord.*, **20** (2), 137–46.

HODGE, A. M., DOWSE, G. K., TOELUPE, P., COLLINS, V. R., IMO, T. and ZIMMET, P. Z. (1994), 'Dramatic increase in the prevalence of obesity in western Samoa over the 13 year period 1978–1991', *Int. J. Obes. Relat. Metab. Disord.*, **18** (6), 419–28.

HOFFSTEDT, J., ERIKSSON, P., HELLSTROM, L., ROSSNER, S., RYDEN, M. and ARNER, P. (2000), 'Excessive fat accumulation is associated with the TNF alpha-308 G/A promoter polymorphism in women but not in men', *Diabetologia*, **43** (1), 117–20.

JAMES, J., THOMAS, P., CAVAN, D. and KERR, D. (2004), 'Preventing childhood obesity by reducing consumption of carbonated drinks: cluster randomised controlled trial', *BMJ*, **328** (7450), 1237.

JEFFERY, R. W., HELLERSTEDT, W. L., FRENCH, S. A. and BAXTER, J. E. (1995), 'A randomized trial of counseling for fat restriction versus calorie restriction in the treatment of obesity', *Int. J. Obes. Relat. Metab. Disord.*, **19** (2), 132–7.

KENDALL, A., LEVITSKY, D. A., STRUPP, B. J. and LISSNER, L. (1991), 'Weight loss on a low-fat diet: consequence of the imprecision of the control of food intake in humans', *Am. J. Clin. Nutr.*, **53** (5), 1124–9.

KIM, O. Y., CHO, E. Y., PARK, H. Y., JANG, Y. and LEE, J. H. (2004), 'Additive effect of the mutations in the beta3-adrenoceptor gene and UCP3 gene promoter on body fat distribution and glycemic control after weight reduction in overweight subjects with CAD or metabolic syndrome', *Int. J. Obes. Relat. Metab. Disord.*, **28** (3), 434–41.

KNOWLER, W. C., PETTITT, D. J., SAAD, M. F. *et al.* (1991), 'Obesity in the Pima Indians: its magnitude and relationship with diabetes', *Am. J. Clin. Nutr.*, **53** (6) Suppl, 1543S–51S.

KOLEHMAINEN, M., VIDAL, H., OHISALO, J. J., PIRINEN, E., ALHAVA, E. and UUSITUPA, M. I. (2002), 'Hormone sensitive lipase expression and adipose tissue metabolism show gender difference in obese subjects after weight loss', *Int. J. Obes. Relat. Metab. Disord.*, **26** (1), 6–16.

KROSNICK, A. (2000), 'The diabetes and obesity epidemic among the Pima Indians', *N. J. Med.*, **97** (8), 31–7.

LARSSON, B., SVARDSUDD, K., WELIN, L., WILHELMSEN, L., BJORNTORP, P. and TIBBLIN, G. (1984), 'Abdominal adipose tissue distribution, obesity, and risk of cardiovascular disease and death: 13 year follow up of participants in the study of men born in 1913', *Br. Med. J. (Clin. Res. Ed)*, **288** (6428), 1401–4.

LEE, G. H., PROENCA, R., MONTEZ, J. M. *et al.* (1996), 'Abnormal splicing of the leptin receptor in diabetic mice', *Nature*, **379** (6566), 632–5.

LEIBEL, R. L. (1997), 'Single gene obesities in rodents: possible relevance to human obesity', *J. Nutr.*, **127** (9), 1908S.

LEUNG, W. Y., NEIL, T. G., CHAN, J. C. and TOMLINSON, B. (2003), 'Weight management and current options in pharmacotherapy: orlistat and sibutramine', *Clin. Ther.*, **25** (1), 58–80.

LINDI, V. I., UUSITUPA, M. I., LINDSTROM, J. *et al.* (2002), 'Association of the Pro12Ala polymorphism in the PPAR-gamma2 gene with 3-year incidence of type 2 diabetes and body weight change in the Finnish Diabetes Prevention Study', *Diabetes*, **51** (8), 2581–6.

LINDI, V., SCHWAB, U., LOUHERANTA, A. *et al.* (2003), 'Impact of the Pro12Ala polymorphism of the PPAR-gamma2 gene on serum triacylglycerol response to n-3 fatty acid supplementation', *Mol. Genet. Metab.*, **79** (1), 52–60.

LISSNER, L. and HEITMANN, B. L. (1995), 'Dietary fat and obesity: evidence from epidemiology', *Eur. J. Clin. Nutr.*, **49** (2), 79–90.

LIU, Y. M., LACORTE, J. M., VIGUERIE, N. *et al.* (2003), 'Adiponectin gene expression in subcutaneous adipose tissue of obese women in response to short-term very low calorie diet and refeeding', *J. Clin. Endocrinol. Metab.*, **88** (12), 5881–6.

LIU, Y. M., MOLDES, M., BASTARD, J. P. *et al.* (2004), 'Adiponutrin: a new gene regulated by energy balance in human adipose tissue', *J. Clin. Endocrinol. Metab.*, **89** (6), 2684–9.

LUAN, J., BROWNE, P. O., HARDING, A. H. *et al.* (2001), 'Evidence for gene–nutrient interaction at the PPARgamma locus', *Diabetes*, **50** (3), 686–9.

LUBRANO-BERTHELIER, C., CAVAZOS, M., DUBERN, B. *et al.* (2003), 'Molecular genetics of human obesity-associated MC4R mutations', *Ann. N. Y. Acad. Sci.*, **994**, 49–57.

LUDWIG, D. S., PETERSON, K. E. and GORTMAKER, S. L. (2001), 'Relation between consumption of sugar-sweetened drinks and childhood obesity: a prospective, observational analysis', *Lancet.*, **357** (9255), 505–8.

LUQUE, C. A. and REY, J. A. (2002), 'The discovery and status of sibutramine as an anti-obesity drug', *Eur. J. Pharmacol.*, **440** (2–3), 119–28.

MACDIARMID, J. I., CADE, J. E. and BLUNDELL, J. E. (1996), 'High and low fat consumers, their macronutrient intake and body mass index: further analysis of the National Diet and Nutrition Survey of British Adults', *Eur. J. Clin. Nutr.*, **50** (8), 505–12.

MAES, H. H., NEALE, M. C. and EAVES, L. J. (1997), 'Genetic and environmental factors in relative body weight and human adiposity', *Behav. Genet.*, **27** (4), 325–51.

MAMMES, O., AUBERT, R., BETOULLE, D. *et al.* (2001), 'LEPR gene polymorphisms: associations with overweight, fat mass and response to diet in women', *Eur. J. Clin. Invest.*, **31** (5), 398–404.

MAMMES, O., BETOULLE, D., AUBERT, R., HERBETH, B., SIEST, G. and FUMERON, F. (2000), 'Association of the G-2548A polymorphism in the 5′ region of the LEP gene with overweight', *Ann. Hum. Genet.*, **64**, Pt 5, 391–94.

MARTINEZ, J. A., CORBALAN, M. S., SANCHEZ-VILLEGAS, A., FORGA, L., MARTI, A. and MARTINEZ-GONZALEZ, M. A. (2003), 'Obesity risk is associated with carbohydrate intake in women carrying the Gln27Glu beta2-adrenoceptor polymorphism', *J. Nutr.*, **133** (8), 2549–54.

MASSON, L. F., MCNEILL, G. and AVENELL, A. (2003), 'Genetic variation and the lipid response to dietary intervention: a systematic review', *Am. J. Clin. Nutr.*, **77** (5), 1098–111.

MEMISOGLU, A., HU, F. B., HANKINSON, S. E. *et al.* (2003), 'Interaction between a peroxisome proliferator-activated receptor gamma gene polymorphism and dietary fat intake in relation to body mass', *Hum. Mol. Genet.*, **12** (22), 2923–9.

MERCER, J. G. (2001), 'Dietary and genetic influences on susceptibility or resistance to weight gain on a high fat diet', *Nutr. Metab. Cardiovasc. Dis.*, **11** (4) Suppl, 114–17.

MEYRE, D., LECOEUR, C., DELPLANQUE, J. *et al.* (2004), 'A genome-wide scan for childhood obesity-associated traits in French families shows significant linkage on chromosome 6q22.31–q23.2', *Diabetes*, **53** (3), 803–11.

MONTAGUE, C. T., FAROOQI, I. S., WHITEHEAD, J. P. *et al.* (1997), 'Congenital leptin deficiency is associated with severe early-onset obesity in humans', *Nature*, **387** (6636), 903–8.

NATIONAL INSTITUTES OF HEALTH (1998), *Clinical Guidelines on the Identification, Evaluation, and Treatment of Overweight and Obesity in Adults*, NIH Publication No. 98-4083.

NEEL, J. V. (1999), 'The "thrifty genotype" in 1998', *Nutr. Rev.*, **57** (5) Pt 2, S2–9.

NEWMAN, D. L., ABNEY, M., DYTCH, H., PARRY, R., MCPEEK, M. S. and OBER, C. (2003), 'Major loci influencing serum triglyceride levels on 2q14 and 9p21 localized by homozygosity-by-descent mapping in a large Hutterite pedigree', *Hum. Mol. Genet.*, **12** (2), 137–44.

NICKLAS, B. J., VAN ROSSUM, E. F., BERMAN, D. M., RYAN, A. S., DENNIS, K. E. and SHULDINER, A. R. (2001), 'Genetic variation in the peroxisome proliferator-activated receptor-gamma2 gene (Pro12Ala) affects metabolic responses to weight loss and subsequent weight regain', *Diabetes*, **50** (9), 2172–6.

NIETERS, A., BECKER, N. and LINSEISEN, J. (2002), 'Polymorphisms in candidate obesity genes and their interaction with dietary intake of *n*-6 polyunsaturated fatty acids affect obesity risk in a sub-sample of the EPIC-Heidelberg cohort', *Eur. J. Nutr.*, **41** (5), 210–21.

NIJENHUIS, W. A., GARNER, K. M., VAN ROZEN, R. J. and ADAN, R. A. (2003), 'Poor cell surface expression of human melanocortin-4 receptor mutations associated with obesity', *J. Biol. Chem.*, **278** (25), 22939–45.

OZATA, M., OZDEMIR, I. C. and LICINIO, J. (1999), 'Human leptin deficiency caused by a missense mutation: multiple endocrine defects, decreased sympathetic tone, and immune system dysfunction indicate new targets for leptin action, greater central than peripheral resistance to the effects of leptin, and spontaneous correction of leptin-mediated defects', *J. Clin. Endocrinol. Metab.*, **84** (10), 3686–95.

PASANISI, F., CONTALDO, F., DE SIMONE, G. and MANCINI, M. (2001), 'Benefits of sustained moderate weight loss in obesity', *Nutr. Metab. Cardiovasc. Dis.*, **11** (6), 401–6.

PELKMAN, C. L., FISHELL, V. K., MADDOX, D. H., PEARSON, T. A., MAUGER, D. T. and KRIS-ETHERTON, P. M. (2004), 'Effects of moderate-fat (from monounsaturated fat) and low-fat weight-loss diets on the serum lipid profile in overweight and obese men and women', *Am. J. Clin. Nutr.*, **79** (2), 204–12.

PERMANA, P. A., DEL PARIGI, A. and TATARANNI, P. A. (2004), 'Microarray gene expression profiling in obesity and insulin resistance', *Nutrition*, **20** (1), 134–8.

PETERS, W. R., MACMURRY, J. P., WALKER, J., GIESE, R. J., JR. and COMINGS, D. E. (2003), 'Phenylethanolamine *N*-methyltransferase G-148A genetic variant and weight loss in obese women', *Obes. Res.*, **11** (3), 415–19.

PETERSEN, M. *et al.* (2003). 'Effect of hypo-caloric low-fat versus medium fat diet on body weight – The NUGENOB EU multicentre, randomised trail'. *Int. J. Obes.* **27** [suppl 1], S25.

POTOCZNA, N. *et al.* (2003), 'Melanocortin-4 receptor gene mutations predict outcome of weight loss treatment in severely obese patients'. *Int. J. Obes.* **27** [suppl 1], S73.

POWELL, J. J., TUCKER, L., FISHER, A. G. and WILCOX, K. (1994), 'The effects of different percentages of dietary fat intake, exercise, and calorie restriction on body composition and body weight in obese females', *Am. J. Health Promot.*, **8** (6), 442–8.

RABEN, A., ANDERSEN, H. B., CHRISTENSEN, N. J., MADSEN, J., HOLST, J. J. and ASTRUP, A. (1994), 'Evidence for an abnormal postprandial response to a high-fat meal in women predisposed to obesity', *Am. J. Physiol.*, **267** (4) Pt 1, E549–59.

RABEN, A., VASILARAS, T. H., MOLLER, A. C. and ASTRUP, A. (2002), 'Sucrose compared with artificial sweeteners: different effects on ad libitum food intake and body weight after 10 wk of supplementation in overweight subjects', *Am. J. Clin. Nutr.*, **76** (4), 721–9.

RAM, V. J. (2003), 'Therapeutic role of peroxisome proliferator-activated receptors in obesity, diabetes and inflammation', *Prog. Drug Res.*, **60**, 93–132.

RAWSON, E. S., NOLAN, A., SILVER, K., SHULDINER, A. R. and POEHLMAN, E. T. (2002), 'No effect of the Trp64Arg beta(3)-adrenoceptor gene variant on weight loss, body composition, or energy expenditure in obese, caucasian postmenopausal women', *Metabolism*, **51** (6), 801–5.

REDONNET, A., BONILLA, S., NOEL-SUBERVILLE, C. *et al.* (2002), 'Relationship between peroxisome proliferator-activated receptor gamma and retinoic acid receptor alpha gene expression in obese human adipose tissue', *Int. J. Obes. Relat. Metab. Disord.*, **26** (7), 920–7.

REILLY, J. J. and DOROSTY, A. R. (1999), 'Epidemic of obesity in UK children', *Lancet*, **354** (9193), 1874–5.

RICHELSEN, B., PEDERSEN, S. B., KRISTENSEN, K. *et al.* (2000), 'Regulation of lipoprotein lipase and hormone-sensitive lipase activity and gene expression in adipose and muscle tissue by growth hormone treatment during weight loss in obese patients', *Metabolism*, **49** (7), 906–11.

ROBITAILLE, J., DESPRES, J. P., PERUSSE, L. and VOHL, M. C. (2003), 'The PPAR-gamma P12A polymorphism modulates the relationship between dietary fat intake and components of the metabolic syndrome: results from the Quebec Family Study', *Clin. Genet.*, **63** (2), 109–16.

ROBITAILLE, J., BROUILLETTE, C., HOUDE, A. *et al.* (2004), 'Association between the PPARalpha-L162V polymorphism and components of the metabolic syndrome', *J. Hum. Genet.*, **49** (9), 482–9.

ROME, S., CLEMENT, K., RABASA-LHORET, R. *et al.* (2003), 'Microarray profiling of human skeletal muscle reveals that insulin regulates approximately 800 genes during a hyperinsulinemic clamp', *J. Biol. Chem.*, **278** (20), 18063–8.

ROSMOND, R., CHAGNON, Y. C., CHAGNON, M., PERUSSE, L., BOUCHARD, C. and BJORNTORP, P. (2000), 'A polymorphism of the 5′-flanking region of the glucocorticoid receptor gene locus is associated with basal cortisol secretion in men', *Metabolism*, **49** (9), 1197–9.

SAKANE, N., YOSHIDA, T., UMEKAWA, T., KOGURE, A., TAKAKURA, Y. and KONDO, M. (1997), 'Effects of Trp64Arg mutation in the beta 3-adrenergic receptor gene on weight loss, body fat distribution, glycemic control, and insulin resistance in obese type 2 diabetic patients', *Diabetes Care*, **20** (12), 1887–90.

SALMON, D. M. and FLATT, J. P. (1985), 'Effect of dietary fat content on the incidence of obesity among ad libitum fed mice', *Int. J. Obes.*, **9** (6), 443–9.

SAMAHA, F. F., IQBAL, N., SESHADRI, P. *et al.* (2003), 'A low-carbohydrate as compared with a low-fat diet in severe obesity', *N. Engl. J. Med.*, **348** (21), 2074–81.

SARIS, W. H., ASTRUP, A., PRENTICE, A. M. *et al.* (2000), 'Randomized controlled trial of changes in dietary carbohydrate/fat ratio and simple vs complex carbohydrates on body weight and blood lipids: the CARMEN study. The Carbohydrate Ratio Management in European National diets', *Int. J. Obes. Relat. Metab. Disord.*, **24** (10), 1310–18.

SCHADT, E. E., MONKS, S. A., DRAKE, T. A. *et al.* (2003), 'Genetics of gene expression surveyed in maize, mouse and man', *Nature*, **422** (6929), 297–302.

SEIDELL, J. C. (1998), 'Societal and personal costs of obesity', *Exp. Clin. Endocrinol. Diabetes*, **106** Suppl 2, 7–9.

SHAH, M., MCGOVERN, P., FRENCH, S. and BAXTER, J. (1994), 'Comparison of a low-fat, ad libitum complex-carbohydrate diet with a low-energy diet in moderately obese women', *Am. J. Clin. Nutr.*, **59** (5), 980–4.

SHIWAKU, K., NOGI, A., ANUURAD, E. *et al.* (2003), 'Difficulty in losing weight by behavioral intervention for women with Trp64Arg polymorphism of the beta(3)-adrenergic receptor gene', *Int. J. Obes. Relat. Metab. Disord.*, **27** (9), 1028–36.

SIMOPOULOS, A. P. (1999), 'Genetic variation and nutrition', *Nutr. Rev.*, **57** (5) Pt 2, S10–19.

SINA, M., HINNEY, A., ZIEGLER, A. *et al.* (1999), 'Phenotypes in three pedigrees with autosomal dominant obesity caused by haploinsufficiency mutations in the melanocortin-4 receptor gene', *Am. J. Hum. Genet.*, **65** (6), 1501–7.

SKOV, A. R., TOUBRO, S., RONN, B., HOLM, L. and ASTRUP, A. (1999), 'Randomized trial on protein vs carbohydrate in *ad libitum* fat reduced diet for the treatment of obesity', *Int. J. Obes. Relat. Metab. Disord.*, **23** (5), 528–36.

SNYDER, E. E., WALTS, B., PERUSSE, L. *et al.* (2004), 'The human obesity gene map: the 2003 update', *Obes. Res.*, **12** (3), 369–439.

SORENSEN, H. T., SABROE, S., GILLMAN, M. *et al.* (1997), 'Continued increase in prevalence of obesity in Danish young men.', *Int. J. Obes.*, **21**, 712–14.

SORENSEN, T. I. A. (2003a), 'Weight loss causes increased mortality: pros', *Obes. Rev.*, **4** (1), 3–7.

SORENSEN, T. I. A. (2003b), 'Interpretation of positive energy balance'. *Int. J. Obes.* **27** [suppl 1], S32.

SORENSEN, T. I. A. and ECHWALD, S. M. (2001), '*Obesity genes*', *BMJ*, **322** (7287), 630–1.

SORENSEN, T. I. A., PRICE, R. A., STUNKARD, A. J. and SCHULSINGER, F. (1989), 'Genetics of obesity in adult adoptees and their biological siblings', *BMJ*, **298** (6666), 87–90.

SORENSEN, T. I. A., HOLST, C. and STUNKARD, A. J. (1992), 'Childhood body mass index – genetic and familial environmental influences assessed in a longitudinal adoption study', *Int. J. Obes. Relat. Metab. Disord.*, **16** (9), 705–14.

SORENSEN, T. I. A. (1996), 'Adoption studies of obesity,' in *Molecular and Genetic Aspects of Obesity*, G. A. Bray and D. H. Ryan, eds., Louisiana State University Press, Baton Rouge and London), 462–9.

STICH, V., HARANT, I., DE, G. I. *et al.* (1997), 'Adipose tissue lipolysis and hormone-sensitive lipase expression during very-low-calorie diet in obese female identical twins', *J. Clin. Endocrinol. Metab.*, **82** (3), 739–44.

STICH, V., MARION-LATARD, F., HEJNOVA, J. *et al.* (2002), 'Hypocaloric diet reduces exercise-induced alpha 2-adrenergic antilipolytic effect and alpha 2-adrenergic receptor mRNA levels in adipose tissue of obese women', *J. Clin. Endocrinol. Metab.*, **87** (3), 1274–81.

STRAUSS, R. S. and POLLACK, H. A. (2001), 'Epidemic increase in childhood overweight, 1986–1998', *JAMA*, **286** (22), 2845–8.

STUBBS, R. J., JOHNSTONE, A. M., HARBRON, C. G. and REID, C. (1998), 'Covert manipulation of energy density of high carbohydrate diets in "pseudo free-living" humans', *Int. J. Obes. Relat. Metab. Disord.*, **22** (9), 885–92.

STUNKARD, A. J., SORENSEN, T. I., HANIS, C. *et al.* (1986), 'An adoption study of human obesity', *N. Engl. J. Med.*, **314** (4), 193–8.

STUNKARD, A. J., HARRIS, J. R., PEDERSEN, N. L. and MCCLEARN, G. E. (1990), 'The body-mass index of twins who have been reared apart', *N. Engl. J. Med.*, **322** (21), 1483–7.

SUVIOLAHTI, E., OKSANEN, L. J., OHMAN, M. *et al.* (2003), 'The SLC6A14 gene shows evidence of association with obesity', *J. Clin. Invest.*, **112** (11), 1762–72.

SWARBRICK, M. M. and VAISSE, C. (2003), 'Emerging trends in the search for genetic variants predisposing to human obesity', *Curr. Opin. Clin. Nutr. Metab. Care*, **6** (4), 369–75.

TABOR, H. K., RISCH, N. J. and MYERS, R. M. (2002), 'Opinion: Candidate-gene approaches for studying complex genetic traits: practical considerations', *Nat. Rev. Genet.*, **3** (5), 391–7.

TEEGARDEN, D. (2003), 'Calcium intake and reduction in weight or fat mass', *J. Nutr.*, **133** (1), 249S–51S.

THOMPSON, D. and WOLF, A. M. (2001), 'The medical-care cost burden of obesity', *Obes. Rev.*, **2** (3), 189–97.

THOMSEN, B. L., EKSTROM, C. T. and SORENSEN, T. I. (1999), 'Development of the obesity epidemic in Denmark: cohort, time and age effects among boys born 1930–1975', *Int. J. Obes. Relat. Metab. Disord.*, **23** (7), 693–701.

UKKOLA, O. and BOUCHARD, C. (2004), 'Role of candidate genes in the responses to long-term overfeeding: review of findings', *Obes. Rev.*, **5** (1), 3–12.

VAISSE, C., CLEMENT, K., GUY-GRAND, B. and FROGUEL, P. (1998), 'A frameshift mutation in human MC4R is associated with a dominant form of obesity', *Nat. Genet.*, **20** (2), 113–14.

VAISSE, C., CLEMENT, K., DURAND, E., HERCBERG, S., GUY-GRAND, B. and FROGUEL, P. (2000), 'Melanocortin-4 receptor mutations are a frequent and heterogeneous cause of morbid obesity', *J. Clin. Invest.*, **106** (2), 253–62.

VAN GAAL, L. F., WAUTERS, M. A. and DE LEEUW, I. H. (1997), 'The beneficial effects of modest weight loss on cardiovascular risk factors', *Int. J. Obes. Relat. Metab. Disord.*, **21** Suppl 1, S5–9.

VAN TILBURG, J. H., SANDKUIJL, L. A., STRENGMAN, E. *et al.* (2003), 'A genome-wide scan in type 2 diabetes mellitus provides independent replication of a susceptibility locus on 18p11 and suggests the existence of novel Loci on 2q12 and 19q13', *J. Clin. Endocrinol. Metab.*, **88** (5), 2223–30.

VIGUERIE, N. and LANGIN, D. (2003), 'Effect of thyroid hormone on gene expression', *Curr. Opin. Clin. Nutr. Metab. Care*, **6** (4), 377–81.

VIGUERIE, N., POITOU, C., CANCELLO, R., STICH, V., CLEMENT, K., and LANGIN, D. (2005a), 'Transcriptomics applied to obesity and caloric restriction', *Biochimie*, **87** (1), 117–23.

VIGUERIE, N., VIDAL, H., ARNER, P., HOLST, C., VERDICH, C., AVIZOU, S., ASTRUP, A., SARIS, W. H., MACDONALD, I. A., KLIMCAKOVA, E., CLÉMENT, K., MARTINEZ, A., HOFFSTEDT, J., SORENSEN, T. I. A. and LANGIN, D. (2005b), 'Adipose tissue gene expression in obese subjects during low-fat and high-fat hypocaloric diets', *Diabetologia*, **48** (1), 123–31.

VINCENT, S., PLANELLS, R., DEFOORT, C. *et al.* (2002), 'Genetic polymorphisms and lipoprotein responses to diets', *Proc. Nutr. Soc.*, **61** (4), 427–34.

VOGLER, G. P., SORENSEN, T. I., STUNKARD, A. J., SRINIVASAN, M. R. and RAO, D. C. (1995), 'Influences of genes and shared family environment on adult body mass index assessed in an adoption study by a comprehensive path model', *Int. J. Obes. Relat. Metab. Disord.*, **19** (1), 40–5.

WADDEN, T. A., FOSTER, G. D. and LETIZIA, K. A. (1994), 'One-year behavioral treatment of obesity: comparison of moderate and severe caloric restriction and the effects of weight maintenance therapy', *J. Consult Clin. Psychol.*, **62** (1), 165–71.

WEST, D. B., WAGUESPACK, J. and MCCOLLISTER, S. (1995), 'Dietary obesity in the mouse: interaction of strain with diet composition', *Am. J. Physiol.*, **268** (3) Pt 2, R658–65.

WEST, D. B. and YORK, B. (1998), 'Dietary fat, genetic predisposition, and obesity: lessons from animal models', *Am. J. Clin. Nutr.*, **67** (3) Suppl, 505S–12S.

WILLIAMS, R. R. (1984), 'The role of genetic analyses in characterizing obesity', *Int. J. Obes.*, **8** (5), 551–9.

WORLD HEALTH ORGANIZATION (1997), *Obesity; Preventing and Managing the Global Epidemic; Report of a WHO Consultation on Obesity; Geneva, 3–5 June 1997*, World Health Organization, Geneva, Geneva.

XINLI, W., XIAOMEI, T., MEIHUA, P. and SONG, L. (2001), 'Association of a mutation in the beta3-adrenergic receptor gene with obesity and response to dietary intervention in Chinese children', *Acta Paediatr.*, **90** (11), 1233–7.

YAMADA, K., YUAN, X., OTABE, S., KOYANAGI, A., KOYAMA, W. and MAKITA, Z. (2002), 'Sequencing of the putative promoter region of the cocaine- and amphetamine-regulated-transcript gene and identification of polymorphic sites associated with obesity', *Int. J. Obes. Relat. Metab. Disord.*, **26** (1), 132–6.

YANAGISAWA, K., HINGSTRUP, L. L., ANDERSEN, G. *et al.* (2003), 'The FOXC2 –512C>T variant is associated with hypertriglyceridaemia and increased serum C-peptide in Danish Caucasian glucose-tolerant subjects', *Diabetologia*, **46** (11), 1576–80.

YANG, D., FONTAINE, K. R., WANG, C. and ALLISON, D. B. (2003), 'Weight loss causes increased mortality: cons', *Obes. Rev.*, **4** (1), 9–16.

YEO, G. S., LANK, E. J., FAROOQI, I. S., KEOGH, J., CHALLIS, B. G. and O'RAHILLY, S. (2003), 'Mutations in the human melanocortin-4 receptor gene associated with severe familial obesity disrupts receptor function through multiple molecular mechanisms', *Hum. Mol. Genet.*, **12** (5), 561–74.

ZEMEL, M. B. (2004), 'Role of calcium and dairy products in energy partitioning and weight management', *Am. J. Clin. Nutr.*, **79** (5), 907S–12S.

ZHANG, Y., PROENCA, R., MAFFEI, M., BARONE, M., LEOPOLD, L. and FRIEDMAN, J. M. (1994), 'Positional cloning of the mouse obese gene and its human homologue', *Nature*, **372** (6505), 425–32.

3

Energy metabolism and obesity

A. Astrup, Royal Agricultural and Veterinary University, Denmark

3.1 Introduction

The first law of thermodynamics states that energy can neither be destroyed nor created. This principle necessitates that body energy stores must remain constant when energy intake equals energy expenditure. This law is a prerequisite for the entire physiology and biochemistry of energy metabolism. An understanding of the physiology of energy expenditure is important for obvious reasons: energy expenditure equals energy requirement of a person, and large differences between subjects in **energy requirements*** can be explained by variations in the determinants of energy expenditure, such as body size and composition, age, physical activity, thyroid hormones, catecholamines, and variants in genes of importance.

Energy intake is defined as the total energy content of foods consumed, as provided by the major sources of dietary energy: carbohydrate (4 **kcal**/g), protein (4 kcal/g), fat (9 kcal/g) and alcohol (7 kcal/g). The energy that is consumed in the form of food and calorie containing drinks can either be stored in the body in the form of fat (the major energy store), glycogen (short-term energy/carbohydrate reserves), or protein (rarely used by the body for energy except in severe cases of starvation and other wasting conditions as discussed later in the chapter), or used by the body to fuel energy requiring events.

Most subjects are likely to have consumed close to one million calories in the last year. Despite this enormous energy intake, most individuals are

* Terms marked with bold on first mention in the text are listed in the glossary.

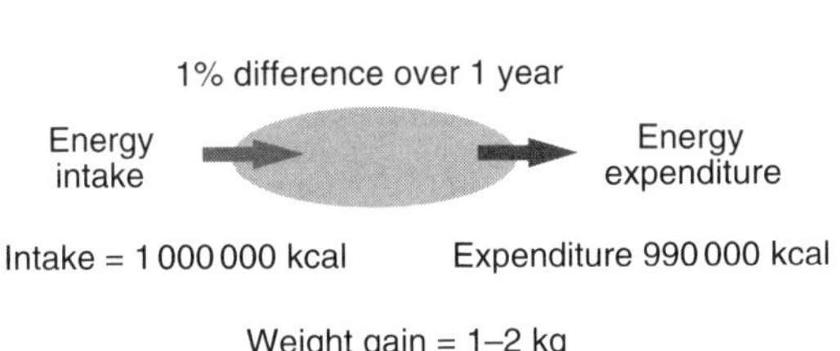

Fig. 3.1 Pictorial diagram representing the balance between energy intake and expenditure.

able to obtain a remarkable balance between how much energy is consumed and how much energy is expended, thus resulting in a state of **energy balance** in the body. The system responsible for this accurate balance between energy intake and energy expenditure is an example of homoeostatic mechanisms that regulate and maintain a constant body weight and body energy stores. This regulation of energy balance is achieved over the long term despite large fluctuations in both energy intake and energy expenditure within and between days. The accuracy and precision by which the body maintains energy balance is highlighted by the fact that even a small permanent error in the system can have detrimental consequences over time. If energy intake chronically exceeds energy expenditure by as little as 50 kcal/day, this is sufficient to explain the substantial weight gain observed in the North American population (Fig. 3.1).

3.2 How to measure energy expenditure

Energy expenditure can be measured by assessment of total heat production in the body (direct calorimetry) or indirectly by measurement of the body's oxygen consumption and carbon dioxide production (indirect calorimetry). The process of energy expenditure and the **oxidation, or combustion, of food** for energy in the body is analogous to a wood-stove which burns wood to release heat in a controlled fashion. In the wood stove analogy, fuel is supplied to the stove and the fuel is gradually combusted in the presence of oxygen to release carbon dioxide, water vapor, and heat. This is similar to what happens in the body when food is consumed. Food is consumed, digested, absorbed, and then oxidised or combusted in the presence of oxygen to release carbon dioxide, water and heat, or, if in excess of requirements, stored. When ingested food is used for energy production, the release and transfer of energy occurs through a series of tightly regulated metabolic pathways in which the potential energy from food is released slowly and gradually over time. This process ensures that the body is provided with a gradual and constant energy store, rather than relying on a sudden release of energy from an immediate combustion of ingested food. As a simple example of how the body uses food for energy, consider the combustion of a simple glucose molecule as follows:

$$C_6H_{12}O_6 + 6O_2 = 6H_2O + 6CO_2 + \text{heat}$$

Similar chemical reactions can be described for the combustion of other sources of energy such as fat, alcohol and other types of carbohydrates. These types of reactions occur continuously in the body and constitute energy expenditure. As discussed previously, the three major sources of energy expenditure in the body are to fuel **resting metabolic rate**, the **thermic effect of meals**, and physical activity. This is discussed in more detail below.

3.2.1 Direct vs. indirect calorimetry

The direct calorimeter was the first used to estimate energy expenditure by measurement of heat production. Direct calorimeters have been built for measuring heat production in humans, but this approach is technically complicated for human studies, and is now infrequently used. Indirect calorimetry measures energy production via respiratory gas analysis. This approach is based on the oxygen consumption and carbon dioxide production that occurs during the combustion (or oxidation) of protein, carbohydrate, fat and alcohol, as shown in the example of glucose combustion. Respiratory gas analysis can easily be achieved in humans over short measurement periods at rest or during exercise using a face mask, mouthpiece, or canopy system for gas collection, and over longer periods of 24 hours (or more) by having subjects live in a metabolic chamber. Resting metabolic rate is typically measured by indirect calorimetry under fasting conditions, while subjects lie quietly at rest in the early morning for 30–40 minutes. The thermic effect of a meal is typically measured by monitoring the changes in metabolic rate by indirect calorimetry for 3–4 hours following consumption of a test meal of known caloric content. The energy expended in physical activity can be measured under laboratory conditions also using indirect calorimetry during standard activities. In addition, free-living physical activity related energy expenditure over extended time periods of up to 2 weeks can be measured by the combination of **doubly labelled water** to measure total energy expenditure (see below), and indirect calorimetry to measure resting energy expenditure and the thermic effect of a meal. Indirect calorimetry has an added advantage in that the ratio of carbon dioxide production to oxygen consumption (the respiratory quotient, or RQ), is indicative of the type of substrate (i.e. fat versus carbohydrate) being oxidised; for example carbohydrate oxidation has an RQ of 1.0, and fat oxidation has an RQ close to 0.7.

3.3 Major components of daily energy expenditure

The energy that is consumed in the form of food is required by the body for cellular, metabolic and mechanical work such as breathing, heart pump function and muscular work, all of which require energy and result in heat production. The body requires energy for a variety of functions. The largest use of energy is needed to fuel **resting** (RMR) **or basal metabolic rate** (BMR), which is the energy expended by the body to maintain basic physiological functions (e.g. heart beat, muscle contraction and function, respiration). BMR is the minimum level of energy expended by the body to sustain life in the woken state. It can be measured after a 12-hour fast while the subject is maintained in a thermoneutral, quiet environment. During sleep metabolic rate is about 5% lower than BMR, because energy expenditure increases above basal levels due to the energy cost of arousal. Because of the difficulty in achieving basal metabolic rate under most measurement situations, resting metabolic rate is frequently measured using the same measurement conditions stated for basal metabolic rate. Thus, the major difference between basal and resting metabolic rate is the slightly higher energy expended during resting metabolic rate (~3%) due to subject arousal and non-fasting. Because of this small difference, the terms, basal and resting metabolic rate are often used interchangeably. Resting metabolic rate occurs in a continual process throughout the 24 hours of a day, and remains relatively constant within individuals over time. In the average adult human resting metabolic rate is approximately 1 kcal/minute. Thus, basal or resting metabolic rate is the largest component of energy expenditure and makes up about two-thirds of total energy expenditure. Because RMR is heavily dependent on the size of the individual's fat-free mass, and fat mass, RMR is often adjusted for differences in fat-free mass and fat mass to allow for comparisons between individuals. The unadjusted RMR is then referred to as the absolute RMR, and the adjusted as the relative RMR.

In addition to resting metabolic rate, there is an increase in energy expenditure in response to food intake. This increase in metabolic rate after food consumption is often referred to as the thermic effect of a meal (or meal induced thermogenesis) and is the energy that is expended in order to digest, metabolise, and store ingested macronutrients. The energy cost associated with meal ingestion is primarily influenced by the composition of the food that is consumed, and is also relatively stable within individuals over time. The thermic effect of a meal usually constitutes ~10% of the caloric content of the meal that is consumed. The third source of energy expenditure in the body is the increase in metabolic rate that occurs during physical activity (this includes exercise as well as all forms of physical activity). Thus **physical activity energy expenditure (or the thermic effect of exercise)** is the term frequently used to describe the increase in metabolic rate that is caused by use of skeletal muscles for any type of muscle movement. Physical activity energy expenditure is the most variable component of

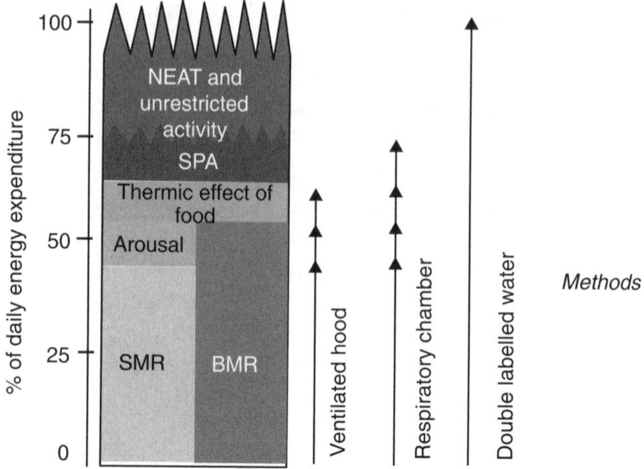

Fig. 3.2 Chart showing components of energy expenditure.

daily energy expenditure and can vary greatly within and between individuals due to the volitional and variable nature of physical activity patterns (Fig. 3.2).

In addition to the three major components of energy expenditure there may also be a requirement for energy for two other minor needs. The energy cost of growth occurs in growing individuals, but is negligible except within the first few months of life. Finally, adaptive thermogenesis is heat production during exposure to reduced temperatures, but rarely occurs in humans except during the initial months of life.

3.3.1 Factors that influence energy expenditure

Each of the components of energy expenditure is determined by various factors. Resting metabolic rate is highly variable between individuals (±25%), but is very consistent within individuals (less than ±5%). Since resting metabolic rate occurs predominantly in muscle and the major organs of the body, the main source of individual variability in resting metabolic rate is an individual's amount of organ and muscle mass.

Body size and composition

Fat-free mass (total mass of the body that is not fat, i.e. predominantly organs and muscle) explains 60–80% of the variation in resting metabolic rate between individuals. Since fat-free mass is a heterogenous mixture of all non-fat body components, the metabolic rate associated with each kilogram of fat free mass is dependent on the quality of the fat-free mass, in terms of hydration and relative contribution of the different organs that make up the fat-free mass. For example, skeletal muscle compromises ~43% of total mass in an adult, but only contributes 22–36% of resting metabolic rate, whereas the brain, which constitutes only ~2% of mass, contributes 20–24% of the resting metabolic rate.

Resting metabolic rate is also influenced by fat mass even though fat mass is generally thought to be metabolically inert. Fat mass contributes in the order of 10–13 kcal/kg to resting metabolic rate. In healthy adults resting metabolic rate declines with age, this decline being greater than would be expected given the age-related decline in fat-free mass. Resting metabolic rate is also influenced by sex, where males have a higher value than females by ~50 kcal/day.

Other factors

More active people tend to have a higher resting metabolic rate than inactive individuals. This difference may be explained in part by the residual effects of chronic exercise on metabolic rate. In other words, resting metabolic rate appears to be elevated because of the long-lasting effects of the thermic effect of exercise. However, other factors are also involved since the higher resting metabolic rate in more active individuals persists long after the last bout of exercise has been completed. Collectively, fat-free mass, fat mass, age, sex and physical activity explain 80–90% of the variance in resting metabolic rate. In addition, a portion of the remaining variance in resting metabolic rate between individuals can be ascribed to differences in thyroid hormone levels, sympathetic nervous system activity, and variants in genes (beta-3, uncoupling proteins, etc).

3.3.2 Predicting BMR

There are a number of prediction equations that have been developed in order to estimate resting metabolic rate from other simple measures. These equations are often useful for making estimates in clinical situations when measurement of resting metabolic rate cannot be achieved, or for estimating energy needs for other individuals. Recent equations have been developed in large groups of subjects and can predict resting metabolic rate from body weight (Table 3.1).

3.3.3 Meal-induced thermogenesis

The **meal-induced thermogenesis or thermic effect of meal** ingestion is primarily influenced by the quantity and macronutrient composition of the ingested calories. The increase in metabolic rate that occurs after meal ingestion occurs over an extended period of at least 5 hours. The cumulative energy cost is equivalent to ~10% of the energy ingested. In other words, if one consumed a mixed meal of 500 kcal, the body would require 50 kcal to digest, process and metabolise the contents of the meal. The

Table 3.1 Simple equations for estimating RMR from body weight[a] according to sex and age

Age (years)	Equation for females	Equation for males
0–3	(60.9 × wt) – 54	(61.0 × wt) – 51
3–10	(22.7 × wt) + 495	(22.5 × wt) + 499
10–18	(17.5 × wt) + 651	(12.2 × wt) + 746
18–30	(15.3 × wt) + 679	(14.7 × wt) + 496
30–60	(11.6 × wt) + 879	(8.7 × wt) + 829
>60	(13.5 × wt) + 487	(10.5 × wt) + 596

[a] Body weight is in kg and RMR is in kcal/day.

thermic effect of feeding is higher for protein (25–30%) and carbohydrate (5–10%) than for fat (1–4%). This is because for fat, the process of energy storage is very efficient, whereas for carbohydrate and protein, additional energy is required for metabolic conversion to the appropriate storage form (i.e. excess glucose converted to glycogen for storage, and excess amino acids from protein, converted to fat for storage).

3.3.4 Physical activity related to energy expenditure

Physical activity energy expenditure encompasses all types of activity including sports and leisure, occupational related activities, general activities of daily living, as well as fidgeting. The metabolic rate of physical activity is determined by the amount or duration of the activity (i.e. time), the type of physical activity (e.g. walking, running, typing), as well as the intensity at which the particular activity is performed. The metabolic cost of physical activities is frequently expressed as metabolic equivalent (METS), which represents multiples of resting metabolic rate. Thus, by definition, sitting quietly after a 12-hour fast is equivalent to 1 MET. The cumulative total daily energy cost of physical activity is highly variable both within and between individuals. Therefore physical activity provides the greatest source of flexibility in the energy expenditure system and is the component through which large changes in energy expenditure can be achieved.

3.3.5 Total energy expenditure

The integrated sum of all components of energy expenditure is termed total energy expenditure. Total energy expenditure is measured over 24 hours or longer in a metabolic chamber, but this environment is artificial and is not representative of the normal daily pattern of physical activity. The doubly labelled water technique allows measurement of the integrated sum of all components of daily energy expenditure, typically over 7–14 days, while subjects are living in their usual environment. The doubly labelled water method requires a person to ingest small amounts of 'heavy' water that is isotopically labelled with deuterium and oxygen-18 (^2H_2O and $H_2{}^{18}O$). In deuterium labelled water the hydrogen is replaced with deuterium, which is an identical form of water except that deuterium has an extra neutron in its nucleus compared to hydrogen, and is thus a heavier form of water. Similarly, oxygen-18 labelled water contains oxygen with an additional two extra neutrons. Thus, these stable isotopes act as molecular tags so that water can be tracked in the body. After a loading dose, deuterium labelled water is washed out of the body as a function of body water turnover. Oxygen-18 is also lost as a function of water turnover, but it is also lost via carbon dioxide production. Therefore, using a number of assumptions, the rate of carbon dioxide production and energy expenditure can be assessed based on the different rates of loss of these isotopes from the body. A major advantage of the doubly labelled water method is that it is non-invasive and non-radioactive, and measurement is performed under free living conditions over 1–2 weeks. Moreover, when BMR is assessed at the same time, physical activity related energy expenditure can be assessed by the difference (i.e. total energy expenditure minus resting metabolic rate, minus the thermic effect of meals = physical activity energy expenditure). Furthermore, assessment of total energy expenditure by the doubly labelled water method can also provide a measure of total energy intake in subjects who are in energy balance. This is because, by definition, in a state of energy balance total energy intake must be equivalent to total energy expenditure. This aspect of the technique has been used as a tool to validate energy intakes using other methods such as food records and dietary recall. For example, it has been known for some time that obese subjects report a lower than expected value for energy intake. At one time it was thought that this may be explained by low energy requirements in the obese due to low energy expenditure and reduced physical activity. However, using doubly labelled water, it has now been established that obese subjects under-report their actual energy intake and actually have a normal energy expenditure, relative to their larger body size. The good accuracy and reasonable precision of the technique allows this method to be regarded as the 'gold standard' measure of total free living energy expenditure in humans.

3.4 Interaction between energy intake and physical activity

How much energy intake is needed to sustain life and maintain our body energy stores? Why do some people require more energy and others less? In other words, what are the energy requirements of different types of people? Based on our earlier definition of energy balance, the energy requirements of the body in order to maintain energy balance must be equal to total daily energy expenditure. Total daily energy expenditure represents the total energy requirements of an individual required to maintain energy balance. With the doubly labelled water technique it is possible to accurately measure total daily energy expenditure, and thus energy needs, in free living humans.

Total energy expenditure is often compared across groups or individuals using the ratio of total energy expenditure to resting metabolic rate, or **physical activity index**. Thus, if one's total energy expenditure is 3000 kcal/day and the resting metabolic rate is 1500 kcal/day, the physical activity index will be 2.0. This value indicates that total energy expenditure is twice the resting metabolic rate. The physical activity index has been assessed in a variety of types of individuals. A low physical activity index indicates a sedentary lifestyle, whereas a high index represents a highly active lifestyle. The highest recorded sustained physical activity index in humans was recorded in cyclists participating in the *Tour de France* road race. These elite athletes were able to sustain a daily energy expenditure that was up to five times their resting metabolic rate over extended periods of time. As stated above, factors such as body weight, fat free mass, and resting metabolic rate account for 40–60% of the variation in total energy expenditure.

3.5 Energy expenditure at different ages

3.5.1 Energy expenditure in infancy and childhood

During the first 12 months of life, energy intake falls from almost 125 kcal/kg per day in the first month of life to a nadir of 95 kcal/kg per day by the eighth month, then rising to 105 kcal/kg per day by the twelfth month. However, total energy expenditure in the first year of life is relatively constant at ~60–70 kcal/kg per day. In infants the large difference between total energy expenditure and energy intake is explained by a **positive energy balance** to account for growth. In the first 3 months of life it is estimated that the energy accretion due to growth is 167 kcal/day or approximately 32% of energy intake, falling to 36 kcal/day or 4% of energy intake by 1 year of age. Individual growth rates and early infancy feeding behaviour are two known factors that would cause variation in these figures.

There is now substantial evidence to suggest that existing recommendations may overestimate true energy needs, based on measurement of total energy expenditure in infants. In the first year of life traditional values of energy requirements overestimate those derived from measurement of total energy expenditure and adjusted for growth by 11%. Between 1 and 3 years of age the discrepancy is more striking, where the traditional values for requirements are 20% higher than those derived from total energy expenditure and adjusted for growth. For example, in 3-year-old children total energy expenditure estimated by doubly labelled water averages 1210 kcal/day, while the currently recommended intake for these children is 1470 kcal/day. Thus, newer estimates of energy needs in infants based on assessment of total energy expenditure data are needed.

In the average 5-year-old child weighing 20 kg total energy expenditure is approximately 1300–1400 kcal/day, which is significantly lower (by ~400–500 kcal/day) than the existing RDAs for energy in children of this age. Thus, as with infants, newer estimates of energy needs in children based on assessment of total energy expenditure data are needed.

3.5.2 Ageing

In one group of the elderly there is a decline in food intake that is associated with dynamic changes in body composition, where there is a tendency to lose fat-free mass that leads to loss in functionality. In another group there is a tendency to gain fat mass, which increases the risk of obesity, cardiovascular disease, and non-insulin dependent diabetes. These two opposing patterns suggest that the ability to self-regulate whole body energy balance may diminish with age. Thus, prescription of individual energy requirements may serve as a useful tool to prevent the age-related deterioration of body composition. Other special considerations in the elderly relate to meeting energy needs in special populations, such as those suffering from Alzheimer or Parkinson disease, which frequently lead to malnourished states and diminished body weight. It was thought that these neurological conditions may lead to body weight loss through an associated hypermetabolic condition in which metabolic rate increases above normal, thus increasing energy needs. However, more recent studies have clearly shown that the wasting, or loss of body weight, often associated with these conditions is explained by a reduction in food intake, probably due to a loss in functionality.

3.5.3 Energy requirements in physically active groups

The doubly labelled water technique has been used to assess energy requirements in highly physically active groups of people. The most extreme case is a study assessing the energy requirements of cyclists performing in the 3-week long *Tour de France* bicycle race. The level of total energy expenditure recorded (5.3 times resting metabolic rate, or approximately 8500 kcal/day) is the highest recorded sustained level in humans. In young male soldiers under training, energy requirements can be 5000 kcal/day (2.6 times predicted resting metabolic rate). Total energy expenditure in free living collegiate swimmers is almost 4000 kcal/day in men and 2600 kcal/day in women.

Regular participation in exercise is traditionally thought to elevate energy requirements due to the additional direct cost of the activity itself as well as through an increase in resting metabolic rate. However, in some situations energy requirements are not necessarily altered by participation in regular physical activity. For example, in a study of an elderly group of healthy volunteers, there was no significant change in total energy expenditure in the last 2 weeks of an 8-week vigorous endurance training programme. The failure to detect an increase in total energy expenditure occurred despite a 10% increase in resting metabolic rate (1596 ± 214 to 1763 ± 170 kcal/day), as well as an additional 150 kcal/day associated with the exercise programme. These increases in energy expenditure were counteracted by a significant reduction in the energy expenditure of physical activity during non-exercising time (571 ± 386 vs. 340 ± 452 kcal/day). The lack of increase in total energy expenditure in this study is probably explained by a compensatory 'energy conserving' adaptation to this vigorous training programme leading to a reduction in spontaneous physical activity and/or a reduction in voluntary physical activities, similar to that observed in several animal studies. Thus, it should not automatically be assumed that energy requirements are elevated by participation in activity programmes and that the ultimate change in energy requirement is dictated by the intensity of the training programme and the net sum of change in the individual components of energy expenditure. An important area of research is to identify the programme of exercise intervention in terms of exercise mode, type, duration and intensity, which has the optimal effect on all components of energy balance.

3.5.4 Energy expenditure in pregnancy and lactation

Pregnancy and lactation are two other examples of healthy human conditions in which energy metabolism is altered in order to achieve positive energy balance. The specific changes in energy requirements during pregnancy are unclear and the various factors affecting this change are complex. Traditional government guidelines suggest that energy requirements are raised by 300 kcal/day during pregnancy. This figure is based on theoretical calculations based on the energy accumulation associated with pregnancy. However, these figures do not include potential adaptations in either metabolic efficiency or physical activity level during pregnancy. In a study that performed measurements in 12 women every 6 weeks during pregnancy the average increase in total energy expenditure was 252 kcal/day. The average energy cost of pregnancy (change in total energy expenditure plus change in energy storage) was 433 kcal/day. However, there was considerable variation among the 12 subjects in the increase in average total energy expenditure (–63 kcal/day to 900 kcal/day) and the average energy cost of pregnancy (35 kcal/day to 1235 kcal/day).

3.6 Energy expenditure and balance in obesity

3.6.1 Why store fat?

A typical normal weight adult with 15 kg of fat carries 135 000 kcal of stored energy. If this person did not eat and was inactive, he might require

2000 kcal/day for survival, and the energy stores would be sufficient for almost 70 days, and this is the limit of human survival without food. Given that glycogen stores require 4 gram to store 1 kcal (3 gram of water plus 1 gram of glycogen = 4 kcal), it can be calculated that 135 kg of weight is required to carry this much energy in the form of glycogen. It is obvious why our body's metabolism favours fat as the preferred energy store. But why does the fat store expand excessively in some subjects and not in others?

3.6.2 Negative and positive energy balance

Energy balance occurs when the energy content of food is matched by the total amount of energy that is expended by the body. An example of energy balance would be the scenario cited at the start of this chapter: in the course of a year the average adult consumes and expends one million calories, resulting in no net change in the energy content of the body. When energy intake exceeds energy expenditure a state of positive energy balance develops. Thus, positive energy balance occurs when excessive overfeeding relative to energy requirements occurs, and the body subsequently increases its overall energy stores. Examples of positive energy balance include periods of time around major seasonal event (e.g. during Christmas) when overeating and inactivity generally prevail, and during pregnancy and lactation when the body purposely increases its stores of energy. When energy intake is lower than energy expenditure a state of **negative energy balance** occurs, e.g. during periods of starvation. It is important to note that energy balance can occur regardless of the levels of energy intake and expenditure. Thus energy balance can occur in very inactive individuals as well as in highly active individuals provided that adequate energy sources are available. It is also important to think of energy balance in terms of the major sources of energy, i.e. carbohydrate, protein and fat. For example, carbohydrate balance occurs when the body balances the amount of carbohydrate ingested with that expended for energy.

3.6.3 Energy balance in obesity

As mentioned above, the sources of energy in the food we eat include the major macronutrients: protein, carbohydrate, and fat, as well as alcohol. Carbohydrate and protein provide 4 kcal of energy for each gram; alcohol provides 7 kcal/g, while fat is the most energy dense, providing 9 kcal/g. One kcal is defined as the amount of heat that is required to raise the temperature of 1 liter of water by 1°C. The energy content of food can be measured by bomb calorimetry. This involves combusting a known weight of food inside a sealed chamber and measuring the amount of heat that is released during this process. One gram of pure fat would release 9 kcal during its complete combustion, while 1 g of pure carbohydrate would release 4 kcal. The values 4, 7, and 9 kcal are rounded and averaged values, after adjusting bomb calorimeter values for typical digestive and metabolic losses.

Thus if the quantities in grams of any type of food are known the energy content can easily be calculated. For example, if a protein rich nutrition snack contains 21 g of carbohydrate, 6 g of fat and 14 g of protein, then the total energy content is $(21 \times 4) + (6 \times 9) + (14 \times 4) = 194$ kcal. The macronutrient composition of food is typically assessed in the percent contribution of each macronutrient to the total number of calories. In our example the carbohydrate content is 21 g, which is 84 kcal or 43% of the total energy in the bar, the fat content is 6 g/54 kcal, equivalent to 28% of the energy, and the protein contributes 14 g/56 kcal, or 29% of the energy (Fig. 3.3).

Stated simply, obesity is the end result of positive energy balance, or an increased energy intake relative to expenditure. However, even the proportion of energy absorbed may vary and be influenced by genetic variability in enzymes responsible for absorption and handling in the enterocyte. Moreover, many dietary factors such as fibre and calcium content, and gut micro flora may significantly influence the extent to which fat and carbohydrate are absorbed from the gastrointestinal channel. It is often stated, or assumed, that obesity is simply the result of overeating or lack of physical activity. However, the aetiology of obesity is not this simple, and many complex and inter-related factors are likely to contribute to the

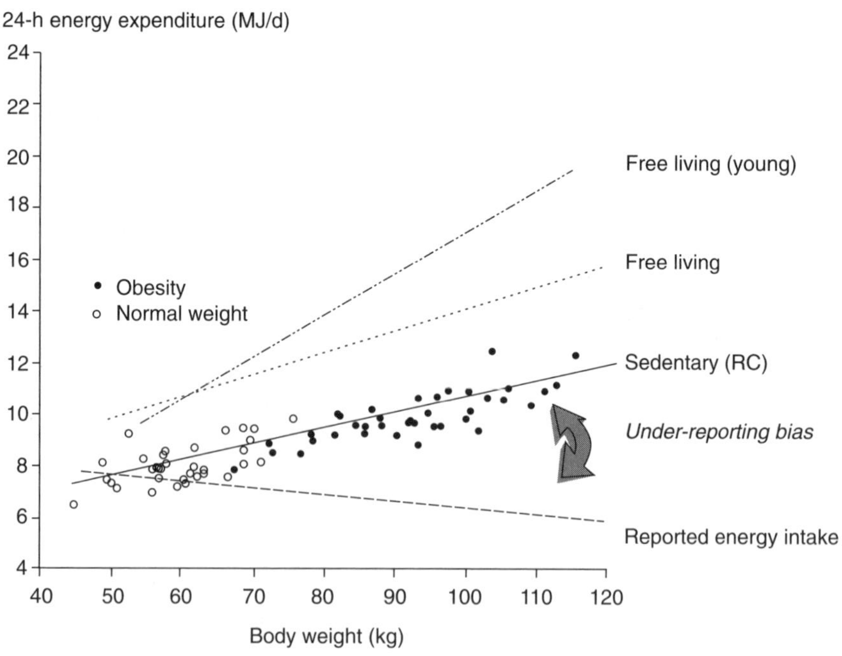

Fig. 3.3 Graph of energy intake vs. expenditure.

development of obesity. It is extremely unlikely that any one single factor causes obesity. Many cultural, behavioural and biological factors drive energy intake and energy expenditure, and contribute to the homoeostatic regulation of body energy stores. In addition, many of these factors are influenced by individual susceptibility, which may be driven by genetic, cultural and/or hormonal factors. Obesity may develop very gradually over time, such that the actual energy imbalance is negligible and undetectable.

Although there are genetic influences on the various components of body weight regulation, and a major portion of individual differences in body weight can be explained by genetic differences, it seems unlikely that the increased global prevalence of obesity has been driven by a dramatic change in the gene pool. It is more likely and reasonable to assume that acute changes in behaviour and environment have contributed to the rapid increase in obesity, and that genetic factors may be important in the individual's susceptibility to these changes. The most striking behavioural changes that have occurred have been an increased reliance on high fat and energy dense fast foods, with larger portion sizes, coupled with an ever increasing sedentary lifestyle. The more sedentary lifestyle is due to an increased reliance on technology and labour saving devices, which has reduced the need for physical activity in everyday activities. Examples of energy saving devices which have resulted in a secular decline in physical activity include: (a) increased use of automated transport rather than walking or biking; (b) central heating and use of automated equipment in the household such as washing machines; (c) reduction in physical activity in the workplace due to computers, automated equipment, electronic mail, which all reduce the requirement for physical activity at work; (d) increased use of television and computers for entertainment and leisure activities; (e) use of elevators and escalators rather than using stairs; (f) increased concern for crime which has reduced the likelihood of outdoor play; (g) poor urban planning which does not provide adequate cycle paths, or even pavements in some communities. Thus, the increasing prevalence of obesity, with the numerous concomitant health risks and astounding economic costs, clearly justify widespread efforts to promote prevention.

The relationship between obesity and lifestyle factors reflects the principle of energy balance. Weight maintenance is the result of equivalent levels of energy intake and energy expenditure. A discrepancy between energy expenditure and energy intake depends on either food intake or energy expenditure, and it is becoming clear that physical activity provides the main source of 'plasticity' in energy expenditure. In addition, lifestyle factors such as dietary and activity patterns are clearly susceptible to behavioural modification, and are likely targets for obesity prevention programmes. A second, yet related, reason why the control of the obesity epidemic is dependent on preventive action is that both the causes and health consequences of obesity begin early in life and track into adulthood. For example, both dietary and activity patterns responsible for the increasing prevalence of obesity are evident in childhood.

3.6.4 Low physical activity or high energy intake in the development of obesity

Although it is a popular belief that a reduced level of energy expenditure leads to the development of obesity, this hypothesis remains controversial and has been difficult to prove. There are certainly good examples of an inverse relationship between physical activity and obesity (e.g. athletes are lean and non-obese individuals), as well as good examples of the positive relationship between obesity and physical inactivity (obese individuals tend to be less physically active). Similar to the results for physical activity, there are some studies suggesting that a low level of energy expenditure predicts the development of obesity, and others which do not support this hypothesis.

Physical activity is supposed to protect the individual from the development of obesity through several mechanisms. Firstly, physical activity, by definition, results in an increase in energy expenditure due to the cost of the activity itself, and is also hypothesised to increase resting metabolic rate. These increases in energy expenditure are likely to decrease the likelihood of positive energy balance. You can simply eat more calories without gaining weight. However, the entire picture of energy balance must be considered, particularly the possibility that increases in one or more components of energy expenditure can result in a compensatory reduction in other components (i.e. resting energy expenditure and activity energy expenditure). Secondly, physical activity has beneficial effects on substrate metabolism, with an increased reliance on fat relative to carbohydrate for fuel utilisation, and it has been hypothesised that highly active individuals can maintain energy balance on a high fat diet.

3.7 Producing a negative energy balance in obese subjects

In almost every overweight and obese patient the diet must be adjusted to reduce energy intake. Dietary therapy consists of instructing patients on how to modify their dietary intake to achieve a decrease in energy intake while maintaining a nutritionally adequate diet. Obese patients have, due to their enlarged body size, higher energy requirements for a given level of physical activity than their normal weight counterparts. Obese diabetics have slightly higher energy requirements than simple obese for a given body size and composition. Reducing the obese patient's total energy intake to that of a normal weight individual will inevitably cause weight loss, consisting of about 75% fat and 25% lean tissue, until weight normalisation occurs at a new energy equilibrium. For patients with class I obesity this requires an energy deficit of 300 to 500 kcal/day, and for patients with class III obesity 500 to 1000 kcal/day.

3.7.1 Does diet composition matter?

There is only little evidence to support that differences in diet composition exert clinically important effects on energy absorption and energy expenditure, so the main mechanism of weight reduction diets is to reduce total energy intake. This can be achieved by setting an upper limit for energy intake. The larger the daily deficit in energy balance the more rapid the weight loss. A deficit of 300 to 500 kcal/day will produce a weight loss of 300 to 500 grams/week, and a deficit of 500 to 1000 kcal/day will produce a weight loss of 500 to 1000 grams/week. Greater initial energy deficits may produce even larger weight loss rates. Total energy expenditure declines and normalises along with weight loss, and total energy intake should therefore be further reduced gradually to maintain the energy deficit. Alternatively, advantage can be taken of the differences in the satiating power of the various dietary components in order to cause a spontaneous reduction in energy intake. This is the principle of the *ad libitum* low-fat diet.

3.7.2 Choosing the dietary energy deficit

Initially the target of a weight loss programme should be to decrease body weight by 10%. Once this is achieved a new target can be set. Patients will generally want to lose more weight, but it should be remembered that even a 5% weight reduction improves risk factors and risk of comorbidities. However, several factors should be taken into consideration, e.g. the patient's degree of obesity, previous weight loss attempts, risk factors, comorbidities, and personal and social capacity to undertake the necessary lifestyle changes.

To prescribe a diet with a defined energy deficit, it is necessary to estimate the patient's actual energy requirements. It would seem natural to estimate the patient's habitual energy intake from self-reported diet registration over 3 to 7 days of weight stability, calculating the energy content of the diet by use of food table programmes. However, these estimates are invalid due to systematic under-reporting of energy intake amounting to 30–40% by obese individuals. Energy requirements should therefore be assessed indirectly by estimation of total energy expenditure. Resting metabolic rate is measured by indirect calorimetry, estimated with great accuracy using equations based on body weight, gender and age (Table 3.1), or, even better, estimated from information on the size of fat-free mass and fat mass. Total energy expenditure (= energy requirement) is estimated by multiplication of RMR (kcal/day) by an activity factor (PAI; physical activity index). The energy level of the prescribed diet is defined as the patient's energy requirement minus the prescribed daily energy deficit.

3.7.3 Theoretical vs. clinical outcome

Translating the physiologically based considerations regarding energy balance and weight loss into clinical practice requires a high degree of compliance, which can be difficult to obtain. Weight loss results tend to be much better in clinical trials conducted in specialised clinics than in trials conducted by non-specialists without sufficient resources and access to auxiliary therapists (dieticians, psychologists, etc.). Compliance and adherence to the diet are the cornerstones of successful weight loss, and are the most complicated part of the dietary treatment of obesity. To improve adherence consideration should be given to the patient's food preferences, as well as to personal, educational, and social factors. Great efforts should be made to see the patient frequently and regularly.

Furthermore, long-term weight reduction is unlikely to succeed unless the patient acquires new eating and physical activity habits. These behavioural changes should be an integral part of the treatment programme.

3.8 Summary

Over the long term most adult humans are able to maintain body energy stores through the process of energy balance, which regulates how much energy is consumed to match how much energy is expended. Energy intake is the calorie or energy content of food. Energy expenditure is required for resting metabolic rate to maintain basic physiological functions (e.g. heart beat, muscle function, respiration), metabolise, digest and store food that is consumed, as well as for physical activity. Resting metabolic rate is the largest component of daily energy expenditure and physical activity related energy expenditure is the most variable. When energy intake exceeds energy expenditure, for example during overfeeding, positive energy balance occurs resulting in increases in body energy stores. Conversely, when energy intake is lower than energy expenditure, for example during periods of starvation, negative energy balance occurs resulting in a depletion of body energy stores.

Energy expenditure occurs when the body's metabolism oxidises, or combusts, food for energy. Energy expenditure can be measured either directly by assessment of heat production, or indirectly via respiratory gas analysis. Free living energy expenditure can be measured over 2 weeks using doubly labelled water. Body energy stores can be measured using various tools for body composition analysis. Body composition consists of fat mass and fat-free mass, with the fat-free mass consisting of a mixture of water, protein, mineral and glycogen.

3.9 Glossary

Doubly labelled water A method for obtaining an integrated measure of all components of daily energy expenditure over extended time periods, typically 7–14 days, while subjects are living in their usual environment.

Energy balance The balance in the body between how much energy is consumed and how much energy is expended.

Energy requirements The energy needs of the body in order to maintain energy balance.

kcal The amount of heat that is required to raise the temperature of 1 liter of water by 1°C.

Meal-induced thermogenesis or thermic effect of a meal The energy that is expended in order to digest, metabolise, and store ingested macronutrients.

Negative energy balance Periods of time in which energy intake is lower than energy expenditure, for example during periods of starvation, resulting in a depletion of body energy stores.

Oxidation or combustion of food The metabolic reactions that utilise oxygen to break down nutrients to release carbon dioxide, water and energy.

Physical activity energy expenditure or the thermic effect of exercise The increase in metabolic rate that is caused by use of skeletal muscles for any type of physical movement.

Physical activity index The ratio of total energy expenditure to resting metabolic rate.

Positive energy balance Periods of time in which energy intake exceeds energy expenditure, for example during overfeeding, resulting in an increase in body energy stores.

Resting or basal metabolic rate The energy expended by the body to maintain basic physiological functions (e.g. heart beat, muscle function, respiration).

3.10 Further reading

ASTRUP, A., BUEMANN, B., FLINT, A. and RABEN, A. (2002), Low-fat diets and energy balance: how does the evidence stand in 2002? *Proc. Nutr. Soc.* **61**, 299–309.

ASTRUP, A., MEINERT LARSEN, T. and HARPER, A. (2004), Atkins and other low-carbohydrate diets: hoax or an effective tool for weight loss? *Lancet* **364**, 897–9.

GORAN, M. I. and ASTRUP, A. (2002), Energy metabolism. In: *Introduction to Human Nutrition*. Eds. Gibney MJ, Vorser HH, Kok FJ. The Nutrition Society, Blackwell Science, Oxford, UK, 30–45.

MUSTAJOKI, P., BJÖRNTORP, P. and ASTRUP, A. (2003), Physical activity and obesity. In *Textbook of Sports Medicine*, eds. Kjær M, Krogsgaard M, Magnussen P, Engebretsen L, Roos H, Takala T, Woo SL-Y. Blackwell Science, London, 481–8.

STUBBS, R. J., HUGHES, D. A., JOHNSTONE, A. M., HORGAN, G. W., KING, N., and BLUNDELL J. E. (2004), A decrease in physical activity affects appetite, energy, and nutrient balance in lean men feeding *ad libitum*. *Am. J. Clin. Nutr.* **79**, 62–9.

4

Physical activity and obesity

K. R. Westerterp, Maastricht University, The Netherlands

4.1 Introduction

Physical activity can be defined as body movement, produced by skeletal muscles, resulting in energy expenditure (Caspersen *et al.*, 1985). Ideally, physical activity is assessed objectively: over periods long enough to be representative for normal daily life and with minimal discomfort to the subject. Furthermore, it is important to identify physical activity patterns (frequency, duration, intensity) as well as activity-induced energy expenditure. Presently there are a large number of techniques for the assessment of physical activity, which can be grouped into five general categories: behavioural observation, questionnaires (including diaries, recall questionnaires and interviews), physiological markers such as heart rate, calorimetry and motion sensors. Validated techniques of estimating habitual physical activity are needed to study the relationship between physical activity and health. The greatest obstacle to validating field methods of assessing physical activity in humans has been the lack of an adequate criterion to which techniques may be compared. The interrelation of various field methods may be of some value, but because there are errors in all methods it is impossible to determine the true validity of any one of them in doing so (Montoye *et al.*, 1996). However, calorimetry, more specifically the doubly labelled water method, is becoming the 'gold standard' for the validation of field methods of assessing physical activity.

Here, activity patterns and activity-induced energy expenditure are related to body weight and obesity. Subsequently, the following aspects will be reviewed: activity-induced energy expenditure and obesity; activity types, level, and obesity; the role of activity in weight loss programmes;

physical activity, physical fitness and weight maintenance; implications and recommendations for physical activity and weight management; future trends; and sources of further information and advice.

4.2 Activity-induced energy expenditure and obesity

Daily energy expenditure generally has three components: basal metabolic rate, diet induced thermogenesis and activity induced energy expenditure. Basal metabolic rate (BMR) covers the energetic costs of the processes essential for life. Diet-induced thermogenesis (DIT) results from the digestion, absorption, and conversion of food. Activity induced energy expenditure (AEE) is the energy expenditure associated with muscular contractions to perform body postures and body movements. Under most circumstances, individual BMR accounts for the largest proportion of total energy expenditure (TEE) and is mainly determined by fat-free body mass. DIT is about 10% of TEE in subjects consuming an average mixed diet that meets energy requirement. AEE is the most variable component of total energy expenditure. Depending on body size and physical fitness, a five- to twenty-fold increase of metabolic rate can be sustained for a few minutes, while a healthy young adult can, if necessary, develop five to eight times the BMR over an 8-hour working day (Bouchard *et al.*, 1993).

Daily energy expenditure increases with body size, as we know since the application of the doubly labelled water technique in humans. Earlier observations of energy intake showed the opposite, a lower reported food

Table 4.1 Characteristics of healthy subjects in the Maastricht doubly labelled database by gender and body mass index category, with the measured energy expenditure

BMI[a] (kg/m^2)	*n*	age (y)	BM (kg)	TEE (MJ/d)	AEE (MJ/d)	AEE (MJ/kg.d)
Women						
<25.0	116	42 ± 22	59 ± 8	9.4 ± 2.0	2.9 ± 1.4	0.05 ± 0.02
25.0–29.9	64	49 ± 21	74 ± 7	9.8 ± 1.5	2.8 ± 1.1	0.04 ± 0.01
30.0–39.9	39	42 ± 11	91 ± 9	11.7 ± 1.6	3.6 ± 1.1	0.04 ± 0.01
>40.0	7	35 ± 11	135 ± 15	14.2 ± 2.0	4.3 ± 1.2	0.03 ± 0.01
Men						
<25.0	138	41 ± 22	70 ± 7	12.4 ± 2.7	4.2 ± 2.0	0.06 ± 0.03
25.0–29.9	102	55 ± 16	84 ± 8	12.6 ± 2.3	3.9 ± 1.7	0.05 ± 0.02
30.0–39.9	41	47 ± 11	105 ± 12	15.8 ± 2.7	5.9 ± 2.3	0.06 ± 0.02
>40	7	38 ± 11	155 ± 28	17.8 ± 2.2	5.1 ± 2.4	0.03 ± 0.02

[a] BMI, body mass index; BM, body mass; TEE, total energy expenditure; AEE, activity-induced energy expenditure.

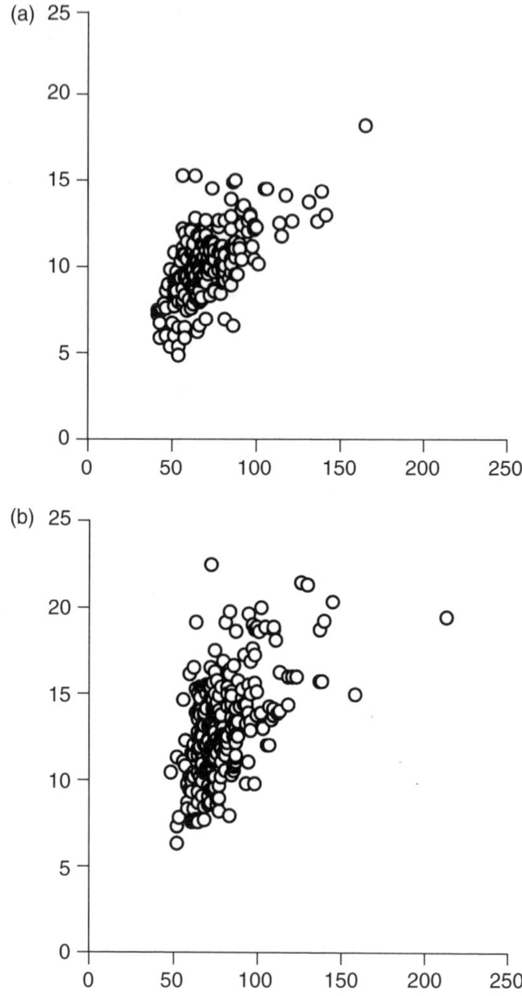

Fig. 4.1 Total energy expenditure (MJ/d) as measured with the doubly labelled water method and plotted as a function of body mass (kg) in healthy adults. (a) women ($n = 226$); (b) men ($n = 288$).

intake in obese than in non-obese subjects. The doubly labelled water method allows accurate measurement of daily energy expenditure under unrestricted conditions over 1- to 3-week intervals depending on the activity level of a subject. In Maastricht we have applied the method since 1983 in humans. Table 4.1 shows data of 524 subjects measured since then in our laboratory, excluding the following characteristics: age <20 years, an intervention in energy intake, an intervention in physical activity including athletic performance, pregnancy, lactation and disease. Data are presented separately for women and for men and by weight category: normal body

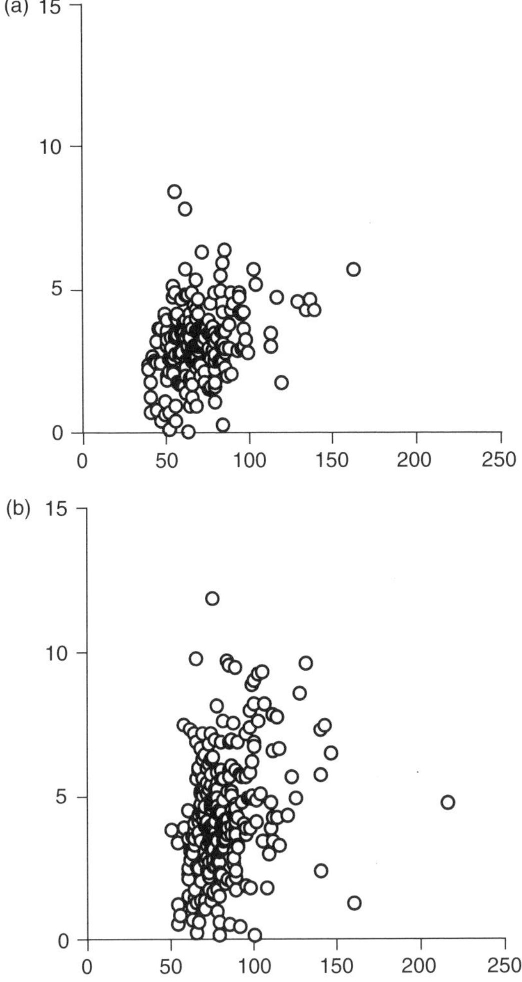

Fig. 4.2 Activity induced energy expenditure (MJ/d) as measured with the doubly labelled water method and plotted as a function of body mass (kg) in healthy adults. (a) women ($n = 226$); (b) men ($n = 288$).

weight, body mass index below 25 kg/m^2; overweight, body mass index from 25 to 29.9 kg/m^2; obese, body mass index from 30 to 39.9 kg/m^2; and morbidly obese, body mass index over 30 kg/m^2. Total energy expenditure is clearly higher in obese subjects and morbid obese subjects. This is not only a consequence of a higher resting energy expenditure as shown by the higher values for AEE in obese and morbidly obese subjects as well. Figure 4.1 shows daily energy expenditure as a function of body mass. It is obvious that the lower limit of energy expenditure, i.e. energy expenditure at a minimal physical activity, increases with body size. The upper limit is set by body size and physical capacity.

Interestingly, there seems to be an upper limit of total energy expenditure, independent of body size, of about 15 MJ/d for women and 20 MJ/d for men. Figure 4.2 shows AEE as a function of body mass for the same subjects. AEE was calculated as daily energy expenditure minus diet induced energy expenditure, assumed to be 10% of daily energy expenditure, and minus BMR. As expected, there is a wide scatter, the activity induced energy expenditure being the most variable component of daily energy expenditure. The mean value (SD) was 3.8 (1.9) MJ/d with a range from 0 to 12 MJ/d. AEE was on average 31(9)% of daily energy expenditure with a range from 1 to 55%. There is a slight but significant increase with body weight ($P < 0.001$) for both genders. The AEE per kg body mass is similar for normal weight, overweight and obese subjects and has a lower value for the morbidly obese, women as well as men. However, the number of morbidly obese subjects was too small to be conclusive at this point.

In conclusion, obese individuals have higher daily energy expenditure, not only as a consequence of higher resting energy expenditure but also by higher values for activity-induced energy expenditure. However, the activity energy expenditure per kilogram bodyweight does not increase with bodyweight and might even be limited in morbidly obese subjects. Here, total energy expenditure seems to reach an upper limit already at a lower value of activity induced energy expenditure.

4.3 Activity types, level and obesity

The AEE of a subject as measured with doubly labelled water reflects the energy expenditure for physical activity but not the amount of physical activities, i.e. body movement. Ekelund *et al.* (2002) compared AEE as well as body movement in obese (BMI > 30) and matched non-obese adolescents where physical activity was measured with doubly labelled water, simultaneously with body movement measurements with an accelerometer. The obese performed less body movement than the non-obese despite no difference in AEE. Thus, body movement does not need to be identical with energy spent on activity. In 1985, an FAO/WHO/UNU expert committee suggested figures for low, moderate and high activity levels, derived from the energy cost and duration of activity (Organization, 1985). The physical activity level was expressed as an index (PAI): daily energy expenditure as a multiple of resting energy expenditure. This expression implied adjustment of daily energy expenditure for body composition leaving the remaining variation for physical activity. Later, analysis of doubly labelled water determined PAI values, confirmed the recommendations adopted by FAO/WHO/UNU. In the general population PAI ranges between 1.2 and 2.2–2.5. At PAI values of ~2.5 subjects have problems maintaining energy balance, often resulting in weight loss (Westerterp, 1998). Recently, it was shown that PAI does not fully adjust for differences in body size. In children, the increase in AEE and PAI during growth does not equate to a higher level of physical activity expressed as body movement (Hoos *et al.*, 2003; Ekelund *et al.*, 2004). An increase in AEE and PAI was more likely due to an increase in body size or body weight, and therefore these estimates were not the best indicators of the total amount of physical activity in comparisons between groups who differ in body size.

The obese have higher energy expenditure for an activity than non-obese subjects, especially for weight bearing activities. Obese and normal-weight subjects who differed in body weight by more than 40 kg did not differ in activity counts obtained during the performance of a standard activity, i.e. walking at 4 km/h, but AEE during this standard activity was significantly higher in the obese group (Ekelund *et al.*, 2002). Additionally, physical activity assessed by accelerometry was significantly lower in the obese group, whereas there was no difference between the obese and normal-weight in AEE under free-living conditions. AEE per kilogram body mass has to be similar to allow the same body movement in an obese as in a non-obese subject. A low physical activity is an important characteristic of the current lifestyle.

Combined observations of the activity pattern with motion sensors and simultaneously doubly labelled water determined PAI values showed the determinants of PAI in healthy non-obese adults (Westerterp, 2001). Subjects were 14 women and 16 men, age 27 ± 5 y, with a similar body mass index of 24.1 ± 2.3 kg/m^2. PAI values ranged from 1.51 to 2.04. Time spent

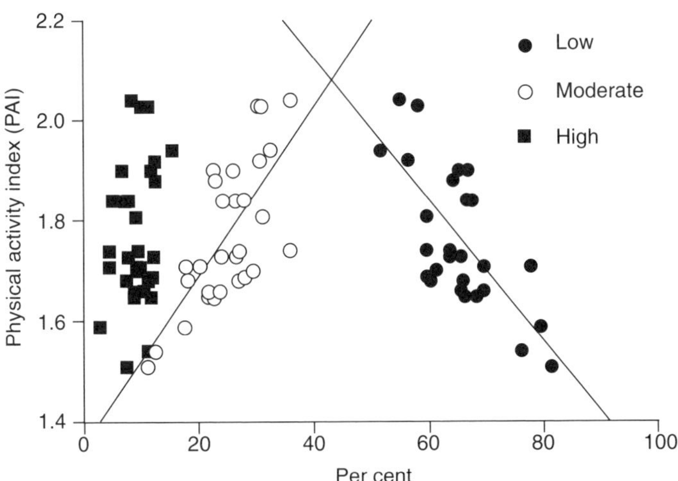

Fig. 4.3 Physical activity index (PAI) as a function of the fraction of daytime hours spent by 30 healthy subjects (with body-mass indexes within the normal range) on activities of low (filled circles), moderate (circles) and high (squares) intensity. Linear regressions are shown for low- and moderate-intensity activity.

on low-intensity activity (e.g. sitting) and on moderate-intensity activity (e.g. walking), as measured with a tri-axial accelerometer for movement registration, was correlated with PAI (Fig. 4.3; $r = -0.67$, $P < 0.0001$; $r = 0.70$, $P < 0.0001$, respectively). PAI was not related to time spent at high-intensity activity (exercise and sports).

In conclusion, within the normal PAI range, the distribution of time spent at activities with low and moderate intensity determines the activity level, and high-intensity activity does not have much impact. This has important implications for the obese, where high-intensity (weight-bearing) activity is limited by body size. High intensity activity is not required to increase the activity energy expenditure.

4.4 The role of activity in weight loss programmes

The addition of exercise to an energy restricted diet results in little further weight loss. Exercise does not reverse the weight loss induced depression of resting metabolic rate and weight loss is not different for groups undergoing dietary restriction and dietary restriction plus exercise. The latter implicates that the direct cost of the exercise training is compensated by a reduction of activity associated energy expenditure outside the training sessions. Two studies compared activity associated energy expenditure before and after dietary restriction and dietary restriction plus exercise, as measured with doubly labelled water. Racette *et al.* (1995) designed diets to promote a weight loss of 1 kg/week by prescribing a diet in the diet-only group and added the calculated energy costs of the exercise for the diet plus exercise group to create a comparable energy deficit. They observed maintenance of daily energy expenditure in the exercise group while daily energy expenditure decreased in the diet-only group. Kempen *et al.* (1995) provided all subjects with an identical low-energy formula diet. They observed a comparable decrease of daily energy expenditure in the diet plus exercise and the diet-only group. Daily energy expenditure dropped significantly, and to a similar extent, at both treatments suggesting no net effect of the exercise training on the activity associated energy expenditure.

Explanations for the relatively minor or non-existent effect of the addition of exercise to an energy-restricted diet are a low compliance to the exercise prescription and/or a negative effect of exercise training on dietary compliance. The overall conclusion was that the size of the exercise intervention only had a minor or no effect on the activity level of the subjects and consequently did not result in additional weight loss. Finally there are studies showing the effect of energy restriction on physical activity. Velthuis-te Wierik *et al.* (1995) observed the effect of a moderately energy-restricted diet on energy metabolism in non-obese men (body mass index, 24.9 ± 1.9 kg/m^2). For 10 weeks subjects received a diet with 67% of their measured daily energy expenditure during weight maintenance. The consequent weight loss was 7.4 ± 1.7 kg and the activity level (PAI) went down from 1.85 ± 0.37 to 1.65 ± 0.29 ($P = 0.06$), i.e. there was a tendency for a reduction of physical activity by reducing energy intake. In conclusion, an exercise intervention, in combination with energy restriction, only has a minor or no effect on the energy expenditure of a subject and consequently does not result in additional weight loss.

4.5 Physical activity, physical fitness and weight maintenance

There is evidence that physical activity is of importance for weight maintenance, especially for the prevention of weight regains after weight loss. Schoeller *et al.* (1997) assessed physical activity energy expenditure in weight-reduced women and found that lower activity levels were associated with greater weight gains at follow-up. Weinsier *et al.* (2002) compared total free–living activity energy expenditure and physical activity level in women successful an unsuccessful at maintaining a normal body weight. Two groups were identified on the basis of extreme weight changes: maintainers had a weight gain ≤2 kg/y and gainers had a weight gain ≥6 kg/y. Gainers had a lower AEE, a lower PAI, and less muscle strength. A lower AEE in the gainers explained ~77% of their greater weight gain after one year.

In conclusion, subjects who maintain a normal body weight are characterised by higher levels of free-living physical activity than subjects who are unsuccessful at weight control.

4.6 Implications and recommendations for physical activity and weight management

The obese spend more energy on physical activity but can perform fewer activities because of a higher body weight, especially weight-bearing activities. Ideally, the obese aim for a similar body movement than the non-obese. The aim is precluded by overweight. Thus, overweight should first be reduced by energy restriction to bring a healthy level of body movement within reach.

In 2002 an expert group of the International Association for the Study of Obesity discussed how much activity is required to prevent unhealthful weight gain (Saris *et al.*, 2003). The consensus statement was: the current physical activity guideline for adults of 30 minutes of moderate intensity activity daily, preferably every day of the week, is of importance for limiting health risks for a number of chronic diseases including coronary heart disease and diabetes. However, for preventing weight gain or regain, this guideline is likely to be insufficient for many individuals in the current environment. There is compelling evidence that prevention of weight regain in formerly obese individuals requires 60–90 minutes of moderate intensity activity or lesser amounts of vigorous intensity activity. Although definitive data are lacking, it seems likely that moderate intensity activity of approximately 45 to 60 minutes per day is required to prevent the transition to overweight or obesity. For children, even more activity time is recommended. A good approach for many individuals to obtain the recommended level of physical activity is to reduce sedentary behaviour by incorporating more incidental and leisure-time activity into the daily routine.

Political action is imperative to effect physical and social environmental changes to enable and encourage physical activity. Settings in which these environmental changes can be implemented include the urban and transportation infrastructure, schools, and workplaces.

4.7 Future trends

The need to be active for survival has largely disappeared in the present society. On the other hand ready access to highly palatable food easily induces a positive energy balance. Strategies to prevent obesity are handicapped by uncertainty as to the aetiology of the problem despite clear statements like 'Evidence suggests that modern inactive lifestyles are at least as important as diet in the aetiology of obesity' (Prentice and Jebb, 1995), and: 'The strongest environmental determinant of total-body and central abdominal fat mass is physical activity level' (Thorburn and Proietto, 2000). Contrary to the suggestion of Prentice and Jebb (1995), that modern inactive lifestyles are at least as important as diet in the aetiology of obesity and possibly represent the dominant factor, excessive energy intake is a more plausible explanation. Man is a discontinuous eater and a continuous metaboliser. A typical human eats three to four times a day to cover total daily energy expenditure. Thus, daily energy intake takes 30 to 60 min for 24-hour energy expenditure, a behaviour selected for during evolution in an environment with a high predation pressure. Nowadays, food is often readily available and can be consumed in a safe environment. Then, the normal eating rate at four to five times the expenditure rate during high intensity exercise results in a high risk for overeating.

It is obvious that the prevention of a positive energy balance with the long-term risk of getting obese is facilitated by a physically active lifestyle. The higher the energy expenditure the more you can eat. Most of the variability in energy expenditure among individuals, independent of differences in body size, is due to variability in the degree of spontaneous moderate intensity physical activity (Westerterp, 2001). Thus, strategies to limit weight gain in the population are focused on the encouragement of spontaneous moderate physical activity as formulated in the consensus statement of the expert group of the International Association for the Study of Obesity

(Saris *et al.*, 2003). However, not many people will know their activity level and are reluctant to take adequate measures for an increase. Spontaneous physical activity has a genetic and an environmental determinant. The genetic determinant was suggested by a more than twofold variation in AEE between individuals in the same confined environment of a respiration chamber and the significant relation with AEE in free-living conditions (Snitker *et al.*, 2001; Westerterp and Kester, 2003). Thus, there are individuals with a predisposition for sedentaryness. They possibly make behavioural choices in line with a minimum AEE.

4.8 Sources of further information and advice

There is ample choice on activity recommendations by different organizations like the Centers for Disease Control and Prevention, the American College of Sports Medicine, the National Institutes of Health, the American Heart Association, the World Health Organization and the Association for the Study of Obesity as mentioned.

4.9 References

BOUCHARD C., SHEPHARD R. and STEPHENS T. (1993), *Physical Activity, Fitness, and Health, Consensus Statement*, Human Kinetics Publishers.

CASPERSEN C. J., POWELL K. E. and CHRISTENSON G. M. (1985), *Public. Health Rep.*, **100**, 126–31.

EKELUND U., AMAN J., YNGVE A., RENMAN C., WESTERTERP K. and SJOSTROM M. (2002), *Am. J. Clin. Nutr.*, **76**, 935–41.

EKELUND U., YNGVE A., BRAGE S., WESTERTERP K. and SJOSTROM M. (2004), *Am. J. Clin. Nutr.*, **79**, 851–6.

HOOS M. B., GERVER W. J., KESTER A. D. and WESTERTERP K. R. (2003), *Int. J. Obes. Relat. Metab. Disord.*, **27**, 605–9.

KEMPEN K. P., SARIS W. H. and WESTERTERP K. R. (1995), *Am. J. Clin. Nutr.*, **62**, 722–9.

MONTOYE H., KEMPER H., SARIS W. and WASHBURN R. (1996), *Human Kinetics*: Champaign.

PRENTICE A. M. and JEBB S. A. (1995), *BMJ*, **311**, 437–9.

RACETTE S. B., SCHOELLER D. A., KUSHNER R. F., NEIL K. M. and HERLING-IAFFALDANO K. (1995) *Am. J. Clin. Nutr.*, **61**, 486–94.

SARIS W. H., BLAIR S. N., VAN BAAK M. A. *et al.* (2003), *Obes. Rev.*, **4**, 101–14.

SCHOELLER D. A., SHAY K. and KUSHNER R. F. (1997), *Am. J. Clin. Nutr.*, **66**, 551–6.

SNITKER S., TATARANNI P. A. and RAVUSSIN E. (2001), *Int. J. Obes. Relat. Metab. Disord.*, **25**, 1481–6.

THORBURN A. W. and PROIETTO J. (2000), *Obes. Rev.*, **1**, 87–94.

VELTHUIS-TE WIERIK E. J., WESTERTERP K. R. and VAN DEN BERG H. (1995), *Int. J. Obes. Relat. Metab. Disord.*, **19**, 318–24.

WEINSIER R. L., HUNTER G. R., DESMOND R. A., BYRNE N. M., ZUCKERMAN P. A. and DARNELL B. E. (2002), *Am. J. Clin. Nutr.*, **75**, 499–504.

WESTERTERP K. R. (1998), *Am. J. Clin. Nutr.*, **68**, 970S-4S.

WESTERTERP K. R. (2001), *Nature*, **410**, 539.

WESTERTERP K. R. and KESTER A. D. (2003), *Obes. Res.*, **11**, 865–8.

WORLD HEALTH ORGANIZATION (1985) *Technical Report Series* 724.

5

Childhood obesity, nutrition and metabolic health

M. Goran, M. Cruz, G. Shaibi, M. Weigensberg and D. Spruijt-Metz, University of Southern California, USA, and C. Ebbeling and D. Ludwig, Children's Hospital, Boston, USA

5.1 Introduction

Over the past 20 years the percentage of overweight adolescents in the United States has increased more than three-fold from 5% to 16% and the percentage of overweight in children aged 6–11 years increased from 5% to 15%. The prevalence of overweight is even more striking among certain ethnic groups. In the United States for example, recent data show that 44% of Latino and 40% of African American adolescents (ages 12–19) are considered overweight (above the 85th percentile for age and gender), which is approximately double the prevalence in Caucasians (Ogden *et al.*, 2002). It is generally agreed that adverse secular changes in diet quality have played an important role in the epidemic of obesity among children, and this will be reviewed. This chapter will also focus on research that contributes to the understanding of the link between obesity and disease risk during childhood and adolescence, especially the mediating role of insulin resistance. This background is essential for understanding the physiological underpinnings needed for the design of more effective treatment and prevention strategies. Finally, we will review studies that have examined various dietary approaches in children. The chapter concludes with the suggestion that a focus on the quality of dietary carbohydrate, and in particular their effects on reducing the postprandial rise in blood glucose and improving insulin resistance, may be an optimal nutritional approach for pediatric obesity management, as it addresses the combined issues of secular/cultural changes in diet and the underlying metabolic problems associated with obesity. Moreover, this approach avoids difficult issues such as a focus on energy restriction, and setting difficult and often unobtainable goals of weight loss.

5.2 Trends in children's diets as a factor in obesity

From 1970 to 2000, total daily energy consumption among adults increased by 270 kcal in women and 168 kcal in men (Wright *et al.*, 2004), an amount sufficient to theoretically explain all of the weight gain during this time in the general population. Among children, daily energy intake appears to have increased in some subpopulations, especially adolescents, and remained stable in others (Troiano *et al.*, 2000; Morton and Guthrie, 1998), though methodology used to obtain these estimates can be problematic. Nevertheless, diet quality among children and adolescents has undergone radical changes in ways that would likely increase risk for obesity. In the sections that follow, we will review changes in beverage consumption, fast food intake, portion sizes and meal patterns as well as related psychosocial aspects of eating behavior in children that have been related to pediatric obesity. Collectively, these phenomenon could interact to promote positive energy balance by stimulating eating in the absence of hunger (e.g. ubiquity of high calorie snack foods), by effects on satiation (i.e. leading to over-consumption at a meal) or by effects on satiety (i.e. causing hunger to return relatively quickly).

5.2.1 Beverage consumption

In the 1970s, children drank one cup of soft drink for every two cups of milk; today, that ratio is reversed, owing to an increase in consumption of soft drinks and a decrease in consumption of milk (Nielsen and Popkin, 2004; French *et al.*, 2003; Jacobson, 2004). Over the past 20 years, soft drink consumption by children aged 6–17 years has increased from a mean of 5 oz to 12 oz per day. Currently, soft drinks constitute the leading source of added sugars in the diets of adolescents (Guthrie and Morton, 2000; Bowman, 1999), amounting to 36.2 grams per day for females and 57.7 grams per day for males, figures that approach or exceed the limits for total added sugar consumption recommended by the USDA (Welsh *et al.*, 1993). Assuming an average sugar content of 11%, these beverages contributed 100 kcal per day more to the diet of adolescent males in 1994 than in 1989, accounting for about 37% of the observed increase in total energy intake in this population according to one report (Morton and Guthrie, 1998).

Soft drinks may cause weight gain, in part, because of the apparently poor satiating properties of sugar in liquid form. Calories from soft drinks appear to increase total energy intake, rather than displace energy from other sources (Mattes, 1996; De Castro, 1993). In addition, children in particular may consume soft drinks for reasons other than to satisfy hunger, including thirst, hedonic reward, or social desirability. Among school-age children, those consuming an average of 9 oz per day or more had total energy intakes that were 188 kcal per day higher than non-consumers (Harnack *et al.*, 1999). Among adults, total energy consumption among 16 subjects was greater on the day that an energy-containing beverage was given at lunch, compared to the preceding day (Mattes, 1996).

Observational studies indicate an independent association between soft drink consumption and body weight. In 548 ethnically diverse middle school students studied over two academic years, each additional serving of sugar-sweetened drink increased the risk of becoming obese by 60%, after controlling for potentially confounding factors (Ludwig *et al.*, 2001). Berkey *et al.* (2004) examined 1-year changes in soft drinks and body weight among 10000 participants in the Growing Up Today Study, reporting direct associations in both boys and girls that were largely explained by total energy intake. These findings are supported by a recent randomized controlled trial using a cluster design, based in six primary schools in southwestern England (James *et al.*, 2004). A targeted programme to reduce soft drink consumption decreased the incidence of obesity in the intervention group by 7.7% compared to control.

5.2.2 Fast food intake

Perhaps no dietary pattern typifies children's eating habits today better than fast food intake. Once an occasional choice, fast food has become regular fare for most American youth. On any given day, one in three children consume fast food (Bowman *et al.*, 2004); three in four do so each week (French *et al.*, 2001). Fast food consumption has increased by a remarkable five-fold among children since the 1970s, now exceeding 10% of total energy intake (Guthrie *et al.*, 2002).

Fast food, as presently marketed, contains numerous unhealthful characteristics, including extraordinarily large portion sizes, very high energy density, high content of refined carbohydrate and *trans*-fatty acids, low content of fiber and micronutrients, and primordial palatability (appealing to innate preferences for sugar, fat and salt). Each of these aspects has been linked to excessive weight gain or obesity-associated co-morbidities (Ebbeling *et al.*, 2002; Prentice and Jebb, 2003).

A nationally representative study by Bowman *et al.* (2004) of approximately 6212 children aged 4 to 18 years found that energy consumption was 187 kcal per day greater on days when fast food was consumed, compared to days without fast food. Studies of adolescents by McNutt *et al.* (1997) and French *et al.* (2001) reached similar conclusions. Moreover, certain individuals may be especially susceptible to the adverse effects of fast food. In 54 lean and overweight adolescents who consumed fast food regularly (Ebbeling *et al.*, 2004), lean individuals compensated appropriately for the large amount of energy in a habitual fast food meal by decreasing consumption of other foods commensurately, whereas overweight subjects did not. On days when the overweight adolescents consumed fast food, energy balance was 409 kcal greater than on days without fast food.

While there are no prospective studies of fast food and obesity in children, we recently examined data from 3031 young adults, ages 18 to 30 years, over a 15-year period (Pereira *et al.*, 2005). Individuals in the highest compared to lowest categories of fast food intake at baseline and follow-up gained an extra 10 pounds, and had a two-fold greater increase in insulin resistance.

5.2.3 Portion sizes

In the 1950s, soft drinks were served in 6.5-oz sizes; today, servings of up to 64 oz (4 pounds!) can be readily obtained (Brownell and Horgen, 2004). This trend towards increasingly large portion sizes seems to have affected virtually all foods prepared outside of the home, from packaged snacks to meals at sit-down restaurants (Nielson and Popkin, 2003).

When adults and children are served large vs. standard portions of food, they eat more food, and total energy intake tends to increase, at least over the short term. Diliberti *et al.* (2004) covertly manipulated the size of a pasta entrée consumed by 180 adults in a cafeteria-style restaurant. Individuals who purchased the large size (377 vs. 248 g) increased their energy intake of the entrée by 43% (172 kcal) and of the entire meal by 25% (159 kcal). Similarly, Levitsky and Youn (2004) found that energy intake increased at a buffet lunch among college students, when portion size was covertly increased. McConahy *et al.* (2004) examined dietary habits and body weight of approximately 5000 children, ages 2 to 5 years, participating in the Continuing Survey of Food Intake by Individuals. Portion size alone accounted for 17% to 19% of the variance in energy intake, whereas body weight explained only 4%. Fisher *et al.* (2003) studied 30 children during two series of lunches in which either age-appropriate or excessively large entrée portion sizes were provided. They found that energy consumption from the entrée and meal increased by 25% and 15%, respectively, when portion size was doubled. Increased food intake was attributed to increases in average bite size.

5.2.4 Meal patterns

The dietary changes discussed above – involving beverages, fast food and portion sizes – are inextricably related to fundamental changes in meal patterns of children. In the 1970s, most food was prepared at home and consumed primarily as regular meals. Today, the proportion of food prepared and eaten away from home has increased to 30% among adolescents (Nicklas *et al.*, 2001), and frequency of snacking has increased markedly among all age groups (Jahns *et al.*, 2001). Not surprisingly, the quality of foods eaten away from home is consistently lower than foods eaten at home (Neumark-Sztainer *et al.*, 2003b; Gillman *et al.*, 2000). At the same time, the prevalence of skipping breakfast, a phenomenon associated with a 4.5-fold higher risk for obesity in adults (Ma *et al.*, 2003), has increased by 13–20% in adolescents (Siega-Riz *et al.*, 1998).

5.2.5 Psychosocial issues

Psychosocial determinants of poor diet can be categorized into individual, social, and environmental determinants. *Individual determinants* of overeating include mood, perceived stress, depressive symptoms, and body dissatisfaction. Each of these determinants has been related to emotional eating, defined as overeating in response to negative mood (Thayer, 2001; Faith *et al.*, 1997). Emotional eating, as well as pressure to be thin, body dissatisfaction, depressive symptoms, and low self-esteem are major risk factors for binge eating in adolescent girls (Stice *et al.*, 2002). Stress alone has been associated with more fatty food intake, less fruit and vegetable intake, more snacking, and a reduced likelihood of daily breakfast consumption, regardless of gender, socioeconomic status and ethnicity (Cartwright *et al.*, 2003).

These individual determinants of overeating may actually interact with overweight status to exacerbate overeating behavior. Stigmatization of overweight and obese children has been documented repeatedly (Kimm *et al.*, 1997; Anesbury and Tiggemann, 2000). These experiences are stressful and have been related to depression, body dissatisfaction and disordered eating (Stunkard *et al.*, 2003). Lack of social support is evident among obese children (Strauss and Pollack, 2003). This is related to increased feelings of body dissatisfaction (Xie *et al.*, 2003), and in turn to overeating and weight gain (Shunk and Birch, 2004). The mechanisms governing the relationship between depression, stress and other psychosocial phenomena with increased caloric intake require further research, although it has been suggested that excessive carbohydrate intake reflects a self-medication that temporarily relieves the depressive symptoms via an increased central serotonergic activity (Moller, 1992; Schlundt *et al.*, 1993).

Interactions with parents and child feeding practices are important social influences on children's food preferences and eating patterns (Birch, 1999). Specific feeding practices, such as dietary restriction by mothers, may be related to overeating in youth (Birch *et al.*, 2003). These practices are more prevalent in mothers of overweight children, who are more likely to restrict palatable foods, which may actually promote eating in the absence of hunger (Birch *et al.*, 2003). Furthermore, mothers who exhibit higher dietary restraint and body image concerns exhibit higher levels of controlling and restrictive child-feeding practices, and parents who display high levels of disinhibited eating, especially when coupled with high dietary restraint may foster the development of obesity in their children (Hood *et al.*, 2000). Nevertheless, increased frequency and quality of family meal times is associated with consumption of healthier foods (Neumark-Sztainer *et al.*, 2003a). Family dinner, for example, has been shown to be associated with consumption of more fruits and vegetables, intake of fewer fried foods and less soda, lower dietary glycemic load, and greater fiber intake (Gillman *et al.*, 2000).

Parents can have an important positive and supportive function in weight control and weight loss. For instance, a recent family-based intervention in children aged 8–12 years showed that parent weight loss directly influenced child weight loss, and overweight youth benefited the most from parents who lost the most weight (Wrotniak *et al.*, 2004). However, a systematic review of randomized trials suggests that while parental involvement was associated with weight loss in children, adolescents achieve better results when treated alone (McLean *et al.*, 2003). Given the evidence that family interactions and habits are extremely influential in energy intake, types of foods eaten, body image perceptions and weight loss, it is evident that incorporation of family into interventions to improve eating habits in children is important if not essential.

5.3 Obesity and chronic disease risk in children and adolescents

Along with the increasing trends in pediatric obesity and the deterioration of nutritional health in children, there has also been an increase in chronic diseases associated with obesity in the pediatric population. This section reviews these developments.

5.3.1 Type 2 diabetes and prediabetes

The incidence of type 2 diabetes has increased among children worldwide (Neufeld *et al.*, 1998; Pinhas-Hamiel *et al.*, 1996; Rosenbloom *et al.*, 1999; Fagot-Campagna *et al.*, 2001), and this is thought to be a consequence of the pediatric obesity epidemic (Ogden *et al.*, 2002; Hedley *et al.*, 2004). According to available estimates, incidence has increased by approximately 20-fold in the last two decades. However, because these estimates are based almost entirely on clinical observations of the number of diagnosed cases of type 1 vs. type 2 diabetes, they should be interpreted with caution. Several small studies have examined the prevalence of type 2 diabetes as well as pre-diabetes in high-risk populations (Paulsen *et al.*, 1968; Sinha *et al.*, 2002b; Goran *et al.*, 2004; Wiegand *et al.*, 2004; Weiss *et al.*, 2004). Among these studies, relatively small numbers of children have been diagnosed with type 2 diabetes (0–6%, despite very high risk in some minority groups and cases severe obesity). In addition, the documentation of type 2 diabetes in pediatric obesity is not a new phenomenon. For example, one study from 1968 found 6% of obese multi-ethnic children had diabetes, presumably type 2 (Paulsen *et al.*, 1968).

Unfortunately, the current overall prevalence of type 2 diabetes in childhood remains unknown. One study in US adolescents aged 12–19 who participated in NHANES III (1988–1994) reported a 0.41% prevalence for all forms of diabetes, approximately one-third of which were considered to represent type 2 (Fagot-Campagna *et al.*, 2001). However, the sample size in this study was too small to provide a stable estimate of diabetes prevalence. In addition, these data preceded more recent reports regarding the rise in obesity (Ogden *et al.*, 2002) in adolescents, and therefore may underestimate the true prevalence of type 2 diabetes in the general pediatric population.

Youth diagnosed with type 2 diabetes are almost always obese, have usually reached puberty, and have a family history of type 2 diabetes (2000). In the USA, the increase in type 2 diabetes appears particularly noteworthy among minority populations such as African-Americans, Latinos, and Native Americans (Fagot-Campagna *et al.*, 2000; Dabelea *et al.*, 1999; Gahagan and Silverstein, 2003), groups that also have the highest prevalence of obesity among North American youth (Ogden *et al.*, 2002; Hedley *et al.*, 2004). Prevalence estimates of type 2 diabetes in higher risk Native American adolescent populations in Canada and the US approach 3–5% (Fagot-Campagna *et al.*, 2000; Dabelea *et al.*, 1999; Gahagan and Silverstein, 2003). Thus, obesity in childhood seems to be a primary risk factor for type 2 diabetes (2000) as it is in adults (Neel *et al.*, 1998; Ferrannini and Camastra, 1998), particularly among high-risk ethnic groups. In adults, the progression from normal glucose tolerance to overt type 2 diabetes involves an intermediate stage of hyperglycemia, characterized by impaired fasting glucose and/or impaired glucose tolerance, now known as pre-diabetes (ADA, 2004).

In a clinic-based population, Caprio *et al.* detected impaired glucose tolerance in 25 per cent of obese children (4 to 10 years of age) and 21 per cent of obese adolescents (11 to 18 years of age); type 2 diabetes was identified in 4 per cent of the obese adolescents (Sinha *et al.*, 2002b). Similarly, in another study, 28% of obese Hispanic children with a positive family history for type 2 had impaired glucose tolerance, with no cases of type 2 diabetes (Goran *et al.*, 2004). An unexpected finding was that the prevalence of children with impaired glucose tolerance was unaffected by overweight severity (Goran *et al.*, 2004). These studies have also revealed another interesting common feature in that pre-diabetes in children and youth is more frequently characterized by impaired glucose tolerance (2-hour glucose $>$ 140 mg/dl), whereas the prevalence of impaired fasting glucose (glucose $\geq$ 110 mg/dl $<$ 125 mg/dl) is typically low (Sinha *et al.*, 2002b; Goran *et al.*, 2004).

5.3.2 The metabolic syndrome

The metabolic syndrome was first described by Reaven (1988), but only recently have both the World Health Organization (1999) and the Adult

Treatment Panel (ATP III) of the National Cholesterol Education Programme proposed clinical definitions (Expert Panel on Detection and Treatment of High Blood Cholesterol in, 2001). The availability of a clinical definition prompted numerous reports on the prevalence of the metabolic syndrome and evidence that this entity places individuals at risk of type 2 diabetes (Laaksonen *et al.*, 2002; Hanson *et al.*, 2002) and cardiovascular disease associated with increased mortality (Isomaa *et al.*, 2001; Lakka *et al.*, 2002).

Although a clinical definition of the metabolic syndrome in children does not currently exist, several large population studies have attempted to establish the prevalence during childhood. Despite differences in definitions and cut points (Laaksonen *et al.*, 2003; Cook *et al.*, 2003; Chen *et al.*, 1999, 2000), these studies suggest that the prevalence of the metabolic syndrome in children and adolescents is relatively low (3–4%) when compared to rates in the adult population. For instance, the age-adjusted prevalence of the metabolic syndrome based on the ATP III definition, in US adults was 23.7% while in adults aged 20–29 years it was 6.7% (Ford *et al.*, 2002). However, the prevalence of the metabolic syndrome is much higher among overweight/obese adolescents. In NHANES III, the prevalence of the metabolic syndrome was 28.7% in overweight adolescents (BMI ≥ 95th percentile) compared to 6.1% in adolescents at risk for overweight (BMI ≥ 85th but lower than 95th percentile) and 0.1% in those with a BMI below the 85th percentile (Cook *et al.*, 2003). Eighty nine per cent of overweight adolescents had at least one abnormality of the metabolic syndrome and more than half (56%) had two abnormalities (Cook *et al.*, 2003). The individual prevalence of abdominal obesity, high triglyceride concentrations, low HDL-cholesterol levels, and high blood pressure in overweight adolescents was: 74.5%, 51.8%, 50% and 11.2%, respectively. Impaired fasting glucose was only present in 2.6% of overweight adolescents. Similarly, several other studies have found a high prevalence of the metabolic syndrome among severely overweight children and adolescents. For example, Cruz *et al.* (2004) described a prevalence of 30% in Hispanic children > 85th percentile for BMI, and Weiss *et al.* (2004) saw prevalences of 39% and 49.7% in obese adolescents above the 97th and 99th percentile for BMI, respectively. Thus, the prevalence of the metabolic syndrome is clearly related to increasing severity of obesity.

5.3.3 Other metabolic issues

Non-alcoholic fatty liver disease (NAFLD) is thought to be the most common liver disease in the US, and obesity is probably the single most important risk factor (Clark *et al.*, 2002). The disorder is being recognized increasingly in the pediatric population (Baldridge *et al.*, 1995; Rashid and Roberts, 2000; Tominaga *et al.*, 1995; Roberts, 2003). A study of 810 schoolchildren from northern Japan showed an overall 2.6% prevalence of fatty liver by ultrasound, with a strong correlation to indices of obesity such as body mass index (Baldridge *et al.*, 1995; Rashid and Roberts, 2000, Tominaga *et al.*, 1995; Roberts, 2003). In obese children screened for elevated serum aminotransferases, this prevalence has been found to be between 10% and 25%. NAFLD in childhood has been shown to occur most commonly in obese or type 2 diabetic children (Schwimmer *et al.*, 2003; Baldridge *et al.*, 1995; Tominaga *et al.*, 1995). Children with biopsy proven NAFLD are almost exclusively obese, hyperinsulinemic and dyslipidemic (Rashid and Roberts, 2000; Schwimmer *et al.*, 2003). In one study, 83% of patients diagnosed with NAFLD were obese, 30% had elevated serum triglycerides and 19% had elevated serum cholesterol (Rashid and Roberts, 2000). Collectively, these studies have brought to light the magnitude of the problem of NAFLD in overweight children as well as the potential for the future burden of liver disease in affected subjects (Rashid and Roberts, 2000; Roberts, 2003). The early development of NASH in childhood may lead to chronic end stage liver disease later in life, most significantly cirrhosis (Bugianesi *et al.*, 2002; Molleston *et al.*, 2002). In fact, a recent case report study documented the development of cirrhosis from NASH in two overweight boys aged 10 and 14 years of age (Molleston *et al.*, 2002).

Polycystic ovary syndrome (PCOS) is a common co-morbidity of obesity in adolescent girls (Gulekli *et al.*, 1993). PCOS is defined as ovulatory dysfunction with evidence of hyperandrogenism not due to other causes (Lewis, 2001). The features of PCOS in adolescents are comparable to those seen in adult women (Gulekli *et al.*, 1993). Menstrual abnormalities may include amenorrhea (primary or secondary), oligomenorrhea, or dysfunctional uterine bleeding. Fertility is significantly reduced. Androgen excess is generally mild to moderate, resulting in hirsutism or acne, but more severe signs of virilization (clitoromegaly, change in voice, increased muscle mass) are less common and generally develop slowly. Acanthosis nigricans is a commonly associated physical finding. Most girls will demonstrate reduced sex hormone binding globulin (Silfen *et al.*, 2003) and elevated free testosterone (Gulekli *et al.*, 1993; Silfen *et al.*, 2003; Lewy *et al.*, 2001; Arslanian *et al.*, 2001), while elevations in total testosterone, androstenedione, and DHEA-sulfate may also be seen (Lewis, 2001; Silfen *et al.*, 2003). Insulin resistance is generally present, and may be higher than in BMI-matched obese controls (Lewy *et al.*, 2001). PCOS affects 5–7% of adult women of reproductive age (Silfen *et al.*, 2003; Gambineri *et al.*, 2002). About half of adult women with PCOS are obese (Gambineri *et al.*, 2002; Franks, 1995; Bringer *et al.*, 1993), and there is a predisposition to central obesity (Hoeger, 2001). Comparable percentages among adolescents are not known, but PCOS can be seen in both obese and non-obese adolescents (Silfen *et al.*, 2003). Women with PCOS have increased incidence of other co-morbidities associated with obesity including prediabetes, type 2 diabetes, hypertension and dyslipidemia (Ehrmann *et al.*, 1999; Wild *et al.*, 2000). With respect to co-morbidities in adolescents, Palmert *et al.* (2002) showed that 33% of overweight, predominantly Caucasian adolescents with

PCOS had either impaired glucose tolerance (8/27), or undiagnosed type 2 diabetes (1/27). The prevalence of impaired glucose tolerance in adolescents with PCOS may approach 50% in some populations (Arslanian *et al.*, 2001).

5.4 Increased body fat and health risk in children

In order to develop effective interventions that reduce chronic disease risk associated with obesity, it is important to understand the physiological underpinnings of why increased adiposity contributes to greater disease risk. This information will be reviewed in this section.

5.4.1 Location of body fat

As in adults, there are several hypotheses that might explain the link between increased body fat and health risk in children (Frayn, 2000). The following sections review these hypotheses and evidence for them in pediatric studies. One of the earlier theories, termed the 'portal theory', links visceral adipose tissue to insulin resistance and is based on the direct effects of free fatty acids on the liver (Frayn, 2000). Numerous studies support a link between body fat, visceral fat, and metabolic risk factors in children (Caprio *et al.*, 1995; Freedman *et al.*, 1987; Gutin *et al.*, 1994; Le Stunff and Bougnäres, 1994). Earlier studies showed the presence of visceral fat in children at an early age (Goran *et al.*, 1995), although to a highly variable degree (Goran *et al.*, 1997), and the gradual expansion of this fat compartment during growth and development (Huang *et al.*, 2001). Due to the high co-linearity between visceral fat, subcutaneous abdominal fat and total body fat, it is challenging to obtain a representative indication of the unique contribution of each of these fat compartments to health risk.

More recently the 'ectopic fat' theory has been proposed (Ravussin and Smith, 2002). This approach suggests that fat deposition outside of adipose tissue (e.g. in muscle or liver) contributes to insulin resistance. Intramyocellular lipid (IMCL), for example, has been shown to be a major determinant of insulin resistance in adults (Kelley and Goodpaster, 2001), as well as obese individuals (Forouhi *et al.*, 1999) including adolescents (Ashley *et al.*, 2002; Sinha *et al.*, 2002a). In addition to IMCL, fat deposition in the liver has also been associated with insulin resistance and hyperinsulinemia in both non-obese normal subjects (Seppala-Lindroos *et al.*, 2002; Nguyen-Duy *et al.*, 2003; Marchesini *et al.*, 2001), and in obese subjects with type 2 diabetes (Kelley *et al.*, 2003; Marchesini *et al.*, 2001), and this seems to be independent of total body adiposity. Liver fat may also be a significant factor in children although there are no studies in this area. In support of both the portal theory and ectopic fat theory, a recent study in adults showed that removal of subcutaneous abdominal fat by liposuction had no metabolic benefits, suggesting that other fat depots may be more clinically relevant (Klein *et al.*, 2004). Thus, the location of body fat deposition seems to be an important factor explaining the link between adiposity and health risk, though more direct evidence of this concept is needed.

5.4.2 Adipose tissue as an endocrine organ

Since the discovery of leptin in 1994 (Zhang *et al.*, 1994), it has become evident that adipose tissue is not an inert tissue but a critical tissue involved with metabolic regulation (Kershaw and Flier, 2004). Adipocytes produce and secrete several important mediators related to insulin resistance, cardiovascular disease, and type 2 diabetes. These mediators, collectively termed 'adipocytokines', exhibit diverse actions at various central (e.g. hypothalamus) and peripheral (e.g. skeletal muscle) sites and may provide insight into the underlying mechanisms linking adiposity with disease risk. Leptin levels correlate with body fat and insulin resistance (Nagy *et al.*, 1997; Haffner *et al.*, 1999), and there is evidence for an inverse relationship between leptin and insulin action *in vivo*, independent of adiposity (Johannsson *et al.*, 1998; Donahue *et al.*, 1999). Baseline leptin levels predicted the development of diabetes in Japanese men (but not women), and this effect was independent of baseline body fat and insulin resistance (McNeely *et al.*, 1999). Adiponectin is the most abundant of the newly described adipokines (reduced by obesity and increased by weight loss) and is associated with insulin sensitivity (Pajvani and Scherer, 2003), including studies in children (Asayama *et al.*, 2003; Stefan *et al.*, 2002a). Changes in adiponectin levels track closely with changes in body fat and precede changes in insulin sensitivity (Stefan *et al.*, 2002b). Adiponectin levels predict the development of diabetes (low levels = increased risk) in Pima Indians (Lindsay *et al.*, 2002) but not changes in body weight (Vozarova *et al.*, 2002). Tumor necrosis factor-alpha (TNF-a) is produced by fat cells and has a well-described action to inhibit insulin signaling, thereby inducing insulin resistance (Hotamisligil, 1999). For Interleukin 6 (IL-6) and C-reactive protein (CRP), there is a large body of literature associating both peptides to obesity and insulin resistance, including studies in children (Weiss *et al.*, 2004). CRP has been reported to be a predictor of development of type 2 diabetes, as well as cardiovascular disease (Pradhan *et al.*, 2001; Ridker *et al.*, 2003), although the cellular mechanism is not well defined.

5.4.3 The role of insulin resistance

Perhaps the most accepted hypothesis linking adiposity to increased chronic disease risk, and one supported by prospective studies, relates to insulin resistance (Reaven, 1988; DeFronzo and Ferrannini, 1991). This section reviews the pediatric evidence relating to the role of insulin resistance in various chronic diseases associated with obesity.

Insulin resistance is one of two primary features in the pathogenesis of type 2 diabetes, the other being impairment of insulin secretion. Prospective longitudinal studies demonstrate that both insulin resistance and diminished insulin secretion are independent predictors of the development of type 2 diabetes in obese adult Mexican American and Pima Indian populations (Weyer *et al.*, 1999; Haffner *et al.*, 1995). Insulin resistance places increased secretory demand on the pancreatic B-cell, resulting in increased compensatory insulin secretion and hyperinsulinemia (DeFronzo *et al.*, 1992). While normoglycemia is maintained as long as compensatory insulin secretion is adequate, a relative failure to compensate for insulin resistance with adequate insulin secretion appears to develop in some individuals over time, leading to impairment in glucose homeostasis (DeFronzo *et al.*, 1992; Buchanan, 2003). The cause of beta cell failure in the face of insulin resistance remains unknown, although it may relate to genetic factors or to physiologic events such as the accumulation of amyloid polypeptide in the pancreatic islets (Hull *et al.*, 2004).

Early evidence indicates that the pathogenesis of type 2 diabetes in youth is likely to be quite similar to that in adults, albeit with an expression over a more accelerated time course. Studies in children have suggested that both insulin resistance and poor beta cell function may be responsible for dysregulation of glucose homeostasis (Goran *et al.*, 2004; Sinha *et al.*, 2002b). In a multiethnic clinic-based study of obese children and adolescents, Sinha *et al.* (2002b) found that insulin sensitivity measured indirectly via the homeostatic model, was decreased in children with impaired fasting glucose compared to children with normal glucose tolerance. In contrast, among overweight Hispanic children, there were no differences in insulin sensitivity (measured via the frequently sampled intravenous glucose tolerance test and minimal modeling) between impaired glucose and normal glucose tolerant obese Hispanic children, but impaired glucose tolerance (Goran *et al.*, 2004; Sinha *et al.*, 2002b) and impaired fasting glucose (Weigensberg *et al.*, 2004) were associated with deteriorating beta cell function. Ongoing longitudinal studies of such childhood cohorts should elucidate the relative risk of future development of type 2 diabetes in overweight children with pre-diabetes.

The role of obesity and insulin resistance in the etiology of the metabolic syndrome has been recently explored in children through cross-sectional and prospective studies (Cruz *et al.*, 2004; Srinivasan *et al.*, 2002; Raitakari *et al.*, 1995). The Cardiovascular Risk in Young Finns Study was one of the first groups to explore the childhood predictors of the metabolic syndrome. To do this, fasting insulin at baseline was related to the development of the metabolic syndrome (defined as having the three following: high triglyceride and high blood pressure (> 75th percentile) and low HDL–cholesterol (< 25th percentile)) after 6 years of follow up in 1865 children and adolescents (6–18 years) (Raitakari *et al.*, 1995). The results from this study showed that baseline insulin concentration was higher in children who subsequently developed the metabolic syndrome, lending support to the view that insulin resistance precedes the development of the metabolic syndrome in childhood. However, this study did not assess whether children and adolescents who developed the metabolic syndrome after the 6-year follow-up period were also more overweight, as might be expected given established associations between obesity and insulin resistance.

More recently, data from the Bogalusa Heart Study (a biracial community-based longitudinal cohort) was used to disentangle the relative contribution of childhood obesity (measured via BMI) vs. insulin resistance (measured via fasting insulin) to the adulthood risk of developing the metabolic syndrome (Srinivasan *et al.*, 2002). Seven hundred and eighteen children aged 8–17 years at baseline, were followed for an average of 11.6 years. The metabolic syndrome was defined as having the following four factors: BMI, fasting insulin, systolic (or mean arterial) blood pressure and triglyceride/HDL ratio in the highest quartile for age, gender, ethnicity and study year (Srinivasan *et al.*, 2002). Significant positive trends were seen between childhood BMI as well as insulin quartiles and the incidence of clustering in adulthood. Children in the top quartile of BMI and insulin vs. those in the bottom quartile were 11.7 and 3.6 times more likely to develop clustering, respectively, as adults. A high childhood BMI was significantly associated with the incidence of clustering in adulthood even after adjustment for childhood insulin levels. However, in this study, adjustment for childhood BMI eliminated the influence of insulin on the incidence of clustering in adulthood. Thus, in this bi-ethnic, community-based study, childhood obesity (measured via BMI) was more closely associated with the presence of the metabolic syndrome in adulthood than was fasting insulin (Srinivasan *et al.*, 2002). These findings suggest that obesity in childhood precedes the development of the metabolic syndrome in adulthood.

Although obesity in childhood may be more closely associated with the development of the metabolic syndrome than insulin resistance, the question remains as to why some obese children develop the metabolic syndrome and others do not. The recent NHANES III data on the prevalence of the metabolic syndrome among US adolescents found that approximately 30% of overweight children (BMI > 95th percentile) have the metabolic syndrome while the remaining 70% did not (Cook *et al.*, 2003). We recently addressed this issue in a cohort (n = 126) of overweight Hispanic adolescents (mean BMI percentile 97 ± 2.9; aged 8–13 years) with a family history for type 2 diabetes (Cruz *et al.*, 2004). We hypothesised that in overweight Hispanic children, insulin resistance would be more closely associated with the metabolic syndrome than overall adiposity. In this study, insulin sensitivity was measured via the frequently sampled intravenous glucose tolerance test and minimal modeling and overall adiposity was measured via dual energy X-ray absorptiometry (DEXA). We found that insulin sensitivity (after adjustment for differences in adiposity) was 62% lower in overweight youth with the metabolic syndrome (defined as having ≥ 3 of the following: hypertriglyceridemia, low HDL–cholesterol, high blood pressure, high waist circumference or impaired glucose tolerance) compared to overweight youth without the metabolic syndrome. Furthermore, in multivariate regression analysis, insulin sensitivity, but not fat mass, was independently and negatively related to triglyceride levels and blood pressure and positively related to HDL–cholesterol concentrations. These results suggest that the effect of adiposity on lipids and blood pressure control is mediated via insulin resistance.

These findings in overweight Hispanic youth are in agreement with previous results in which directly measured insulin sensitivity has been shown to be independently associated to the separate components of the metabolic syndrome (Sinaiko *et al.*, 2001; Cruz *et al.*, 2002; Jiang *et al.*, 1995). Collectively, these findings in pediatric studies, suggest that obesity, coupled with insulin resistance, may contribute to the development of the metabolic syndrome in childhood.

In adults, insulin resistance is regarded as an essential factor for the development of NAFLD and in turn, NAFLD is considered a feature of the metabolic syndrome (Kelley *et al.*, 2003; Marchesini *et al.*, 2001). Peripheral insulin resistance may lead to steatosis through increased adipose tissue lipolysis and delivery of fatty acids to the liver (Sanyal *et al.*, 2001). In turn excess delivery of free fatty acids to the liver may lead to hepatic insulin resistance, as has been observed in adults with NAFLD (Kelley *et al.*, 2003; Marchesini *et al.*, 2001). Supporting a central role of insulin resistance in NASH is a recent report that treatment with the insulin sensitizer, pioglitazone, was associated with improvements in biochemical and histological features of NASH (Promrat *et al.*, 2004). In addition, the majority of both obese and non-obese women with PCOS are insulin resistant, and the insulin resistance tends to be greater in obese women (Dunaif *et al.*, 1987). Obese adolescents with PCOS show greater insulin resistance than those without PCOS matched for total body and abdominal adiposity (Lewy *et al.*, 2001). The relationship of obesity and insulin resistance to the pathogenesis of PCOS is still incompletely understood. The prevailing hypothesis is that insulin resistance resulting in increased compensatory insulin secretion and hyperinsulinemia, leads to the hyperandrogenism seen in PCOS through multiple, complex mechanisms.

Influence of ethnicity on insulin resistance

Detailed studies comparing ethnic differences in metabolic risk factors have been helpful in understanding why certain sub-groups of the population may be at increased disease risk. Studies in children are of increased significance because they allow examination of potentially underlying biological differences across sub-groups of the population to be performed in the absence of potential confounding factors such as smoking, alcohol, aging and menopausal status. Data from the Bogalusa Heart study provided the first evidence of increased insulin resistance in African-American compared to Caucasian children based on measures of fasting insulin (Freedman *et al.*, 1987). Subsequently, other studies, have demonstrated greater insulin resistance and a greater acute insulin response in African-American than in Caucasian children (Arslanian *et al.*, 1997; Gower *et al.*, 1999), and these differences were independent of body fat, visceral fat, dietary factors, and physical activity. Previous studies have shown that African-American children have a higher than expected acute insulin response to glucose than Caucasian children (Goran, 1997), and the higher insulin levels in African-Americans are partly attributable to increased secretion and a lower hepatic extraction (Gower *et al.*, 2002; Uwaifo *et al.*, 2002), and may have a genetic basis (Gower *et al.*, 2003).

Studies of obesity, insulin resistance, insulin secretion and the beta-cell response in the Hispanic population are limited, even in adults. Only a few studies have examined the relationship between obesity and insulin resistance among Hispanics. Hispanic adults have greater fasting and post-challenge insulin (Haffner *et al.*, 1996), and greater insulin resistance (Haffner *et al.*, 1990, 1995) than non-Hispanic whites. One study (Chiu *et al.*, 2000) assessed insulin action using the hyperglycemic clamp in healthy (glucose tolerant), non-obese, young adults including 16 Mexican Americans. There was no ethnic difference in fasting insulin, but Mexican Americans were more insulin resistant and had an appropriately higher second phase insulin response than Caucasians.

We recently showed that Hispanic and African-American children are equally more insulin resistant than Caucasian children (Goran *et al.*, 2002). The compensatory response to the same degree of insulin resistance was different in Hispanic compared to African-American children. African-American children compensated with a higher acute insulin response to glucose, and this effect was in part due to a reduction in hepatic insulin extraction. Hispanic children compensated to the same degree of insulin resistance with greater second phase insulin secretion (Goran *et al.*, 2002). This difference may be the basis that could explain ethnic differences in disease risk profile.

The well-documented ethnic differences in insulin action and secretion could be explained by either genetic or environmental factors. We have been unable to explain the lower insulin sensitivity and higher acute insulin response in African-American compared to Caucasian children by factors such as diet, physical activity and socioeconomic status (Ku *et al.*, 2000; Lindquist *et al.*, 2000). More recently, we have examined whether genetic admixture, determined from approximately 20 ancestry informative markers, explained these ethnic differences (Gower *et al.*, 2003). The analysis indicated that greater African-American genetic admixture was independently related to lower insulin sensitivity ($P < 0.001$) and higher fasting insulin ($P < 0.01$), providing initial evidence that these ethnic differences may have a genetic basis.

In summary, there are distinct biological differences between high-risk ethnic groups, and we have only really begun to scratch the surface of this concept. One clear finding is that minority children are more insulin resistant and this seems to be independent of adiposity and other biological and behavioral factors, and could have a genetic basis. From the limited evidence that is available it seems that the pathophysiology of obesity related metabolic conditions, and in particular the compensatory responses to insulin resistance may be different across the various ethnic groups. These differences are likely to have implications for the development of effective intervention strategies that may need to be ethnic specific, and/or target specific metabolic factors.

The influence of puberty on insulin resistance

Puberty is associated with rapid and dynamic changes in various metabolic systems, including hormonal regulation, changes in body fat and fat distribution, as well as transient changes in insulin resistance. Several studies have demonstrated that insulin sensitivity decreases at the onset of puberty and recovers by the end of the maturation process (Amiel *et al.*, 1986; Goran and Gower, 2001; Moran *et al.*, 1999, Cook *et al.*, 1993). In Caucasian children, decreased insulin sensitivity during puberty is accompanied by increased insulin secretion that normalizes as insulin resistance improves near the end of puberty (Caprio *et al.*, 1989). In a large cross-sectional study (Sinaiko *et al.*, 2001) insulin sensitivity (measured using the euglycemic–hyperinsulinemic clamp) was highest in Tanner stage I, lowest in Tanner stage III (~20% lower than stage I) and near pre-pubertal levels in Tanner stage V. Using a longitudinal design, we have previously observed (Goran and Gower, 2001) that the pubertal transition from Tanner stage I to III was associated with a 32% reduction in insulin sensitivity (measured by the intravenous glucose tolerance test) in Caucasian and African-Americans, and this change was consistent across a range of body fatness.

Putting it all together: the additive effects

The prior sections have reviewed the multiple factors that influence insulin resistance (including greater body fat, especially muscle, liver and visceral fat, adipocytokines, ethnicity and puberty). These factors seem to have additive and independent effects on insulin resistance. To understand the physiological impact of insulin resistance, Bergman *et al.* (2002) (Bergman, 1989) proposed the disposition index that characterizes the hyperbolic relationship between insulin resistance and insulin secretion (Fig. 5.1). Thus, as insulin sensitivity of tissues decreases (i.e. greater insulin resistance), beta-cells in the pancreas have to work harder to secrete more insulin. This relationship is characterized by a hyperbola. Figure 5.1 demonstrates hypothetical examples in the pediatric population at various degrees of insulin resistance. At the tail-end of the hyperbola, very large decreases in insulin sensitivity are associated with very small requisite increases in insulin secretion. At the other end of the extreme, the same relative reduction in insulin sensitivity requires a huge increase in insulin secretion. Thus,

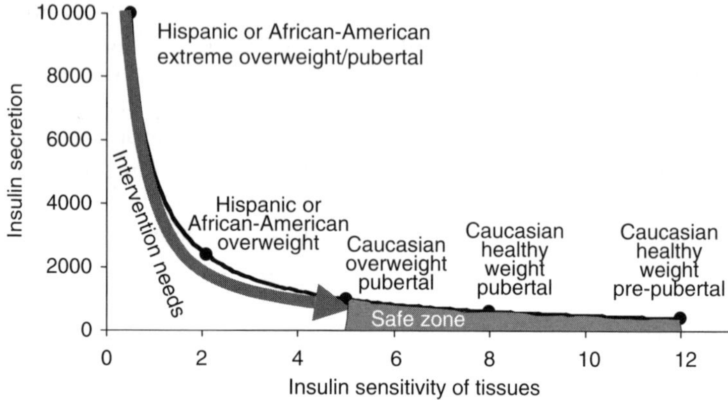

Fig. 5.1 Hyperbolic relationship between insulin secretion (μU/ml) and insulin sensitivity ($\times 10^{-4}\,min^{-1}/(\mu U/ml)$). This figure demonstrates examples at various degrees of insulin resistance and the focus of interventions to improve insulin resistance and secretion.

overweight minority children are operating in the zone of the hyperbola where periods of exposure to insulin resistance (e.g. due to more weight gain or due to puberty) will have a significant impact on insulin secretion. Hypothetically, these requisite increases in insulin secretion may lead to beta-cell exhaustion over time in pre-disposed individuals.

Figure 5.1 also demonstrates that effective interventions to improve metabolic health must focus on decreasing insulin resistance to move individuals into the 'safe zone' of the hyperbola. In the sections that follow, we review various strategies to accomplish this aim that move beyond traditional energy balance/weight loss strategies.

5.5 Nutrition-based prevention and treatment of obesity and related disease risk

Nutrition-based interventions are going to be a critical element of interventions to prevent and treat obesity and to reduce chronic disease risk among already overweight/obese children and adolescents. Nutrition interventions need to therefore address the following critical elements: (a) the secular changes in nutritional health outlined in Section 5.2; (b) provide a healthful diet that supports growth and development but yet is also likely to result in negative energy balance; and (c) reduce the burden of obesity in terms of lowering chronic disease risk typically associated with excess adiposity.

Despite the obvious role for nutrition in addressing the health problem, there are actually very few examples of intervention studies designed to specifically address the underlying metabolic abnormalities and chronic disease risk. Most typical 'weight management' programmes for youth have been based on the traditional 'energy balance' model and used restrictive diets, behavior modification techniques, physical activity, and/or drugs, but these approaches have generally not been successful and don't necessarily address insulin resistance and the underlying risks beyond weight loss. In addition, a recent study shows that dieting approaches are generally ineffective in children and adolescents and may actually promote weight gain (Field *et al.*, 2003). Thus, as was concluded in a recent Cochran review, conventional approaches targeting weight management in children have not been effective (Summerbell *et al.*, 2003). The purpose of the discussion that follows is to review nutrition based intervention studies that have addressed metabolic abnormalities related to obesity and aimed to reduce chronic disease risk beyond weight reduction.

The most successful long-term studies of obesity reduction in children have been reported by Epstein *et al.* (2001). The dietary component of these family-based behavioral interventions have used what is called the 'Traffic Light Diet, Food Guide Pyramid' that differentiates food choices primarily based on energy density and fat content. Other expert dietary recommendations for children have been non-specific and have promoted well-balanced, healthful meals based on the Food Pyramid (Barlow and Dietz, 2002) and nutritionally balanced meals to support optimal growth (Committee on Nutrition, 1998), with a general emphasis on reducing dietary fat and consuming complex carbohydrate rather than focusing on types of fat or carbohydrate in the diet. Current clinical treatment guidelines are therefore generally based on limited empirical evidence and expert opinion (Barlow and Dietz, 1998).

Remarkably few studies have examined nutritional approaches for reducing obesity and chronic disease risk factors in children. Most studies have focused on diet and weight loss and have been conducted in Caucasian children. In terms of risk reduction, most previous studies have examined dietary intervention for lipid improvement in children. The Dietary Intervention Study in Children (DISC) examined the effects of nutrition education on lipid profiles in 663 mostly Caucasian children over 3 years (Obarzanek *et al.*, 2001). There was a small but significant 8% reduction in LDL-cholesterol that was sustained 2 years after the intervention ended. However, there was a general trend of increasing triglyceride levels in both control and intervention groups indicating that alternative dietary combinations may have more beneficial effects on multiple risk factors. Another large trial (CATCH: Child and Adolescent Trial for Cardiovascular Health), sought to improve diet and physical activity in a national study involving 5000 children from almost 100 schools. Despite improvements in diet and physical activity in schools there were very limited effects on overall dietary intake and physical activity and no significant changes in obesity measures, blood pressure or cholesterol (Luepker *et al.*, 1996).

Based on our review of the literature, we conclude that more specific, targeted, and individualized dietary approaches are needed for risk reduction in overweight children. Specifically, there is good evidence to suggest that modification of the quality, as well as the quantity, of carbohydrates in the diet may be effective for improving insulin sensitivity and reducing insulin secretion and may also contribute to weight loss. This dietary strategy may be more effective than previous interventions to reduce caloric intake and/or severely restrict carbohydrate consumption (Hu *et al.*, 2001). In particular, diets containing whole grain, rather than refined, products and foods higher in fiber have been shown to have beneficial effects, possibly owing to attenuation of postprandial blood glucose responses. In a cross-sectional study in adolescents, whole grain intake was associated with a lower body mass index as well as improved insulin sensitivity (Steffen *et al.*, 2003a). In addition, epidemiological studies show that intake of whole grains is associated with protection from type 2 diabetes (Murtaugh *et al.*, 2003) as well as coronary artery disease (Steffen *et al.*, 2003b). Dietary fiber, especially soluble fiber (e.g. psyllium), has beneficial effects on blood glucose control and blood lipids (Jenkins *et al.*, 2002; Davidson *et al.*, 1998; Ludwig, 2002). Fiber intake also has beneficial effects on regulating food intake at the levels of both satiation and satiety (Ebbeling and Ludwig, 2001), and can improve glycemic control and reduce lipids (Ludwig *et al.*, 1999b).

These carbohydrate effects may work by lowering glycemic load (GL, a measure of how blood glucose changes after ingestion of a particular food). Foods with a low glycemic value have been hypothesized to be beneficial for reducing risk for type 2 diabetes because they reduce the demand for high levels of insulin secretion (Ebbeling and Ludwig, 2001; Hu *et al.*, 2001). Adult studies have consistently indicated less hunger and voluntary energy intake in response to decreases in GL achieved by dietary manipulations affecting carbohydrate quality or quantity (i.e. carbohydrate amount), as previously reviewed (Ebbeling and Ludwig, 2001). Three studies substantiate these findings in children. The effects of three different breakfast meals that contained the same amount of energy but varied in GL (high, moderate, low) were compared in obese adolescents under controlled conditions (Ludwig *et al.*, 1999a). Two of the breakfasts had identical macronutrient composition (64% carbohydrate, 20% fat and 16% protein) but varied in GI owing to different carbohydrate sources (i.e. high-GI instant oatmeal vs. moderate-GI steel-cut oats). The third breakfast, a vegetable omelet, achieved a low GL by reduction in both carbohydrate amount (40%) and GI. Hunger ratings and cumulative voluntary energy intake over the 5-hour postprandial period were highest following the high GL meal, intermediate following the moderate GL meal, and lowest following the low GL meal. Moreover, the interval between completion of the meal and initiation of voluntary energy intake from foods on a buffet platter was shortest following the high GL breakfast. Using a similar study design, Ball *et al.* (2003)

also observed less prolonged satiety in obese adolescents following high- vs. low-GL meal replacements that were controlled for energy and macronutrient composition (43–45% carbohydrate, 29–32% fat, 25–27% protein) but varied in GI. In a study of preadolescent children ranging from normal weight to obese, Warren *et al.* (2003) fed breakfasts matched for energy but differing in GI due to variations in types of cereal and bread. They subsequently observed food intake during lunch in the naturalistic setting of a school cafeteria. Hunger ratings and voluntary energy intake at lunchtime were higher following the high- vs. low-GI breakfasts. Taken together, these studies provide consistent evidence that GL has a significant effect on energy intake over the short term.

Reducing GL seems to be a promising weight management strategy based on several short-term intervention studies that relied on outpatient counseling to foster changes in dietary intake (Bouche *et al.*, 2002; Slabber *et al.*, 1994). However, relatively few intervention studies have been conducted in the pediatric population. In an outcomes assessment study of 107 patients attending a pediatric obesity clinic, Spieth *et al.* (2000) prescribed either an *ad libitum* low glycemic load diet (45–50% carbohydrate, 30–35% fat, 20–25% protein) emphasizing low-GI carbohydrate sources or an energy-restricted low-fat diet (55–60% carbohydrate, 25–30% fat, 15–20% protein). Patients on the low glycemic load diet lost more weight, resulting in a group difference of $-1.5\,kg/m^2$ for change in body mass index (BMI) over a mean of 4 months. Long-term efficacy was examined in one small-scale study of 16 obese adolescents who were randomly assigned to a low GL diet or a low fat diet (Ebbeling *et al.*, 2003). The low GL treatment encouraged consumption of low- to moderate-GL meals and snacks, with 45–50% of energy from carbohydrate and 30–35% of energy from fat (particularly healthful sources such as olive oil); while the reduced fat treatment emphasized intake of low-fat products, with 55–60% of energy from 'complex' carbohydrate and 25–30% from fat. At 12 months, BMI had decreased more in the low GL group compared to the low fat group (−1.3 vs. $+0.7\,kg/m^2$). Based on these data, an *ad libitum* reduced GL diet, focusing on GI and without strict limitation on carbohydrate intake, appears to be a promising alternative to a conventional energy-restricted diet. To our knowledge, this is the only study of diet composition in children in which differences between intervention groups persisted at 12 months of follow-up. These findings require confirmation with a larger number of subjects and in other populations.

As noted above (Ebbeling *et al.*, 2003), the GL of a conventional low-fat, high-carbohydrate diet is typically reduced by replacing high-GI carbohydrate-containing foods with low-GI alternatives and sources of healthful fat. Thus, we can not dismiss the possibility that the quality of dietary fat may have contributed to long-term weight control in our adolescent efficacy study (Ebbeling *et al.*, 2003). Indeed, data from a mouse model reported by Wang *et al.* (2002) suggest that polyunsaturated fatty acids may protect against obesity via beneficial effects on hypothalamic neuropeptides regulating energy balance. Perhaps, individuals can succeed with weight management on *ad libitum* diets varying widely in macronutrient composition when adequate attention is directed towards dietary quality with respect to both carbohydrate and fat (Ludwig and Jenkins, 2004). Further mechanistic research is warranted to address this topic.

Although limited data exist on the relationship between dietary intake and disease processes in children, most epidemiologic studies of adults (Buyken *et al.*, 2001; Ford and Liu, 2001; Frost *et al.*, 1999; Liu *et al.*, 2000, 2001; Salmeron *et al.*, 1997a, 2001; Schulze *et al.*, 2004), but not all (Meyer *et al.*, 2000; Stevens *et al.*, 2002; van Dam *et al.*, 2000), provide evidence that the quality of dietary carbohydrate and fat influences risk. Dietary GI (Buyken *et al.*, 2001; Ford and Liu, 2001; Frost *et al.*, 1999) and GL (Ford and Liu, 2001; Liu *et al.*, 2001) are inversely associated with HDL–cholesterol concentrations, and GL has a stronger (direct) association with triglyceride levels than either GI or carbohydrate amount (Liu *et al.*, 2001). Moreover, individuals in the highest categories of GL appear to be at substantially increased risk for incident coronary heart disease (Liu *et al.*, 2000) and type 2 diabetes (Salmeron *et al.*, 1997a, b; Schulze *et al.*, 2004). Regarding the quality of dietary fat, partially hydrogenated (*trans*) fat – frequently contained in commercial bakery products and fast foods (Litin and Sacks, 1993) – increases risk for CVD (Hu *et al.*, 1997) and type 2 diabetes (Salmeron *et al.*, 2001), while unsaturated fats from vegetable and marine sources decrease risk (Hu *et al.*, 1997; Salmeron *et al.*, 2001).

Another important consideration specific to children's nutrition is the role of the family. Factors in the home environment, such as the availability of healthful foods, methods of food preparation and involvement of other family members, specifically the parent or caregiver, are extremely influential in promoting or inhibiting eating behavior linked to excessive weight gain in the child. Numerous studies report that parental involvement in obesity treatments for children are superior to traditional approaches targeting child only (Epstein *et al.*, 1981, 1987; Robinson, 1999; Pronk and Boucher, 1999). Most notably, in a longitudinal study of obese 6- to 12-year-old children over 10 years, Epstein *et al.* (1990) found a greater reduction in percentage overweight among those who received an intervention targeting the parent and child compared to their counterparts who were assigned to a group in which the child was the primary target. Another study of 9–13-year-old children found that both children in the parent–child group and child-only group lost weight after a 9-week intervention but by 1 year, children in the parent–child group continued to lose weight, while children in the child–only group showed a trend in weight gain (Kirschenbaum *et al.*, 1984). However, many of these weight loss studies showing the positive influences of educating children with their parent(s) target primarily Caucasian children under 13 years of age. Brownell *et al.* (1983) demonstrated the beneficial effects of weight loss interventions with older children educating the child and parent(s) separately. In this study, 42 obese adolescents, 12–16 years of age, were assigned to one of three treatment groups: (a) mother–child together, (b) mother–child separately, and (c) child alone. The mother–child separately group lost more weight than the other two groups and was the only group that was able to maintain the weight loss for 1 year.

5.6 Summary and implications: multiple targets for treatment and prevention

Most prior interventions for treating and preventing obesity in children have traditionally targeted body weight/body mass index through conventional approaches based on the energy balance model. Several arguments against this approach can be made, especially as it relates to the pediatric population. For example, it may take generations to reverse the population BMI trend, short-term weight loss may be effective but not usually sustainable, and weight loss per se does not necessarily address health and metabolic risk factors. Finally, a focus on body weight/energy restriction in children and adolescents may not support healthy growth and development and emerging evidence suggests that this approach is not effective and may actually be harmful. In a large cohort study, children who reported more dieting attempts were more likely to gain weight over a 3-year period (Field *et al.*, 2003). Thus, the risks of a focus on weight loss in children and adolescents may include greater weight gain, lower self-esteem (due to repeated failures), and body image and eating disorders. Finally, a focus on weight alone in children is too simplistic of an approach given the underlying changes that are expected to occur due to growth in fat and fat free mass (e.g. fat free mass would be expected to increase due to growth). Therefore, a focus on the relative change in fat relative to lean mass acquisition is a much stronger indication of the dynamic changes in body composition. A reasonable goal would be a reduction in fat mass, or in the relative accumulation of fat relative to lean mass.

Interventions designed to target specific metabolic factors/health outcomes may be more effective, especially in high-risk groups with elevated metabolic risk factors. One approach based on the centrally mediating role of insulin resistance, for example, is to identify interventions for improvement in insulin sensitivity and reducing insulin secretion. Improvement in insulin resistance may be an efficient intervention strategy because it addresses multiple risk factors, targeted through one common mechanism. However, whether improvement of insulin resistance can lead to reduced risk of type 2 diabetes and cardiovascular disease over and above any effects on risk reduction through weight loss warrants further investigation.

Alternative dietary strategies can be designed around this concept. For example, traditional dietary approaches (reduced calorie, low fat, low carbohydrate) have generally been designed to lead to weight loss and have failed to recognize the data suggesting that the quality and type of fats and carbohydrates affect metabolic outcomes. For fat, replacing foods high in saturated fat and trans fatty with foods rich in plant based sources (MUFAs and PUFAs; nuts, avocado, soya) may be effective for improving risk factors associated with obesity. For carbohydrate, data are beginning to show that replacing foods based on simple/processed carbohydrates with foods high in whole grain/unprocessed carbohydrates, fiber and low glycemic index value may be effective, not only for weight loss but for disease risk reduction.

The purpose of this review has, therefore, been to summarize the negative health outcomes associated with obesity during childhood and to review the case for insulin resistance as a potential mediating factor in this relationship. We present existing data showing the efficacy of intervention strategies that also address risk factor reduction, beyond weight loss. Our general premise is not at the exclusion of any focus on body weight, but rather we propose a focus on multiple targets. Indeed, the emphasis on risk reduction (rather than weight reduction) may be more effective in the long term because it may help patients to take the focus off of body weight reduction, for which self-efficacy and outcome expectancy (and actual outcomes) may not be optimal.

5.7 References

ADA (2000), *Pediatrics*, **105**, 671–80.

ADA (2004), *Diabetes Care*, **27**, S5–10.

AMIEL, S. A., SHERWIN, R. S., SIMONSON, D. C., LAURITANO, A. A. and TAMBORLANE, W. V. (1986), *N. Engl. J. Med.*, **315**, 215–19.

ANESBURY, T. and TIGGEMANN, M. (2000), *Health Educ. Res.* **15**, 145–52.

ARSLANIAN, S., SUPRASONGSIN, C. and JANOSKY, J. E. (1997), *J. Clin. Endocrinol. Metab.*, **82**, 1923–7.

ARSLANIAN, S. A., LEWY, V. D. and DANADIAN, K. (2001), *J. Clin. Endocrinol. Metab.*, **86**, 66–71.

ASAYAMA, K., HAYASHIBE, H., DOBASHI, K. *et al.* (2003), *Obes. Res.*, **11**, 1072–9.

ASHLEY, M. A., BUCKLEY, A. J., CRISS, A. L. *et al.* (2002), *Pediat. Res.*, **51**, 81–6.

BALDRIDGE, A. D., PEREZ-ATAYDE, A. R., GRAEME-COOK, F., HIGGINS, L. and LAVINE, J. E. (1995), *J. Pediatr.*, **127**, 700–4.

BALL, S. D., KELLER, K. R., MOYER-MILEUR, L. J., DING, Y. W., DONALDSON, D. and JACKSON, W. D. (2003), *Pediatrics*, **111**, 488–94.

BARLOW, S. E. and DIETZ, W. H. (1998), *Pediatrics*, **102**, E29.

BARLOW, S. E. and DIETZ, W. H. (2002), *Pediatrics*, **110**, 236–8.

BERGMAN, R. N. (1989), *Diabetes*, **38**, 1512–27.

BERGMAN, R. N., ADER, M., HUECKING, K. and VAN CITTERS, G. (2002), *Diabetes*, **51** Suppl 1, S212–20.

BERKEY, C. S., ROCKETT, H. R., FIELD, A. E., GILLMAN, M. W. and COLDITZ, G. A. (2004), *Obes. Res.*, **12**, 778–88.

BIRCH, L. L. (1999), *Ann. Rev. Nutr.*, **19**, 41–62.

BIRCH, L. L., FISHER, J. O. and DAVISON, K. K. (2003), *Am. J. Clin. Nutr.*, **78**, 215–20.

BOUCHE, C., RIZKALLA, S. W., LUO, J. *et al.* (2002), *Diabetes Care*, **25**, 822–8.

BOWMAN, B. A., GORTMAKER, S. L., EBBELING, C. B., PEREIRA, M. A. and LUDWIG, D. S. (2004), *Pediatrics*, **113**, 112–18.

BOWMAN, S. A. (1999), *Fam. Econ. Nutr. Rev.*, **12**, 31–8.

BRINGER, J., LEFEBVRE, P., BOULET, F. *et al.* (1993), *Ann. NY. Acad. Sci.*, **687**, 115–23.

BROWNELL, K., KELMAN, J. and STUNKARD, A. (1983), *Pediatrics*, **71**, 515–23.

BROWNELL, K. D. and HORGEN, K. B. (2004), *Food Fight*, Contemporary Books, Chicago, IL.

BUCHANAN, T. A. (2003), *Clin. Therap.* **25** Suppl B, B32–46.

BUGIANESI, E., LEONE, N., VANNI, E. *et al.* (2002), *Gastroenterology*, **123**, 134–40.

BUYKEN, A. E., TOELLER, M., HEITKAMP, G. *et al.* (2001), *Am. J. Clin. Nutr.*, **73**, 574–81.

CAPRIO, S., HYMAN, L. D., LIMB, C. *et al.* (1995), *Am. J. Physiol.: Endocrinol. Metab.*, **269**, E118–26.

CAPRIO, S., PLEWE, G., DIAMOND, M. P. *et al.* (1989), *J. Pediatr.*, **114**, 963–7.

CARTWRIGHT, M., WARDLE, J., STEGGLES, N., SIMON, A. E., CROKER, H. and JARVIS, M. J. (2003), *Health Psychol.*, **22**, 362–9.

CHEN, W., SRINIVASAN, S. R., ELKASABANY, A. and BERENSON, G. S. (1999), *Am. J. Epidemiol.*, **150**, 667–74.

CHEN, W., BAO, W., BEGUM, S., ELKASABANY, A., SRINIVASAN, S. R. and BERENSON, G. S. (2000), *Diabetes*, **49**, 1042–8.

CHIU, K. C., COHAN, P., LEE, N. P. and CHUANG, L. M. (2000), *Diabetes Care*, **23**, 1353–8.

CLARK, J. M., BRANCATI, F. L. and DIEHL, A. M. (2002), *Gastroenterology*, **122**, 1649–57.

COMMITTEE ON NUTRITION, A. A. O. P. (1998), American Academy of Pediatrics, Oak Grove, IL.

COOK, J. S., HOFFMAN, R. P., STENE, M. A. and HANSEN, J. R. (1993), *J. Clin. Endocrinol. Metab.*, **77**, 725–30.

COOK, S., WEITZMAN, M., AUINGER, P., NGUYEN, M. and DIETZ, W. H. (2003), *Arch. Pediatr. Adolesc. Med.*, **157**, 821–7.

CRUZ, M. L., HUANG, T. T. K., JOHNSON, M. S., GOWER, B. A. and GORAN, M. I. (2002), *Hypertension*, **40**, 18–22.

CRUZ, M. L., WEIGENSBERG, M. J., HUANG, T., T-K BALL, G. D. C., SHAIBI, G. Q. and GORAN, M. I. (2004), *J. Clin. Endocrinol. Metab.*, **89**, 108–13.

DABELEA, D., PETTITT, D. J., JONES, K. L. and ARSLANIAN, S. A. (1999), *Endocrinol. Metab. Clin. N. Am.*, **28**, 709–29.

DAVIDSON, M. H., MAKI, K. C., KONG, J. C. *et al.* (1998), *Am. J. Clin. Nutr.*, **67**, 367–76.

DE CASTRO, J. M. (1993), *Physiol. Behav.*, **53**, 1133–44.

DEFRONZO, R. A. and FERRANNINI, E. (1991), *Diabetes Care*, **14**, 173–94.

DEFRONZO, R. A., BONADONNA, R. C. and FERRANNINI, E. (1992), *Diabetes Care*, **15**, 318–68.

DILIBERTI, N., BORDI, P. L., CONKLIN, M. T., ROE, L. S. and ROLLS, B. J. (2004), *Obes. Res.*, **12**, 562–8.

DONAHUE, R. P., PRINEAS, R. J., DONAHUE, R. D. *et al.* (1999), *Diabetes Care*, **22**, 1092–6.

DUNAIF, A., GRAF, M., MANDELI, J., LAUMAS, V. and DOBRJANSKY, A. (1987), *J. Clin. Endocrinol. Metab.*, **65**, 499–507.

EBBELING, C. B. and LUDWIG, D. S. (2001), *Adv. Pediatr.*, **48**, 179–212.

EBBELING, C. B., PAWLAK, D. B. and LUDWIG, D. S. (2002), *Lancet*, **360**, 473–82.

EBBELING, C. B., LEIDIG, M. M., SINCLAIR, K. B., HANGEN, J. P. and LUDWIG, D. S. (2003), *Arch. Pediatr. Adolesc. Med.*, **157**, 773–9.

EBBELING, C. B., SINCLAIR, K. B., PEREIRA, M. A., GARCIA-LAGO, E., FELDMAN, H. A. and LUDWIG, D. S. (2004), *JAMA*, **291**, 2828–33.

EHRMANN, D. A., BARNES, R. B., ROSENFIELD, R. L., CAVAGHAN, M. K. and IMPERIAL, J. (1999), *Diabetes Care*, **22**, 141–6.

EPSTEIN, L. H., WING, R. R., KOSESKE, R., ANDRASIK, F. and OSSIP, D. J. (1981), *J. Cons. Clin. Psychol.*, **49**, 675–85.

EPSTEIN, L. H., WING, R. R., KOESKE, R. and VALOSKI, A. (1987), *J. Cons. Clin. Psychol.*, **55**, 91–5.

EPSTEIN, L. H., VALOSKI, A., WING, R. R. and MCCURLEY, M. A. (1990), *J. Am. Med. Assoc.*, **264**(19), 2519–23.

EPSTEIN, L. H., ROEMMICH, J. N. and RAYNOR, H. A. (2001), *Pediatr. Clin. North Am.*, **48**, 981–93.

EXPERT PANEL ON DETECTION, E. and TREATMENT OF HIGH BLOOD CHOLESTEROL IN, A. (2001), *J. Am. Med. Assoc.*, **285**, 2486–97.

FAGOT-CAMPAGNA, A., PETTITT, D. J., ENGELGAU, M. M. *et al.* (2000), *J. Pediatr.*, **136**, 664–72.

FAGOT-CAMPAGNA, A., FLEGAL, K. M., SAADDINE, J. B. and BECKLES, G. L. A. (2001), *Diabetes Care*, **5**, 837.

FAITH, M. S., ALLISON, D. B. and GELIEBTER, A. (1997), In *Overweight and Weight Management: The Health Professional's Guide to Understanding and Practice* (Ed, Dalton, S.) Aspen Publishers, Gaithersburg, MD, pp. 439–65.

FERRANNINI, E. and CAMASTRA, S. (1998), *Eur. J. Clin. Invest.*, **28** Suppl 2, 3–6.

FIELD, A. E., AUSTIN, S. B., TAYLOR, C. B. *et al.* (2003), *Pediatrics*, **112**, 900–6.

FISHER, J. O., ROLLS, B. J. and BIRCH, L. L. (2003), *Am. J. Clin. Nutr.*, **77**, 1164–70.

FORD, E. S. and LIU, S. (2001), *Arch. Intern. Med.*, **161**, 572–6.

FORD, E. S., GILES, W. H. and DIETZ, W. H. (2002), *J. Am. Med. Assoc.*, **287**, 356–9.

FOROUHI, N., JEKINSON, G., THOMAS, E. *et al.* (1999), *Diabetologia*, **42**, 932–5.

FRANKS, S. (1995), *N. Engl. J. Med.*, **333**, 853–61.

FRAYN, K. N. (2000), *Br. J. Nutr.*, **83**, S71–7.

FREEDMAN, D. S., SRINIVASAN, S. R., BURKE, G. L. *et al.* (1987), *Am. J. Clin. Nutr.*, **46**, 403–10.

FRENCH, S. A., LIN, B.-H. and GUTHRIE, J. F. (2003), *J. Am. Diet. Assoc.*, **103**, 1326–31.

FRENCH, S. A., STORY, M., NEUMARK-SZTAINER, D., FULKERSON, J. A. and HANNAN, P. (2001), *Int. J. Obes.*, **25**, 1823–33.

FROST, G., LEEDS, A. A., DORE, C. J., MADEIROS, S., BRADING, S. and DORNHORST, A. (1999), *Lancet*, **353**, 1045–8.

GAHAGAN, S. and SILVERSTEIN, J. (2003), *Pediatrics*, **112**, e328.

GAMBINERI, A., PELUSI, C., VICENNATI, V., PAGOTTO, U. and PASQUALI, R. (2002), *Int. J. Obes. Relat. Metab. Disord.*, **26**, 883–96.

GILLMAN, M. W., RIFAS-SHIMAN, S. L., FRAZIER, A. L. *et al.* (2000), *Arch. Fam. Med.*, **9**, 235–40.

GORAN, M. I. (1997), *Proc. Nutr. Soc.*, **56**, 195–209.

GORAN, M. I. and GOWER, B. A. (2001), *Diabetes*, **50**, 2444–50.

GORAN, M. I., KASKOUN, M. C. and SHUMAN, W. P. (1995), *Int. J. Obes.*, **19**, 279–83.

GORAN, M. I., NAGY, T. R., TREUTH, M. T. *et al.* (1997), *Am. J. Clin. Nutr.*, **65**, 1703–9.

GORAN, M. I., CRUZ, M. L., BERGMAN, R. N. and WATANABE, R. M. (2002), *Diabetes Care*, **25**, 2184–90.

GORAN, M. I., BERGMAN, R. N., AVILA, Q. *et al.* (2004), *J. Clin. Endocrinol. Metab.*, **89**, 207–12.

GOWER, B. A., NAGY, T. R. and GORAN, M. I. (1999), *Diabetes*, **48**, 1515–21.

GOWER, B. A., GRANGER, W. M., FRANKLIN, F., SHEWCHUK, R. M. and GORAN, M. I. (2002), *J. Clin. Endocrinol. Metab.*, **87**, 2224.

GOWER, B. A., FERNANDEZ, J. R., BEASLEY, T. M., SHRIVER, M. D. and GORAN, M. I. (2003), *Diabetes*, **52**, 1047–51.

GULEKLI, B., TURHAN, N. O., SENOZ, S., KUKNER, S., ORAL, H. and GOKMEN, O. (1993), *Gynecol. Endocrinol.*, **7**, 273–7.

GUTHRIE, J. F. and MORTON, J. F. (2000), *J. Am. Diet. Assoc.*, **100**, 43–51, quiz 49–50.

GUTHRIE, J. F., LIN, B.-H. and FRAZAO, E. (2002), *J. Nutr. Educ. Behav.*, **34**, 140–50.

GUTIN, B., ISLAM, S., MANOS, T., CUCUZZO, N., SMITH, C. and STACHURA, M. E. (1994), *J. Pediat.*, **125**, 847–52.

HAFFNER, S. M., STERN, M. P., HAZUDA, H. P., MITCHELL, B. D. and PATTERSON, J. K. (1990), *J. Am. Med. Assoc.*, **263**, 2893–8.

HAFFNER, S. M., MIETTINEN, H., GASKILL, S. P. and STERN, M. P. (1995), *Diabetes*, **44**, 1386–91.

HAFFNER, S. M., D'AGOSTINO, R., SAAD, M. F. *et al.* (1996), *Diabetes*, **45**, 742–8.

HAFFNER, S. M., MYKKANEN, L., RAINWATER, D. L., KARHAPAA, P. and LAAKSO, M. (1999), *Obes. Res.*, **7**, 164–9.

HANSON, R. L., IMPERATORE, G., BENNETT, P. H. and KNOWLER, W. C. (2002), *Diabetes*, **51**, 3120–7.

HARNACK, L., STANG, J. and STORY, M. (1999), *J. Am. Diet. Assoc.*, **99**, 436–41.

HEDLEY, A. A., OGDEN, C. L., JOHNSON, C. L., CARROLL, M. D., CURTIN, L. R. and FLEGAL, K. M. (2004), *J. Am. Med. Assoc.*, **291**, 2847–50.

HOEGER, K. (2001), *Obstet. Gynecol. Clin. N. Am.*, **28**, 85–vii.

HOOD, M. Y., MOORE, L. L., SUNDARAJAN-RAMAMURTI, A., SINGER, M., CUPPLES, L. A. and ELLISON, R. C. (2000), *Int. J. Obes. Relat. Metab. Disord.*, **24**, 1319–25.

HOTAMISLIGIL, G. S. (1999), *J. Intern. Med.*, **245**, 621–5.

HU, F. B., STAMPFER, M. J., MANSON, J. E. *et al.* (1997), *N. Engl. J. Med.*, **337**, 1491–9.

HU, F. B., VAN DAM, R. M. and LIU, S. (2001), *Diabetologia*, **44**, 805–17.

HUANG, T.-K., JOHNSON, M. S., FIGUEROA-COLON, R., DWYER, J. H. and GORAN, M. I. (2001), *Obes. Res.*, **9**, 283–9.

HULL, R. L., WESTERMARK, G. T., WESTERMARK, P. and KAHN, S. E. (2004), *J. Clin. Endocr. Metab.*, **89**, 3629–43.

ISOMAA, B., ALMGREN, P., TUOMI, T. *et al.* (2001), *Diabetes Care*, **24**, 683–9.

JAHNS, L., SIEGA-RIZ, A. M. and POPKIN, B. M. (2001), *J. Pediatr.*, **138**, 493–8.

JAMES, J., THOMAS, P., CAVAN, D. and KERR, D. (2004), *BMJ.*, **328**, 1237.

JENKINS, D. J., KENDALL, C. W., VUKSAN, V. *et al.* (2002), *Am. J. Clin. Nutr.*, **75**, 834–9.

JIANG, X., SRINIVASAN, S. R., WEBBER, L. S., WATTIGNEY, W. A. and BERENSON, G. S. (1995), *Arch. Intern. Med.*, **155**, 190–6.

JOHANNSSON, G., KARLSSON, C., LONN, L. *et al.* (1998), *Obes. Res.*, **6**, 416–21.

KELLEY, D. E. and GOODPASTER, B. H. (2001), *Diabetes Care*, **24**, 933–41.

KELLEY, D. E., MCKOLANIS, T. M., HEGAZI, R., KULLER, L. and KALHAN, S. (2003), *Am. J. Phyiol.*, **285**, E906–16.

KERSHAW, E. E. and FLIER, J. S. (2004), *J. Clin. Endocrinol. Metab.*, **89**, 2548–56.

KIMM, S. Y., BARTON, B. A., BERHANE, K., ROSS, J. W., PAYNE, G. H. and SCHREIBER, G. B. (1997), *Ann. Epidemiol.*, **7**, 550–60.

KIRSCHENBAUM, D. S., HARRIS, E. S. and TOMARKEN, A. J. (1984), *Behav. Ther.*, **15**, 485–500.

KLEIN, S., FONTANA, L., YOUNG, V. L. *et al.* (2004), *N. Engl. J. Med.*, **350**, 2549–57.

KU, C. Y., GOWER, B. A., HUNTER, G. R. and GORAN, M. I. (2000), *Obes. Res.*, **8**, 506–15.

LAAKSONEN, D. E., LAKKA, H. M., LYNCH, J. *et al.* (2003), *Diabetes Care*, **26**, 2156–64.

LAAKSONEN, D. E., LAKKA, H. M., NISKANEN, L. K., KAPLAN, G. A., SALONEN, J. T. and LAKKA, T. A. (2002), *Am. J. Epidemiol.*, **156**, 1070–7.

LAKKA, H. M., LAAKSONEN, D. E., LAKKA, T. A. *et al.* (2002), *J. Am. Med. Assoc.*, **288**, 2709–16.

LE STUNFF, C. and BOUGNÄRES, P. (1994), *Diabetes*, **43**, 696–702.

LEVITSKY, D. A. and YOUN, T. (2004), *J. Nutr.*, **134**, 2546–9.

LEWIS, V. (2001), *Obstet. Gynecol. Clin. N. Am.*, **28**, 1–20.

LEWY, V. D., DANADIAN, K., WITCHEL, S. F. and ARSLANIAN, S. (2001), *J. Pediatr.*, **138**, 38–44.

LINDQUIST, C. H., GOWER, B. A. and GORAN, M. I. (2000), *Am. J. Clin. Nutr.*, **71**, 725–32.

LINDSAY, R. S., FUNAHASHI, T., HANSON, R. L. *et al.* (2002), *Lancet*, **360**, 57–8.

LITIN, L. and SACKS, F. (1993), *N. Engl. J. Med.*, **329**, 1969–70.

LIU, S., MANSON, J. E., STAMPFER, M. J. *et al.* (2001), *Am. J. Clin. Nutr.*, **73**, 560–6.

LIU, S., WILLETT, W. C., STAMPFER, M. J. *et al.* (2000), *Am. J. Clin. Nutr.*, **71**, 1455–61.

LUDWIG, D. S. (2002), *J. Am. Med. Assoc.*, **287**, 2414–23.

LUDWIG, D. S. and JENKINS, D. J. (2004), *Am. J. Clin. Nutr.*, **80**, 797–8.

LUDWIG, D. S., MAJZOUB, J. A., AL-ZAHRANI, A., DALLAL, G. E., BLANCO, I. and ROBERTS, S. B. (1999a), *Pediatrics*, **103**, e26.

LUDWIG, D. S., PEREIRA, M., KROENKE, C. *et al.* (1999b), *J. Am. Med. Assoc.*, **282**, 1539–46.

LUDWIG, D. S., PETERSON, K. E. and GORTMAKER, S. L. (2001), *Lancet*, **357**, 505–8.

LUEPKER, R. V., PERRY, C. L., MCKINLAY, S. M. *et al.* (1996), *J. Am. Med. Assoc.*, **275**, 768–76.

MA, Y., BERTONE, E. R., STANEK, E. J., 3RD *et al.* (2003), *Am. J. Epidemiol.*, **158**, 85–92.

MARCHESINI, G., BRIZI, M., BIANCHI, G. *et al.* (2001), *Diabetes*, **50**, 1844–50.

MATTES, R. D. (1996), *Physiol. Behav.*, **59**, 179–87.

MCCONAHY, K. L., SMICIKLAS-WRIGHT, H., MITCHELL, D. C. and PICCIANO, M. F. (2004), *J. Am. Diet. Assoc.*, **104**, 975–9.

MCLEAN, N., GRIFFIN, S., TONEY, K. and HARDEMAN, W. (2003), *Int. J. Obes. Relat. Metab. Disord.*, **27**, 987–1005.

MCNEELY, M. J., BOYKO, E. J., WEIGLE, D. S. *et al.* (1999), *Diabetes Care*, **22**, 65–70.

MCNUTT, S. W., HU, Y., SCHREIBER, G. B., CRAWFORD, P. B., OBARZANEK, E. and MELLIN, L. (1997), *J. Adolesc. Health*, **20**, 27–37.

MEYER, K. A., KUSHI, L. H., JACOBS, D. R., SLAVIN, J., SELLERS, T. A. and FOLSOM, A. R. (2000), *Am. J. Clin. Nutr.*, **71**, 921–30.

MOLLER, S. E. (1992), *Pharmacol Toxicol*, **71** Suppl 1, 61–71.

MOLLESTON, J. P., WHITE, F., TECKMAN, J. and FITZGERALD, J. F. (2002), *Am. J. Gastroenterol.*, **97**, 2460–2.

MORAN, A., JACOBS, D. R. J., STEINBERGER, J. *et al.* (1999), *Diabetes*, **48**, 2039–44.

MORTON, J. F. and GUTHRIE, J. F. (1998), *Fam. Econ. Nutr. Rev.*, **11**, 44–57.

MURTAUGH, M. A., JACOBS, D. R., JR., JACOB, B., STEFFEN, L. M. and MARQUART, L. (2003), *Proc. Nutr. Soc.*, **62**, 143–9.

NAGY, T. R., GOWER, B. A., TROWBRIDGE, C. A., DEZENBERG, C., SHEWCHUK, R. M. and GORAN, M. I. (1997), *J. Clin. Endocrinol. Metab.*, **82**, 2148.

NEEL, J. V., WEDER, A. B. and JULIUS, S. (1998), *Perspect. Biol. Med.*, **42**, 44–74.

NEUFELD, N. D., RAFFEL, L. J., LANDON, C., CHEN, Y.-D. and VADHEIM, C. M. (1998), *Diabetes Care*, **21**, 80–6.

NEUMARK-SZTAINER, D., HANNAN, P. J., STORY, M., CROLL, J. and PERRY, C. (2003a) *J. Am. Diet. Assoc.*, **103**, 317–22.

NEUMARK-SZTAINER, D., HANNAN, P. J., STORY, M., CROLL, J. and PERRY, C. (2003b) *J. Am. Diet. Assoc.*, **103**, 317–22.

NGUYEN-DUY, T. B., NICHAMAN, M. Z., CHURCH, T. S., BLAIR, S. N. and ROSS, R. (2003), *Am. J. Physiol.*, **284**, E1065–71.

NICKLAS, T. A., BARANOWSKI, T., CULLEN, K. W. and BERENSON, G. (2001), *J. Am. Coll. Nutr.*, **20**, 599–608.

NIELSON, S. J. and POPKIN, B. M. (2003), *J. Am. Med. Assoc.*, **289**, 450–3.

NIELSEN, S. J. and POPKIN, B. M. (2004), *Am. J. Prev. Med.*, **27**, 205–10.

OBARZANEK, E., KIMM, S., BARTON, B. A. *et al.* (2001), *Pediatrics*, **107**, 256–64.

OGDEN, C. L., FLEGAL, K. M., CARROLL, M. D. and JOHNSON, C. L. (2002), *J. Am. Med. Assoc.*, **288**, 1728–32.

PAJVANI, U. B. and SCHERER, P. E. (2003), *Curr. Diab. Rep.*, **3**, 207–13.

PALMERT, M. R., GORDON, C. M., KARTASHOV, A. I., LEGRO, R. S., EMANS, S. J. and DUNAIF, A. (2002), *J. Clin. Endocrinol. Metab.*, **87**, 1017–23.

PAULSEN, E. P., RICHENDERFER, L. and GINSBERG-FELLNER, F. (1968), *Diabetes*, **17**, 261–9.

PEREIRA, M. A., KARTASHOV, A. I., EBBELING, C. B. *et al.* (2005), *Lancet*, **365** (9453), 36–42.

PINHAS-HAMIEL, O., DOLAN, L. M., DANIELS, S. R., STANDIFORD, D., KHOURY, P. R. and ZEITLER, P. (1996), *J. Pediat.*, **128**, 608–15.

PRADHAN, A. D., MANSON, J. E., RIFAI, N., BURING, J. E. and RIDKER, P. M. (2001), *J. Am. Med. Assoc.*, **286**, 327–34.

PRENTICE, A. M. and JEBB, S. A. (2003), *Obes. Rev.* **4**, 187–94.

PROMRAT, K., LUTCHMAN, G., UWAIFO, G. I. *et al.* (2004), *Hepatology*, **39**, 188–96.

PRONK, N. P. and BOUCHER, J. (1999), *Int. J. Obes. Rel. Metab. Disord.*, **23**, 38–42.

RAITAKARI, O. T., PORKKA, K. V. K., RONNEMAA, T., KNIP, M., UHARI, M. and AKERBLOM, H. K. (1995), *Diabetologia*, **38**, 1042–50.

RASHID, M. and ROBERTS, E. A. (2000), *J. Pediatr. Gastroenterol. Nutr.*, **30**, 48–53.

RAVUSSIN, E. and SMITH, S. R. (2002), *Ann. NY. Acad. Sci.*, **967**, 363–78.

REAVEN, G. M. (1988), *Diabetes*, **37**, 1595–607.

RIDKER, P. M., BURING, J. E., COOK, N. R. and RIFAI, N. (2003), *Circulation*, **107**, 391–7.

ROBERTS, E. A. (2003), *Curr. Gastroenterol. Rep.*, **5**, 253–9.

ROBINSON, T. (1999), *Int. J. Obes. Rel. Metab. Disord.*, **23**, S52–7.

ROSENBLOOM, A. L., JOE, J. R., YOUNG, R. S. and WINTER, W. E. (1999), *Diabetes Care*, **22**, 345–54.

SALLIS, J. F., HASKELL, W. L., WOOD, P. D. *et al.* (1985), *Am. J. Epidemiol.*, **121**, 91–106.

SALMERON, J., ASCHERIO, A., RIMM, E. B. *et al.* (1997a), *Diabetes Care*, **20**, 545–50.

SALMERON, J., MANSON, J. E., STAMPFER, M. J., COLDITZ, G. A., WING, A. L. and WILLETT, W. C. (1997b), *J. Am. Med. Assoc.*, **277**, 472–7.

SALMERON, J., HU, F. B., MANSON, J. E., STAMPFER, M. J., COLDITZ, G. A., RIMM, E. B. and WILLETT, W. C. (2001), *Am. J. Clin. Nutr.*, **73**, 1019–26.

SANYAL, A. J., CAMPBELL-SARGENT, C., MIRSHAHI, F. *et al.* (2001), *Gastroenterology*, **120**, 1183–92.

SCHLUNDT, D. G., VIRTS, K. L., SBROCCO, T., POPE-CORDLE, J. and HILL, J. O. (1993), *Addict. Behav.*, **18**, 67–80.

SCHULZE, M. B., LIU, S., RIMM, E. B., MANSON, J. E., WILLETT, W. C. and HU, F. B. (2004), *Am. J. Clin. Nutr.*, **80**, 348–56.

SCHWIMMER, J. B., DEUTSCH, R., RAUCH, J. B., BEHLING, C., NEWBURY, R. and LAVINE, J. E. (2003), *J. Pediatr.*, **143**, 500–5.

SEPPALA-LINDROOS, A., VEHKAVAARA, S., HAKKINEN, A. M. *et al.* (2002), *J. Clin. Endocrinol. Metab.*, **87**, 3023–8.

SHUNK, J. A. and BIRCH, L. L. (2004), *J. Am. Diet. Assoc.*, **104**, 1120–6.

SIEGA-RIZ, A. M., POPKIN, B. M. and CARSON, T. (1998), *Am. J. Clin. Nutr.*, **67**, 748S–56S.

SILFEN, M. E., DENBURG, M. R., MANIBO, A. M. *et al.* (2003), *J. Clin. Endocrinol. Metab.*, **88**, 4682–8.

SINAIKO, A. R., JACOBS, D. R. JR., STEINBERGER, J. *et al.* (2001), *J. Pediatr.*, **139**, 700–7.

SINHA, R., DUFOUR, S., PETERSEN, K. F. *et al.* (2002a), *Diabetes*, **51**, 1022–7.

SINHA, R., FISCH, G., TEAGUE, B. *et al.* (2002b), *N. Engl. J. Med.*, **346**, 802–10.

SLABBER, M., BARNARD, H. C., KUYL, J. M., DANNHAUSER, A. and SCHALL, R. (1994), *Am. J. Clin. Nutr.*, **60**, 48–53.

SPIETH, L. E., HARNISH, J. D., LENDERS, C. M. *et al.* (2000), *Arch. Pediatr. Adol. Med.*, **154**, 947–51.

SRINIVASAN, S. R., MYERS, L. and BERENSON, G. S. (2002), *Diabetes*, **51**, 204–9.

STEFAN, N., BUNT, J. C., SALBE, A. D., FUNAHASHI, T., MATSUZAWA, Y. and TATARANNI, P. A. (2002a), *J. Clin. Endocrinol. Metab.*, **87**, 4652–6.

STEFAN, N., VOZAROVA, B., FUNAHASHI, T. *et al.* (2002b), *Diabetes*, **51**, 1884–8.

STEFFEN, L. M., JACOBS, D. R. JR., MURTAUGH, M. A. *et al.* (2003a), *Am. J. Epidemiol.*, **158**, 243–50.

STEFFEN, L. M., JACOBS, D. R., JR., STEVENS, J., SHAHAR, E., CARITHERS, T. and FOLSOM, A. R. (2003b), *Am. J. Clin. Med.*, **78**, 383–90.

STEVENS, J., AHN, K., JUHAERI HOUSTON, D., STEFFAN, L. and COUPER, D. (2002), *Diabetes Care*, **25**, 1715–21.

STICE, E., PRESNELL, K. and SPANGLER, D. (2002), *Health Psychology*, **21**, 131–8.

STRAUSS, R. S. and POLLACK, H. A. (2003), *Arch. Pediatr. Adolesc. Med.*, **157**, 746–52.

STUNKARD, A. J., FAITH, M. S. and ALLISON, K. C. (2003), *Biol. Psychiatry*, **54**, 330–7.

SUMMERBELL, C., ASHTON, V., CAMPBELL, K., EDMUNDS, L., KELLY, S. and WATERS, E. (2003), *Cochrane Database of Systematic Reviews*, **3**, CD001872.

THAYER, R. (2001), *Calm Energy: How People Regulate Mood with Food and Exercise*, Oxford University Press, Oxford.

TOMINAGA, K., KURATA, J. H., CHEN, Y. K. *et al.* (1995), *Dig. Dis. Sci.*, **40**, 2002–9.

TROIANO, R. P., BRIEFEL, R. R., CARROLL, M. D. and BIALOSTOSKY, K. (2000), *Am. J. Clin. Nutr.*, **72**, 1343S–53S.

UWAIFO, G. I., NGUYEN, T. T., KEIL, M. F. *et al.* (2002), *J. Pediatr.*, **140**, 673–80.

VAN DAM, R. M., VISSCHER, A. W. J., FESKENS, E. J. M., VERHOEF, P. and KROMHOUT, D. (2000), *Eur. J. Clin. Nutr.*, **54**, 726–31.

VOZAROVA, B., STEFAN, N., LINDSAY, R. S. *et al.* (2002), *Diabetes*, **51**, 2964–7.

WANG, H., STORLIEN, L. H. and HUANG, X. F. (2002), *Am. J. Physiol. Endocrinol. Metab.*, **282**, E1352–9.

WARREN, J. M., HENRY, C. J. and SIMONITE, V. (2003), *Pediatrics*, **112**, e414.

WEIGENSBERG, M. J., BALL, G., SHAIBI, G. Q., CRUZ, M. L. and GORAN, M. I. (2004), *Obes. Res.*, **12**, A120;467-P.

WEISS, R., DZIURA, J., BURGERT, T. S. *et al.* (2004), *N. Engl. J. Med.*, **350**, 2362–74.

WELSH, S., SHAW, A. and DAVIS, C. (1994), *Crit. Rev. Food. Sci. Nutr.*, **34** (5–6), 441–51.

WEYER, C., BOGARDUS, C., MOTT, D. M. and PRATLEY, R. E. (1999), *J. Clin. Invest.*, **104**, 787–94.

WIEGAND, S., MAIKOWSKI, U., BLANKENSTEIN, O., BIEBERMANN, H., TARNOW, P. and GRUTERS, A. (2004), *Europ. J. Endocrinol.*, **151**, 199–206.

WILD, S., PIERPOINT, T., MCKEIGUE, P. and JACOBS, H. (2000), *Clin. Endocrinol. (Oxf).*, **52**, 595–600.

WORLD HEALTH ORGANIZATION (1999), pp. 31–3.

WRIGHT, J., KENNEDY-STEPHENSON, J., WANG, C., MCDOWELL, M. and JOHNSON, C. (2004), *Morbid. Mortal. W. Rep.*, **53**, 80–2.

WROTNIAK, B. H., EPSTEIN, L. H., PALUCH, R. A. and ROEMMICH, J. N. (2004), *Arch. Pediatr. Adolesc. Med.*, **158**, 342–7.

XIE, B., LIU, C., CHOU, C. P. *et al.* (2003), *J. Adolesc. Health*, **33**, 202–10.

ZHANG, Y., PROENCA, R., MAFFEL, M., BARONE, M., LEOPOLD, L. and FRIEDMAN, J. M. (1994), *Nature*, **372**, 425–32.

6

The psychology of overeating

C. P. Herman, J. Polivy and T. Leone, University of Toronto, Canada

6.1 Introduction

Everyone knows that overeating is a serious problem in developed countries. What everyone doesn't know is what exactly overeating is. Overeating is . . . well, eating more than you should. But how much should you eat? From the standpoint of nutrition, you should eat only as much as is necessary to offset the caloric demands made on your body. That calculation quickly gets complicated. For one thing, people differ in their basic metabolic rate, so that one person's overeating may be another person's adequate intake. Second, people differ in their activity levels, so that adequate intake for one (particularly active) person may be overeating for another (less active) person, even holding metabolic factors constant.[1] In fact, adequate intake for one person on a given (particularly active) day may be overeating for that same person on another (more lethargic) day. And who is to say that the day is the proper unit of analysis? Nutritionists and almost everyone else do their calculations in diurnal units, but there is something profoundly arbitrary about that choice. Whether or not you overeat on a particular day may be irrelevant if the unit of temporal analysis is the week, and you have the opportunity to compensate on Wednesday for what you (over)ate on Tuesday. Lest you imagine that this example of weekly analysis of overeating is meant as pedantic hairsplitting, consider the following: when people say that they have overeaten, more often than

[1] The old joke – 'I'm not overweight; I'm just underheight' – has its parallel here: 'I don't overeat; I just underexercise.' There is some truth buried in these facetious claims.

not they are referring to a single eating episode (typically a meal). Indeed, one often gets the impression that most instances of overeating are judged (by the perpetrators, at least) in the context of a meal rather than in the context of a day. And who is to say that they are not correct? It may well be that the meal is the appropriate unit of analysis, inasmuch as excess caloric intake at a given meal may well end up unbalancing the regulatory system (Woods, 1991).

How do people determine that they have overeaten at a meal? Usually, this calculation is no calculation at all; often it is a sense of distention or grogginess, combined with a recognition that one has eaten something – or several somethings – that one should not have eaten.[2] These excessive morsels are usually consumed either because they are simply too tempting to resist or because the eater is barely aware of how much is being eaten. Much of this chapter will explore these two types of overeating.

For the moment, though, let us return to definitional matters. Perhaps more to the point, let us concede that there really is no good definition of overeating. Even those who eat just enough to offset the caloric demands of the body may be overeating, after all; for all we know, these people are overweight, and if by staying in caloric balance they fail to bring their weight back down to where it should be – there's that pesky word 'should' again! – they may be overeating while eating normally. In fact, it's technically possible to overeat while undereating, if one doesn't undereat by enough to achieve the goal of normal weight. Ultimately, we may have to accept a colloquial definition of overeating: 'I may not know exactly what overeating is, but I know when I've overeaten!'

6.2 Historical overview

There is scant evidence that overeating existed prior to the twentieth century. Needless to say, there were people who, prior to 1900, ate prodigious amounts of food, amounts that nowadays we would all concur are excessive. The difference is that a concern with weight was largely absent – or more accurately, the notion of overweight did not exist as a cultural and

[2] There is some evidence that overindulgence may be more a qualitative than quantitative matter. Oakes (2005), for instance, demonstrated that people consider a 'bad' food (such as a miniature Snickers bar) to be more fattening than a 'good' food (such as a snack of cottage cheese, carrots, and pears), even when the Snickers bar contains only 47 calories and the 'good' snack contains 569 calories. Similarly, laboratory research (e.g. Knight and Boland, 1989) has demonstrated that forced consumption of 'bad' food (e.g. an ice-cream bar) will induce dieters to overeat (presumably because their diets are 'blown' and there is little point in continuing to diet), whereas forced consumption of a 'good' food (e.g. cottage cheese and fruit) with the same number of calories will not induce dieters to overeat, presumably because their diets are still intact.

public-health concern as it does now. One of us fondly remembers a grandmother, who was already a married woman by 1906, and who used to comment about a friend of ours: 'He's such a nice boy, but why does he have to be so skinny?' In centuries past, a weight problem was usually a matter of insufficient weight; indeed, emaciation was the condition most often associated with the (largely infectious) diseases of which grandmothers were so fearful. Life expectancy was short enough so that the diseases of corpulence rarely had a chance to manifest themselves; death from heart disease in one's 60s was considered a relative blessing. Now, with the virtual eradication of infectious diseases in the developed world, life expectancy has been prolonged to the point where the diseases thought to be associated (accurately or not) with overweight or obesity are taking a larger proportionate toll. Slimness is associated with health rather than disease; as a consequence, we have developed a sensitivity to the possibility of eating too much, of being too heavy. This sensitivity would have amused the wealthier classes of the nineteenth century and earlier, for whom a stout physique was a sign of prosperity and even good health. President Taft (1908–1912) happily tipped the scales at over 300 pounds; and even later, Winston Churchill would have scoffed at the idea of eating sparingly – and perhaps he would have been justified, given that he died in his tenth decade. It is probably worth noting here that there are many places in the world where food is scarce enough and life is short enough that overeating is 'feasting', something that one does whenever one can; indeed, in these circumstances, can one really overeat?

In the first half of the twentieth century, some tentative efforts were made to identify and explain overeating. For the most part, these early analyses focused on the 'compulsive' aspect of overeating as the problem (rather than its implications for weight and physical health). The psychoanalysts, for instance, were quick to seize upon the symbolic aspects of overeating and find its roots in unconscious motives, often based on a vaguely identified 'oral fixation'. Overeating might represent a form of gratification otherwise lacking in one's life (Fenichel, 1945). Robert Lindner, in his classic '*Fifty-Minute Hour*' (1962), tells the story of someone whom we would now call a bulimic. Lindner traced her apocalyptic binges back to a deeply sexual (and naturally, unconscious) source. The symbolic focus of the psychoanalysts was not always on eating, though. Obesity might have its own symbolic meanings (e.g. pregnancy, power), with overeating serving simply as a means of getting to that symbolic end (Fenichel, 1945). Bruch (1961) developed a variation on the psychoanalytic doctrine, arguing that the developing child's internal sensations (including hunger and satiety) were subject to misinterpretation by the caregiver (i.e. mother) and were consequently vulnerable to learned misinterpretation by the growing child herself. Thus, an unfortunate upbringing might produce a child who cannot clearly distinguish between sensations of hunger and satiety, on the one hand, and emotional disturbance, on the other. The result is someone who may (over)eat for emotional reasons. (It is worth noting that Bruch did not argue that such emotional eating was satisfying in any way; after all, the attempt to assuage distress by eating was fundamentally misguided, in her opinion.)

Kaplan and Kaplan (1957) provided yet another analysis of the connection between distress and overeating. Their unfortunately named 'psychosomatic hypothesis' argued (a) that some (not all) people tend to overeat when they get upset, and (b) that distress-induced overeating can serve to counteract distress. The 'psychosomatic hypothesis', then, was actually two separate hypotheses that have been commonly conflated ever since.

One other approach to 'morbid' overeating that has been around for the better part of a century, and that is likely to remain with us indefinitely, might be termed the 'glandular' approach. The notion here is that overeating is driven by an intense (non-metaphorical) hunger that is dissociated from normal bodily functioning. An extreme example would be a hypothalamic tumor or lesion which might induce prodigious overeating either by constantly stimulating the 'hunger centre' or by interfering with the functioning of the 'satiety centre' (Hetherington and Ranson, 1940). Variations on this theme have spanned the range from hormonal abnormalities to the absence or presence of various blood-borne elements that interfere with normal caloric regulation. We are always hearing about the identification of these hunger/satiety chemicals (e.g. leptin; Campfield, 2002), usually with a promise that a 'cure' for overeating is just around the corner.

6.3 Modern theories of overeating and its causes

The year 1968 was revolutionary in many ways, political and cultural; it was also the year in which our understanding of overeating underwent a revolutionary change. In 1968, Stanley Schachter (see Schachter, 1968) published a series of experiments supporting his novel analysis of the determinants of eating and overeating. The most significant aspect of Schachter's approach was his argument that overeating is not primarily under the control of internal states. That is, most people who overeat do not do so because molecules in their bloodstream affect their hypothalamus, which in turn drives them to eat (or to not stop eating). Also, people who overeat do not do so because of internal psychological states, either; distress, in Schachter's view, is not the culprit. The culprit, rather, is palatable food cues. Of course, insofar as palatable food cues are ubiquitous, they do not provide a compelling explanation of why some people overeat in their presence while others do not. To account for individual differences – for the fact that of two people in the same situation, one may overeat while the other does not – Schachter posited that some people are 'external', or particularly responsive to food cues as a determinant of eating. An external individual, when confronted with a large amount of palatable food, will be inclined to eat a lot – potentially, all of it – because the external individual's eating is 'stimulus bound' or under the control of those food cues. A normal individual, on the other hand, is responsive to the regulatory influences of (internal) hunger and satiety cues, which for some reason are ineffective in external people.

Once Schachter had postulated the existence of 'externality', he was in a position to account for overeating simply in terms of exposure to plentiful, palatable food. His laboratory studies showed that some people were indeed more responsive than were others to external food cues, most notably the mere presence of salient, attractive food. A close examination of Schachter's thinking, however, reveals that he did not really start with externality and move from there to overeating. Rather, he started with overeating and moved 'backward' toward externality. In fact, he did not even start with overeating, but rather with overweight, which he (like most researchers, then and now) assumed was the consequence of overeating. Schachter divided his research samples into overweight and normal-weight segments, and proceeded to demonstrate that the overweight people were particularly responsive to external cues. A typical study of this type (e.g. Nisbett, 1968) showed that when people were given a plate with either one sandwich or three sandwiches on it (with more sandwiches available in the nearby refrigerator), overweight people were more affected by the initial number of sandwiches on the plate than were normal-weight people. That is, whereas normal-weight people ate on average just under two sandwiches each, no matter how many sandwiches were put on their plates, overweight people ate on average 1.48 sandwiches when initially presented with one sandwich and 2.32 sandwiches when initially presented with three sandwiches. This study seemed to demonstrate that the food cues themselves controlled intake for overweight people but not for normal-weight people. It was a short step from studies such as these (for a review see Schachter and Rodin, 1974) to the conclusion that chronic exposure to palatable food cues would lead certain people to overeat substantially. Note that Schachter identified his 'external' people on the basis of their degree of overweight rather than in terms of an independent index of externality. He was thus engaged in somewhat circular reasoning, in that he was using externality as the explanation of overweight (mediated by overeating) while at the same time he used overweight (and presumptive overeating) as the means of identifying who was external. Eventually, he argued that externality was the overt reflection of an underlying hypothalamic dysfunction, possibly a 'functional lesion' of the ventromedial hypothalamus (VMH) (Schachter, 1971). Nisbett (1972) pushed this argument a little further, arguing that the functional lesion of the VMH was a consequence of weight suppression, common among fat people. Thus, if you were fat, and undertook to suppress your weight, your brain would react by (defensively) suppressing the activity of your 'satiety centre' (the VMH), so that you would eat more and restore the lost weight. Nisbett started with the notion that some people were effectively 'born' fat and became external when they tried to become thin. Schachter believed that some people were 'born' external and became fat when exposed (as we all are) to palatable food cues. The differences between these theories are less important than is the recognition that both theories argued that enhanced responsiveness to palatable food cues was the proximate cause of overeating. Both theories also argued that such overeating in response to palatable food cues was a characteristic of only some people, rendering only some people fat (Schachter) or reflecting the fact that only some people are destined to be fat (Nisbett).

6.4 Types of overeating

In the three-plus decades since Schachter and Nisbett speculated about individual differences in responsiveness to palatable food cues, a large literature has accumulated testing their ideas, as well as other approaches to understanding controls on eating and why such controls frequently appear to be weak or absent. Our assessment of this literature, to oversimplify things only slightly, is that there are two major types of overeating. One type is based on over-responsiveness to environmental factors that promote overeating. The second type is based on the acute release of inhibitions, with external cues playing a relatively minor role. Ironically, it now appears that the type of overeating that emphasizes responsiveness to external cues (as in Schachter/Nisbett) does not emphasize individual differences (as Schachter/Nisbett did), but instead suggests that everyone is vulnerable to cue-based overeating. On the other hand, the 'disinhibition' type of overeating, in which external cues play only a minor role, emphasizes the sort of individual differences in which Schachter and Nisbett were so interested. We will now explore these various types of overeating.

6.4.1 Type 1 overeating: environmental pressures

Brownell (2002) and Brownell and Horgen (2003) have argued that the developed world has become a 'toxic environment' promoting obesity. Brownell notes that demands and incentives for exercise in daily life have declined, but his major emphasis is on the tremendous growth in the availability and marketing of food, much of which is of dubious nutritional value. The basic assumption underlying Brownell's characterization of the food environment as 'toxic' is that exposure to food cues and cues promoting food consumption drives eating, and that exposure to an excess of such cues drives overeating. The individual is seen as relatively helpless to resist the allure of palatable food and the insistence of advertisers that one consume such food.

There are various elements in the toxic environment that conduce to overeating. For purposes of this chapter, we will focus on two such elements, one well known, the other less so; both, however, have been the subject of considerable empirical work, and their impact on eating is large and indisputable.

Portion size

The better-known element in the toxic environment, one that Brownell and others have implicated in the recent acceleration in the fattening of the citizenry of developed countries, is portion size (see Rolls, this volume). The recent rise in obesity corresponds, at least in a rough way, with a rise in the size of complete meals and their individual components, especially as served at restaurants and by other commercial food purveyors (Nielsen and Popkin, 2003). Of course, this correlation does not prove that larger portion sizes are responsible for the current obesity epidemic. It is possible that fat people demand larger portions, or that obesity and larger portions are both the result of greater prosperity. Demonstrating that portion size directly affects food intake requires experimentation.

The experiments that have been conducted, manipulating portion size and examining its effect on eating, have been conclusive. Rolls, Morris, and Roe (2002) found that people ate in direct proportion to the size of the portion (of macaroni and cheese) that they were served. (This finding did not reflect a ceiling effect, with those served a small portion unable to eat as much as they wanted: There was always more food available in a readily accessible container). It is worth dwelling on some implications of this experiment. First and foremost, it appears that an environmental factor (an arbitrary portion size) overrides biologically based nutritional considerations. People eat more when they are served more, and less when they are served less, pretty much regardless of their initial level of hunger/satiety. This finding highlights not only the power of the environmental cue but also the weakness of the internal cues (hunger/satiety) that have long been regarded as the most important determinants of food intake (see Herman, 1996, for an elaboration of this argument). Insofar as environmental cues are strong and biological cues are weak, we have the ideal scenario for the development of overeating, with plenty of 'go' signals (emanating from the food itself) and a paucity of 'stop' signals (which should emanate from the gut or midbrain).

A second important feature of the Rolls *et al.* (2002) experiment is the apparent absence of individual differences. Recall that Schachter and Nisbett postulated that (over)responsiveness to external/environmental food cues would be a salient characteristic of the obese, but would be effectively absent in normal-weight individuals. It is now well over two decades since Rodin (1981) rejected Schachter's simple association of externality with obese people and internality with normal-weight people, but studies such as Rolls *et al.*'s have gone well beyond Rodin to demonstrate that (over)responsiveness to portion-size cues is something that appears to be virtually universal. Fat or thin, male or female, committed to dieting or not, people show the standard 'portion-size effect', eating more as portion size increases. Wansink and Park (2001) and Edelman *et al.* (1986) provide further examples of the basic portion-size effect, albeit with some minor qualifications. The implication here is that the pressures exerted by palatable and ubiquitous food cues affect everybody, and that there is no need to search for individual differences or dispositions in order to account for the effect.

Still, the fact that portion size has a direct effect on food intake is not self-explanatory, even if we are all personally familiar with the phenomenon. Why do people eat more just because they start with more food on their plate? The fact that more food is available does not logically imply that one should eat more of it, does it? Why not simply eat in concert with one's nutritional needs and leave the rest?

Our view (see also Wansink, 2004, for a similar position) is that people are at best barely aware of their nutritional needs, because internal signals about nutritional deficit and surfeit are usually weak and unattended to; moreover, such signals, if they manifest themselves at all, do so after a significant temporal delay, so that by the time we realize that we have eaten too much, it's too late to do anything about it. Because people cannot rely on internal signals to start and stop eating, they become dependent on alternative signals suggesting when and how much to eat. In short, because the body is an ineffective source of information regarding what is an appropriate amount to eat, the person develops a reliance on the environment to indicate appropriate consumption norms.

Portion size is an exemplary source of consumption norms. That is, people assume that the portion that they have been served is an appropriate amount to eat – after all, why would they be given this amount of food if it was not meant to be eaten? – and they eat accordingly, at least within certain limits. (If the portion is preposterously small or large, we imagine, people might be tempted to regard the portion as an unsuitable indicator of appropriateness and reject it, overriding the basic portion-size effect. Research testing this proposition has yet to be conducted.) In our view, then, portion size affects eating through the intermediary step of providing people with a sense of what is the 'correct' amount to eat. Once people are convinced that they have discovered the 'correct' amount to eat, they will eat that amount – or perhaps just a little less (see our discussion of social influences, below).

The reader may object that the view that everyone is vulnerable to the portion-size effect is contradicted by the Nisbett (1968) study that we described above, in which only obese people seemed to be affected by the manipulation of the number of sandwiches (1 vs. 3) served initially. Although it appears that this manipulation of portion size was ineffective for normal-weight people, we believe that our analysis in terms of appropriateness holds, and can even 'explain away' Nisbett's data that normal-weight people ate just under two sandwiches, on average, regardless of whether they were initially served one sandwich or three sandwiches. Our solution to this problem hinges on the fact that while people do not necessarily know *how much* they should eat when served sandwiches, people (at least normal-weight people) do know *how many* sandwiches it is appropriate to eat. When male undergraduates are served relatively small sandwiches – as was the case in the Nisbett study (personal communication with R. E. Nisbett, 2004) – they understand that two sandwiches is the normative number to eat. (Obese people, who struggle to eat less, often eat more, and probably have only a vague idea of how many sandwiches would be normatively consumed in such a situation, would be more vulnerable to the manipulation of sandwich number). We suggest that had Nisbett varied the *size* of the sandwiches rather than their number, he would have obtained the standard portion-size effect even with normal-weight people. That is, if normal-weight people had been served one small sandwich or three small sandwiches or one large sandwich or three large sandwiches, they would probably have ended up eating just under two sandwiches on average, as Nisbett found. But if we examine how much was consumed in these various conditions, we would have found that in the large-sandwich conditions, people would have eaten much more than in the small-sandwich conditions. People would have eaten about two sandwiches regardless, but two large sandwiches could have contained many more calories than two small sandwiches. Thus, while normal-weight males know that two sandwiches is about the right amount to eat for lunch, they do not have a clear idea of how large those sandwiches should be. Manipulations of portion size (rather than portion number) would therefore exert a strong influence on them. (This study, too, has yet to be conducted).

Before we leave portion size as an example of the power of environmental influences on eating, we should emphasize a couple of extrapolations that are necessary to get us from these laboratory studies to real-world instances of overeating and obesity. The first, more trivial extrapolation, concerns the fact that laboratory studies of eating are usually time-limited and involve relatively modest amounts of food. The portion-size effect is easily demonstrable, and statistically quite significant; but the actual amount of food eaten, even in the large-portion condition, is usually not extravagant in absolute terms. Thus, in extrapolating from the laboratory to the restaurant, we must make certain assumptions about the duration of the eating episode and the amounts of food that may be consumed. On balance, we believe that portion-size effects in the real world are substantial and can produce true overeating on a given occasion. The second, more significant, extrapolation concerns the frequency of overeating. Laboratory studies are typically confined to a single eating episode. The argument that portion-size effects are responsible for the obesity epidemic requires the assumption that episodic overeating becomes chronic for many people, with the result that excess calories consumed on single occasions cumulate over time (and eating episodes) in a way that can plausibly account for significant or even morbid weight gain. In principle, a well-regulated system would compensate for overeating on a particular occasion by making provision for a compensatory decrease in caloric intake on the next eating occasion. The evidence in rats, however, suggests that consuming more calories at a particular meal delays the onset of the next meal, rather than decreasing the size of the next meal (Le Magnen, 1985). That would work if people could, or would, delay their next meal until they were really hungry. In our society, however, as in most societies, meal times are not dictated primarily by hunger but by a variety of familial, social and occupational constraints. People eat the next meal even if they are not yet truly hungry, and the size of that next meal does not reflect the size of the previous meal. Looking at the situation from a broader perspective, we must acknowledge that the exquisitely regulated negative-feedback model of food intake that nature perhaps intended for us has not been working very well. We don't compensate very well for previous excessive meals, and when between-meal snacks are added to the equation, the notion of precise caloric regulation seems antiquated. Our overall caloric intake (as a society) is clearly increasing; and combined with the societal decline in physical activity, we are observing a strong upsurge in the extent of obesity. The extent to which this upsurge is attributable to larger portion sizes is debatable, but no doubt larger portion sizes are part of the problem.

Social influence

Portion size is one example of an environmental influence that can promote overeating, but it is not the only one. Another strong influence, albeit one that is not as widely recognized (and editorialized against), is social influence. Like portion size, social influence appears to affect just about everyone, but its effects depend on the specific kind of social influence. Herman *et al.* (2003) subdivided social influences into three separate categories, each of which displays the potential for inducing overeating. We shall discuss these three categories in decreasing order of their impact on overeating.

Social facilitation refers to the empirical finding that people in groups tend to eat more than do individuals eating alone. This effect is quite strong (as much as 50% greater intake by individuals eating in groups) and is derived largely from food diaries completed by people in the 'real world', transcending some problems associated with lab studies (although raising problems of self-report) (de Castro and de Castro, 1989; Patel and Schlundt, 2001). Laboratory studies have corroborated the basic effect (Berry *et al.*, 1985; Clendenen *et al.*, 1994; Edelman *et al.*, 1986). De Castro and Brewer (1992) concluded that the social facilitation effect is a direct (power) function of the number of people present, such that the addition of another group member makes a greater difference in a small group than in a large group, but Clendenen *et al.* have challenged this exponential claim without challenging the basic finding that individuals in groups eat more than do solo individuals.

The explanation for the social-facilitation effect remains uncertain. de Castro has proposed a 'time-extension' explanation: People spend longer eating when they eat in groups and therefore consume more food. This explanation is not entirely satisfying. First, the fact that you spend a longer time at the table does not logically require that you eat more. Moreover, this proposal does not explain where the extra food comes from to support socially-facilitated eating. We (Herman *et al.*, 2003) have proposed an explanation based on the same sort of normative model that we invoked above to explain the portion-size effect. Our explanation starts with the premise that eating in a group is generally a more pleasant experience than is eating alone, so people are motivated to eat with others. Once they are with others, the amount that others eat becomes a normative cue indicating how much one should eat. (We assume that when the food is palatable, people are eager to eat more of it, and that social norms act as a constraint, in the sense that social norms establish the permissible upper limit of appropriate consumption). In a group, it is easy to lose track of exactly how much one has eaten, and how much the others have eaten, with the result that individuals may perceive the consumption norm as relatively high and eat more than they otherwise would have. This additional eating may in turn stimulate (or permit) others to eat more, in a positive feedback loop.

Social facilitation of eating does not obtain in all circumstances. It appears to be reduced, for instance, when one eats with strangers (Clendenen *et al.*, 1994; de Castro, 1994; Shide and Rolls, 1991). This suppression of social facilitation effect is probably a matter of people trying harder to make a positive impression on strangers than on people who already know them well (Tice *et al.*, 1995), along with the assumption that eating sparingly conveys a positive impression (L. Vartanian, C. P. Herman and J. Polivy, unpublished review). It is important to note, though, that this qualification does not mean that there are individual differences in social facilitation. Eating with friends and family promotes social facilitation, and (virtually) everyone has friends and family. The constraint here is a matter of situation, rather than of chronic individual differences.

A legitimate individual difference in social facilitation of eating is the finding that social facilitation is more prevalent among males than among females (Klesges *et al.*, 1984; Shide and Rolls, 1991). Also, it is important to note that de Castro excluded dieters from his diary studies. Women and dieters, then, may be more cautious about allowing their food intake to spiral upward. Women and dieters, of course, are a largely overlapping set, representing those for whom suppressing food intake is a major concern. Even so, women do show social facilitation of eating, if not to the same extent as do men.

The fact that we tend to eat our meals in the presence of other people means that social facilitation of intake is perhaps a regular occurrence in our society, where abundant food is available to fuel facilitated intake. We are unaware of anyone suggesting that socially facilitated overeating is a major public health concern, but the possibility remains intriguing. Nor are we suggesting that socially facilitated eating has increased recently in the same way that portion sizes have increased, but insofar as people make their eating occasions social occasions, they do increase the likelihood of overeating.

Modeling refers to the fact that individuals tend to follow the lead of others when it comes to eating. A large number of laboratory studies have demonstrated that when experimental confederates eat a lot (or only a little), naive experimental participants tend to go along, eating a lot (or only a little) (e.g. Conger *et al.*, 1980; Nisbett and Storms, 1974; Roth *et al.*, 2001). Again, we believe (Herman *et al.*, 2003) that the confederate serves a norm-setting role, establishing an upper limit for the naive eater regarding what is an appropriate amount to eat. In this literature, naive eaters often eat a little less than does the confederate, to guarantee that their intake is not excessive; but insofar as the confederate eats a lot, naive eaters will eat a lot. Indeed, manipulations of hunger in the naive eaters do not limit the social-influence effect. Hungry eaters will eat minimally when the confederate eats minimally (Goldman *et al.*, 1991) and sated eaters will continue to eat when the confederate eats a great deal (Herman *et al.*, 2004). The powerful effect of models does not appear to depend much on the type of person exposed to the influence (Polivy *et al.*, 1979), suggesting that virtually everyone is likely to follow the example set by the confederate.

Obviously, eating in the presence of other people who eat a lot may induce overeating in individuals who might not otherwise have overeaten. Whether such 'bad influences' can be blamed for the overeating that appears to be endemic in our society is debatable, but eating in the company of others who are eating prodigiously is more likely to promote overeating than to provoke contrarian undereating. Part of the toxic environment that we face is our eating companions, whose excessive eating makes our own excessive eating seem simply normal.

Impression management, the third category of social influence identified by Herman *et al.* (2003), refers to changes in food intake designed to convey a positive impression to one's eating companions. By and large, this category refers to people's apparent suppression of their food intake when eating with others or when in the presence of one or more non-eating observers. At first glance, it would appear that suppression of food intake when eating with others directly contradicts the well-documented phenomenon of social facilitation of eating. The contradiction is more apparent than real, however. Recall that social facilitation of eating is strongest in the presence of people who know you well – that is, the people on whom you are least likely to be trying to make a positive impression. Impression management studies of eating tend to focus on situations in which the eater is paired with someone (e.g. a date, a prospective employer) who does not know the eater well and whose opinion, often based on a first impression, is of great importance. In such circumstances, where one's food intake is thought to be under intense scrutiny, people generally tend to eat less than they otherwise might. Mori *et al.* (1987), for instance, found that people ate least when paired with opposite-sex individuals. Even more dramatic suppression of food intake occurs when one eats in the presence of a non-eating observer (Conger *et al.*, 1980; Roth *et al.*, 2001).

It is not immediately obvious how impression management might produce overeating. No empirical studies have used an impression-management interpretation to explain overeating. Still, it is conceivable that in the right circumstances, impression-management concerns might lead to overeating (eating contests aside). For instance, we are occasionally pressured to eat more, even excessively, by other people who have a vested interest in our overindulgence. If the chef is present, it may be impolite to confine oneself to a normal helping.

As we noted earlier, social influences are not often cited as a cause of overeating and obesity. To a large extent, this minimization of the effect of social influence is attributable to the fact that people are simply unaware of how powerful social influences are. The effects of social facilitation and modeling manipulations often equal or exceed the effects of palatability or hunger manipulations. Acknowledging the power of social influence, however, may not lead to the same prescriptions for social engineering that other culprits (like portion size) attract. It is one thing for us to 'demand' that food purveyors reduce portion sizes, but how many of us would insist that people eat in isolation so as to avoid the risk of socially induced overeating?

6.4.2 Type 2 overeating: disinhibition

Portion size and social influence represent two examples drawn from the category of broad influences on eating that affect virtually everyone. Insofar as people in general are eating more and getting fatter, it is that category that deserves our epidemiological attention. There is another major category of influences on eating that can provoke substantial overeating, however. This category of factors promoting overeating applies only to a certain segment of the population, but that segment is large enough to warrant our consideration. We are referring here to people who chronically attempt to suppress their food intake, but who occasionally 'lose control' and overeat. This overeating no doubt contributes to the weight problems that these people are concerned about – it is this concern that causes them to attempt to suppress their eating in the first place – but because this overeating occurs in the context of generally restrained eating, it probably is not as significant a contributor to the obesity epidemic as are the 'toxic' environmental factors such as portion size. We shall discuss a small number of examples of factors that trigger overeating in otherwise restrained eaters.

Distress is a widely acknowledged cause of binge-like eating. Indeed, clinically diagnosed binge eaters rate distress as among the most prominent triggers of their binges (Polivy and Herman, 1993). Even among apparently normal eaters, however, distress is a common precursor of overeating. Closer inspection of the data, however, reveals that distress does not cause overeating in a general way, the way that large portion sizes do. Rather, distress triggers overeating specifically among people who are restrained eaters, deliberately attempting to curtail their food intake. In people who are unconcerned about restraining their eating, distress does not produce overeating (and may even decrease intake).

Herman and Polivy (1975) demonstrated that distress – the anticipation of electric shock – had opposite effects on restrained and unrestrained eaters. Restrained eaters (identified by means of a questionnaire focused on eating habits and weight fluctuations indicative of chronic dieting) ate somewhat more, whereas unrestrained eaters ate substantially less. This pattern was similar to what Schachter *et al.* (1968) had found with obese and normal-weight eaters, respectively; this parallel was interpreted by Herman and Polivy as reflecting the fact that obese people are more likely than are normal-weight people to be concerned about their weight.

Several elements of the Herman and Polivy (1975) study warrant attention. First, because distress affected only some people (dieters), the explanation of the effect must take into account the peculiar psychology of dieters. Unlike portion size or social influence, distress does not induce overeating across the board; in fact, in many people, it induces undereating. (On strictly physiological grounds, distress should make people eat less, insofar as distress has sympathomimetic effects, releasing energy stores into the bloodstream; an increase in blood glucose should suppress, not enhance, eating). Herman and Polivy focused on the fact that dieters, almost by definition, attempt to inhibit their eating; and in the absence of distress, restrained eaters did in fact eat less than did unrestrained eaters. When they were upset, however, it was as if their ability to maintain an inhibitory stance toward food was undermined. Chronically deprived (or so they believe themselves to be), these dieters were now 'released' from their inhibitions and able to eat freely, which (to them) meant overeating.

Various explanations have been offered for why distress disinhibits eating in restrained eaters, but the general pattern of results has been found time and time again. The ability of distress to provoke overeating in dieters appears to be greater when the distress is 'personal' rather than 'physical' (Heatherton *et al.*, 1991), such that more overeating is seen when experimental participants experience depression (Baucom and Aiken, 1981; Frost *et al.*, 1982), or general negative affect (Ruderman, 1985), than when they are threatened physically (e.g. by electric shock), but the precise means by which distress releases inhibitions and produces overeating remains controversial (for review see Herman and Polivy, 2004). Distress may lead dieters to abandon their long-term goals and immerse themselves in immediate sensory experiences (e.g. salient food), according to Heatherton and Baumeister (1991). Dieters may break their diets, deliberately upsetting themselves, so as to provide a more manageable reason for their being upset than the personal threat that is really bothering them (Herman and Polivy, 1988). Or perhaps the effort of coping with distressing emotions depletes thc dieter's reserve of energy available for other self-control tasks (Kahan *et al.*, 2003; Vohs & Heatherton, 2000).

Craving[3] is a subjective state often associated with overeating; indeed, a large majority of bulimics blame their binges on cravings (Mitchell *et al.*, 1985), although it should be noted that cravings and distress are not mutually exclusive when it comes to triggering binges. Insofar as people develop strong cravings, we can expect them to overeat, unless they are particularly abstemious dieters. The fact is, though, that cravings are not distributed equally through the population. Certain types of people (e.g. premenstrual or pregnant women) are especially likely to experience cravings. Indeed, one group especially likely to experience cravings is dieters (Fedoroff *et al.*, 1997, 2003; Gendall *et al.*, 1998, 1999; Pelchat, 1997). The prevalence of craving among dieters might mean that those who happen to experience cravings – and especially those who capitulate to the cravings – must of necessity try to limit their food intake. Another possibility is that dieting itself – or at least the objective or subjective deprivation that dieters experience – induces craving (Polivy *et al.*, 2004).

Craving is an especially interesting phenomenon because it appears to arise in response to both internal and external cues. Polivy *et al.* (2004) demonstrated that a recent deprivation accentuates craving. Fedoroff *et al.* (1997, 2003) demonstrated that exposure to food cues accentuates craving. It seems likely that both of these sources of craving might be mediated by thoughts or images of the craved food. Moreover, it seems reasonable to predict that cravings will be more intense when the cued food corresponds to the food that has been missing during the deprivation experience. Deprivation alone might stimulate craving (as when we dream of what we have been missing); and exposure alone might stimulate craving (as when we crave a highly palatable food without having been deprived of it); but the

[3] The craving construct continues to elude precise definition. Researchers often assess craving by self-report (where 'craving' is indistinguishable from strong liking or other subjective terms), but this approach, even when bolstered with a facade of quantification, is acknowledged to be flawed. Is one person's craving equivalent to another's? Occasionally craving is operationalized in terms of the amount eaten, or the speed of eating, but this approach, while more objective, is highly dubious, if only because of its inherent circularity. Why does she eat so much? Because she strongly craves the food. And how do we know that she strongly craves the food? Because she eats so much. Attempts to assess craving psychophysiologically also seem more objective at first glance, but measures such as salivation are responsive to a variety of factors (including the mere anticipation of consumption), rendering them inadequate as valid and distinctive measures of craving. Multiple (non-perfect) measures may provide converging evidence of craving, but what if they do not converge?

combination seems likely to have a multiplicative effect. In any case, the evidence seems to favor the notion that cravings are more prevalent in dieters, perhaps because they are more deprived, or perhaps because they are more intently focused on available food cues, or perhaps because of both. Overeating based on craving is a widespread phenomenon; even if dieting exacerbates craving, it remains a danger for almost everyone. Even if it applies to some extent to everyone, like the Type I factors of portion size or social influence, craving nevertheless displays one noticeable difference: People are acutely aware that they are experiencing a craving, whereas when the Type I factors induce overeating, they appear to do so without necessarily reaching consciousness. We may overeat when served a large portion without even thinking about it; when we crave a food, though, we think about little else.

Preloading represents a final example of a trigger for overeating that applies only to dieters. The term 'preload' refers to a portion of food that an experimental participant is required to consume in its entirety (on some pretext). In a typical preloading experiment, the researchers are interested in how consuming the preload affects participants' subsequent intake when they are given access to another food that they are allowed to eat in an *ad lib* fashion. Like distress, preloading ought to suppress intake, strictly on physiological grounds; after all, calories consumed at Time 1 should reduce the need for calories at Time 2 in a well-regulated system. In normal non-dieters, preloading does in fact suppress *ad lib* intake (Herman and Mack, 1975; Schachter *et al.*, 1968). In dieters, though, preloading appears to reverse normal regulation, producing 'counter-regulation'. Herman and Mack, for instance, found that, whereas preloading non-dieters with 0, 1, or 2 milkshakes led to successively less *ad lib* ice cream consumption, dieters ate significantly more after being preloaded with 1 or 2 milkshakes than after no preload. Their interpretation was similar to the interpretation offered by Herman and Polivy (1975). Preloading, like distress, serves to disinhibit eating in dieters. Why? Herman and Mack speculated that dieters, having consumed a large, rich, forced preload, would regard their diets as 'blown' for the day and no longer worth maintaining (the 'what-the-hell' effect). In the absence of a preload, the dieter's diet remains intact, and so continued restraint is in order.

Several features of this experimental paradigm are worth noting. First, the preload need not be high in calories as long as it is perceived to be high in calories. Researchers who have separated the perceived calories in the preload from the actual calories (e.g. Knight and Boland, 1989; Polivy, 1976) have found that it is the perceived calories that drives the effect. If dieters think that the preload has ruined their diet for the day, then they become disinhibited. Because people are often so irrational in their caloric calculations (see Oakes, 2005), we may legitimately wonder whether a 47-calorie miniature candy bar may act as a disinhibiting preload while a 567-calorie snack of cottage cheese, carrots, and pears may leave the diet intact. Indeed, studies such as Oakes's and Knight and Boland's suggest that calories per se may not be the operative variable; rather, consuming something 'bad' may produce disinhibition in dieters, whereas eating something 'good' may leave the diet intact, caloric considerations notwithstanding.

Insofar as the preload-disinhibition effect operates by ruining the dieter's diet for the day, we may also ask: Why are diets designed in terms of days? If the diet were designed on a yearly basis, for instance, then it seems unlikely that a milkshake or two would ruin the diet; over the course of the year, there would be plenty of opportunity to compensate for the rich preload without compromising the diet (and creating conditions ripe for disinhibited eating). Perhaps it is precisely because a diet organized on an annual basis is so forgiving that we do not organize diets that way (see Herman and Polivy, 2003, for a discussion). Nutritionally, there is nothing special about the day as the fundamental dietary unit; and yet dieters think in diurnal units, such that diets tend to start 'first thing tomorrow' rather than right away, and when disinhibition occurs, the diet does not resume until the next day.

Given that the diet is comprehended and calculated by the dieter on a daily basis, it is possible that the failure of a diet may be prospective, rather than retrospective. A rich preload at Time 1 may disinhibit eating at Time 2, because there is no chance that the daily diet may be salvaged; but it is also conceivable that the anticipation of a rich preload at Time 3 (later that same day) may disinhibit eating at Time 2. Ruderman *et al.* (1985) and Tomarken and Kirschenbaum (1984) both found that dieters overeat when they expect that their diets will be ruined later in the day.

Rich preloads are associated with disinhibited eating on the same day, and with the resumption of dieting on the following day. So just as the anticipation of a rich preload on the same day may produce disinhibited eating, so may the anticipation of restrained eating on the following day produce disinhibited eating. Urbszat, Herman, and Polivy (2003) found that dieters overate when they expected to start a diet on the following day. (Such overeating was not observed in dieters not anticipating a next-day diet, nor was it observed in nondieters regardless of their expectations).

6.5 Implications for reducing obesity

We have surveyed a few salient examples of environmental, cognitive, and emotional factors that contribute to overeating. Our separation of these factors into two broad classes (environmental factors and disinhibitory factors) has immediate consequences. Because these factors operate in different ways, policy implications will differ according to the type of factor considered. For instance, portion size, arguably the best known of the factors that we have examined, may submit to certain initiatives. We have already seen a fairly impressive public hue and cry about portion size in the media recently. McDonald's has to some extent eliminated 'super-sizing', although the non-super-size portions are considerably larger than they were decades ago. As psychologists who are perhaps understandably skeptical about the likelihood of vested interests serving the needs of public health, we are naturally eager to attack the problem of growing portion sizes by making people more aware. There is no reason why people cannot take some responsibility for their behavior. As things stand now, the individual is portrayed as a passive automaton, eating in direct response to cues such as portion size, and blindly assuming that whatever portion is served is appropriate. It is time to put the onus on the individual, by raising the issue of portion size in a public way. Rather than clamoring for McDonald's or any other food purveyor to reduce portion sizes, we should be clamoring for people to take the issue of portion size into their own hands and make independent, informed decisions about how much to eat. People needn't wait for McDonald's to reduce the portions it serves before reducing the portions that they consume. If it is true that a larger portion of fries is more 'economical' than is a smaller portion of fries, it is nevertheless just as true that the smaller portion of fries is still less expensive than the larger portion in absolute terms. People must come to realize that they are not getting a 'bargain' by eating as much as they can. Rather than campaign against the food industry, we should be campaigning for education of the citizenry – starting in the early school years – about what constitutes proper nutrition. Such a campaign would be expensive, no doubt, but it is preferable to arm people with knowledge and responsibility than to perpetuate the notion that 'they can't help what they eat' and therefore we must engineer the environment so that they will eat properly without realizing what they are doing. Such environmental engineering simply will not succeed in the face of the powerful food and restaurant industries (see Critser, 2003).

When it comes to social influence, we have no choice but to make an educational effort. There is no insidious corporate conspiracy that we can legislate away – unless we consider advertising that features people enjoying meals in a social context as a cynical ploy by the food industry. Social influence powerfully affects eating, but people do not realize the extent of that influence. Only by enlightening people as to how they are affected by the behavior of others can we hope to combat that influence. We have no evidence that knowing that you are affected by others lessens that influence, but there seems to be little alternative to trying this consciousness-raising route.

Dieters are at particular risk of overeating. Not only are they subject to the same broad influences as everyone else, but because of their efforts to suppress their intake, they are prone to periodic bouts of overeating when their inhibitions are released. And because their inhibitions are maintained by a relatively fragile 'resolve', disinhibition-fueled overeating is a common occurrence in dieters (Heatherton *et al.*, 1991). We have long argued that dieting is more a problem than a solution (Polivy and Herman, 1983), and we continue to urge alternatives to weight control (Polivy and Herman, 2002). Again, railing against the diet industry seems to be a doomed cause; and trying to convince people not to pursue strenuous diets does not appear to be a much more hopeful enterprise; but we are better served when we educate people than when we try to simply manipulate them.

Overeating will not soon disappear as a public health problem; the (commercial and psychological) forces that promote overeating are extremely strong. Looked at from the historical perspective of our understanding of the causes of overeating, we should perhaps recognize that we are still in the infancy of our explanatory efforts. There is a felt urgency to deal with the problem immediately, on account of the 'obesity epidemic' that is threatening our society. We must remain patient, however, and work to develop a clear understanding of the roots of the problem while informing the potential victims about how they can protect themselves by recognizing the factors that are likely to make them overeat.

6.6 References

BAUCOM, D. H. and AIKEN, P. A. (1981), Effects of depressed mood on eating among obese and nonobese dieting and nondieting persons. *Journal of Personality and Social Psychology*, **41**, 577–85.

BERRY, S. L., BEATTY, W. W. and KLESGES, R. C. (1985), Sensory and social influences on ice-cream consumption by males and females in a laboratory setting. *Appetite*, **6**, 41–5.

BROWNELL, K. D. (2002), The environment and obesity. In C. G. Fairburn and K. D. Brownell (Eds.). *Eating Disorders and Obesity: A Comprehensive Handbook.* New York: Guilford, pp. 433–8.

BROWNELL, K. D. and HORGEN, K. B. (2003), *Food Fight: The Inside Story of the Food Industry, America's Obesity Crisis, and What We Can Do about It.* New York: McGraw-Hill.

BRUCH, H. (1961), Transformation of oral impulses into eating disorders: a conceptual approach. *Psychiatric Quarterly*, **35**, 458–81.

CAMPFIELD, L. A. (2002), Leptin and body weight regulation. In C. G. Fairburn and K. D. Brownell (Eds.). *Eating Disorders and Obesity: A Comprehensive Handbook.* New York: Guilford, pp. 32–6.

CLENDENEN, V. I., HERMAN, C. P. and POLIVY, J. (1994), Social facilitation of eating among friends and strangers. *Appetite*, **23**, 1–13.

CONGER, J. C., CONGER, A. J., COSTANZO, P. R., WRIGHT, K. L. and MATTER, L. A. (1980), The effect of social cues on the eating behavior of obese and normal subjects. *Journal of Personality*, **48**, 258–71.

CRITSER, G. (2003), *Fat Land: How Americans Became the Fattest people in the World.* New York: Houghton Mifflin.

DE CASTRO, J. M. (1994), Family and friends produce greater social facilitation of food intake than other companions. *Physiology and Behavior*, **56**, 445–55.

DE CASTRO, J. M. and DE CASTRO, E. S. (1989), Spontaneous meal patterns of humans: influence of the presence of other people. *American Journal of Clinical Nutrition*, **50**, 237–47.

DE CASTRO, J. M. and BREWER, E. M. (1992), The amount eaten in meals by humans is a power function of the number of people present. *Physiology and Behavior*, **51**, 121–5.

EDELMAN, B., ENGELL, D., BRONSTEIN, P. and HIRSCH, E. (1986), Environmental effects on the intake or overweight and normal-weight men. *Appetite*, **7**, 71–83.

FEDOROFF, I., POLIVY, J. and HERMAN, C. P. (1997), The effect of pre-exposure to food cues on the eating behavior or restrained and unrestrained eaters. *Appetite*, **28**, 33–47.

FEDOROFF, I., POLIVY, J. and HERMAN, C. P. (2003), The specificity of restrained versus unrestrained eaters' responses to food cues: General desire to eat, or craving for the cued food? *Appetite*, **41**, 7–13.

FENICHEL, O. (1945), *The Psychoanalytic Theory of the Neuroses*. New York: Norton.

FROST, R. O., GOOLKASIAN, G. A., ELY, R. J. and BLANCHARD, F. A. (1982), Depression, restraint and eating behavior. *Behavior Research and Therapy*, **20**, 113–21.

GENDALL, K. A., JOYCE, P. R. and ABBOTT, R. M. (1999), The effects of meal composition on subsequent craving and binge eating. *Addictive Behaviors*, **24**, 305–15.

GENDALL, K. A., JOYCE, P. R., SULLIVAN, P. F. and BULIK, C. M. (1998), Food cravers: Characteristics of those who binge. *International Journal of Eating Disorders*, **23**, 353–60.

GOLDMAN, S. J., HERMAN, C. P. and POLIVY, J. (1991), Is the effect of a social model attenuated by hunger? *Appetite*, **17**, 129–40.

HEATHERTON, T. F. and BAUMEISTER, R. F. (1991), Binge eating as escape from self-awareness. *Psychological Bulletin*, **110**, 86–108.

HEATHERTON, T. F., HERMAN, C. P. and POLIVY, J. (1991), Effects of physical threat and ego threat on eating behavior. *Journal of Personality and Social Psychology*, **60**, 138–43.

HEATHERTON, T. F., POLIVY, J. and HERMAN, C. P. (1991), Restraint, weight loss, and variability of body weight. *Journal of Abnormal Psychology*, **100**, 78–83.

HERMAN, C. P. (1996), Cognitive is more important than physiological in the regulation of appetite – pro. In A. Angel *et al.* (Eds.) *Progress in Obesity Research*. London: John Libbey and Co., pp. 379–83.

HERMAN, C. P. and MACK, D. (1975), Restrained and unrestrained eating. *Journal of Personality*, **43**, 647–60.

HERMAN, C. P. and POLIVY, J. (1975), Anxiety, restraint, and eating behavior. *Journal of Abnormal Psychology*, **84**, 666–72.

HERMAN, C. P. and POLIVY, J. (1988), Studies of eating in normal dieters. In B. T. Walsh (Ed.), *Eating Behavior in Eating Disorders*. Washington, DC: American Psychiatric Association Press, pp. 95–112.

HERMAN, C. P. and POLIVY, J. (2003), Dieting as an exercise in behavioral economics. In G. Loewenstein, D. Read and R. F. Baumeister (Eds.), *Time and Decision: Economic and Psychological Perspectives on Intertemporal Choice*. New York: Russell Sage Foundation, pp. 459–90.

HERMAN, C. P. and POLIVY, J. (2004), The self-regulation of eating: theoretical and practical problems. In R. F. Baumeister and K. D. Vohs (Eds.) *Handbook of Self-regulation: Research, Theory, and Applications*. New York: Guilford Press, pp. 492–508.

HERMAN, C. P., POLIVY, KAUFFMAN, N. and ROTH, D. A. (2004), Is the effect of a social model on eating attenuated by satiety? Unpublished manuscript, University of Toronto.

HERMAN, C. P., ROTH, D. A. and POLIVY, J. (2003), Effects of the presence of others on food intake: a normative interpretation. *Psychological Bulletin*, **129**, 873–86.

HETHERINGTON, A. W. and RANSON, S. W. (1940), Hypothalamic lesions and adiposity in the rat. *Anatomical Record*, **78**, 149–72.

KAHAN, D., POLIVY, J. and HERMAN, C. P. (2003), Conformity and dietary disinhibition: a test of the ego-strength model of self-regulation. *International Journal of Eating Disorders*, **33**, 165–71.

KAPLAN, H. I. and KAPLAN, H. S. (1957), The psychosomatic concept of obesity. *Journal of Nervous and Mental Diseases*, **125**, 181–201.

KLESGES, R. C., BARTSCH, D., NORWOOD, J. D., KAUTZMAN, D. and HAUGRUD, S. (1984), The effects of selected social and environmental variables on the eating behavior of adults in the natural environment. *International Journal of Eating Disorders*, **3**, 35–41.

KNIGHT, L. J. and BOLAND, F. J. (1989), Restrained eating: an experimental disentanglement of the disinhibiting variables of perceived calories and food type. *Journal of Abnormal Psychology*, **98**, 499–503.

LEMAGNEN, J. (1985), *Hunger*. Cambridge, UK: Cambridge University Press.

LINDNER, R. M. (1962), *The Fifty-Minute Hour*. New York: Transworld Publishers.

MITCHELL, J. E., HATSUKAMI, D., ECKERT, E. D. and PYLE, R. L. (1985), Characteristics of 275 patients with bulimia. *American Journal of Psychiatry*, **142**, 482–5.

MORI, D., CHAIKEN, S. and PLINER, P. (1987), 'Eating lightly' and the self-presentation of femininity. *Journal of Personality and Social Psychology*, **53**, 693–702.

NIELSEN, S. J. and POPKIN, B. M. (2003), Patterns and trends in food portion sizes, 1977–1998. *Journal of the American Medical Association*, **289**, 450–3.

NISBETT, R. E. (1968), Determinants of food intake in human obesity. *Science*, **159**, 1254–5.

NISBETT, R. E. (1972), Hunger, obesity, and the ventromedial hypothalamus. *Psychological Review*, **79**, 433–53.

NISBETT, R. E. and STORMS, M. D. (1974), Cognitive and social determinants of food intake. In H. London and R. E. Nisbett (Eds.), *Thought and Feeling: Cognitive Alteration of Feeling States*. Chicago: Aldine, pp. 190–208.

OAKES, M. E. (2005). Beauty or beast: does categorical thinking about foods contribute to overeating? *Food Quality and Preference.*

PATEL, K. A. and SCHLUNDT, D. G. (2001), Impact of moods and social context on eating behavior. *Appetite*, **36**, 111–18.

PELCHAT, M. L. (1997), Food cravings in young and elderly adults. *Appetite*, **28,** 103–13.

POLIVY, J. (1976), Perception of calories and regulation of intake in restrained and unrestrained subjects. *Addictive Behaviors*, **1**, 237–43.

POLIVY, J., COLEMAN, J. and HERMAN, C. P. (2004), The effect of deprivation on food craving and eating behavior in restrained and unrestrained eaters. *International Journal of Eating Disorder* in press.

POLIVY, J. and HERMAN, C. P. (1983), *Breaking the Diet Habit: The Natural Weight Alternative*. New York: Basic Books.

POLIVY, J. and HERMAN, C. P. (1993), Etiology of binge eating: psychological mechanisms. In C. G. Fairburn and G. T. Wilson (Eds.) *Binge Eating: Nature, Assessment and Treatment*. New York: Guilford, 173–205.

POLIVY, J. and HERMAN, C. P. (2002), If at first you don't succeed: false hopes of self-change. *American Psychologist*, **57**, 677–89.

POLIVY, J., HERMAN, C. P., YOUNGER, J. C. and ERSKINE, B. (1979), Effects of a model on eating behavior: Induction of a restrained eating style. *Journal of Personality*, **47**, 100–17.

RODIN, J. (1981), Current status of the internal–external hypothesis for obesity. *American Psychologist*, **36**, 361–72.

ROLLS, B. J., MORRIS, E. L. and ROE, L. S. (2002), Portion size of food affects energy intake in normal weight and overweight men and women. *American Journal of Clinical Nutrition*, **76**, 1207–13.

ROTH, D. A., HERMAN, C. P., POLIVY, J. and PLINER, P. (2001), Self-presentational conflict in social eating situations: a normative perspective. *Appetite*, **36**, 165–71.

RUDERMAN, A. J. (1985), Dysphoric mood and overeating. *Journal of Abnormal Psychology*, **94**, 78–85.

RUDERMAN, A. J., BELZER, L. J. and HALPERIN, A. (1985), Restraint, anticipated consumption, and overeating. *Journal of Abnormal Psychology*, **94**, 547–55.

SCHACHTER, S. (1968), Obesity and eating. *Science*, **161**, 751–6.

SCHACHTER, S. (1971), Some extraordinary facts about obese humans and rats. *American Psychologist*, **26**, 129–44.

SCHACHTER, S., GOLDMAN, R. and GORDON, A. (1968), The effects of fear, food deprivation, and obesity on eating. *Journal of Personality and Social Psychology*, **10**, 91–7.

SCHACHTER, S. and RODIN, J. (1974), *Obese Humans and Rats*. Potomac, MD: Lawrence Erlbaum Associates.

SHIDE, D. J. and ROLLS, B. J. (1991), Social facilitation of caloric intake in humans by friends but not by strangers. *International Journal of Obesity*, **15** (Suppl.3), 8 (Abstract).

TICE, D. M., BUTLER, J. L., MURAVEN, M. B. and STILLWELL, A. M. (1995), When modesty prevails: Differential favorability of self-presentation to friends and strangers. *Journal of Personality and Social Psychology*, **69**, 1120–38.

TOMARKEN, A. J. and KIRSCHENBAUM, D. S. (1984), Effects of plans for future meals on counterregulatory eating by restraiend eaters. *Journal of Abnormal Psychology*, **93**, 458–72.

URBSZAT, D., HERMAN, C. P. and POLIVY, J. (2003), Eat, drink, and be merry, for tomorrow we diet: Effects of anticipated deprivation on food intake in restrained and unrestrained eaters. *Journal of Abnormal Psychology*, **111**, 396–401.

VARTANIAN, L., HERMAN, C. P. and POLIVY, J. Consumption stereotypes and impression management: how you are what you eat. Unpublished manuscript, University of Toronto.

VOHS, K. D. and HEATHERTON, T. F. (2000), Self-regulatory failure: a resource-depletion approach. *Psychological Science*, **11**, 249–54.

WANSINK, B. (2004), Environmental factors that unknowingly increase food consumption by consumers. *Annual Review of Nutrition*, **24**, 455–79.

WANSINK, B. and PARK, S. B. (2001), At the movies: How external cues and perceived taste impact consumption volume. *Food Quality and Preference*, **12**, 69–74.

WOODS, S. C. (1991), The eating paradox: How we tolerate food. *Psychological Review*, **98**, 488–505.

7

Sensory responses, food intake and obesity

C. de Graaf, Wageningen University, The Netherlands

7.1 Introduction

The relevance for studying and understanding sensory responses and food acceptance in relation to obesity is that sensory preferences have a major impact on food choice and food intake. Our senses tell us which foods are good (like) and which are bad to ingest (dislike). They also guide us with respect to the amount of food to eat. The availability of a large variety of good-tasting foods with a high energy density tempt many of us to ingest more energy than we expend.

One basic human trait is that, in the first years of life, we very quickly learn to like those flavours/tastes that are associated with energy (fat and carbohydrates), and presumably with the relief from hunger (e.g. Birch *et al.*, 1990; Kern *et al.*, 1993). This notion is clear from the transformation of a crying baby miserable with hunger to a happy satiated baby after the ingestion of some milk. It seems much more difficult to learn to like flavours/tastes that are associated with a low energy content (e.g. Lowe *et al.*, 1998; Wardle *et al.*, 2003). It is difficult for children to learn to like the taste of vegetables. Our senses drive us to like and ingest foods with a high energy content (Drewnowski, 1998). The abundant food environment in growing parts of world facilitates these basic drives.

This chapter starts with a short overview about the sensory perception of foods and on the impact of liking/preferences on food intake and choice. Preferences are not stable over time and can decrease or increase with repeated exposure. The decline of preference while eating a food is called sensory-specific satiety. Sensory-specific satiety contributes to the drive for variety in the diet, and the absence of variety may be one of the important working mechanisms of some popular weight loss diets, such as the Atkins diet.

In the 1970s and 1980s, researchers started to investigate whether or not obese subjects differed in their sensory responses to food to normal weight subjects. Although in general there are no big differences between obese and normal weight subjects in sensory preferences, we do see that obese people show a higher preference for high fat/high energy dense foods. Another important issue is that obese subjects tend to be more responsive to the hedonic value of foods (externality) than normal weight subjects. The heightened responsiveness to the hedonic value may relate to differences in sensitivity with respect to sensory-specific satiety. Another related issue concerns the taste responsiveness after weight loss, where after weight loss our senses make food even more attractive. The chapter ends with a discussion on how we can make weight control foods more attractive to consumers.

7.2 Sensory perception, preference and food intake

7.2.1 Sensory perception

The sensory systems guide us through the outside world. In the framework of nutrition, they constitute the connecting principle between the food that we eat and the physiological processes of digestion and substrate utilisation. The sensory perception of food involves vision, smell, taste, touch, audition, the trigeminal system for sensing irritation (CO_2/bubbles in drinks, pepper) and temperature (Lawless and Heyman, 1999).

With our eyes we see the appearance, the colour, size and shape of foods, and we recognise its identity. With our sense of smell we can 'smell' the volatile compounds of foods 'orthonasally' by sniffing with our nose just above the foods. When we move/break down the foods within our mouth, we also perceive the volatile compounds within foods. These compounds are transported retronasally to the olfactory epithelium after swallowing parts of the food. The sense of taste mainly located at the tongue is responsible for the sensations sweet, salt, bitter, sour and umami (the taste of glutamate, Ve-Tsin). The texture of foods is perceived by a variety of senses, we perceive the hardness, the viscosity, the roughness and many other texture attributes. With some crispy foods, auditory senses play a role in sensory perception. Another important attribute is the temperature.

7.2.2 Sensory preference, liking in relation to arousal

The sensory perception of foods is not the primary point of interest of most consumers. The most important characteristic of a food is whether we like it or not. The initial response to a food is whether we like or not. Do we eat/drink more of it or not? The liking of a food can be considered as the positive and/or negative evaluation of the sensory attributes of a particular

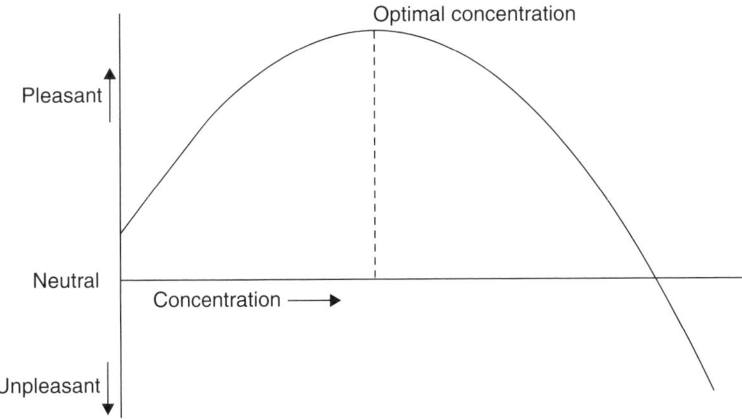

Fig. 7.1 Example of a Wundt curve, or single peaked preference curve, relating concentration to pleasantness. The concentration that concurs with the highest pleasantness is the optimal concentration.

food. With most sensory attributes, there is an optimal level of arousal (concentration, intensity), which is most liked. An arousal level high above the optimal levels may cause aversion. This optimal level of arousal is nicely reflected in the Wundt curve (Fig. 7.1), through the nineteenth century psychologist who discovered this principle. Wundt curves are interesting, because they may differ from person to person, and within subject from moment to moment. Differences in sensory preferences between groups (e.g. between men and women, young and old; normal weight and obese) can be investigated through the comparison (concentration/arousal-preference) of Wundt curves for different groups (e.g. de Graaf *et al.*, 1996).

7.2.3 Sensory preference, liking and intake

Liking generally refers to the degree/amount of sensory pleasure that is derived from tasting or eating a particular product. Preference refers to a choice between two or more foods, where liking generally plays an important role. However, there are also many situations where people prefer a less liked food over a more liked food because of various other motives that are involved, e.g. health, convenience, price, etc.

Liking has a positive effect on food intake; the more a food is liked, the more will be eaten from it. In many strictly controlled experimental studies, it has been shown that ratings about the liking of a food are strongly correlated with the *ad libitum* intake of a food (e.g. Bellisle *et al.*, 1984; Bobroff and Kissileff, 1986; Guy-Grand *et al.*, 1994; Helleman and Tuorila, 1991; Zandstra *et al.*, 1999). For example, Zandstra *et al.* (1999) showed that the liking ratings during consumption of yoghurt with various sugar concentrations had an average within-subject correlation of 0.8 with actual *ad*

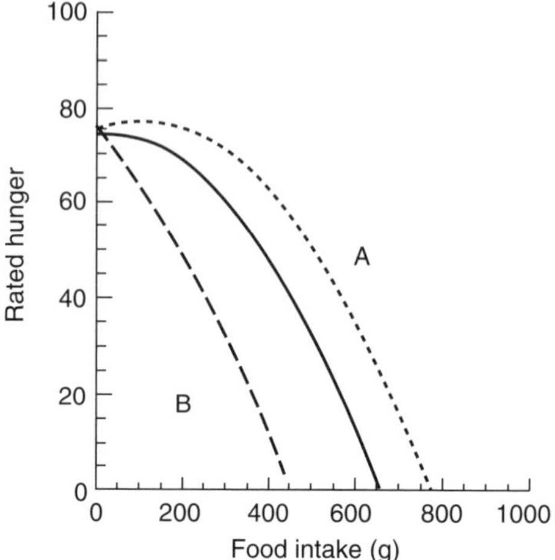

Fig. 7.2 Changes in rated hunger for normal weight men eating a 'palatable' (A, - - - - - -), bland (——), or overly strong flavoured (B, – – – –) test meal (*Source*: Yeomans, 1996).

libitum intake. A large number of other studies have found similar relationships between liking rating and intakes in laboratory conditions. According to Yeomans, liking affects intake through the enhancement of the desire to eat a food, particularly at the start of the meal. He called this the appetiser effect (Yeomans, 1996; Yeomans *et al.*, 2004; see Fig. 7.2).

The relationship between liking and intake also holds outside the laboratory. In a recent paper on a series of four field studies with US Army men and women (de Graaf *et al.*, 2005a), it was shown that the correlation between ratings on a nine-point hedonic scale and intake ranged between 0.22 and 0.62 for main dishes and between 0.13 and 0.56 for snacks. When the rating of a particular food was lower than 5 (the neutral point; neither like, nor dislike) on the nine-point scale, subjects consumed on average less than 87% of the meal, and with ratings above 7 on this scale subjects consumed on average 100% of the provided main dishes.

Although liking has a strong positive effect on intake, the sensory hedonic dimension is not the only driver for intake. Mattes *et al.* (1990) showed that people with taste and smell disturbances still have a drive to eat, and do not necessarily eat less than people with a normal sense of smell and taste. Without sensory stimulation, people still have a strong appetite, i.e. the internal drive to search, choose and ingest foods.

7.2.4 Sensory preference and choice

If presented with two foods, people will generally choose the most liked food. This point also holds across foods and across people. In a canteen, the average market share of different products will tend to co-vary with the average liking scores of different products (Pilgrim and Kamen, 1963). In a recent paper with US Army men and women it was shown that the chance of selecting a meal a second time was positively related to the hedonic rating on the first time that a product was tasted (de Graaf *et al.*, 2005b).

7.2.5 The role of appropriateness (eating context)

Although it is clear that liking has a strong effect on intake and choice, we do not always eat the most liked food on each occasion. If someone's favourite food is beefsteak, he will not eat beefsteak every day. It is also improbable that he will eat beefsteak at breakfast or during a coffee break. This issue is related to the notion of 'appropriateness' (Schutz, 1988; Cardello and Schutz, 1996). We develop eating patterns, where many foods get a particular fitness for use for particular eating occasions. In the USA many people eat turkey for Thanksgiving, and in the Netherlands, people consume 'oliebollen' at New Year's Eve. Appropriateness is linked to the various religious, symbolic and emotional roles that foods can play.

Appropriateness interferes in the relationship between preference/liking and intake and choice. Some foods that are very special need special occasions on which they can be eaten; very common foods need common eating occasions.

7.3 Changing sensory responses to food intake

7.3.1 Sensory-specific satiety

The pleasantness of foods varies over time. For many people, the first cup of coffee in the morning tastes very good, but a second of coffee immediately after the first one tastes less good. The pleasantness of the 'taste' decreases as a function of exposure to that 'taste'. This phenomenon is called sensory-specific satiety (Rolls *et al.*, 1981a). Sensory-specific satiety is often defined as the decline of the pleasantness/desire to eat a particular food after eating that food compared to the decline in pleasantness of uneaten foods (Rolls *et al.*, 1981a). Sensory-specific satiety occurs within 2 minutes after eating a particular food, and can last up until at least 90–120 min after consumption (Rolls *et al.*, 1981a,b; Rolls *et al.*, 1982; de Graaf *et al.*, 1993).

Sensory-specific satiety can be conceived as a major driving force for the appreciation and search for variety within the diet. This drive makes sense from a Darwinistic/evolutionary point of view, as it promotes the intake from a variety of foods, and limits the intake of one food. Taking a variety of foods increases the chance of having an adequate intake of the various micronutrients, and reduces the risk of a toxic overload of one substance in one food.

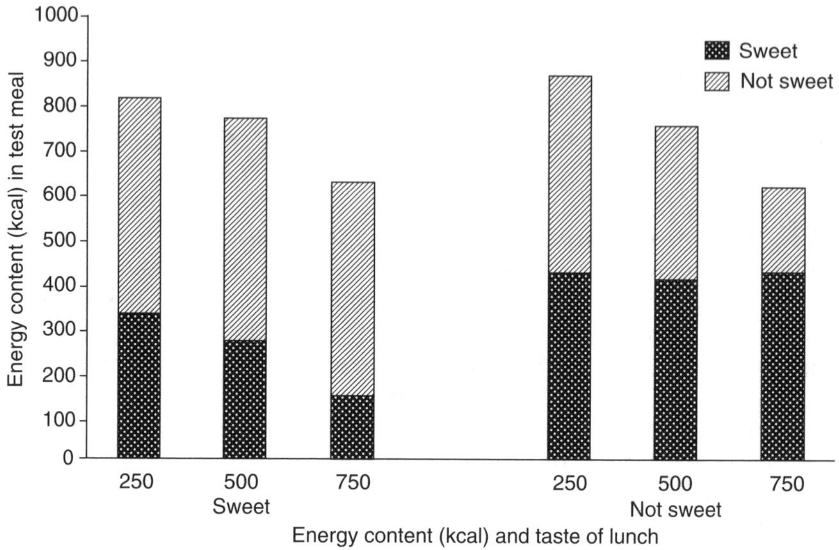

Fig. 7.3 Illustration of the effect of sensory-specific satiety: energy intake at a test meal 2h after consumption of a lunch (preload) that varied in energy content and taste (sweet and non-sweet). The preloads with equal energy content were matched with respect to weight, fat, protein, fibre and carbohydrate content. The energy intake in the test meal is divided into energy intake from sweet foods and the energy intake from non-sweet foods (*Source*: de Graaf *et al.*, 1993)

Sensory-specific satiety has been shown to occur for various foods in relation to the taste, odour and texture of foods. In the original studies in the beginning of the 1980s, sensory-specific satiety was shown for sausages vs. cheese on crackers, various types of pasta shapes (Rolls *et al.*, 1982), different sandwich fillings (Rolls *et al.*, 1981a), and fruit-flavoured yoghurts (Rolls *et al.*, 1981a). This effect was apparent both in terms of ratings as well as in food consumption data. Figure 7.3 shows the *ad libitum* intake in test meal with sweet and savoury foods after the consumption of preloads with sweet foods, and after preloads with savoury foods. After eating sweet foods, the intake of sweet foods declines, and the intake of savoury foods remains stable, and vice versa (de Graaf *et al.*, 1993). Guinard showed a similar effect for hard and soft textures. After subjects ate bread with a hard crust, the pleasantness of hard crusted bread did not decrease, while the pleasantness of soft crusted bread remained intact (Guinard and Brun, 1998).

Olfactory stimulation is sufficient to produce sensory-specific satiety. When subjects had olfactory stimulation by either vanilla or banana, this decreased the pleasantness rating of the exposed odour (Rolls and Rolls, 1997). The decrease also led to a lower intake. The time frame of occurrence and the notion that olfactory stimulation are sufficient to produce sensory-specific satiety suggest that the nutritional composition has little effect on sensory-specific satiety. This idea is confirmed in a number of studies, where it was shown that macronutrient content has no effect on sensory-specific satiety (e.g. Rolls, 1986).

7.3.2 Variety, monotony and boredom

Sensory-specific satiety operates on a short time frame; its effect is already apparent 2 minutes after consumption. It has mainly been studied within meals, where it contributes to within meal variety. However, a decline in acceptance after repeated exposure can also occur across meals over days. In the tradition of the literature on this issue, this phenomenon has been called 'monotony'. Monotony is the decrease in pleasantness of foods after repeated exposure. In a number of more recent studies monotony has also been related to boredom and to a sense of 'craving' for other foods than the exposed food (Pelchat and Schaefer, 2000).

The study on monotony started in the 1950s with soldiers in the US Army (Schutz and Pilgrim, 1958; Siegel and Pilgrim, 1958). It was observed that a monotonous diet of a few available foods/day across a time period of more than 3 weeks resulted in a declined acceptance. Increasing the number of available foods to a number of four different menus/day was enough to counteract monotony (Siegel and Pilgrim, 1958).

Another interesting observation in the early US Army studies was that some foods were more resistant to boredom than others. Staple foods with more neutral tastes appeared to be resistant to boredom, whereas other foods like vegetables, fruits and canned meats produced boredom/monotony more easily. In a recent study of Meiselman *et al.* (2000) in which subjects were served the same lunch across 5 days, it was shown that the vegetable part of the meal (green beans in this case) was the most boring, whereas the staple part (mashed potatoes) was not boring at all (Meiselman *et al.*, 2000). The meat part in this study took an intermediary positition with respect to its boredom-generating potential. Hetherington *et al.* (2000) showed that repeated exposure to chocolate led to a decline in pleasantness ratings, whereas repeated exposure to bread and butter did not. In a recent study of Zandstra *et al.* (2000), it was shown that even a consumption frequency of once/week can lead to a considerable decline in acceptance. Repeated consumption of the same flavour of a particular meat sauce across a period of 10 weeks led to a decline in acceptance and *ad libitum* intake of that sauce (Zandstra *et al.*, 2000).

The notion that different foods have different boredom potential led to investigations about the sensory properties of foods that are related to boredom. Based on the work of Berlyne (1970), it was argued that the attributes 'intensity' and 'complexity' may play a role in this. Intuitively, this makes sense. Staple foods which are characterised by a low taste intensity are resistant to boredom. Many vegetables that have a very distinct taste are very sensitive to boredom. More complex foods (such as wine and cheese) may allow the consumer to focus on different sensations during tasting. This may prevent boredom.

Several studies have been done on the effects of complexity and intensity on product boredom; however, in most studies with little success yet. In one study of Vickers and Holton (1998) it was shown that tea with a high intensity leads to boredom faster than tea with a lower taste intensity. Studies of Porcherot and Issanchou (1998) and Zandstra *et al.* (2004) did not show an effect of complexity on boredom after repeated exposure.

7.3.3 Variety and food intake

The effect of sensory-specific satiety on actual food intake is clear in laboratory studies. In many studies it has been shown, that giving a variety of foods within a (test-)meal leads to higher intakes than when giving a single food (e.g. Raynor and Epstein, 2001; Rolls, 1986). One could argue that sensory-specific satiety is a laboratory phenomenon, and that it does not play a major role in food intake in real-life situations. As soon as one gets bored with the taste of one particular item, subjects will shift to another food, which still has a reward value. Generally, in real life, subjects will try to avoid sensory-specific satiety. In present day society most subjects have ample opportunity to shift from one food to many other foods, and therefore have ample opportunity to avoid sensory-specific satiety. This may contribute to overeating.

The effect of variety across meals on actual food and energy intake is clear from many animal studies (for an overview see Raynor and Epstein, 2001), and from some experimental studies in humans. Stubbs *et al.* (2001) showed across a period of 7 days that increasing the variety of sensorially distinct foods that are virtually identical in composition can increase food and energy intake. When subjects had continuous *ad libitum* access to 15 different foods, they consumed, on average, 2 MJ (= 12 MJ) more than when they access to five different foods. The results of a cross-sectional study of McCrory *et al.* (1999) suggested that a high variety of sweets, snacks, condiment main dishes and carbohydrates promotes long-term increases in energy intake and body fatness. In an 18 month, longitudinal study, Raynor *et al.* (2004) concluded that 'changing variety in specific food groups may help in adopting and sustaining a diet low in energy and fat, producing better weight loss and weight loss maintenance'.

The effects of monotony on food intake and energy balance is also clear from the early US-Army studies, where soldiers did not eat enough to maintain their energy balance and lost weight on a monotonous diet (Schutz and Pilgrim, 1958; Siegel and Pilgrim, 1958). Considerable body weight loss (3 kg) on a monotonous diet was later confirmed by Cabanac and Rabe (1976), who fed subjects vanilla-flavoured beverages only, for a time period of 3 weeks.

The issue of monotony may also play a role in current popular diet regimens such as the Atkins diet (Atkins, 2002) or the Montignac diet (Montignac, 1997), whose books appeared on US and European bestseller lists for some years. In the Atkins diet, major sources of carbohydrates are removed from the meal/diet. A major source of carbohydrates are the staple foods like bread, potatoes, rice or pasta which, in general, have a neutral taste. In the Montignac diet, one is allowed to consume both fat and carbohydrates, but not within the same meal. In effect, this has the same consequences as the Atkins diet; one removes many neutral tasting foods from the meal. The result is that the meal only contains the more flavoured items, such as the meat part and vegetable part. These products cause earlier sensory-specific satiety and/or monotony, probably because of their more intense taste. This early sensory satiety/monotony results in a lower *ad libitum* food intake.

In line with this reasoning, one could argue that any monotonous diet, a fruit diet, a bread diet, a chocolate diet, or a whipped cream diet, would lead to a low food and energy intake. It is a challenge to find out whether or not monotony is one of the working mechanisms of the current popular diets.

7.4 Sensory responses, intake and obesity

7.4.1 Sensory (intensity) perception and obesity

There are no indications that obese subjects have a different sensory perception of foods than normal weight subjects. Their threshold and suprathreshold sensitivity to various tastes (sweet, salt, bitter, sour) is not different from normal weight individuals. There have been some studies that have tried to link obesity with PROP sensitivity, but these attempts have led to mixed results, with the far majority of the studies showing no relationship between PROP status and BMI (Mattes, 2004). There is little information available with respect to odour sensitivity and obesity, but *a priori* there does not seem a compelling reason why odour perception should be different in obese and normal weight individuals.

One area regarding sensory perception, which might be of interest to study in relation to obesity, is fat perception. Fat is a texture attribute, and humans are not very well able to discriminate between small changes in fat concentrations in foods. People are much more sensitive to relative changes in sugar/salt concentrations than to fat. Mattes (2001, 2002) showed that oral exposure to free fatty acids in foods leads to elevated post-prandial triacylglycerol blood levels. These findings indicate that free fatty acids are 'sensed' on the tongue, and that they have metabolic consequences in terms of the postprandial lipid profile.

In relation to this observation form, there are studies with rats from Gilbertson *et al.*, 1998, who showed that specific strains of rats are more or less sensitive to the taste of linoleic acid. The insensitivity to taste of linoleic acid was inversely related to dietary preferences for fat. Kamphuis recently tried to distinguish between linoleic acid tasters and non-tasters in humans. They also tried to relate this sensitivity to food intake and fat preferences in humans. Its relevance of this phenomenon for human taste perception remains to be elucidated (Kamphuis, 2003).

7.4.2 Sensory preferences and obesity

In the 1970s it was thought that obese individuals were characterised by a sweet tooth, i.e. a liking for high sweetness levels in foods. The rationale behind this idea is simple and attractive. Obese subjects ingest more energy than lean subjects; sweetness is the outspoken biological signal for the energy content of foods; a higher liking for higher sugar levels in obese individuals would then be a driver for a higher energy intake. Empirical studies on this hypothesis did not confirm this idea. This failure to find any effect of weight status on sweetness preferences is very consistent across a large number of studies Drewnowski (1987), Frijters (1984), Esses and Herman (1984), Thompson *et al.* (1977), Rodin *et al.* (1977), and Rissanen *et al.* (2002).

Although it is clear that, on average, obese and normal weight subjects do not differ in preferences for sugar, there are several studies that suggest that there is a difference in the preference for fat. Studies from Drewnowski (1987) on optimal sugar and fat levels in fat–sugar mixtures showed that obese subjects preferred higher fat levels than normal weight subjects. A study of Mela and Sacchetti (1991) showed a positive association between body fat percentage and the average optimal preferred fat levels in ten different foods across a group of 30 subjects. In a more recent study of Fisher and Birch (1995) with 18 3–5-year-old children it was shown that fat preferences as measured by a sensory test predicted fat intake from a standard menu. The fat preferences/intakes in the children were also positively associated with their parents' BMI. In a large survey study with 428 4–5-year-old children, Wardle *et al.* (2001) observed that the children from the obese/overweight families had a higher preference for fatty foods in a taste test and a lower liking for vegetables.

Data from Rissanen *et al.* (2002) provide an additional interesting perspective. In a survey study with 23 pairs of monozygotic twins with discordant BMIs, the obese twins expressed a much higher preference for high fat foods than their lean counterparts. The obese twins also reported that they had a higher tendency to overeat from sandwiches, pastries and ice-cream, but not from sweets and soft drinks. The authors concluded that the acquired preference for fatty foods is associated with obesity.

In line with the data on a higher fat preference, there are results of studies that suggest that obese subjects have a relatively higher intake of foods with a higher energy density than normal weight subjects. Using data from a British national food survey, MacDiarmid *et al.* (1996) showed that obese subjects had a higher consumption of high-fat/high sugar food than subjects with a lower BMI. In a study with 41 lean subjects and 35 obese subjects, Cox *et al.* (1999) found that the obese subjects appear to consume a diet higher in energy density, which was particularly associated with intakes of salty/savoury food items. In a study with 34 obese and 34 normal weight subjects, Westerterp-Plantenga (2004) showed that the obese subjects had a relatively higher intake from energy dense foods (15–22.5 kJ/g), and a relatively lower intake from low energy dense foods (<0–7.5 kJ/g). Le Noury *et al.* (2002) as cited by Yeomans *et al.* (2004) reported that obese subjects consumed greater amounts of high fat foods in a test-meal than their normal weight counterparts, and reported greater feelings of pleasantness and satisfaction with high-fat foods.

As far as the author is aware, there are not many other data concerning differences in sensory preferences of obese and normal weight subjects. There seems to be no obvious reason why the sensory preferences of obese are different from that of normal weight subjects. The issues around preferences for high fat/high energy dense foods in obese subjects warrant further study. One of the central questions in this respect is how these preferences develop, and how these preferences translate into actual eating behaviour.

7.4.3 Responsiveness to palatability with respect to intake in obese consumers

In a fascinating paper in the journal *Science* in 1968, Schachter presented a number of new ideas about obesity and eating behaviour (Schachter, 1968). He suggested that eating behaviour of obese and normal weight subjects was differentially affected by internal and external cues. Schachter argued that obese individuals were more responsive to external cues not directly related to hunger, whereas normal weight subjects were more responsive to internal cues. External cues are signal related to emotional state (fear, stress, arousal), external environmental circumstances (e.g. easy–difficult access, time of day), and the palatability (unpleasant vs. pleasant) of food. In this paper, Schachter reported a series of experiments, of which the results supported the idea that obese subjects were more responsive to external signals whereas lean subjects 'listened' better to hunger signals. This theory was called the 'externality hypothesis'.

After the presentation of the externality hypothesis, a large number of studies were done to test this idea. Then, it appeared that there was not such a clear distinction between obese and normal weight subjects with respect to internal–external sensitivity. Obese subjects also responded to internal cues (such as hunger/deprivation time) and normal weight subjects also responded to external cues such as the palatability of foods. Also, the definition of an 'external signal' was not clear. Is arousal or anxiety an external signal? In addition, a large number of studies failed to replicate the internal–external difference between overweight and normal weight subjects. This was particularly the case for issues such as deprivation time, the effects of arousal, and cognitive and social cues (Spitzer and Rodin, 1981). These 'failures' to confirm the original ideas led in 1981 to a paper by Rodin (1981), with the title 'Current status of the internal–external hypothesis for obesity – what went wrong?'. After this paper, it became silent with respect to this idea for some time. However, the basic idea behind the externality hypothesis, i.e. that people are responsive to external cues, such as environmental circumstances/cues (social facilitation, portion sizes) and sensory stimulation is now at the centre of many theories about overeating and the high prevalence of obesity (see also the chapter by Herman in this volume). Ideas with respect to the 'obesogenic environment' are a reflection of this concept (Finkelstein *et al.*, 2005).

In his paper Schachter also reported the results of two experiments (Hashim and van Itallie, 1965; Nisbett, 1968) which were related to taste. In the study of Hashim and van Itallie (1965) it was shown that obese subjects showed a dramatic decrease in food intake when put on an unpalatable bland liquid diet regime, whereas normal weight subjects maintained their intakes at levels sufficient for energy balance. In the study of Nisbett (1968) two types of ice cream were used, one 'delicious' ice cream, and one ice cream with added quinine (called vanilla bitter). The results showed that the overweight subjects consumed more of the palatable ice cream, but not of the unpalatable ice cream. The results of these two experiments suggested that obese subjects eat less of unpalatable food than normal weight subjects, but eat more of palatable food, i.e. the hedonic value of a food had a stronger effect on food intake of obese individuals than of normal weight subjects.

Unlike with the other 'external' factors, this finding was later consistently replicated in a number of other studies (Hill, 1974; Hill and McCutcheon, 1975 (see Fig. 7.4); Rodin, 1975; Rodin *et al.*, 1977; Spiegel *et al.*, 1989). This finding was also replicated with normal weight and obese children (Ballard *et al.*, 1980).

In conclusion, the general hypothesis of a higher external responsiveness of obese subjects to external cues cannot be maintained in all its dimensions. However, there are quite a number of studies that have confirmed the stronger effect of palatability on intake in obese subjects compared to normal weight subjects. This is one of the most consistently observed differences in eating behaviour between normal weight and obese subjects. The higher sensitivity to palatability could be related to the idea that eating palatable foods is more rewarding (reinforcing) for obese subjects than for normal weight subjects.

7.4.4 Food reward and weight status

Ice-cream sales are higher in the summer than they are in the winter. In the ski-season in the Alps, many consumers show a high desire for a product

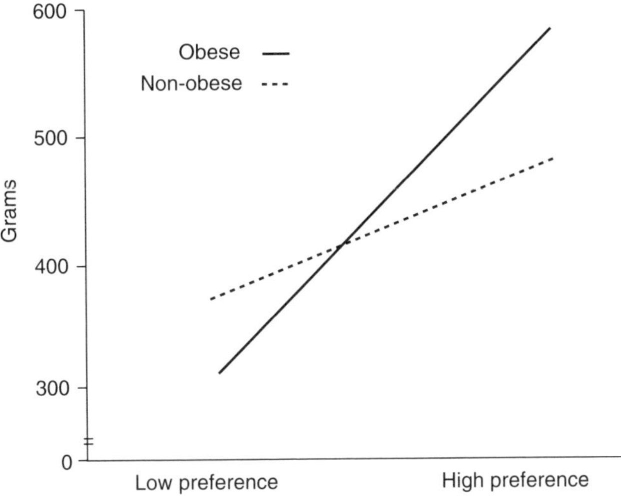

Fig. 7.4 Illustration of the externality effect. Mean grams of food eaten by seven obese and seven normal weight subjects during two low preference and two high preference dinner meals. Mean preference scores on an 11-point scale were 3.9 for the low preference meals and 8.6 for the high preference meals (*Source*: Hill and McCutcheon, 1975).

called *Glüh-wein*, a product that makes you feel warm. The pleasantness of these sensations relates to the 'physiological usefulness' in relation to the setpoint for body temperature (Cabanac, 1975).

Cabanac (1971) argued that body weight also has its setpoint, and that the body defends this setpoint by changing the hedonics of foods, i.e. liking is modulated by the 'need-state' of the individual. The setpoint does not need to be on a body weight which is optimal from an aesthetic or health point of view. The idea of a setpoint is widely supported by many animal studies (Woods and Seeley, 2002), showing that animals depending on genetic make-up and environmental circumstances defend a particular body weight. This idea also explains the observations in many human studies where, after weight loss/starvation and/or short-term food deprivations, most people return to their original body weight through increased energy consumption (Jeffery *et al.*, 2004). The question within the framework of this chapter is whether or not the return to setpoint-weight is guided by changes in the hedonic responses to food.

In one of Cabanac's original papers he showed that 'hungry' people before a preload of 50 g glucose showed an increased liking response to increasing sugar concentrations (Cabanac *et al.*, 1973; Duclaux *et al.*, 1973). After the preload there was an optimal preferred sugar concentration, above which the pleasantness of the sugar concentration decreased. This latter observation is in line with the idea of the normal Wundt curve for sensory stimulation (see paragraph 7.2.2 on liking in relation to arousal). In the *Science* paper in 1971, Cabanac (1971) showed that people (three subjects) below their setpoint weight continued to like strong tasting/smelling solutions, even after a preload of 50 g glucose. The implication was that, when people are below their setpoint weight, food intake during a meal will not satiate as quickly as when people are at, or above, their setpoint, i.e. food maintains its rewarding properties. This observation is in line with the idea that compensatory behaviour after weight loss works through increases in meal size (Woods and Seeley, 2002).

Although Cabanac's idea is attractive and appealing, there have been only a very few studies that actually produced data from humans in line with this idea. Fantino *et al.* (1983) showed that overfed people (three North African women who were overfed before their marriage) expressed a lower liking for sweetness. A study from Raynor and Epstein (2003) found that the relative-reinforcing value of food increases after short-term (13 h) food deprivation. However, it is not clear whether or not the reinforcing value of food is directly/linearly related to the hedonic value of the food. Kleifeld and Lowe (1991) found no increase in sweetness liking after weight loss. Another study of Kaufman *et al.* (1995) showed that 20 h deprived subjects ate more of good-tasting foods, but less of bad-tasting foods, i.e. 'mild' food deprivation made subjects more finicky about the food they ate. This latter observation is not in line with the concept of liking as a straightforward function of physiological usefulness.

The reinforcing/rewarding value of foods has two components, which are sometimes difficult to distinguish in humans, i.e. 'liking', and 'wanting' (Berridge, 2004). Liking refers to the sensory-hedonic dimension, whereas wanting reflects the drive to ingest a particular food. A high wanting level does not necessarily coincide with a high liking level and vice versa. Pizza may be one's favourite food, most people do not want it for breakfast. Similarly, water is probably not the 'drink' with the highest hedonic value, but it is drunk in large quantities. To summarise, it seems clear that liking in humans is not always dependent on need state (Yeomans *et al.*, 2004). It is also not clear that the hedonic value of a food increases when subjects are in a negative energy balance. More data and better theories are necessary to understand the effects of palatability on intake, and also to understand the effects of weight status on palatability and intake.

7.4.5 Sensory-specific satiety, sensory cues and obesity

As discussed above, there are quite a number of studies that suggest that obese subjects are more responsive to the hedonic value of foods than normal weight subjects. One of the potential mechanisms that could explain this observation is the hypothesis that obese subjects are less sensitive to sensory-specific satiety than normal weight subjects. This would manifest itself in a lower decline in the reward value of foods during consumption, i.e. obese subjects would continue to get reward from tasting a food compared to normal weight subjects. This leads to the postponement of meal termination, i.e. larger meals and higher energy intake. On the other hand, one could also make a case for the hypothesis that obese subjects are more sensitive to sensory-specific satiety (Raynor and Epstein, 2001). A higher sensitivity may lead to earlier switching between foods/flavours during and/or across meals. The resulting high variety of foods may lead to a higher energy intake.

There are some experimental data that support the hypothesis of a lower sensitivity to sensory-specific satiety in obese subjects compared to normal weight subjects. In a study of Epstein *et al.* (1996) both 10 obese and 10 normal weight subjects were repeatedly (10×) stimulated to palatable food cues (lemon yoghurt). The dependent variable in this study was the salivary response which can be considered as a measure for the desire to eat. The obese women showed a significantly slower decline in salivation than non-obese subjects. More recent data from Jansen *et al.* (2003), with obese and normal weight children, showed that, after intense olfactory exposure, normal weight children decreased their intake during a test-meal, whereas obese children over-ate. So, in both studies, the sensory exposure reduced the desire to eat in normal weight subjects but failed to do so in obese subjects.

The idea that obese subjects are less sensitive to sensory-specific satiety was recently tested in a study with 21 obese and 23 normal weight women, matched for age, and restrained eating behaviour (Snoek *et al.*, 2004). Food intake, appetite ratings and liking scores were measured before and after an *ad libitum* lunch. The experimental products differed in fat content (low, high) and taste (sweet, savoury). The study comprised two experiments, one with sandwiches, and one with snacks. The results showed that the obese and non-obese subjects did not differ with respect to sensory-specific satiety, i.e. the decline in liking ratings were about equal for obese and normal weight subjects. However, appetite ratings for something sweet and something savoury after lunch were consistently higher for the obese than for the normal weight subjects. This finding shows that, even after eating until satiation, obese subjects still expressed a higher wanting level to eat foods.

Apparently, obese subjects are not less sensitive to sensory-specific satiety, but they do have a higher tendency to continue to eat. One hypothesis could be that obese subjects are more responsive to sensory cues, even after they are 'physiologically satiated'. This hypothesis is partly reflected in the theory of cue-reactivity of Nederkoorn and Jansen (2002) with respect to eating binges. This theory states that 'when a person regularly has eating binges, and these binges are reliably preceded by certain cues (e.g. the sight, smell and taste of the food, environment, cognitions, emotions), these cues becomes predictors of a binge' (Nederkoorn and Jansen, 2002).

The continued interest in sensory reward during a meal might be an attractive hypothesis why obese people have bigger meals than normal weight subjects. Much more work seems needed in this area.

7.4.6 Food addiction and obesity

The cue-reactivity model for eating disorder and obesity bears various similarities with models of drug addiction. Drug addicts are often tempted to a relapse in response to environmental/sensory cues that were related to regular drug use (Woods, 1991). In this way, eating binges can be conceived as a conditioned response to certain food related cues. There is strong evidence that both drug addictions and food cravings are mediated by the dopimanergic neurotransmitter system. In this sense there are many similarities between food consumption and drug consumption (Pelchat, 2002).

The analogy between drug use and the excessive consumption of high energy density foods such as hamburgers or chocolate has brought some people to accuse the food industry of a conspiracy to produce addictive foods. However, not eating chocolate or not eating a hamburger does not lead to the specific physical and psychological withdrawal symptoms compared to not drinking alcohol for an alcoholic, or not smoking for a smoking addict.

As the hedonic value of a food is so important for its selection/choice, it seems only logical that food companies will launch the best-tasting products on the market. This is a simple Darwinistic process, where the best-tasting product on the market will survive. As discussed earlier in this chapter, after a first exposure people will generally choose the best-tasting item for a repeat choice (de Graaf *et al.*, 2005b). As also indicated earlier in this chapter, humans are born with the trait to learn to like those taste/flavours that are associated with a high energy density. This applies over a large range of foods (Drewnowksi, 1998), but also within the the group of fruit/vegetables for children (Gibson and Wardle, 2003). This is the reason why we like pizzas and hamburgers, and why we do not have a strong liking response for vegetables. From this perspective it can be predicted that food with a higher energy density will probably have a higher hedonic value than foods with a lower energy density. So, one does not need a conspiracy theory to explain why a hamburger/pizza chain of restaurants is more likely to be profitable than a chain of vegetable grocery stores.

7.5 Making weight control foods more attractive to consumers

Foods differ in their satiating capacity per kJ. There is substantial evidence for the hierarchy from high to low satiating capacity for the order: protein, carbohydrates, fat, alcohol. High energy dense foods have a lower satiating capacity than lower energy dense foods. Fibres contribute to the satiating efficiency of foods, and solid foods have been shown to have a higher satiating capacity than liquid foods. With respect to taste, one could also hypothesise that stronger tasting foods will lead to earlier sensory-specific satiety than weaker tasting foods. From this perspective, it is clear that solid foods with an outspoken taste and a low energy density have a high satiating capacity. Producing low energy, high satiating foods with pleasant tastes seems to be the best way to make weight control foods attractive for consumers.

Many studies have shown that covert manipulations of energy density are not easily sensed by consumers, even after continued exposure. In general, people do not compensate if high energy foods are replaced by low energy foods with similar sensory properties (de Graaf *et al.*, 2004). This is true for fat-replacers and for sugar-replacers. Considering the primary interest in taste, convenience and price, it is clear that convenient low energy foods with a reasonable price and a good taste will be attractive for consumers. The making of these products is an important responsibility of the food industry.

Within the framework of the study on the regulation of food intake, there is rapidly expanding knowledge with regard to the hormonal and neural signalling pathways with respect to hunger and satiety. It is also clear that the composition of foods (including taste/odour components) have an effect on these signalling pathways. For example, whey proteins have a stronger effect on satiety than casein proteins, and this effect is possibly mediated through the release of CCK and GLP-1 (Hall *et al.*, 2003). Fibres like guar gum have been shown to form a gel in the stomach, and increase satiety (Hoad *et al.*, 2004). Knowledge about these effects with regard to biomarkers of satiety may result in new products with higher satiating capacity (de Graaf *et al.*, 2004).

Some authors have argued on theoretical (and some empirical) grounds that low energy dense foods with similar tastes as high energy dense foods, e.g. diet/light cola vs. regular cola may undermine our 'natural' appetite system. One study from Davidson and Swithers (2004) with rat pups just after birth gives interesting data on this issue. In this study there were two groups, one control group got foods with sugar as sweetener, and the experimental group got foods with saccharin as sweetener. The sucrose sweetener group 'learned' that sweetness was associated with energy, whereas the saccharin group did not learn to associate sweetness with energy. Later on, both groups participated in a preload-testmeal study, in which they were served a sucrose containing preload after which they could eat *ad libitum*. The rats who were used to sucrose reduced their intake in the testmeal, whereas the rats with saccharin did not reduce their intake in the testmeal response to the sucrose in the preload. Their appetite system had been corrupted by saccharin. It could be argued that this would also happen in humans in response to light/diet products. One argument could be raised against this position. The study with Davidson was done with rat pups just after birth. The similar time frame in humans would be just after birth. Newborn humans are not fed with artificial sweeteners. All conditioning studies in humans that have been successful have been done with children (Birch *et al.*, 1990; Kern *et al.*, 1993). In well-fed adults in the present day industrialised society it is difficult to show caloric conditioning effects (Zandstra *et al.*, 2002). So, it is unlikely that a similar effect as in rat pups would occur in adult humans, who already have a long-standing experience with many foods and many flavours.

In a similar way, it could also be argued that, in the long run, low energy foods may lose their attractiveness because of the lack of reinforcement (Stubbs and Whybrow, 2004). However, there is little empirical evidence for this observation. In the studies of Mela *et al.* (1993), Stubenitsky *et al.* (1999), and Zandstra *et al.* (2002) longer-term exposure of low energy dense foods did not lead to a lower pleasantness of these foods.

7.6 Implications, recommendations and future trends

Consumers want a large variety of good-tasting products with a high convenience value and a reasonable price. From the point of view of the regulation of food intake, the large variety of convenient and good-tasting products will lead to a higher intake. As we are programmed to like energy dense foods, the high availability of cheap energy dense foods adds to the burden of our normal drive to consume more than we expend (Drewnowski and Specter, 2004). Obesity is a normal response in an abnormal environment.

The understanding of the regulation of food intake may yield new ways to limit our food intake, while maintaining the enjoyment we get from foods. New ingredients may come from our understanding of how molecules determine sensory and metabolic satiety. This is a vast and new exciting area of research, to establish how ingredients of food affect our short-term and long-term food intake and energy balance (see also de Graaf *et al.*, 2004).

The food industry is now producing a large array of food items with lower fat levels, lower sugar levels and higher fibre levels, than the original formulas of the food. This is a positive development, and it is recommended to proceed with these efforts. More specific knowledge on how specific proteins, carbohydrates, fat or new ingredients affect appetite may yield attractive food items with higher satiating efficiencies per unit of energy. These products could have a high added value. It is very attractive for many consumers to consume a breakfast food with a moderate energy content that leads to a sustaining comfortable satiety feeling until lunch.

7.7 References

ATKINS, R. C. (2002), *Dr. Atkins New Diet Revolution.* Avon Books, New York.

BALLARD, B. D., GIPSON, M. T., GUTTENBERG, W. and RAMSEY, K. (1980), Palatability of food as a factor influencing obese and normal-weight children's eating habits. *Behav. Res. Therapy.*, **18**, 598–600.

BELLISLE, F., LUCAS, F., AMRANI, R. and LEMAGNEN, J. (1984), Deprivation, palatability and the microstructure of meals in human subjects. *Appetite*, **5**, 85–94.

BERLYNE, D. E. (1970), Novelty, complexity and hedonic value. *Percept. Psychophys.*, **8**, 279–86.

BERRIDGE, K. C. (2004), Motivation concepts in behavioural neuroscience. *Physiol. Behav.*, **81**, 179–209.

BIRCH, L. L., MCPHEE, L., STEINBERG and SULLIVAN, S. (1990), Conditioned flavor preferences in young children. *Physiol. Behav.*, **47**, 501–5.

BOBROFF, E. M. and KISSILEFF, H. R. (1986), Effects of changes in palatability on food intake and the cumulative food intake curve in man. *Appetite.*, **7**, 85–96.

CABANAC, M. (1971), Physiological role of pleasure. *Science.*, **173**, 1103–7.

CABANAC, M. (1975), Temperature regulation. *Annu. Rev. Physiol.*, **37**, 415–39.

CABANAC, M. and RABE, F. (1976), Influence of a monotonous food on body weight regulation in humans. *Physiol. Behav.*, **17**, 675–8.

CABANAC, M., PRUVOST, M. and FANTINO, M. (1973), Negative alliesthesia for sweet stimuli after varying ingestions of glucose. *Physiol. Behav.*, **11**, 345–8.

CARDELLO, A. V. and SCHUTZ, H. G. (1996), Food appropriateness measures as an adjunct to consumer preference/acceptability evaluation. *Food. Qual. Prefer.*, **7**, 239–49.

COX, D. N., PERRY, L., MOORE, P. B., VALLUS, L. and MELA, D. J. (1999), Sensory and hedonics associations with macronutrient and energy intake of lean and obese consumers. *Int. J. Obes.*, **23**, 403–10.

DAVIDSON, T. L. and SWITHERS, S. E. (2004), A Pavlovian approaxh to the problem of obesity. *Int. J. Obes. Relat. Metab. Disord.*, **28**, 933–5.

DE GRAAF, C., SCHREURS, A. and BLAUW, Y. H. (1993), Short-term efects of different amounts of sweet and nonsweet carbohydrates on satiety and energy intake. *Physiol. Behav.*, **54**, 833–43.

DE GRAAF, C., VAN STAVEREN, W. A. and BUREMA, J. A. (1996), Psychophysical and psychohedonic functions of four common food flavours in elderly subjects. *Chem. Senses.*, **21**, 293–302.

DE GRAAF, C., BLOM, W. A. M., SMEETS, P., STAFLEU, A. and HENDRIKS, H. F. J. (2004), Biomarkers of satiation and satiety. *Am. J. Clin. Nutr.*, **79**, 946–61.

DE GRAAF, C., CARDELLO, A. V., KRAMER, F. M., LESHER, L. L., MEISELMAN, H. L. and SCHUTZ, H. G. (2005a), A comparison between liking ratings obtained under laboratory and field conditions: the role of choice. *Appetite.*, **44**, 15–22.

DE GRAAF, C., KRAMER, F. M. and MEISELMAN, H. L. *et al.* (2005b), Food acceptability in field studies with US Army men and women: relationship with food intake and food choice after repeated exposures. *Appetite.*, **44**, 23–31.

DEL PARIGI, A., CHEN, K., SALBE, A. D., REIMAN, E. M. and TATARANNI, P. A. (2003), Are we addicted to food? *Obes. Res.*, **11**, 493–5.

DREWNOWKSI, A. (1987), Body weight and sensory preferences for sugar and fat. *Can. Inst. Food. Sci. Technol. J.*, **20**, 327–30.

DREWNOWSKI, A. (1998), Energy density, palatability, and satiety: implications for weight control. *Nutr. Rev.*, **56**, 347–53.

DREWNOWSKI, A. and SPECTER, S. E. (2004), Poverty and obesity: the role of energy density and energy costs. *Am. J. Clin. Nutr.*, **79**, 6–16.

DUCLAUX, R., FEISTHAUER, J. and CABANAC, M. (1973), Effects of a meal on the pleasantness of food and non-food odors in man. *Physiol. Behav.*, **10**, 1029–33.

EPSTEIN, L. H., PALUCH, R. and COLEMAN, K. J. (1996), Differences in salivation to repeated food cues in obese and nonobese women. *Psychosom. Med.*, **58**, 160–4.

ESSES, V. M. and HERMAN, C. P. (1984), Palatability of sucrose before and after glucose ingestion in dieters and nondieters *Physiol. Behav.*, **32**, 711–15.

FANTINO, M., BAIGTS, F., CABANAC, M. and APFELBAUM, M. (1983), Effects of an overfeeding regimen-the affective component of a sweet sensation. *Appetite.*, **4**, 155–64.

FISHER, J. O. and BIRCH, L. L. (1995), Fat preferences and fat consumption of 3- to 5-year-old children are related to parental adiposity. *J. Am. Diet. Assoc.*, **95**, 759–64.

FINKELSTEIN, E. A., RUHM, C. J. and KOSA, K. M. (2005), Economic causes and consequences of obesity. *Ann. Rev. Public. Health.*, **26**, 239–57.

FRIJTERS, J. E. R. (1984), Sweetness intensity perception and pleasantness in women varying in reported restraint of eating. *Appetite.*, **5**, 102–8.

GIBSON, E. L. and WARDLE, J. (2003), Energy density predicts preferences for fruits and vegetables in 4-year old children. *Appetite.*, **41**, 97–8.

GILBERTSON, T. A., LIU, L., YORK, D. A. and BRAY, G. A. (1998), Dietary fat preferences are inversely correlated with peripheral fatty acid sensitivity. *Ann. NY Acad. Sci.*, **855**, 165–8.

GRINKER, J., HIRSCH, J. and SMITH, D. V. (1972), Taste sensitivity and suspectibility to external influence in obese and normal weight subjects. *J. Person. Soc. Psychol.*, **22**, 320–5.

GUINARD, J.-X. and BRUN, P. (1998), Sensory-specific satiety: comparison of taste and texture effects. *Appetite*, **31**, 141–57.

GUY-GRAND, B., LEHNERT, V., DOASSANS, M. and BELLISLE, F. (1994), Type of test-meal affects palatability and eating style in humans. *Appetite.*, **22**, 125–34.

HALL, W. L., MILLWARD, D. J., LONG, S. J. and MORGAN, L. M. (2003), Casein and whey exert different effects on plasma amino acid profiles, gastrointestinal hormone secretion and appetite. *Br. J. Nutr.*, **89**, 239–48.

HASHIM, S. A. and VAN ITALLIE, B. (1965), Studies in normal and obese subjects with a monitored food dispensing device. *Ann. NY Acad. Sci.*, **131**, 654–91.

HELLEMAN, U. and TUORILA, H. (1991), Pleasantness ratings and consumption of open sanfwiches with varying NaCl and acid contents. *Appetite.*, **17**, 229–38.

HETHERINGTON, M. M. (1995), Sensory-specific satiety and its importance in meal termination. *Neurosci. Biobehav. Rev.*, **20**, 113–17.

HETHERINGTON, M. M., PIRIE, L. M. and NABB, S. (2000), Stimulus satiation: effects of repeated exposure to foods on pleasantness and intake. *Appetite.*, **38**, 19–28.

HILL, S. W. (1974), Eating responses of humans during dinner meals. *J. Compar. Physiol. Psychol.*, **86**, 652–7.

HILL, S. W. and MCCUTCHEON, N. B. (1975), Eating responses of obse and nonobese humans during dinner meals. *Psychosom. Med.*, **37**, 395–401.

HOAD, C. L., RAYMENT, P., SPILLER, R. C. *et al.* (2004), In vivo imaging of intragastric gelation and its effect on satiety in humans. *J. Nutr.*, **134**, 2293–300.

JANSEN, A., THEUNISSEN, N., SLECHTEN, K. *et al.* (2003), Overweight children after exposure to food cues. *Eating. Behav.*, **4**, 197–209.

JEFFERY, R. W., KELLY, K. M., ROTHMAN, A. J., SHERWOOD, N. E. and BOUTELLE, K. N. (2004), The weight loss experience: a descriptive analysis. *Ann. Behav. Med.*, **27**, 100–6.

KAMPHUIS, M. (2003), The sense of dietary fat: food intake and body weight regulation. PhD thesis, University Maastricht, Datawyse, Universitaire Pers Maastricht, the Netherlands.

KAUFFMAN, N. A., HERMAN, C. P. and POLIVY, J. (1995), Hunger-induced finickiness in humans. *Appetite.*, **24**, 203–18.

KERN, D. L., MCPHEE, L., FISHER, J., JOHNSON, S. and BIRCH, L. L. (1993), The postingestive consequences of fat condition preferences for flavours associated with high dietary fat. *Physiol. Behav.*, **54**, 71–6.

KLEIFELD, E. I. and LOWE, M. R. (1991), Weight loss and sweetness preferences: the effects of recent vs. past weight loss. *Physiol. Behav.*, **49**, 1037–42.

LAWLESS, H. T. and HEYMAN, H. (1999), *Sensory Evaluation of Food: Principles and Practices.* Kluwer Academic Publishers, Dordrecht, the Netherlands.

LE NOURY, J. C., LAWTON, C. and BLUNDELL, J. E. (2002), Food choice and hedonic responses: difference between overweight and lean high fat phenotypes. *Int. J. Obes.*, **26**, S125.

LOWE, C. E., DOWEY, A. J. and HORNE, P. J. (1998), Changing what children eat. In *The Nation's Diet: The Social Science of Food Choice*, ed. A. Murcott. London: Longman. pp 57–80.

MACDIARMID, J. I., CADE, J. E. and BLUNDELL, J. E. (1996), High and low fat consumers, their macronutrient intake and body mass index: further analysis of the National Diet and Nutrition Survey of British Adults. *Eur. J. Clin. Nutr.*, **50**, 505–12.

MATTES, R. D. (2001), The taste of fat elevates postprandrial triacylglycerol. *Physiol. Behav.*, **74**, 343–8.

MATTES, R. D. (2002), Oral fat exposure increases the first phase triacylglycerol concentration due to release of stored lipid in humans. *J. Nutr.*, **132**, 3656–62.

MATTES, R. D. (2004), PROP status: dietary modifier, marker or misleader. In Prescott J., Tepper B. *Genetic Variation in Taste Sensitivity.* Marcel Dekker, Inc., NY, pp. 229–50.

MATTES, R. D., COWART, B. J., SCHIAVO, M. A., ARNOLD, C., GARRISON, B., KARE, M. R. and LOWRY, L. D. (1990), Dietary evaluation of patients of with smell and/or taste disorders. *Am. J. Clin. Nutr.*, **51**, 233–40.

MCCRORY, M. A., FUSS, P. J., MCCALLUM, J. E. *et al.* (1999), Dietary variety within food groups: association with energy intake and body fatness in men and women. *Am. J. Clin. Nutr.*, **69**, 440–7.

MCKENNA, R. J. (1972), Some effects of anxiety level and food cues on the eating behaviour of obese and normal weight subjects: a comparison of the Schachterian and psychosomatic conceptions. *J. Personal. Soc. Psychol.*, **22**, 311–19.

MEISELMAN, H. L., DE GRAAF, C. and LESHER, L. L. (2000), The effects of variety and monotony on food acceptance and intake at a midday meal. *Physiol. Behav.*, **70**, 119–25.

MELA, D. J. and SACCHETTI, D. A. (1991), Sensory preferences for fats: relationships with diet and body composition. *Am. J. Clin. Nutr.*, **53**, 908–15.

MELA, D. J., TRUNCK, F. and AARON, J. I. (1993), No effect of extended home use on linking for sensory characteristic of reduced-fat foods. *Appetite.*, **21**, 117–29.

MONTIGNAC, M. (1997), *Eat Yourself Thin.* Michel-Ange Publishing.

NEDERKOORN C. and JANSEN A. Cue reactivity and regulation of food intake. *Eat. Behav.*, **3**, 61–72.

NISBETT, R. E. (1968), Taste, deprivation, and weight determinants of eating behaviour. *J. Personal. Soc. Psychol.*, **10**, 107–16.

PELCHAT, M. L. (2002), Of human bondage: food craving, obsession, compulsion, and addiction. *Physiol. Behav.*, **76**, 347–52.

PELCHAT, M. L. and SCHAEFER, S. (2000), Dietary monotony and food cravings in young and elderly adults. *Physiol. Behav.*, **68**, 353–9.

PILGRIM, F. J. and KAMEN, J. M. (1963), Predictors of human food consumption. *Science*, **355**, 501–2.

PORCHEROT, C. and ISSANCHOU, S. (1998), Dynamics of liking for flavoured crackers: test of predictive value of a boredom test. *Food Qual. Pref.*, **9**, 21–9.

RAYNOR, H. A. and EPSTEIN, L. H. (2001), Dietary variety, energy regulation, and obesity. *Psychol. Bull.*, **127**, 325–41.

RAYNOR, H. A. and EPSTEIN, L. H. (2003), The relative-reinforcing value of food deprivation and restriction. *Appetite*, **40**, 15–24.

RAYNOR, HA., JEFFERY, R. W., TATE, D. F. and WING, R. R. (2004), Relationship between changes in food group variety, dietary intake, and weight during obesity treatment. *Int. J. Obes. Rel. Metab. Disord.*, **28**, 813–20.

RISSANEN, A., HAKALA, P., LISSNER, L., MATTLAR, C. E., KOSKENVUO, M. and RONNER, T. (2002), Acquired preference especially for dietary fat and obesity: a study of weight-disconcordant monozygotic twin pairs. *Int. J. Obes. Relat. Metab. Disord.*, **26**, 973–7.

RODIN, J. (1975), Effects of obesity and set point on taste responsiveness and ingestion in humans. *J. Compar. Physiol. Psychol.*, **89**, 1003–9.

RODIN, J. (1981), Current status of the internal-external hypothesis for obesity, what went wrong. *Am. Psychol.*, **36**, 361–72.

RODIN, J., SLOCHOWER, J. and FLEMING, J. (1977), Effects of degree of obesity, age of onset and weight less on responsiveness to sensory and external stimuli. *J. Compar. Physiol. Psychol.*, **91**, 586–97.

ROLLS, B. J. (1986), Sensory-specific satiety. *Nutr. Rev.*, **44**, 93–101.

ROLLS, B. J., ROLLS, E. T., ROWE, E. A. and SWEENEY, K. (1981a), Sensory-specific satiety in man. *Physiol. Behav.*, **27**, 137–42.

ROLLS, B. J., ROWE, E. A., ROLLS, E. T., KINGSTON, B., MEGSON, A. and GUNARY, R. (1981b), Variety in a meal enhances food intake in man. *Physiol. Behav.*, **26**, 251–5.

ROLLS, B. J., ROWE, E. A., and ROLLS, E. T. (1982), How sensory properties of food effect feeding behaviour. *Physiol. Behav.*, **29**, 409–17.

ROLLS, E. T. and ROLLS, J. H. (1997), Olfactory sensory-specific satiety in humans. *Physiol. Behav.*, **61**, 461–73.

SAELENS, B. E. and EPSTEIN, L. H. (1996), Reinforcing value of food in obese and non-obese women. *Appetite*, **27**, 41–50.

SALBE, A. D., DELPARIGI, A., PRATLEY, R. E., DREWNOWSKI, A. and TATARANNI, P. A. (2004), Taste preferences and body weight changes in an obesity-prone population. *Am. J. Clin. Nutr.*, **79**, 372–8.

SCHACHTER, S. (1968), Obesity and eating. *Science.*, **161**, 751–6.

SCHUTZ, H. G. and PILGRIM, F. J. (1958), A field study of monotony. *Psycholog. Rep.*, **4**, 559–65.

SCHUTZ, H. G. (1988), Beyond preference: appropriateness as a measure of contextual acceptance of food. In *Food Acceptability*, ed. Thomson DMH. Elsevier, New York, pp.115–134.

SIEGEL, P. S. and PILGRIM, F. J. (1958), The effect of monotony on the acceptance of food. *Am. J. Psychol.*, **71**, 756–9.

SNOEK, H. M., HUNTJENS, L., VAN GEMERT, L. J., DE GRAAF, C. and WEENEN, H. (2004), Sensory-specific satiety in obese and normal-weight women. *Am. J. Clin. Nutr.*, **80** (4), 823–31.

SORENSON, L. B., MOLLER, P., FLINT, A., MARTENS, M. and RABEN, A. (2003), Effect of sensory perception of foods on appetite and food intake: a review of studies on humans. *Int. J. Obes.*, **27**, 1152–66.

SPIEGEL, T. A., SHRAGER, E. E. and STELLAR, E. (1989), Responses of lean and obese subjects to preloads, deprivation, and palatability. *Appetite.*, **13**, 45–69.

SPIEGEL, T. A. and STELLAR, E. (1990), Effects of variety on food intake of underweight, normal-weight and overweight women. *Appetite.*, **15**, 47–61.

SPITZER, L. and RODIN, J. (1981), Human eating behaviour: a critical review of studies in normal weight and overweight individuals. *Appetite*, **2**, 293–329.

STUBBS, R. J., JOHNSTONE, A. M., MAZLAN, N., MBAIWA, S. E. and FERRIS, S. (2001), Effect of altering the variety of sensorially distinct foods, of the same macronutrient content on food intake and body weight in men. *Eur. J. Clin. Nutr.*, **55**, 19–28.

STUBBS, R. J. and WHYBROW, S. (2004), Energy density, diet composition and palatability: influences on overall food energy intake in humans. *Physiol. Behav.*, **81**, 755–64.

STUBENITSKY, K., AARON, J. I., CATT, S. L. and MELA, D. J. (1999), Effect of information and extended use on the acceptance of reduced-fat product. *Food. Qual. Pref.*, **10**, 367–76.

TEPPER, B. J. (1992), Dietary restraint and responsiveness to sensory-based food cues as measured by cephalic phase salivation and sensory-specific satiety. *Physiol. Behav.*, **52**, 305–11.

THOMPSON, D. A., MOSKOWITZ, H. R. and CAMPBELL, R. G. (1977), Taste and olfaction in human obesity. *Physiol. Behav.*, **19**, 335–7.

VICKERS, Z. and HOLTON, E. (1998), A comparison of taste test rating, repeated consumption, and postconsumption ratings of different strengths of iced tea. *J. Sensory. Stud.*, **13**, 199–212.

WARDLE, J., GUTHRIE, C., SANDERSON, S., BIRCH, L. L. and PLOMIN, R. (2001), Food and activity preferences in children of lean and obese parents. *Int. J. Obes.*, **25**, 971–7.

WARDLE, J., HERRERA, M.-L., COOKE, L. and GINSON, E. L. (2003), Modifying children's food preferences: the effects of exposure and reward on acceptance of an unfamiliar vegetable. *Eur. J. Clin. Nutr.*, **57**, 341–8.

WESTERTERP-PLANTENGA, M. S. (2004), Effects of energy density of daily food intake on long-term energy intake. *Physiol. Behav.*, **81**, 765–71.

WOODS, S. C. (1991), The eating paradox: how we tolerate food. *Psychol. Rev.*, **98**, 488–505.

WOODS, S. C. and SEELEY, R. J. (2002), Understanding the physiology of obesity: review of recent development in obesity research. *Int. J. Obes. Rel. Metab. Disord.*, **26** Suppl 4: S8–S10.

YEOMANS, M. R. (1996), Palatability and the microstructure of feeding humans: the appetizer effect. *Appetite*, **27**, 119–33.

YEOMANS, M. R., BLUNDELL, J. E. and LESHEM, M. (2004), Palatability: response to nutritional need or need-free stimulation of appetite? *Br. J. Nutr.*, **92**, Suppl. **1**, S3–S14.

ZANDSTRA, E. H., DE GRAAF, C., VAN TRIJP, H. C. M. and VAN STAVEREN, W. A. (1999), Laboratory hedonic rating as predictors of consumption. *Food. Qual. Pref.*, **10**, 414–18.

ZANDSTRA, E. H., DE GRAAF, C. and VAN TRIJP, H. C. (2000), Effects of variety and repeated in-home consumption on product acceptance. *Appetite*, **35**, 113–19.

ZANDSTRA, E. H., STUBENITSKY, K., DE GRAAF, C. and MELA, D. J. (2002), Effects of learned flavour cues on short-term regulation of food intake in realistic setting. *Physiol. Behav.*, **75**, 83–90.

ZANDSTRA, E. H., WEEGELS, M. F., VAN SPRONSEN, A. A. and KLERK, M. (2004), Scoring or boring? Predicting boredom through repeated in-home consumption. *Food. Quality Pref.*, **15**, 549–57.

8

Portion size and food intake[1]

B. Rolls, J. Ello-Martin and J. Ledikwe, The Pennsylvania State University, USA

8.1 Introduction: the growth in portion sizes

Obesity is a rapidly growing, world-wide public health problem. In recent decades, there has been a significant increase in the prevalence of obesity. The World Health Organization estimates that globally there are over 1 billion adults and 17 million children who are overweight or obese (World Health Organization, 2004). It is unlikely that our biology could have changed in several decades, so other explanations for this surge in obesity rates must be found. One possible reason for the increase is that the environment in Westernized societies has altered, so that overconsumption of energy has become easier. At the same time, opportunities for physical activity have declined. Thus, it is increasingly difficult for individuals to match energy intake to energy output in order to maintain a healthy body weight. Some of the changes in the eating environment that encourage overeating are the increasing availability of inexpensive high-energy-dense (kJ/g) foods, the wide variety of palatable foods, the increasing frequency of meals consumed outside of the home, and the rise in portion sizes. While all of these changes may stimulate excess intake, we will present data suggesting that large portion sizes, particularly of energy-dense foods, are contributing to the epidemic of obesity, and we will present constructive measures that could help to improve the eating environment.

[1] Supported by NIH grants R37DK039177 and R01DK059853.

8.1.1 Increasing portion sizes

Studies of food portions offered at fast food outlets, chain restaurants, and convenience stores indicate that portion sizes of many items have increased (Young and Nestle, 2002). According to Nestle (2003), this trend began in the USA as early as the 1970s, with portion sizes increasing sharply in the 1980s and continuing to rise. Data from Denmark show similar trends (Matthiessen *et al.*, 2003). The growth of portion sizes has been most evident in fast food restaurants where the 'supersizing' of some menu items is relatively common (Harnack *et al.*, 2000). Items available at fast food restaurants are estimated to be two to five times larger than two decades ago (Young and Nestle, 2003). In general, food packaging and common portion sizes of popular dishes are 25% larger in the USA than in France where rates of obesity are lower (Rozin *et al.*, 2003). With the availability of many foods in larger sizes, it is not surprising that epidemiological studies indicate people are consuming larger portions of food (Smiciklas-Wright *et al.*, 2003).

8.2 Studies showing that portion size affects energy intake

8.2.1 Adults

Although the increase in the size of portions and the prevalence of overweight and obesity have occurred in parallel, a crucial step in assessing a causal relationship between portion size and obesity is to determine experimentally whether portion size affects energy intake. Recent controlled studies clearly show that portion size does affect energy intake. When we tested how adults responded to four different portions of macaroni and cheese served on different days, we found that the bigger the portion, the more participants ate (Rolls *et al.*, 2002). They consumed 30% more energy (676 kJ) when offered the largest portion (1000 g) compared to the smallest portion (500 g). The effect was seen both when the portion on the plate was determined by the investigator and when the participants served themselves from bowls containing different size portions. Of particular interest was the finding that, despite the difference in intake, participants reported similar ratings of hunger and fullness after eating. The results were not affected by subject characteristics including sex, body mass index, or concern about food intake or body weight. After the study was over, less than half (45%) of the subjects reported noticing that there were differences in the portions served. It is surprising that, in a controlled laboratory setting where the main focus was food and eating, many participants in the study appeared to be unaware of the changes in the amount of food offered and the subsequent effect on their intake, hunger, and satiety. It seems likely that, when individuals are in situations where there are more distractions, such as when eating out, they would be even less aware of portion size.

It could be argued that the effects of portion size on intake are specific to foods like macaroni and cheese that are amorphous or have no defined shape. The portion size of such foods has been shown to be particularly difficult to judge, especially when the portions are large (Slawson and Eck, 1997). We conducted further studies to test whether intake can also be influenced by the portion size of other types of foods, such as those with clearly defined shapes or units.

People tend to eat in units. That is, if they are offered a food that comes in a preportioned unit, such as a cookie, most people will eat the whole cookie (Siegel, 1957). One of the most common unit foods is the sandwich. In most fast food establishments there is a choice of sandwich sizes; often the larger sandwiches are purchased because the consumers perceive them as better value in that they get more food for their money (National Alliance for Nutrition and Activity, NANA, 2002). A key question is, if consumers choose a larger sandwich, are they likely to eat more? To test this, on four different days, we offered men and women submarine sandwiches that varied in size: 6, 8, 10, and 12 inches (15, 20, 25, 30 cm) (Rolls *et al.*, 2004e). We found a systematic and significant effect of portion size on intake for both men and women (Fig. 8.1). When served the 12-inch sandwich compared to the 6-inch sandwich, women consumed 31% more energy (665 kJ) and men consumed 56% more energy (1485 kJ). Ratings of hunger and fullness after lunch did not differ significantly when subjects were served the 8-, 10-, and 12-inch (20-, 25-, 30-cm) sandwiches, despite the increase in energy intake. It appears that, when served bigger portions, consumers override or adjust their level of satiety to accommodate greater energy intakes.

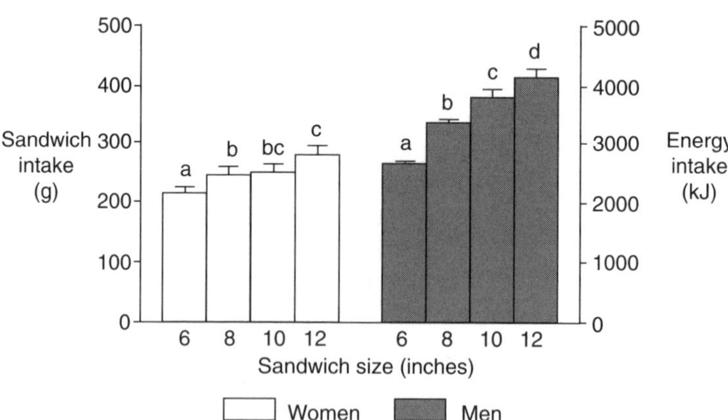

Fig. 8.1 On separate days, adults were served a 6-, 8-, 10-, or 12-inch sandwich for lunch. For both men ($n = 38$) and women ($n = 37$), energy intake increased as sandwich size increased. Within each sex, means with different letters are significantly different ($P < 0.025$).

The amount of food in a package or container may also influence how much is eaten. Some prepackaged foods come in a wide variety of sizes; for example, bags of potato chips range from 28 g single-serving bags to 560 g family-size bags. To test how the size of the bag affects intake, on five occasions we served men and women an afternoon snack that consisted of 28, 42, 85, 128 or 170 g of potato chips in a plain, unlabelled foil bag (Rolls *et al.*, 2004b). Participants ate directly from the bag so that they had few visual cues to guide consumption. The results showed that portion size had a significant effect on snack intake for both the men and the women (Fig. 8.2). For example, when served the 170 g package, women ate 18% (200 kJ) more and men ate 37% (511 kJ) more than when served the 85 g package. As subjects increased their snack intake with increasing package size, they also reported feeling fuller; however, they did not adjust their intake at the subsequent dinner meal to compensate for the increased energy intake and fullness. Thus, bigger portions of a prepackaged snack increased energy intake in the short term. It is not clear that all prepackaged foods will have a similar effect. It is possible that the effect will be greatest for highly palatable foods, such as chips, that people find difficult to stop eating.

Additional studies conducted in a variety of situations confirm that the package or container size of a variety of foods can affect how much food

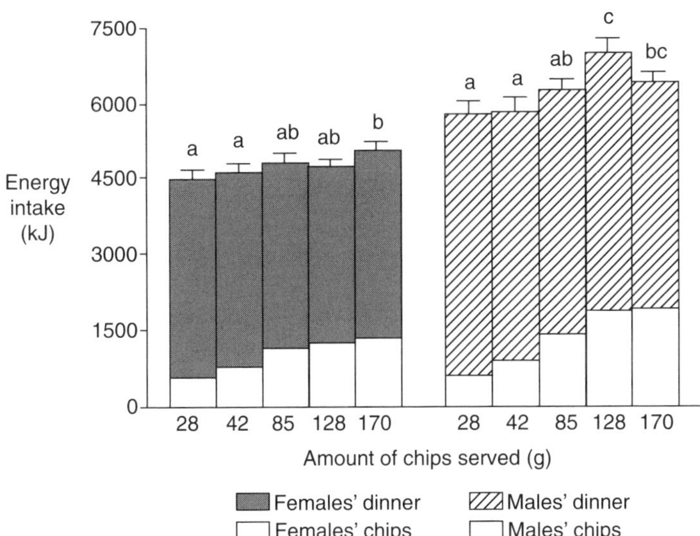

Fig. 8.2 At a mid-afternoon snack on different days, men ($n = 26$) and women ($n = 34$) were offered one of five package sizes containing different portions of potato chips (crisps). Both men and women increased their intake of chips as the package size increased; furthermore, subjects did not significantly adjust their intake at dinner for the excess energy consumed with the snack. Means within each sex with different letter are significantly different ($P < 0.02$).

is prepared and eaten (Wansink, 1996). When women were given a 2 lb box of spaghetti and asked to take out enough to make a dinner for two, they removed an average of 302 strands. But when given a 1 lb box, they removed only 234 strands. When frying chicken, women poured 4.3 ounces (126 ml) of cooking oil from a 32-oz bottle, but only 3.5 ounces (103 ml) from a 16-oz bottle. When people were asked how many chocolate candies they would eat while watching a movie by themselves, participants poured 63 from a small package that contained 114 candies, 103 from a package double in size, and 122 from a package triple in size. That is, they poured about twice as much from a jumbo bag, a difference of about 1046 kJ (Wansink, 1996). In a cinema, consumers were given either a medium (120 g) or large (240 g) bucket of popcorn. Subjects rated the taste of the popcorn, and were divided into two groups depending upon whether they perceived the taste as favorable or unfavorable. The results showed an effect of the portion size of popcorn on intake regardless of how the taste of popcorn was rated (Wansink and Park, 2001). Thus, it is not just the palatability of foods that is driving intake up when large portions are available.

A number of controlled studies show that both in the laboratory and in more naturalistic settings, the portion size and package size of a variety of foods can affect energy intake in adults in the short term. It is possible that, after a bout of overeating stimulated by large portions, compensatory mechanisms will limit subsequent intake. We tested this in a study in which the portion size was increased for all foods served to men and women over a 2-day period (Rolls *et al.*, in press). The results showed a significant effect of portion size on energy intake over the 2 days. When the portions of all foods were doubled, energy intake on both days increased for all subjects by a mean of 26% (2218 kJ/d for women and 3402 kJ/d for men) (Fig. 8.3). Although subjects reported feeling more full after they consumed the larger portions, they did not compensate for the excess energy eaten over the course of the first day by reducing their intake on the second day. Thus, these results show that the effects of portion size can persist over several days and are associated with significant increases in daily intakes. Studies of longer term effects of portion size on energy intake are in progress.

8.2.2 Children

While it has been clearly shown that adults respond to increasing portions by eating more, they probably did not start life responding in this way. A recent analysis of food survey data over a 20-year period indicates that, despite changes in the eating environment, there has been remarkable stability in the average portion size of foods consumed by children in the second year of life (McConahy *et al.*, 2002). A controlled laboratory study that we conducted confirms that, in young children, intake is relatively unaffected by environmental cues such as portion size. When we fed 3-year-olds three different portions of macaroni and cheese at three separate lunches,

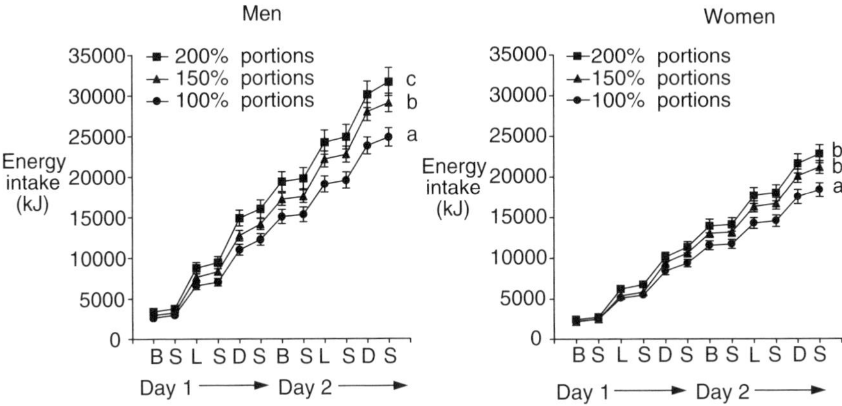

Fig. 8.3 Cumulative energy intakes (mean ± SEM) by condition of portion size (100, 150, 200%) of all foods consumed for men ($n = 16$) and women ($n = 16$) over 2 consecutive days. B, breakfast, L, lunch, D, dinner, S, snack. The effect of portion size on energy intake persisted over 2 days. Means within each sex with different letters are significantly different.

they ate the same amount at each meal. Their intake was therefore unaffected by portion size. In contrast, 5-year-old children responded as adults do, in that they ate significantly more as the portions increased. This response to portion size occurred even though their hunger did not differ at the start of the meals (Rolls *et al.*, 2000). Similarly, Fisher and colleagues (2003) found that 4-year-old children ate 25% more when they were served an entrée that was twice the size of an age-appropriate portion. In this study, the children who increased their intake the most when served large portions were those who had been identified as more likely to eat in the absence of hunger.

It is not clear why children are more influenced by portion size as they age. Data suggest that early experiences lead to the development of behaviors that shape eating habits. In one study, 4-year-old children who were rewarded for cleaning their plates increased their energy intake. On the other hand, children who were taught to focus on satiety cues, indicated by the fullness in their stomachs, ate an appropriate amount of food (Birch *et al.*, 1987). Thus, the response to portion size by children could be a learned behavior which leads to a shift of attention away from internal hunger and satiety cues toward food cues in the external environment. A lack of response to satiety signals may predispose children to overeat in an environment in which large portions of palatable foods are readily available (Barkeling *et al.*, 1992; Birch and Fisher, 1998). The influence of large portions on intake, however, has been shown to be moderated simply by allowing children to serve themselves. One study demonstrated that children ate 25% less of a large entrée when they decided for themselves how much food to put on their plates, compared to when they were served the large portion of the entrée by an adult (Fisher *et al.*, 2003).

8.3 Eating out and portion size

Although there is some evidence that portions consumed at home are increasing (Nielsen and Popkin, 2003; Young and Nestle, 2002), the large portions served in restaurants may be a bigger problem for weight management. The increase in the prevalence of obesity since the 1970s coincides with an increase in the number of meals eaten outside the home (Harnack *et al.*, 2000; Lin *et al.*, 1999). Today, Americans are 40% more likely to consume meals from restaurants three or more times a week as they were in the late 1980s (Kant and Graubard, 2004).

A number of studies indicate that meals consumed away from home have a lower diet quality and are higher in energy than at-home foods (Bowman *et al.*, 2004; Clemens *et al.*, 1999; French *et al.*, 2001; Kant and Graubard, 2004; Paeratakul *et al.*, 2003). Furthermore, in both adolescents and adults, the frequency of eating out is associated with an increase in energy and fat intake (Clemens *et al.*, 1999; French *et al.*, 2001; Kant and Graubard, 2004). For example, women who eat out frequently (more than six times a week) have been shown to have daily energy intakes approximately 1200 kJ higher than those who eat at restaurants less often (Clemens *et al.*, 1999).

In addition to high energy intakes, data show a relationship between eating out and weight status (Binkley *et al.*, 2000; Cho *et al.*, 2003; French *et al.*, 2000; Kant and Graubard, 2004; McCrory *et al.*, 1999). Nationally representative data indicate that the proportion of food consumed from fast-food restaurants is positively associated with body mass index (BMI) in both men and women (Binkley *et al.*, 2000). One prospective study found that, over 3 years, an increase in the frequency of fast food consumption was associated with an increase in body weight (French *et al.*, 2000).

The high availability of large portions of energy-dense foods in restaurants may provide an explanation for the association between eating out and increased body weight. A cross-cultural analysis revealed that the portion sizes of popular restaurant dishes were 25% larger in the USA than in France, a country with substantially lower rates of obesity (Rozin *et al.*, 2003). Restaurants have found that customers appreciate good value, and this translates into large portions at a low price. Since food is only a small percentage of the cost of a restaurant meal, giving customers more food is an excellent economic strategy if it increases total sales. This is possible because agricultural subsidies have helped to reduce the cost of some foods and commodities, such as vegetable oil and sugar, which have become very inexpensive (Drewnowski and Specter, 2004; Nestle, 2003). Thus the practice of 'supersizing' (giving customers a lot more food and energy for only a small additional cost) is widespread, particularly in fast food establishments.

Restaurants may be giving consumers what they want in terms of value, but a crucial issue is whether people can adjust their energy intake to their energy needs when tempted with large portions of energy-dense, palatable foods. The American Institute of Cancer Research has provided data that offer insight into how individuals view portion size when dining out (American Institute for Cancer Research, 2003). In a survey of more than 1000 adults, 69% indicated that, when dining out, they finish their entrées all or most of the time. Of those adults, 30% reported that they would have been satisfied with a smaller portion. This suggests that, when eating out, many adults ignore satiety signals and eat beyond the point of noticeable fullness. Additionally, a number of survey respondents (42%) reported that they determine the amount of food to eat according to what they are used to eating. Thus, the portion sizes that individuals customarily eat may be related to frequent exposure to large portions over time.

A recent study demonstrates that the portions served in restaurants can directly affect how much is eaten. We tested how increasing the portion size of a popular dish, while keeping the price the same, would affect intake in a restaurant setting (Diliberti *et al.*, 2004). An entrée, baked ziti, was offered ten times over 5 months and 180 adult customers purchased the dish during that period. On different days, the portion was varied between a standard portion (248 g, 1766 kJ) and a large portion (377 g, 2647 kJ). Results showed that portion size had a significant impact on intake, such that mean intake of the standard portion was 1671 kJ and of the larger portion was 2390 kJ. Thus when customers were served 50% more they ate 43% more, equivalent to 719 kJ. A survey filled out by the customers showed no difference in ratings of the appropriateness of the two portions. Thus, in restaurants as well as in the laboratory, portion size has a significant impact on energy intake, and it is likely that the consumers are often unaware of this effect.

8.4 Portion size, energy intake and obesity

When eating out, portion size is one of a number of variables that could affect consumption. Having a wide variety of palatable foods, eating in a convivial atmosphere with friends, and the consumption of alcohol may also increase energy intake. The high energy density (kJ/g) of restaurant meals is likely to promote excess intake. A systematic series of studies indicates that individuals consistently consume more energy when presented with foods having a higher energy density than with similar foods having a lower energy density (Bell *et al.*, 1998; Rolls *et al.*, 1999a,b). Prentice and Jebb (2003) recently compiled the energy density values of foods from well-known fast food outlets in Britain, finding that the energy density of *the entire menu* (beverages were not included) from these restaurants was

12.0 kJ/g. Further work is needed to determine the average energy density of fast food meals and to examine the influence of the new, popular salad options on meal energy density at these establishments. For comparative purposes, the energy density of the US diet, based on all foods consumed over two days, was found to be 7.8 kJ/g (Ledikwe *et al.*, 2005). The relatively high energy density of fast food can facilitate the overconsumption of energy. For example, when served a fast food meal with extra large portions in a food court, adolescents consumed over 6908 kJ in one meal, which was about 62% of their estimated daily energy requirements (Ebbeling *et al.*, 2004). It seems likely that both the large portions and the high energy density of the foods in fast food outlets contribute to excessive energy intakes, but it is important to determine whether these two influences on intake interact or simply add together.

Several recent studies have investigated how the combined effects of energy density and portion size influence energy intake. In a controlled laboratory study, Kral *et al.* (2004) served a main lunch entrée at two energy density levels (5.23 kJ/g and 7.32 kJ/g), in three different portion sizes (500 g, 700 g, 900 g) on different days. Subjects consumed 925 kJ more (56%) when served the largest portion of the high-energy-dense entrée, compared to when served the smallest portion of the low-energy-dense entrée. Interestingly, there was no interaction between the effects of energy density and portion size, indicating that both factors acted independently to affect energy intake. When increased simultaneously, the effects of energy density and portion size added together to increase energy intake (Fig. 8.4).

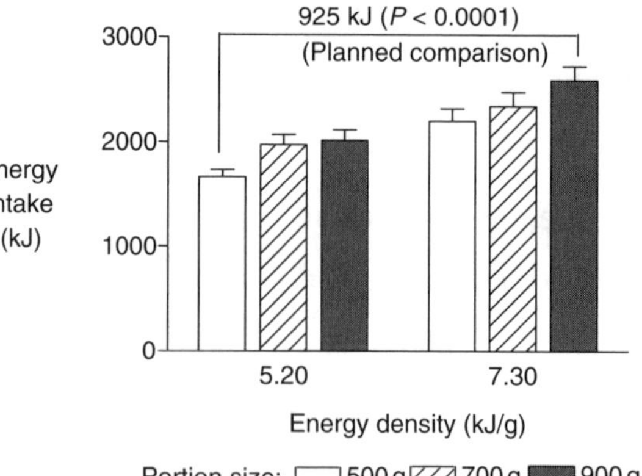

Fig. 8.4 Energy intakes (mean ± SEM) for women ($n = 39$) by energy density and portion size. The effects of portion size and energy density add together to influence energy intake. Reproduced with permission by the *American Journal of Clinical Nutrition* © *Am J Clin Nutr*. American Society for Clinical Nutrition (Kral *et al.*, 2004).

Another study in which the additive effects of energy density and portion size were examined over two days showed that the effects persisted beyond a single meal and that larger portions of higher-energy-dense foods had the greatest impact on energy intake (Rolls *et al.*, 2004c). Thus, both in the short term and over 2 days, the effects of portion size and energy density added together to influence *ad libitum* intake.

In some situations, however, consumption of large portions can decrease overall energy intake if the food has a low energy density. A recent controlled study showed that consumption of a large portion of a food low in energy density at the start of a meal can decrease energy intake at the rest of the meal (Rolls *et al.*, 2004d). On different days, subjects were required to consume a first course salad, which was varied in portion size (150 and 300 g) and energy density (1.38, 2.80, and 5.56 kJ/g); the first course was followed by a main course of pasta that was consumed *ad libitum*. Compared to having no first course, consuming the low-energy-dense salads reduced meal energy intake (by 7% for the small portion and 12% for the large), and consuming the high-energy-dense salads increased intake (by 8% for the small portion and 17% for the large). When two salads with the same number of calories were compared, meal intake was decreased more when the larger portion of the lower-energy-dense salad was consumed (Fig. 8.5). It has also been shown that consuming a low-energy-dense soup at the start of a meal reduced overall meal intake (Rolls *et al.*, 1999b).

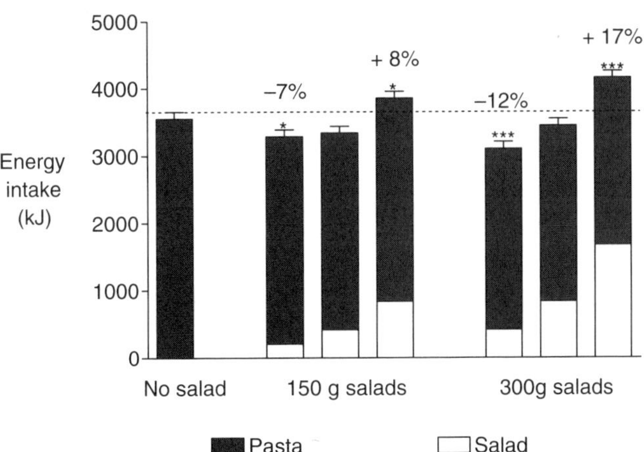

Fig. 8.5 Energy intakes (mean ± SEM) for women (n = 42) after consumption of compulsory first course salads differing in portion size (g) and energy density (kJ/g). Difference in meal intake compared to consuming no salad: * $P < 0.05$; *** $P < 0.0001$. Intake was influenced by both energy density and the portion of salad. Reprinted with permission from the American Dietetic Association (Rolls *et al.*, 2004d).

These studies indicate that energy density and portion size work together to influence energy intake and satiety and suggest several different strategies that can help to lower energy intake and increase satiety (Ello-Martin *et al.*, 2005). When choosing entrées to be consumed *ad libitum*, reductions in both energy density and portion size can significantly decrease energy intake while maintaining fullness. In contrast, when choosing a first course, the greatest enhancement of satiety and reduction in overall meal intake was seen with large portions of foods low in energy density such as salad or soup. Understanding how energy density and portion size work together can lead to more effective nutrition education messages than simply to 'eat less'. Instead, messages may be focused on encouraging the consumption of satisfying portions of foods with a low energy density. Strategies to lower the energy density of meals involve reducing fat and adding water-rich foods, such as soups, vegetables and fruits (Rolls, 2005; Rolls and Barnett, 2003; Rolls *et al.*, 2004a).

8.4.1 Are large portions making us obese?

There are few studies on the relationship between food portion size and weight status, and even fewer studies that also address dietary energy density. Nationally representative data for children indicate that portion size alone accounted for 17 to 19% of the variance in energy intake (McConahy *et al.*, 2004); in other words, larger portions were associated with higher intakes. In addition, children with a higher BMI consumed portions of foods that were as much as 100% larger than those consumed by children with a lower BMI (McConahy *et al.*, 2002). These analyses, however, did not also examine the energy density of the foods consumed. This last point is important because large portions of low-energy-dense foods would likely be associated with a lower weight status. A small study in the Netherlands that examined both portion size and energy density indicated that obese women consume larger portions of high-energy-dense foods and smaller portions of low-energy-dense foods, as compared to non-obese women (Westerterp-Plantenga *et al.*, 1996). While calculating dietary energy values in large groups of free-living individuals can be a complex task (Ledikwe *et al.*, 2005), there is a need for nationally representative epidemiological studies examining relationships between food portion size and weight status that take energy density into account.

Even though the trend toward larger portion sizes coincided with an increase in the prevalence of obesity, this does not prove a causal link. Similarly, data indicating that large portion sizes increase energy intake do not show a definitive relationship between portion size and weight status; nevertheless, the available data do support the hypothesis that portion size could play a role in the obesity epidemic.

8.5 Strategies to moderate the influence of portion size on energy intake

A number of recent reports have included statements regarding food portion sizes (US Department of Health and Human Services, 2001; World Health Organization, 2003). The Food and Drug Administration (FDA) Report, entitled 'Calories Count' (2004), recommended that foods be labeled as a single-serving if they could be reasonably consumed at one sitting because part of the problem people have identifying appropriate food portions may arise from difficulties in interpreting the information on food labels (Seligson, 2003). The report also encouraged food manufactures to use appropriate comparative labeling statements and urged the restaurant industry to provide point of purchase information. The 2005 Dietary Guidelines Advisory Committee acknowledged the importance of energy density in making food choices (Dietary Guidelines Advisory Committee, 2005), and suggested that limiting portion sizes, especially of energy-dense foods, could help to reduce calorie intake. On the other hand, consumption of low-energy dense foods that are nutrient-dense 'provides individuals a way to meet nutrient needs while avoiding the overconsumption of calories' (US Department of Health and Human Services and US Department of Agriculture, 2005). Research is needed to determine if adding information about energy density to food packages could be a useful tool for helping consumers to choose appropriate portions and to rapidly compare the energy content of similar foods.

One approach to limiting the intake of energy-dense foods is to impose penalties, such as 'sin taxes' on beverages and foods high in fat and energy (Horgen and Brownell, 2002). However, determining which items should be taxed is problematic and it is not clear whether foods with large portion sizes should also be taxed. In addition, there are no data on whether such taxes would significantly impact food choices. An alternative approach would be through incentives to provide healthful, low-energy-dense foods and to provide reasonable portions. The FDA considered pilot testing the use of their name and logo on menus and advertisements as an incentive for restaurants to provide patrons with voluntary point-of-purchase nutrition information (Food and Drug Administration's Obesity Working Group, 2004). This would allow patrons to make informed decisions. It would also provide the food industry with motivation to provide a greater range of portion sizes and to make smaller portions more appealing. While it is not feasible for restaurants to serve portions based on an individual customer's energy needs, the restaurant industry can provide a variety of choices that would make it easier for customers to eat less. More attractive pricing strategies (French, 2003; Horgen and Brownell, 2002) could be used to promote the selection of smaller portion sizes.

However, smaller portions or 'eating less' may not always be an effective solution since it is not just large portion sizes that increase energy intake, but rather, large portions of energy-dense foods. Instead, foods could be modified to give consumers satisfying portions and good taste as well as less energy at a reasonable price. One strategy is to decrease the energy density of menu items. Reductions in energy density are unlikely to affect customer satisfaction if palatability is not compromised and cost is not increased. A combination of fat reduction along with the addition of water-rich vegetables could reduce the energy density of popular foods such as burgers, sandwiches and pizza. It is likely that, with unit foods such as these, patrons will order and consume their usual portion size, but will ingest less energy while feeling just as full and satisfied (Rolls *et al.*, 2004e). In one study, a fish dish was substantially reduced in fat and energy, with no effect on how much people liked the dish, how well it matched their expectations, and how likely they would be to purchase it again (Stubenitsky *et al.*, 2000). Even small reductions in energy density are likely to have a big impact at a population level. For example, using an alternative method for cooking French fries in fast food restaurants, which decreases fat absorption, could lead to a significant reduction in per capita energy consumption (Morley-John *et al.*, 2002).

There is a need for extensive funding to deliver effective educational messages that not only emphasize limiting intake of foods with a high energy density, but also encourage consuming foods with a low energy density, such as fruits and vegetables. Organizations that have been successful at increasing consumption of foods low in energy density, such as the Produce for Better Health Foundation (Foerster *et al.*, 1995), should be rewarded with larger budgets. Policy makers need to organize a well-funded campaign using marketing and psychological techniques, as sophisticated as those being used by industry, to help consumers understand the long-term health effects of eating large portions of energy-dense foods (Tillotson, 2002). This can help consumers equip themselves with the knowledge and skills to adequately determine portions that are appropriate to their energy requirements. When faced with large portions of energy-dense, palatable foods in restaurants, people should adopt strategies to limit their intake, such as ordering reduced-sized portions, saving part of the entrée for another meal, or sharing with a friend. Consumers also need to encourage the food industry to provide high quality, low-energy-dense foods. It is important that consumers purchase these items when available so that the food industry has an economic incentive to provide tasty, healthful options that can be consumed in reasonable portions without promoting excessive energy intake.

8.6 The future: the eating environment and obesity

There is increasing evidence that excessive food portions, particularly of energy-dense foods, contribute to the overconsumption of energy. Telling people to simply 'eat less' is not likely to be an effective solution, since it is not just large portion sizes that increase energy intake, but rather, large portions of energy-dense foods. Large portions of foods low in energy density such as vegetables, fruits and broth-based soups can aid weight management by providing satisfying portions with few calories (Rolls, 2005; Rolls and Barnett, 2003). There is a need to deliver effective educational messages that combine the principles of portion size and energy density. The development and intensive marketing of appealing, low-energy-dense foods can help create an environment in which consumers are better able to maintain a healthy weight. Successful strategies will not only require cooperation among the food and restaurant industries, policy makers, and scientists, but will also require consumers to understand and accept the importance of eating reasonable food portions for better health.

8.7 References

2005 DIETARY GUIDELINES ADVISORY COMMITTEE (2005), 'Report of the Dietary Guidelines Advisory Committee on the Dietary Guidelines for Americans, 2005', http://www.health.gov/dietaryguidelines/dga2005/report/, accessed August 19, 2004.

AMERICAN INSTITUTE FOR CANCER RESEARCH (2003), 'Awareness and action: AICR surveys on portion size, nutrition and cancer risk', http://www.aicr.org/press/awarenessandaction_03conf.pdf, (accessed 17 September 2004).

BARKELING, B., ELKMAN, S. and ROSSNER, S. (1992), 'Eating behaviour in obese and normal weight 11-year-old children', *Int. J. Obes. Relat. Metab. Disord.*, **16**, 355–60.

BELL, E. A., CASTELLANOS, V. H., PELKMAN, C. L., THORWART, M. L. and ROLLS, B. J. (1998), 'Energy density of foods affects energy intake in normal-weight women', *Am. J. Clin. Nutr.*, **67**, 412–20.

BINKLEY, J. K., EALES, J. and JEKANOWSKI, M. (2000), 'The relation between dietary change and rising US obesity', *Int. J. Obes.*, **24**, 1032–9.

BIRCH, L. L. and FISHER, J. O. (1998), 'Development of eating behaviors among children and adolescents', *Pediatrics*, **101**, 539–49.

BIRCH, L. L., MCPHEE, L., SHOBA, B. C., STEINBERG, L. and KREHBIEL, R. (1987), 'Clean up your plate: effects of child feeding practices on the conditioning of meal size', *Learn. Motiv.*, **18**, 301–17.

BOWMAN, S. A., GORTMAKER, S. L., EBBELING, C. B., PEREIRA, M. A. and LUDWIG, D. S. (2004), 'Effects of fast-food consumption on energy intake and diet quality among children in a national household study', *Pediatrics*, **113**, 112–18.

CHO, S., DIETRICH, M., BROWN, C. J., CLARK, C. A. and BLOCK, G. (2003), 'The effect of breakfast type on total daily energy intake and body mass index: results from the third National Health and Nutrition Examination Survey (NHANES III)', *J. Am. Coll. Nutr.*, **22**, 296–302.

CLEMENS, L. H. E., SLAWSON, D. L. and KLESGES, R. C. (1999), 'The effect of eating out on quality of diet in premenopausal women', *J. Am. Diet. Assoc.*, **99**, 442–4.

DILIBERTI, N., BORDI, P., CONKLIN, M. T., ROE, L. S. and ROLLS, B. J. (2004), 'Increased portion size leads to increased energy intake in a restaurant meal', *Obes. Res.*, **12**, 562–8.

DREWNOWSKI, A. and SPECTER, S. E. (2004), 'Poverty and obesity: the role of energy density and energy costs', *Am. J. Clin. Nutr.*, **79**, 6–16.

EBBELING, C. B., SINCLAIR, K. B., PEREIRA, M. A., GARCIA-LAGO, E., FELDMAN, H. A. and LUDWIG, D. S. (2004), 'Compensation for energy intake from fast food among overweight and lean adolescents', *JAMA*, **291**, 2828–33.

ELLO-MARTIN, J. A., LEDIKWE, J. H. and ROLLS, B. J. (2005), 'The influence of food portion size and energy density on energy intake: implications for weight management', *Am. J. Clin. Nutr.*, (in press).

FISHER, J. O., ROLLS, B. J. and BIRCH, L. L. (2003), 'Children's bite size and intake of an entrée are greater with large portions than with age-appropriate or self-selected portions', *Am. J. Clin. Nutr.*, **77**, 1164–70.

FOERSTER, S. B., KIZER, K. W., DISOGRA, L. K., BAL, D. G., KRIEG, B. F. and BUNCH, K. L. (1995), 'California's "5 a day – for better health!" campaign: an innovative population-based effort to effect large-scale dietary change', *Am. J. Prev. Med.*, **11**, 124–31.

FOOD AND DRUG ADMINISTRATION'S OBESITY WORKING GROUP (2004), US Food and Drug Administration. Center for Food Safety and Applied Nutrition.

FRENCH, S. A. (2003), 'Pricing effects on food choices', *J. Nutr.*, **133**, 841S–3S.

FRENCH, S. A., HARNACK, L. and JEFFERY, R. W. (2000), 'Fast food restaurant use among women in the Pound of Prevention study: dietary, behavioral and demographic correlates', *Int. J. Obes.*, **24**, 1353–9.

FRENCH, S. A., STORY, M., NEUMARK-SZTAINER, D., FULKERSON, J. A. and HANNAN, P. (2001), 'Fast food restaurant use among adolescents: associations with nutrient intake, food choices and behavioral and psychosocial variables', *Int. J. Obes.*, **25**, 1823–33.

HARNACK, L. J., JEFFERY, R. W. and BOUTELLE, K. N. (2000), 'Temporal trends in energy intake in the United States: an ecologic perspective', *Am. J. Clin. Nutr.*, **71**, 1478–84.

HORGEN, K. B. and BROWNELL, K. D. (2002), 'Comparison of price change and health message interventions in promoting healthy food choices', *Health Psychol.*, **21**, 505–12.

KANT, A. K. and GRAUBARD, B. I. (2004), 'Eating out in America, 1987–2000: trends and nutritional correlates', *Prev. Med.*, **38**, 243–9.

KRAL, T. V. E., ROE, L. S. and ROLLS, B. J. (2004), 'Combined effects of energy density and portion size on energy intake in women', *Am. J. Clin. Nutr.*, **79**, 962–8.

LEDIKWE, J. H., BLANCK, H. M., KETTEL-KHAN, L. *et al.* (2005), 'Dietary energy density determined by eight calculation methods in a nationally representative United States population', *J. Nutr.*, **135**, 273–8.

LIN, B.-H., GUTHRIE, J. and FRAZAO, E. (1999), 'Nutrient contribution of food away from home', in Frazao, E, *America's Eating Habits: Changes and Consequences*, US Department of Agriculture/Economic Research Service, 213–42.

MATTHIESSEN, J. FAGT, S., BILTOFT-JENSEN, A., BECK, A. M. and OVESEN, L. (2003), 'Size makes a difference', *Public Health Nutr.*, **6**, 65–72.

MCCONAHY, K. L., SMICIKLAS-WRIGHT, H., BIRCH, L. L., MITCHELL, D. C. and PICCIANO, M. F. (2002), 'Food portions are postively related to energy intake and body weight in early childhood', *J. Pediatr.*, **140**, 340–7.

MCCONAHY, K. L., SMICIKLAS-WRIGHT, H., MITCHELL, D. C. and PICCIANO, M. F. (2004), 'Portion size of common foods predicts energy intake among preschool-aged children', *J. Am. Diet. Assoc.*, **104**, 975–9.

MCCRORY, M. A., FUSS, P. J., HAYS, N. P., VINKEN, A. G., GREENBERG, A. S. and ROBERTS, S. B. (1999), 'Overeating in America: association between restaurant food consumption and body fatness in healthy adult men and women ages 19–80', *Obes. Res.*, **7**, 564–71.

MORLEY-JOHN, J., SWINBURN, B. A., METCALF, P. A. and RAZA, F. (2002), 'Fat content of chips, quality of frying fat and deep-frying practices in New Zealand fast food outlets', *Aust. NZ J. Public Health*, **26**, 101–6.

NATIONAL ALLIANCE FOR NUTRITION AND ACTIVITY (NANA) (2002), 'From wallet to waistline: the hidden costs of super sizing'. http://www.cspinet.org/w2w.pdf, accessed July 2, 2002.

NESTLE, M. (2003), 'Increasing portion sizes of American diets: more calories, more obesity', *J. Am. Diet. Assoc.*, **103**, 39–40.

NIELSEN, S. J. and POPKIN, B. M. (2003), 'Patterns and trends in food portion sizes, 1977–1998', *J. Am. Med. Assoc.*, **289**, 450–3.

PAERATAKUL, S., FERDINand, D. P., CHAMPAGNE, C. M., RYAN, D. H. and BRAY, G. A. (2003), 'Fast-food consumption among US adults and children: dietary and nutrient intake profile', *J. Am. Diet. Assoc.*, **103**, 1332–8.

PRENTICE, A. M. and JEBB, S. A. (2003), 'Fast foods, energy density and obesity: a possible mechanistic link', *Obes. Rev.*, **4**, 187–94.

ROLLS, B. (2005), *The Volumetrics Eating Plan*, New York, HarperCollins Publishers, Inc.

ROLLS, B. and BARNETT, R. A. (2003), *The Volumetrics Weight-Control Plan: Feel Full on Fewer Calories*, New York, HarperTorch.

ROLLS, B. J., BELL, E. A., CASTELLANOS, V. H., CHOW, M., PELKMAN, C. L. and THORWART, M. L. (1999a), 'Energy density but not fat content of foods affected energy intake in lean and obese women', *Am. J. Clin. Nutr.*, **69**, 863–71.

ROLLS, B. J., BELL, E. A. and THORWART, M. L. (1999b), 'Water incorporated into a food but not served with a food decreases energy intake in lean women', *Am. J. Clin. Nutr.*, **70**, 448–55.

ROLLS, B. J., ENGELL, D. and BIRCH, L. L. (2000), 'Serving portion size influences 5-year-old but not 3-year old children's food intakes', *J. Am. Diet. Assoc.*, **100**, 232–4.

ROLLS, B. J., MORRIS, E. L. and ROE, L. S. (2002), 'Portion size of food affects energy intake in normal-weight and overweight men and women', *Am. J. Clin. Nutr.*, **76**, 1207–13.

ROLLS, B. J., ELLO-MARTIN, J. A. and TOHILL, B. C. (2004a), 'What can intervention studies tell us about the relationship between fruit and vegetable consumption and weight management?' *Nutr. Rev.*, **62**, 1–17.

ROLLS, B. J., ROE, L. S., KRAL, T. V. E., MEENGS, J. S. and WALL, D. E. (2004b), 'Increasing the portion size of a packaged snack increases energy intake in men and women', *Appetite*, **42**, 63–9.

ROLLS, B. J., ROE, L. S. and MEENGS, J. S. (2004c), 'Reducing the energy density and portion size of foods decreases energy intake over two days', *Obes. Res.*, **12**, A5.

ROLLS, B. J., ROE, L. S. and MEENGS, J. S. (2004d), 'Salad and satiety: energy density and portion size of a first course salad affect energy intake at lunch', *J. Am. Diet. Assoc.*, **104**, 1570–6.

ROLLS, B. J., ROE, L. S., MEENGS, J. S. and WALL, D. E. (2004e), 'Increasing the portion size of a sandwich increases energy intake', *J. Am. Diet. Assoc.*, **104**, 367–72.

ROLLS, B. J., ROE, L. S. and MEENGS, J. S. (in press), 'The effect of increased portion size on energy intake is sustained over two days'. *J. Am. Diet. Assoc.*

ROZIN, P., KABNICK, K., PETE, E., FISCHLER, C. and SHIELDS, C. (2003), 'The ecology of eating: smaller portion sizes in France than in the United States help explain the French paradox', *Psychol. Sci.*, **14**, 450–4.

SELIGSON, F. H. (2003), 'Serving size standards: can they be harmonized?' *Nutr. Today*, **38**, 247–53.

SIEGEL, P. S. (1957), 'The completion compulsion in human eating', *Psychol. Rep.*, **3**, 15–16.

SLAWSON, D. L. and ECK, L. H. (1997), 'Intense practice enhances accuracy of portion size estimation of amorphous foods', *J. Am. Diet. Assoc.*, **97**, 295–7.

SMICIKLAS-WRIGHT, H., MITCHELL, D. C., MICKLE, S. J., GOLDMAN, J. D. and COOK, A. (2003), 'Foods commonly eaten in the United States, 1989–1991 and 1994–1996: are the portion sizes changing?' *J. Am. Diet. Assoc.*, **103**, 41–7.

STUBENITSKY, K., AARON, J. I., CATT, S. L. and MELA, D. J. (2000), 'The influence of recipe modification and nutritional information on restaurant food acceptance and macronutrient intakes', *Public Health Nutr.*, **3**, 201–9.

TILLOTSON, J. E. (2002), 'We're fat and getting fatter! What is the food industry's role?' *Nutr. Today*, **37**, 136–8.

US DEPARTMENT OF HEALTH AND HUMAN SERVICES (2001), *The Surgeon General's Call to Action to Prevent and Decrease Overweight and Obesity*, Rockville, MD, US Department of Health and Human Services, Public Health Service, Office of the Surgeon General.

US DEPARTMENT OF HEALTH AND HUMAN SERVICES AND US DEPARTMENT OF AGRICULTURE (2005), *Dietary Guidelines for Americans 2005*, Washington, DC.

WANSINK, B. (1996), 'Can package size accelerate usage volume?' *J. Marketing*, **60**, 1–14.

WANSINK, B. and PARK, S. B. (2001), 'At the movies: how external cues and perceived taste impact consumption volume', *Food Qual. Prefer.*, **12**, 69–74.

WESTERTERP-PLANTENGA, M. S., PASMAN, W. J., YEDEMA, M. J. W. and WIJCKMANS-DUIJSENS, N. E. G. (1996), 'Energy intake adaptation of food intake to extreme energy densities of food by obese and non-obese women', *Eur. J. Clin. Nutr.*, **50**, 401–7.

WORLD HEALTH ORGANIZATION (2003), World Health Organization (WHO Technical Report Series, No. 916). Geneva, Switzerland.

WORLD HEALTH ORGANIZATION (2004), 'Obesity and overweight', http://www.who.int/dietphysicalactivity/publications/facts/obesity/en/, (accessed 4 October 2004).

YOUNG, L. R. and NESTLE, M. (2002), 'The contribution of expanding portion sizes to the US obesity epidemic', *Am. J. Public Health*, **92**, 246–9.

YOUNG, L. R. and NESTLE, M. (2003), 'Expanding portion sizes in the US marketplace: implications for nutrition counseling', *J. Am. Diet. Assoc.*, **103**, 231–4.

Part II

Macronutrient influences on weight loss

9

Energy density and weight control

S. Whybrow, The Rowett Research Institute, UK, N. Mazlan, International Islamic University of Malaysia and R.J. Stubbs, The Rowett Research Institute, UK

9.1 Introduction

The diet we eat has changed considerably since the Second World War. Fat contributes more to the diet now than in the 1930s, although recently it appears to be decreasing slightly (Stephen and Sieber, 1994; DEFRA, 2001). Consumption of sugars added to the diet has increased steadily (Johnson and Frary, 2001). The way we eat has also changed, with restaurant meals, processed foods and soft-drinks being a bigger part of the diet than previously (Cavadini *et al.*, 2000; Zizza *et al.*, 2001). These changes have contributed to a food environment that contains a wider range of relatively inexpensive, highly palatable and energy dense foods than ever before. It is frequently considered axiomatic that the ready availability of these foods is, at least partly, responsible for the current secular trends in increasing prevalence of obesity. In the last two decades a large amount of work has been conducted examining the role of diet composition in appetite and energy balance control (Stubbs, 1998). We now have a clearer idea of the nutritional attributes of the diet that tend to elevate energy intakes. The increased availability of readily assimilated carbohydrates mixed with dietary fat appears to have some role in elevating energy intakes (Stubbs *et al.*, 2001). Recently considerable attention has focused on how the energy density of the diet is involved in these processes (Prentice and Poppitt, 1996; Rolls and Bell, 1999; Stubbs *et al.*, 2000). The purpose of this chapter is to consider the role of energy density in the control of body weight in humans, and its importance in human energy balance. These issues are be-devilled by what is often deemed to be common sense or anecdotally obvious relationships between energy density, diet composition, food choice, the amount of food eaten and how fat we are.

We aim to disentangle some of these issues by breaking down the main theme into a number of discrete considerations. These are (i) how diet composition influences energy density (ii) the relationships between food composition, energy density and energy intake, (iii) the relationship between obesity, food choice and energy density, (iv) implications for the global food industry and public health strategies.

9.2 Definitions

For the purposes of this chapter, diet is defined as water ($g \cdot day^{-1}$), protein ($MJ \cdot day^{-1}$), carbohydrate ($MJ \cdot day^{-1}$), fat ($MJ \cdot day^{-1}$), energy ($MJ \cdot day^{-1}$), energy density ($MJ \cdot kg^{-1}$) and amount of food eaten ($kg \cdot day^{-1}$). Energy density can be calculated a number of different ways, and different methods can give different apparent relationships between energy density and, for example, the diets of lean and obese subjects (Cox and Mela, 2000). Here energy density is defined as the energy per kg of wet weight of ready to eat food.

There is considerable debate as to the definition of palatability. The reader is referred to an in-depth discussion of this issue (Kissileff, 1990; Ramirez, 1990; Rogers, 1990). Here, palatability is defined as the momentary subjective oro-sensory pleasantness of food.

9.3 Influence of diet composition on energy density

As macronutrients come in the diet, fat is more energy dense ($37 kJ \cdot g^{-1}$) than either carbohydrate ($16 kJ \cdot g^{-1}$) or protein ($17 kJ \cdot g^{-1}$), while alcohol is $29 kJ \cdot g^{-1}$ (Holland *et al.*, 1991).

The fat content of foods and energy density are strongly associated (Drewnowski, 1998; Stubbs *et al.*, 2000; Yao and Roberts, 2001; Crowe *et al.*, 2004). Because of its high energy density, increasing or decreasing the fat content of foods has a pronounced effect on the energy density of these foods while achieving similar sensory properties and, once consumers have become accustomed to them, being equally acceptable. Margarine, for example, is considerably more energy dense than some low-fat spreads (30 compared to $11 kJ \cdot g^{-1}$).

There is a weak negative association between the contribution of carbohydrate, expressed as a percentage of the energy content of foods, and energy density (Stubbs *et al.*, 2000). However, when expressed as a percentage of energy content, some high-carbohydrate foods such as 'low-fat' confectionery can be highly energy dense (at around $18 kJ \cdot g^{-1}$), whereas others, such as fruit and sucrose-sweetened beverages, can have a relatively low energy density (around $1.5 kJ \cdot g^{-1}$).

As they are consumed, foods with a high protein content tend to also have a high moisture content and this lowers their overall energy density, such as meat and fish, which are approximately 4–7 $kJ \cdot g^{-1}$ (Holland *et al.*, 1991). The effect of protein on the energy density of foods is similar to that of carbohydrate, with a weak positive correlation when expressed as grams of protein per unit weight of food, and a weak negative correlation when the energy contribution of protein is expressed as a percentage of energy (Stubbs *et al.*, 2000).

Of importance is whether beverages are included when calculating the energy density of diets. Beverages consumed in more than small quantities can produce a disproportionate effect on energy density, especially artificially-sweetened soft drinks because of their effectively zero energy content, but moderate weight and volume per serving. Beverages are excluded to varying degrees in the literature when calculating the energy density of diets. For example, Gibson calculated weight in three ways, including all drinks, excluding tap water and excluding soft drinks (Gibson, 2000).

Even spirits, such as whisky, are by weight mostly water, and the energy density of alcoholic drinks ranges from approximately 1 to 9 $kJ\,g^{-1}$ for beers and spirits respectively (Holland *et al.*, 1991). In moderate drinkers the effects of alcohol on energy density are not likely to be great, although there appears to be little published data on this.

Dietary fibre and inorganic constituents can also influence energy density; some fibre is fermented in the gut to provide energy as short-chain fatty acids, but fibre also reduces the metabolisable energy of fat and protein. When consumed in typical Western mixed diets the net energy value of fibre is likely to be negligible (Baer *et al.*, 1997). Furthermore, fibre makes up only a small proportion of the typical Western diet (DoH, 1991; Howarth *et al.*, 2001).

An analysis of 1032 ready to eat foods from the British food composition tables shows that the primary determinants of energy density are water and fat (Fig. 9.1).

Fat elevates energy density and water decreases energy density. Protein and carbohydrates contribute very little to dietary energy density *per se* (Blundell and Stubbs, 1999). Thus, the energy density of foods is mainly determined by a fat–water seesaw. If high-protein, high-carbohydrate and high-fat foods are selected so that the two remaining macronutrients are equally represented (in MJ), then high-protein foods are less energy-dense than high carbohydrate foods, which are less energy-dense than high fat foods. There is about 50% overlap in energy density between each category (Stubbs *et al.*, 2000) (Fig. 9.2).

When the same relationships were examined in 73 adults self recording their own food intakes for 7 days, similar features prevailed (Fig. 9.3).

Thus, the primary factor decreasing the energy density of food is water. Dietary fat content is the main factor increasing the energy density of foods.

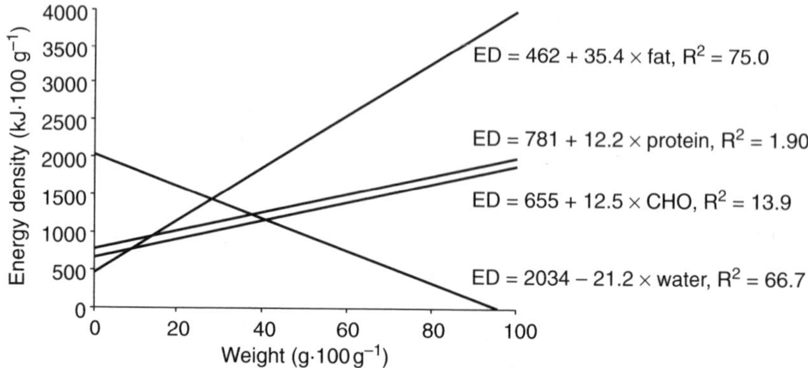

Fig. 9.1 Relationship between percentage of energy from dietary macronutrients and water (in grams) (predictor variables) and energy density (outcome variable) of 1032 ready to eat foods, taken from the British food composition tables (Holland *et al.*, 1991).

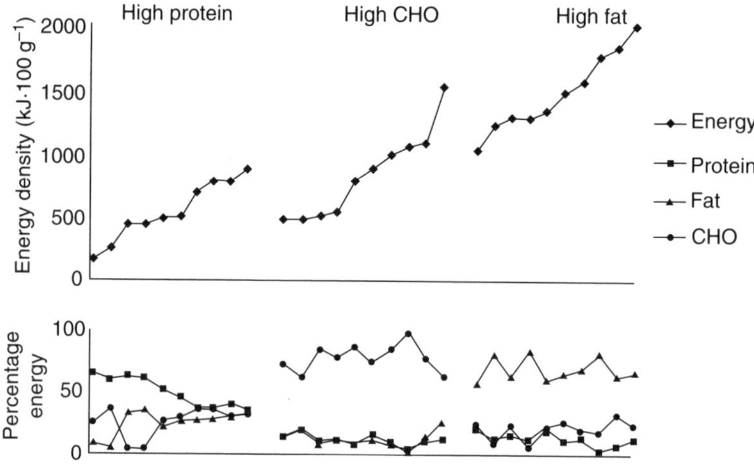

Fig. 9.2 Energy density of high-protein, high-carbohydrate and high-fat foods.

The energy density of 'snack' foods is perhaps a case of some current interest. Commercially available snack foods tend to be highly energy dense because they are dry mixtures of fats and readily assimilated carbohydrates, and which are low in protein and fibre. This can be seen in Fig. 9.4.

Commercially available snack foods are, on average, considerably more energetically dense than most foods in our diets, and the average of the overall diet (Cox and Mela, 2000; Gibson, 2000; Westerterp-Plantenga, 2001). Many 'lower-fat' alternatives of foods are of a similar energy density to their more traditional counterparts, because in these products fats are

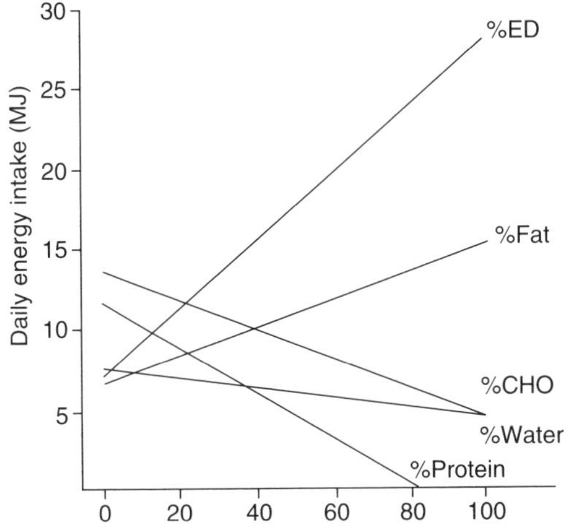

Fig. 9.3 Relationships between mean daily energy intake and percentage energy density, percentage of energy from fat, CHO and protein, and water intake as a percentage of each subject's maximum daily water intake, as predictor variables.

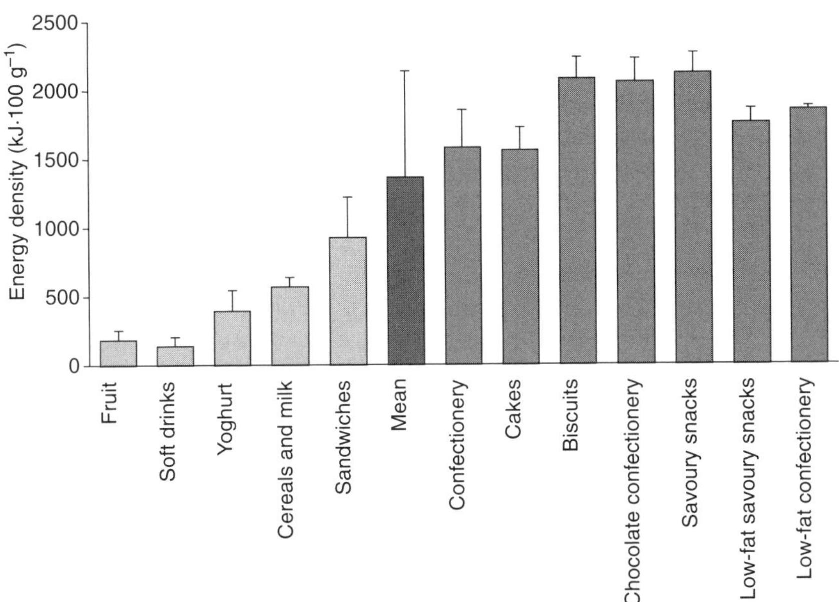

Fig. 9.4 Energy density of some common snack foods.

largely replaced by readily assimilated starches and disaccharides. This has been suggested as a potential explanation for the failure of the introduction of lower-fat alternative foods to significantly reduce energy intakes (McCrory *et al.*, 2000).

9.4 Relationships between food composition, energy density and energy intake

9.4.1 Sources of evidence

There is very little direct evidence showing how the ingestion of specific foods or food components has led any person to become obese. There are a number of sources of data that can be referred to, and all are imperfect, that suggest relationships between diet composition and an increased risk of weight gain.

Epidemiological and diet survey studies

These have the advantage of using large numbers of subjects who are going about their everyday activities in their natural setting. The ecological validity is therefore theoretically high. However, there are methodological problems associated with these types of studies that must be taken into account and which inevitably weaken the conclusions derived from them. Firstly, the errors in data collection are high and are not necessarily random, such as apparently greater underreporting of energy intake in the obese (Schoeller, 1990; Black *et al.*, 1991; Goldberg *et al.*, 1991). Secondly, in many studies subjects are not randomly selected and therefore the sample is not necessarily totally representative of the general population. Thirdly, many epidemiological studies are cross sectional and assume that the processes influencing the phenomena under investigation are uniform over time and hence age groups. This is not always the case. Finally, consideration should be given to the problem of misreported dietary intakes and the likely impact of on observed dietary patterns. The results of diet survey and epidemiological studies should therefore be treated with some caution.

Laboratory-based studies

The laboratory setting allows the effects of diet composition on energy intake to be studied with greater control. But experiments typically use small numbers of non-randomly selected subjects in an artificial environment and employing protocols and techniques that are often unfamiliar to the subject. It is also important to understand the limitations of the laboratory approach when attempting to extrapolate results from the laboratory (where the signal to noise ratio may be artificially elevated) to everyday life. For instance, a common feature is that, when obese subjects are studied in the laboratory, they typically lose a little weight when ostensibly feeding *ad libitum*.

Intervention studies
Interventions often represent a good compromise between the artificiality of the laboratory and the lack of control over both manipulation and measurement that occurs in epidemiological studies. Typically, subjects adhere to a given manipulation (for example, consuming *ad libitum* a number of low-fat foods made available by the investigator) but go about their normal lives so that the impact of the manipulation can be assessed.

Because each approach has its advantages and limitations, it is important to examine the effects of diet composition, energy density and palatability on energy intake in each experimental environment. If broadly similar phenomena are apparent in each experimental condition, it is reasonable to accept that the phenomenon under scrutiny is robust and not an artefact of the experimental conditions themselves. This is especially so for energy density, which has a huge effect on energy intake in short-term laboratory studies but a far weaker effect in the long term, and in real life.

9.4.2 The effects of macronutrients on motivation to eat and energy intake

Weststrate has summarised the effects of macronutrients on satiety from a number of studies in which preloads of increasing energy were given as protein, carbohydrates and fats (Weststrate, 1992). Above a dose of 1 to 1.5 MJ, protein is more satiating than carbohydrate, which is in turn more satiating than fat. Macronutrients thus exert hierarchical effects on satiety and in suppressing subsequent energy intake (Stubbs, 1998). In free feeding humans, self-recording their dietary intakes, protein induces super-caloric compensation; carbohydrate leads to approximately caloric compensation; fat generates sub-caloric compensation and hence promotes excess energy intakes. Alcohol stimulates intake (see Blundell and Stubbs, 1997). When energy density is controlled, protein is still more satiating than either carbohydrate or fat (de Castro, 1987; Stubbs, 1998), and the differences between carbohydrate and fat is more subtle – with carbohydrate tending to exert a more acute effect on satiety than does fat. Specific subtypes of individual macronutrients also exert significant effects on satiety. These issues have been considered elsewhere (Stubbs *et al.*, 2000).

9.4.3 The effects of energy density on energy intake

In the laboratory, energy density exerts a very large effect on energy intake (Prentice and Poppitt, 1996; Bell *et al.*, 1998; Stubbs *et al.*, 1998b). This is because, in laboratory studies, where dietary energy density is covertly manipulated, people appear to eat a relatively constant amount of food across different dietary treatments. This is especially so when many learning cues have been removed from experimental foods, which are often unfamiliar or covertly manipulated. Under these conditions, energy density accounts for a very significant proportion of the variability in energy intake. By using covertly modified mixed diets in our laboratory, six lean men were in energy balance over 14 days when consuming a diet of $549\,kJ \cdot 100\,g^{-1}$, gained 0.95 kg on a $737\,kJ \cdot 100\,g^{-1}$ diet and lost 1.2 kg on a $377\,kJ \cdot 100\,g^{-1}$ diet – a decrease in energy density of 33% compared to the relatively normal diet (Stubbs *et al.*, 1998b). In this study, the weight of food consumed changed with changing energy density of the diet, but this was insufficient to achieve energy balance. It has been assumed that energy density is also the main determinant of energy intake in people consuming their normal diets in the real world (McCrory *et al.*, 2000; Prentice and Jebb, 2003).

It has been variously assumed or claimed that volume, weight, energy content, macronutrient proportion and energy density may all be monitored and constitute the source of specific satiation or satiety signals (Blundell and Stubbs, 1997). These may be divided into general factors (e.g. weight and volume), which apply to all foods, and specific factors (nutrient content, taste and smell) that depend on the particular food consumed. Why should weight appear as an important feature that affects food intake in some studies, especially when covertly manipulated diets are used? Weight or amount of food consumed is a learned cue with high functional validity (proximal cues that correlate well with more distal cues such as hormone release, contact with gastrointestinal receptors, etc.). This is why weight often appears to be an important monitored variable (rather than energy or nutrient content) when the nutritional composition of food has been surreptitiously manipulated (Blundell and Stubbs, 1997). The system is operating sensibly according to its previous experience; but it does not mean that weight is fundamentally more important than energy content. In the laboratory, factors such as energy density may have an over-riding effect on energy intake, whereas each of these effects is considerably diminished in real life. The apparent constancy of food intake appears to be a more robust effect in the laboratory than real life (Stubbs *et al.*, 2000).

In real life the determinants of energy intake are multifactorial (de Castro, 2000, 2001b; Stubbs *et al.*, 2000; Westerterp-Plantenga, 2001; de Castro and Plunkett, 2002). Each individual dietary determinant of energy intake explains only a small proportion of the total variance. When considering the dietary determinants of energy intake in 73 adults, self-recording their food intake over seven days, the relationships depicted in Fig. 9.3 are apparent (Stubbs *et al.*, 2000). Hierarchical relationships are evident with energy density having the greatest potential contribution to an increase in energy intake, but this only explains around 7% of the variance. It is also apparent from Fig. 9.3 that large changes in water intake have little effect on energy intake. Furthermore, in real-life, unlike in the laboratory, increases in the energy density of the diet elevate energy intakes but also decrease food intake (Stubbs *et al.*, 2000). Westerterp-Plantenga has analysed the relationship between energy density and *ad libitum* food and drink consumption. She found that average daily energy intake was related to dietary energy density when energy density was influenced by specific macronutrients (i.e. if foods contained little water). However, when energy density was strongly influenced by the weight of water, it was not related to energy intake (Westerterp-Plantenga, 2001). Thus, the water content of the overall diet tends to blur the relationship between energy density and energy intake, because it has a relatively large (negative) effect in determining the energy density of the overall diet, but a relatively small (positive) effect in determining energy intake.

As the majority of soft-drinks are of considerably lower energy density than most foods, and of the overall diet, an increased beverage consumption will lower overall dietary energy density. This does not, however, mean that increasing consumption of beverages will result in lower energy intakes (Rolls *et al.*, 1999). This can also be seen in Fig. 9.3. Water consumed with a meal can affect feelings of hunger and satiety during the meal, but the effect is not maintained (Lappalainen *et al.*, 1993), presumably because it empties from the stomach rapidly without slowing the gastric emptying of foods.

With the shift away from full-fat to reduced-fat milks, there are currently few high-fat beverages on the market; most non-alcoholic beverages are solutions of sugars and starches. Despite the low energy density of these beverages, they do not induce compensatory reductions in food intake as effectively as the same amount of carbohydrate contained in solid foods (DiMeglio and Mattes, 2000). This may be, in part, because of the rate, timing and density at which the energy is ingested. Furthermore, the sensory properties of most beverages are selected to encourage their consumption.

The extent to which the dietary determinants of energy intake are multifactorial is evident from the multiple regression equations calculated from 73 adults, self-recording their food intake over seven days (Stubbs *et al.*, 2000). Equations were calculated for the overall diet (including the contribution of drinks) and for food only (after excluding drinks).

Food and drinks

$$\begin{aligned}\text{Energy intake (MJ)} = &-2.83 + \text{subject effect} + 0.10\%\ \text{water}\\ &+ 0.66\%\ \text{energy density} - 0.032\%\ \text{CHO}\\ &- 0.044\%\ \text{protein}\ R^2 = 82.8\%\end{aligned}$$

Food only

$$\begin{aligned}\text{Energy intake (MJ)} = &-4.62 + \text{subject effect} + 0.097\%\ \text{water}\\ &+ 0.48\%\ \text{energy density} - 0.024\%\ \text{protein}\\ &R^2 = 86.5\%\end{aligned}$$

The amount of variance in energy intake explained was similar for each of the macronutrients, energy density and water, with no single main determinant when the analysis included drinks. Furthermore, no single component explained a large proportion of the variance. These analyses suggest that, unlike in the laboratory, energy density *per se* does not explain a large proportion of the variance in energy intake when subjects are consuming their normal diets. There are a considerable number of situational and behavioural factors that influence food and energy intake, such as the number of people present at a meal, and the same is true for these; each can explain a large proportion of the variance in energy intake in the laboratory, but a much smaller proportion in real-life (de Castro and Plunkett, 2002).

Having considered the role of diet composition in influencing energy intake, it is important to consider why energy density has a much bigger effect on energy intake in the laboratory than in real life. Part of the explanation is in the role of learning.

A number of factors influence the nature and extent of compensatory feeding responses to changes in the composition or energy density of the diet. It is pertinent to mention them here because some major differences between the feeding responses detected in the laboratory and real-life may be heavily influenced by these factors (Stubbs *et al.*, 1998c). Firstly, it has been argued above that, if the diet is systematically manipulated, the manipulation itself places a constraint on the compensatory feeding responses of human subjects. In sum, the more systematic a dietary manipulation the fewer degrees of freedom given to the subject to respond, the more blunted any compensatory response is likely to be. Caloric compensation appears to be facilitated when subjects can select from a range of familiar food items. It should also be remembered that humans tend to compensate better for prior decrements than for increments in energy intake, particularly over longer periods (Garrow, 1988).

Knowledge of the nature of the dietary manipulation can exert important influences on feeding responses, particularly in certain groups of people who are sensitive to health and diet-related issues, such as restrained eaters. Several studies have suggested that the response of restrained eaters to dietary manipulations is at least as heavily influenced by the knowledge of a dietary manipulation as by the nature of the manipulation itself (Miller *et al.*, 1998; Westerterp-Plantenga *et al.*, 1998).

It appears that learning plays a role in the feeding responses of a range of species (Forbes, 1995) and humans are no exception (Booth *et al.*, 1976). Here learning refers to associative conditioning of hunger or appetite for specific foods rather than information gleaned from external sources or any form of long-term conscious self-monitoring by the subject; these are additional forms of learning that can also affect feeding behaviour. In diet selection studies in non-human mammals the subject animal learns much more rapidly to select a diet that meets a physiological need, or alleviates a physiological stress, if the different diets from which they select are clearly distinguished by visual or olfactory cues (Forbes, 1995; Cairns *et al.*, 2002). The animal appears to associate the physiological consequences of ingesting a food with the sensory characteristics of that food. Similarly, in carefully controlled conditioning experiments, young children increase their preference for flavours associated with more energy-dense versions of foods (Johnson *et al.*, 1991; Kern *et al.*, 1993). Under these conditions, the experimenter is providing strong clues that accelerate the learned association between the food and its post-ingestive consequences. In the laboratory subjects often feed *ad libitum* from, or between, foods that have been covertly modified to differ only in the nutrient of interest while maintaining almost identical flavours, textures and odours. If subjects are given totally novel diets, then they may show very little compensatory responses in the short-to-medium term, simply because they have not had time to begin to learn to associate the post-ingestive consequences of eating novel foods with the sensory attributes of the foods themselves. In real life the foods they ingest are often familiar through years of experience.

There appears to be little experimental evidence demonstrating that adult humans also learn to associate the sensory properties of new foods with the food's energy content or energy density. This may be because of insufficient, and inconsistent, exposure that allows re-educating of learned associations. This would suggest that 'lower-fat' versions of foods, and acaloricaly sweetened versions of beverages, would have a greater impact on reducing energy intakes than they generally appear to (Gatenby *et al.*, 1995; de Graaf *et al.*, 1997). However, consumers' perceptions of foods are also an influence – in the laboratory restrained eaters consume more of a food when it is described as 'low-fat' than when the same food carries a 'high-fat' label (Shide and Rolls, 1995; Miller *et al.*, 1998). It could be argued that the 'low-fat' label effectively shortcircuits the learning process by providing a strong cue as to the food's energy content.

People are often able to anticipate the effects of familiar foods on their motivation to eat. For instance, most people will appreciate from past experience alone that adding cheese to a salad sandwich will 'fill them up for longer'. If foods are novel, subjects cannot refer to experience accurately in order to anticipate the post-ingestive consequences of eating those foods.

Sensory factors are also potent influences on the acceptability and selection of foods. Sensory factors can be of overriding importance in determining the intake of a particular food during a given bout of feeding (Drewnowski, 1992). As discussed below, sensory factors are not entirely dissociated from the post-ingestive consequences of having consumed a given food.

9.5 Relationship between obesity, food choice and energy density

A number of studies have found that high-fat, energy dense foods induce higher levels of energy intake than lower fat, less energy dense foods. Blundell has termed this 'passive overconsumption' (Blundell and

Macdiarmid, 1997). This term appears appropriate because it reflects the notion that the high-fat, energy-dense diet is not increasing motivation to eat or actual food intake. Thus food choice can be critically important in relation to energy density. Consumers should understand that by altering the energy density of foods they consume they can increase (or decrease) energy intake without altering the amount of food they consume at all.

It is known that the obese tend to select a diet that contains a greater percentage of foods that are more energy dense (Cox *et al.*, 1999; Stookey, 2001) and that the increasing number of new, energy-dense, foods introduced into the market in recent decades (McCrory *et al.*, 1999) has almost certainly raised the energy density of the average diet. There is evidence that we actually tend to prefer more energy dense foods (Drewnowski, 1998). Why should this be so? To appreciate the influence of energy density on food choice, and hence obesity, the influence of energy density on the palatability of foods should be considered.

Figure 9.5 shows meal size as a function of palatability from 564 US adults, self-recording their food intake for 7 days (de Castro *et al.*, 2000b). The figure illustrates a number of important features of the relationship

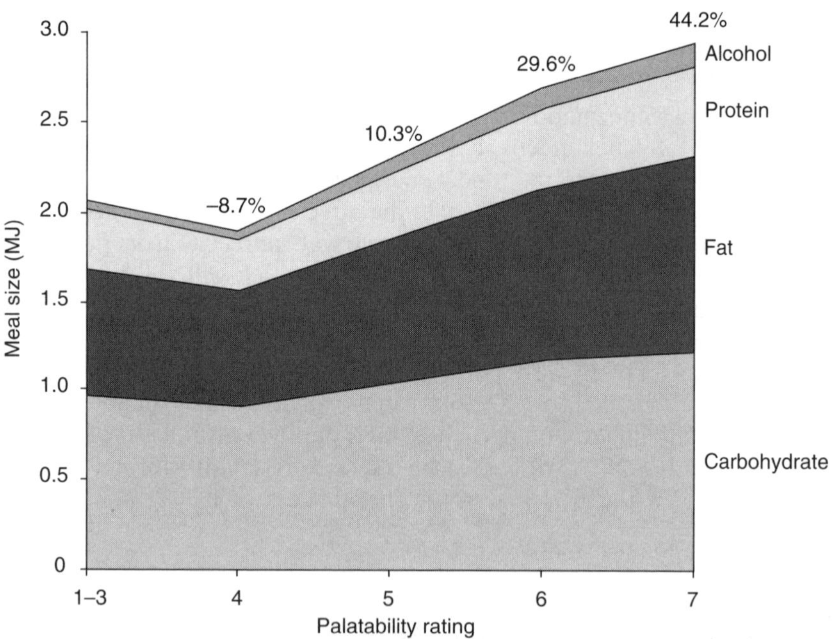

Fig. 9.5 Meal size as a function of palatability in 564 American adults, self reporting their food intakes for 7 days. The values above the lines represent the percentage increase in overall meal size relative to meals rated 1 to 3 (from *Castro et al.*, 2000).

between palatability and meal size in free living humans. Firstly, it is important to note that there were very few meals with a palatability rating 1–3 on a 7-point scale. This suggests a possible threshold effect on whether people will consider a food sufficiently palatable to actually ingest in real life. People eat what they like and avoid what they dislike. As the palatability of meals increased, so did energy intake. Furthermore, as the palatability of a meal increased intake of fat, protein and alcohol was higher. de Castro, Bellise and Dalix found the same relationships in 54 French adults self-recording food intake for 7 days (de Castro *et al.*, 2000a).

While the palatability of a food is related to energy intake, a number of other factors relate to the palatability of foods. Fat, protein, and alcohol all contribute to palatability of foods. Meal-time has a large effect on ratings of hunger and palatability, such that palatability ratings are higher for meals later in the day. Level of self-rated elation was also strongly related to palatability (de Castro *et al.*, 2000b). This illustrates the multidimensional nature of relationships in real-life (de Castro, 2000, 2001a; de Castro and Plunkett, 2002). It has also been shown that the palatability of foods is related to subjective appetite and the amount of food eaten in the laboratory (Hill *et al.*, 1984; Yeomans, 1996, 1998; Yeomans *et al.*, 1997). It appears that there is a positive correlation between subjectively rated palatability of foods and the amount of those foods eaten. However, de Castro has noted that while the regression lines for the relationships between palatability and energy intake are often characterized by steep slopes, they explained very little (~2%) of the variability in energy intake (de Castro *et al.*, 2000b). This is characteristic of real world models of the determinants of energy intake (de Castro and Plunkett, 2002). Not only do a number of factors relate to palatability, they inter-correlate. How then, do energy density and palatability of foods relate to each other and to energy intake?

Firstly it should be pointed out that because of the post-ingestive consequences of consuming foods and the learning that relates these consequences to perceived pleasantness of foods (see following sections), the short-term effects of energy density on energy intake do not extrapolate into longer term effects (Stubbs *et al.*, 2000; Westerterp-Plantenga, 2001). In the few longer-term human interventions that have been conducted, compensation is greater than seen in short term experiments (see Stubbs *et al.*, 2000 for detailed discussion).

Meiselman *et al.* noted a positive relationship between the energy density of foods habitually eaten and mean food preferences expressed by US army personnel (Meiselman *et al.*, 1974). Holt, in short-term studies has noted a positive relationship between satiety and the weight of a serving consumed (Holt *et al.*, 1995). From these observations, and those concerning the short-term effects of energy density on energy intake made above, Drewnowski has suggested that people prefer more energy dense foods over less energy dense foods (Drewnowski, 1998). He further argues that more energy dense foods are more palatable, and that as foods of a high energy density promote excess energy intakes, relative to foods of a lower energy density, they are therefore less satiating in energetic terms (i.e. per MJ of energy ingested).

These arguments are based on the observations of others that, in laboratory studies, people appear to eat a relatively constant weight of food, suggesting that 'weight or volume of food' may be an important regulatory signal in the control of energy intake (see above). Recently, this argument has been strongly promoted (Rolls and Bell, 2000; Prentice and Jebb, 2003). For instance, Drewnowski observes a growing viewpoint among some authors that 'energy density as opposed to the macronutrient content of foods, is currently thought to be the key factor in the regulation of food intake' (Drewnowski, 1998). It has been thus suggested that, since people seem to eat a constant weight of food, changes in dietary energy density are likely to be the main factor determining energy intake. It is argued here that such a conclusion is perhaps premature, for the following reasons. As noted in the analyses above, energy density is only one small part of the picture that predicts energy intake. Most of the studies in which a constant weight of food eaten appears as a major feature are short-term laboratory studies, laboratory studies conducted using systematically manipulated diets or cross sectional diet records of a short duration (see above). Our analysis of the dietary intakes of free-living subjects (with subjects reporting implausibly low energy intake values removed) suggests that increases in dietary energy density predict decreases in food intake to a greater extent than increases in energy intake. Under these conditions, where subjects are being studied in their normal environment, food-based learning cues are largely intact. The role of food-based learning cues in weight control has been given too little attention in recent years.

It is important to qualify the view that the most preferred foods are the least satiating and the most energy dense, and *vice versa*. It appears that animals (Reed *et al.*, 1990; Tordoff and Reed, 1991) and children (Johnson *et al.*, 1991; Kern *et al.*, 1993; Birch, 1998) acquire sensory preferences for energy-rich foods. Furthermore, preference conditioning experiments have shown that metabolic reinforcement of a sensory signal is far more effective at conditioning preference that the sensory stimulus alone. This implies that people will tend to prefer energy-rich foods to their low calorie counterparts. Nevertheless if energy density simply correlated with palatability and inversely correlated with satiety, the Western diet would appear to be a recipe for a positive feedback in energy intake, which would be reflected in a rapid monotonic body weight gain in many individuals. In reality we do not do this. Western adults appear to gain weight at around 0.2–2.0 kg a year (Kant *et al.*, 1995). In considering the relationships between energy density, palatability and energy intake it is important to ask: if energy dense foods are less satiating and more palatable, why does the relationship not develop into a positive feedback and promote monotonic rises in body weight? Why do we not preferentially select diets that are sufficiently energy dense that they elevate energy intake to 20 or 40 MJ a day. Such rampant hyperphagia only appears to be apparent in cases of severe protein energy malnutrition (Keys *et al.*, 1950), genetically determined leptin deficiency (Farooqi *et al.*, 2002) or intermittently in the case of some eating disorders (Hetherington *et al.*, 1994; Cooke *et al.*, 1997). All of the above considerations and the available evidence to date suggest that in longer term interventions weight changes are a mere fraction of those predicted by short-term experiments. This indicates that there is considerable amelioration of the extent to which energy density levers energy intake. Put more simply, people seem to compensate more in the longer term (Stubbs *et al.*, 2000).

9.6 Energy density and learned aspects of satiety

What enables us to learn to control intake to some extent when consuming more energy dense foods? The palatability of a food can be thought of as its sensory capacity to stimulate ingestion of that food (Mela and Rogers, 1998). This definition takes account of the fact that the palatability of the food is jointly determined by the nature of the food (smell, taste, texture and state), the sensory capabilities and metabolic state of the subject, and the environment in which the food and subject interact. Palatability is therefore not stable; indeed the palatability of a food typically declines as its own ingestion proceeds. This has been called sensory-specific satiety (Le Magnen, 1971; Rolls *et al.*, 1981). Satiety is said to be sensory-specific in relation to foods because the palatability of a food declines as its ingestion proceeds while unsampled foods do not change in perceived pleasantness (O'Doherty *et al.*, 2000). It may well be, however, that part of the specificity of satiety relates to the post-ingestive consequences of consuming a specific food. Some people may learn, or be inherently more susceptible to linking, the post-ingestive consequences of consuming certain foods with the reward-based responses associated with nutrient digestion, absorption, metabolism and storage.

9.7 Energy density in the context of other influences on intake

Considerable attention has recently focused on the issue of how the macronutrient composition of the diet can influence the current epidemic of obesity in Western society (Blundell and Stubbs, 1997; Stubbs *et al.*, 2000). Ingestion of dietary fat does appear to be a risk factor for subsequent weight gain (Lissner and Heitmann, 1995; Bray and Popkin, 1998; Sherwood *et al.*, 2000), although it is also possible to gain weight on a high carbohydrate diet (Stubbs *et al.*, 1998a). In particular, certain types of carbohydrates may interact with fat to facilitate higher levels of intake. Mela and Sacchetti (1991) have produced data suggesting that fatter people prefer fattier foods. There is little direct evidence that preference *per se* will influence quantitative intake (i.e. how much food is eaten) to an extent that will influence body weight. It is, however, very likely that preference influences qualitative food intake, i.e. which foods are eaten. This is important because the phenomenon of passive overconsumption of energy on high fat diets is not an issue of quantitative increases in food intake but of qualitative selection of high-fat, energy dense foods. In the 1950s Jean Mayer highlighted the need to distinguish between the dynamic period of rapid weight gain and the stable plateau that body weight appears to reach in obesity. The truth is we are remarkably ignorant of exactly how and at what rate different people gain weight (Mayer, 1955). It appears from laboratory experiments that satiation, post-ingestive satiety and hunger are influenced by food intake in a similar way in the obese as in lean people (Hill and Blundell, 1989). Spitzer and Rodin (1981) also note that the majority of studies on eating behaviour in normal weight and overweight individuals conducted between 1969 and 1981 were 'impressive in their demonstration of the lack of clear overweight-normal weight differences in eating behaviour'. The situation has not changed much today. They did note, however, that in short-term studies palatability appeared to be the most consistent variable in producing overweight-normal differences in amount of food eaten. It is also worth noting that obesity is a generic category which, like skin colour, identifies an obvious recognisable feature of individuals, but explains little of the behaviour of those individuals. Furthermore, there are many 'routes to obesity' (Blundell and Cooling, 2000).

The physiological features and psychological profiles that characterise the obese, and may be involved in the maintenance of the obese state, may not necessarily be the same features that led to obesity in the first place. Understanding the factors that produce sustained increases in energy intake over expenditure and the time-course over which this occurs is crucial for understanding the aetiology of obesity. There are likely to be a number of different factors that individually or together influence body weight. For instance, it is well known that not all obese subjects are restrained eaters. Similarly, not all obese subjects are insulin resistant. Since it is presently difficult to categorise which 'type' of obesity a person belongs to or indeed how many 'types' there are it is equally difficult to identify the factors bringing about these characteristics. Thus, while there is abundant evidence that certain aspects of diet composition, such as dietary fat, are risk factors for weight gain, weight gain on a high fat diet is not a biological inevitability. It should be noted that often ~40–50% of the variance in energy intake or subjective appetite in a group of subjects is due to differences between the subjects themselves (Ferris *et al.*, 2001).

This raises the issue of phenotypes (Cooling and Blundell, 1998). We have recently examined the contribution of dietary and phenotypic deter-

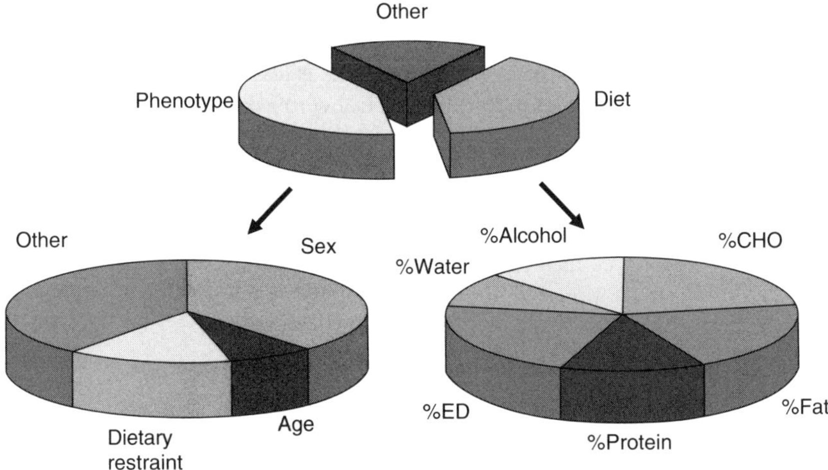

Fig. 9.6 Summary of the variance in reported energy intake explained by dietary and phenotypic determinants.

minants of energy intake in 102 free-living subjects self-recording their own food intake over seven days (Fig. 9.6).

Diet and phenotype explained similar amounts of the total variability in energy intake, and combined explained all but approximately 20% (Ferris *et al.*, 2001). However, the closer we tend to focus on any aspect of diet the more it fragments into specific components each explaining a smaller proportion of the variance. For instance diet explains approximately 40% of the total variability in energy intake. In the laboratory energy density also explained approximately 40% of the variability in energy intake when we covertly manipulated the energy density of the diet. In real-life energy density only explains about 7% of the total variability in energy intake. This is because in the laboratory we strip out all of the other influences on energy intake that are apparent in real life (Blundell and Stubbs, 1997). The effects of energy density alone can be subdivided into the effects of fat elevating energy density and water decreasing it (Blundell and Stubbs, 1999). In considering fat, it can be subdivided into different types of fat (degree of saturation, degree of esterification, chain length and triglyceride structure). Several aspects of fat structure are known to exert small but significant influences on energy intake (Stubbs and Harbron, 1996; Lawton *et al.*, 2000). This exercise could be repeated for all of the dietary constituents. The same general principle is true for the phenotype and its components.

It is not only the nutritional properties of foods that influence their selection and ingestion. Mass manufactured, processed, foods tend to be considerably less expensive in terms of energy per dollar, pound or Euro than fresh fruits and vegetables. They also tend to be more energy dense

(Drewnowski, 2004), and highly palatable and desirable – simply because unpalatable foods will not survive long in the market place. Thus, almost counter intuitively, a highly energy dense diet is less expensive for the consumer than one of lower energy density (Drewnowski, 2004). The necessary frequent purchasing, and cost, of fruits and vegetables are perceived as barriers to their consumption (Anderson *et al.*, 1998), and are likely to be real barriers for low income families. The high cost of a relatively low energy dense diet will mean a greater proportion of highly energy dense foods will tend to be selected, especially by those with low incomes. Drewnowski concluded that part of the explanation of the inverse relationship between poverty and obesity in America is economic.

9.8 Implications for the global food industry and public health strategies

Energy density is not the only determinant of energy intake, but it is clear from the previous discussion that highly energy dense foods present a risk of overconsumption. Lowering the energy density of the diet has been suggested as a way of passively lowering energy intake (Rolls *et al.*, 1998; McCrory *et al.*, 1999; Rolls and Bell, 1999), and there are several ways that this could be achieved.

The large contribution of dietary fat to the energy density of foods makes reducing the fat content of foods likely to be an effective way of lowering overall dietary energy density. Manufactured foods tend to be mixtures of refined carbohydrates and fats, and are potentially good candidates for fat reduction, and hence energy density reduction, strategies. However, in many 'lower-fat' versions of these foods most of the fat is replaced by starches and sugars, and they are not necessarily of low energy density (Stubbs *et al.*, 2001). The few intervention studies that have examined the impact of lower-fat foods on energy intakes over several weeks or more have provided little evidence that increasing consumption of lower-fat foods generally leads to any marked lowering of energy intake (Gatenby *et al.*, 1995) except in individuals reporting initially high fat intakes (de Graaf *et al.*, 1997). High-carbohydrate and high-fat snacks have similar effects in increasing energy intake when their energy density is similar, under laboratory (Johnstone *et al.*, 2000; Mazlan *et al.*, 2001) and free-living conditions (Whybrow *et al.*, 2004). Altering the ratio of fats to sugars in highly energy dense foods, without greatly lowering the energy density, is unlikely to help consumers lose weight through a passive lowering of energy intakes.

We generally acquire sensory preferences for energy dense foods, and will therefore tend to prefer energy dense foods over their low-energy (and often lower-fat) counterparts. But cognition can also influence food choice, for example when 'low-fat' is perceived as 'healthier' or fashionable. It is a challenge for the food industry to lower the fat content, and the energy density, of foods while either maintaining sufficient sensory appeal, or finding a sufficiently strong marketable angle, that we will buy them. Fat adds important sensory and textural properties to foods, and it is difficult to greatly reduce the fat content of most foods without altering the properties of the foods; very low fat spreads, while of a much lower energy density than margarine, are unsuitable for cooking with. Alternatively, low fat versions of some commonly available foods have been so successful that they now dominate the market, for example skimmed and semi-skimmed milks. A few fat mimetics have been developed that possess some or all of fat's sensory properties but which have about half the energy density of fat, or have no metabolisable energy. But, there is currently only a limited range of foods in which these can be used (Stubbs, 2001).

Leveille and Finley note that sucrose can be replaced by an intense sweetener in many drinks since the bulk is largely provided by water. However, replacement of sugars and starches in solid foods is more difficult because of the contribution these carbohydrates make to the physical and sensory properties of foods (Leveille and Finlay, 1997). The use of carbohydrate substitutes will not nearly impact on the energy density of the diet as effectively as replacement of fat with fat substitutes, except for the use of intense sweeteners in soft drinks. The effectiveness of intense sweeteners in reducing energy intakes by reducing carbohydrate intakes is the subject of some controversy. How the use of carbohydrate substitutes will develop in the current 'low-carb revolution', and how this will impact on the energy density of foods and of the overall diet is currently unclear.

The long-term effects of dissociating the sensory cues of foods from their post-ingestive effects are unknown. If foods that maximise the sensory stimulation to eat but contain few calories are effective at achieving weight loss, they may undermine their own purpose. People may learn to dislike these foods because they will become associated with the relatively unpleasant sensations induced by weight loss. Furthermore, using 'low energy density' as a marketing angle may also be counter productive, in much the same way that 'low fat' is regarded by some as a licence to over consume (Shide and Rolls, 1995; Miller *et al.*, 1998). A critical challenge for the food industry is to understand how to maximise postingestive feedback from foods in a way that they enhance satiety but do not decrease learned palatability in the longer term. To do so will require a great quantitative understanding of the way diet composition influences palatability and satiety and how both relate to total energy intake.

It is obvious that adding water to any food will reduce its energy density. However, what is less obvious is the effect that this procedure may have on appetite and feeding behaviour. It appears that a critical factor is the extent to which the water remains bound to the food matrix in the gut (D. Mela, personal communication). The exact effect that fluid intake exerts on food and energy intake is currently unclear and is an area that requires investigation.

The composition and properties of unmodified low-fat (high-carbohydrate) foods have remained stable over time. People will have learned to associate the taste, texture and flavour of such foods with the post-ingestive consequences of having regularly ingested them. The sensory qualities of these foods reliably inform of the post-ingestive consequences of their ingestion, and conditioned (or learned) appetites for these foods are likely to be stable. Fruits and vegetables are, with a few exceptions, low in both fat and energy density. Furthermore, there is weak evidence that increased fibre intake has mild to moderate effects on reducing motivation to eat and increasing satiety (Levine and Billington, 1994; Delargy *et al.*, 1997). Finding ways of increasing the contribution of fruits and vegetables to Western type diets remains a public health holy grail.

Manufactured foods tend to be energy dense, and therefore palatable, for the simple reason that we like them and are prepared to buy them. Obviously the food industry cannot market unpalatable foods, but consumers could be guided towards foods that are less likely to elevate energy intakes. One option that is suggested occasionally is to make 'unhealthy' food choices less attractive by introducing a 'fat-tax'. It is currently difficult to see this being implemented, at least at a sufficient level to impact on the cost difference between, for example, processed convenience foods, and fruits and vegetables. Such a tax is likely to be too unpopular with the food industry and consumers.

9.9 Conclusions

The main factors that influence the energy density of individual foods, and the overall diet, are fat and water content. Dietary energy density influences energy intake, but the large effects seen in controlled laboratory experiments are diminished when people are consuming normal, unmodified, foods in the wild. Although we tend to prefer the more energy dense foods, partly because they tend to be more palatable, we learn to consume them in smaller portions or less frequently. However, there is still an elevated risk of overconsumption on a highly energy dense diet. This, when combined with the current, Western, environment with its vast range of inexpensive, energy dense and highly palatable foods is contributing to the current secular trend of increasing levels of obesity.

9.10 References

ANDERSON, A. S., COX, D. N., MCKELLAR, S., REYNOLDS, J., LEAN, M. E. and MELA, D. J. (1998), Take Five, a nutrition education intervention to increase fruit and vegetable intakes: impact on attitudes towards dietary change. *British Journal of Nutrition* **80**, 133–40.

BAER, D. J., RUMPLER, W. V., MILES, C. W. and FAHEY, G. C. (1997), Dietary fiber decreases the metabolizable energy content and nutrient digestibility of mixed diets fed to humans. *Journal of Nutrition* **127** (4), 579–86.

BELL, E. A., CASTELLANOS, V. H., PELKMAN, C. L., THORWART, M. L. and ROLLS, B. J. (1998), Energy density of foods affects energy intake in normal-weight women. *American Journal of Clinical Nutrition* **67**, 412–20.

BIRCH, L. L. (1998), Development of food acceptance patterns in the first years of life. *Proceedings of the Nutrition Society* **57** (4), 617–24.

BLACK, A. E., GOLDBERG, G. R., JEBB, S. A., LIVINGSTONE, M. B. E., COLE, T. J. and PRENTICE, A. M. (1991), Critical-evaluation of energy-intake data using fundamental principles of energy physiology. 2. Evaluating the results of published surveys. *European Journal of Clinical Nutrition* **45** (12), 583–99.

BLUNDELL, J. E. and COOLING, J. (2000), Routes to obesity: phenotypes, food choices and activity. *British Journal of Nutrition* **83**, S33–8.

BLUNDELL, J. E. and MACDIARMID, J. I. (1997), Passive overconsumption. Fat intake and short-term energy balance. *Annals of the New York Academy of Science* **827**, 392–407.

BLUNDELL, J. E. and STUBBS, R. J. (1997), Diet and food intake in Humans. *International Handbook of Obesity*, ed. G. A. Bray, C. Bouchard and W. P. T. James. New York, Marcel Dekker Inc.: 243–72.

BLUNDELL, J. E. and STUBBS, R. J. (1999), High and low carbohydrate and fat intakes: limits imposed by appetite and palatability and their implications for energy balance. *European Journal of Clinical Nutrition* **53** (Suppl. 1), S148–65.

BOOTH, D., LEE, M. and MCALEAVEY, C. (1976), Acquired sensory control of satiation in man. *British Journal of Psychology* **67**, 137–47.

BRAY, G. A. and POPKIN, B. M. (1998), Dietary fat intake does affect obesity! *American Journal of Clinical Nutrition* **68** (6), 1157–73.

CAIRNS, M. C., COOPER, J. J., DAVIDSON, H. P. B. and MILLS, D. S. (2002), Association in horses of orosensory characterstics of foods with their-post-ingestive consequences. *Animal Science* **75**, 257–65.

CAVADINI, C., SIEGA-RIZ, A. M. and POPKIN, B. M. (2000), US adolescent food intake trends from 1965 to 1996. *Western Journal of Medicine* **173** (6), 378–83.

COOKE, E. A., GUSS, J. L., KISSILEFF, H. R., DEVLIN, M. J. and WALSH, B. T. (1997), Patterns of food selection during binges in women with binge eating disorder. *International Journal of Eating Disorders* **22** (2), 187–93.

COOLING, J. and BLUNDELL, J. E. (1998), Are high-fat and low-fat consumers distinct phenotypes? Differences in the subjective and behavioural response to energy and nutrient challenges. *European Journal of Clinical Nutrition* **52**, 193–201.

COX, D. N. and MELA, D. J. (2000), Determination of energy density of freely selected diets: methodological issues and implications. *International Journal of Obesity* **24** (1), 49–54.

COX, D. N., PERRY, L., MOORE, P. B., VALLIS, L. and MELA, D. J. (1999), Sensory and hedonic associations with macronutrient and energy intakes of lean and obese consumers. *International Journal of Obesity* **23** (4), 403–10.

CROWE, T. C., LA FONTAINE, H. A., GIBBONS, C. J., CAMERON-SMITH, D. and SWINBURN, B. A. (2004), Energy density of foods and beverages in the Australian food supply: influence of macronutrients and comparison to dietary intake. *European Journal of Clinical Nutrition* **58** (11), 1485–91.

DE CASTRO, J. M. (1987), Macronutrient relationships with meal patterns and mood in the spontaneous feeding-behavior of humans. *Physiology and Behavior* **39** (5), 561–9.

DE CASTRO, J. M. (2000), Eating behavior: Lessons from the real world of humans. *Nutrition* **16** (10), 800–13.

DE CASTRO, J. M. (2001a), Heritability of diurnal changes in food intake in free-living humans. *Nutrition* **17** (9), 713–20.

DE CASTRO, J. M. (2001b), Palatability and intake relationships in free-living humans: the influence of heredity. *Nutrition Research* **21** (7), 935–45.

DE CASTRO, J. M., BELLISLE, F. and DALIX, A. M. (2000a), Palatability and intake relationships in free-living humans: measurement and characterization in the French. *Physiology and Behavior* **68** (3), 271–7.

DE CASTRO, J. M., BELLISLE, F., DALIX, A. M. and PEARCEY, S. M. (2000b), Palatability and intake relationships in free-living humans: characterization and independence of influence in North Americans. *Physiology and Behavior* **70** (3–4), 343–50.

DE CASTRO, J. M. and PLUNKETT, S. (2002), A general model of intake regulation. *Neuroscience and Biobehavioral Reviews* **26** (5), 581–95.

DE GRAAF, C., DRIJVERS, J. J. M. M., ZIMMERMANNS, N. J. H. *et al.* (1997), Energy and fat compensation during long-term consumption of reduced fat products. *Appetite* **29**, 305–23.

DEFRA (2001), *National Food Survey 2000*, Department for Environment, Food and Rural Affairs.

DELARGY, H. J., O'SULLIVAN, K. R., FLETCHER, R. J. and BLUNDELL, J. E. (1997), Effects of amount and type of dietary fibre (soluble and insoluble) on short-term control of appetite. *International Journal of Food Science and Nutrition* **48**, 67–77.

DIMEGLIO, D. P. and MATTES, R. D. (2000), Liquid versus solid carbohydrate: effects on food intake and body weight. *International Journal of Obesity* **24** (6), 794–800.

DOH (1991), *Dietary Reference Values for Food Energy and Nutrients for the United Kingdom*. London, HMSO.

DREWNOWSKI, A. (1992), Cognitive aspects of taste and food preferences. *International Journal of Psychology* **27** (3–4), 182.

DREWNOWSKI, A. (1998), Energy density, palatability, and satiety: implications for weight control. *Nutrition Reviews* **56** (12), 347–53.

DREWNOWSKI, A. (2004), Obesity and the food environment. Dietary energy density and diet costs. *American Journal of Preventative Medicine* **27** (S3), 154–62.

FAROOQI, I. S., MATARESE, G., LORD, G. M. *et al.* (2002), Beneficial effects of leptin on obesity, T cell hyporesponsiveness, and neuroendocrine/metabolic dysfunction of human congenital leptin deficiency. *Journal of Clinical Investigation* **110** (8), 1093–103.

FERRIS, S., WHYBROW, S. and STUBBS, R. J. (2001), Dietary and phenotypic determinants of energy intake 102 UK adults. *International Journal of Obesity* **25** (Suppl2), S56.

FORBES, J. M. (1995), *Voluntary Food Intake and Diet Selection in Farm Animals.* Oxon, CAB International.

GARROW, J. S. (1988), Is obesity an eating disorder. *Journal of Psychosomatic Research* **32**, 585–90.

GATENBY, S. J., AARON, J. I., MORTON, G. M. and MELA, D. J. (1995), Nutritional implications of reduced-fat food use by free-living consumers. *Appetite* **25** (3), 241–52.

GIBSON, S. A. (2000), Associations between energy density and macronutrient composition in the diets of pre-school children: sugars *vs.* starch. *International Journal of Obesity* **24** (5), 633–8.

GOLDBERG, G. R., BLACK, A. E., JEBB, S. A., COLE, T. J., MURGATROYD, P. R., COWARD, W. A. and PRENTICE, A. M. (1991), Critical-evaluation of energy-intake data using fundamental principles of energy physiology. 1. Derivation of cutoff limits to identify under-recording. *European Journal of Clinical Nutrition* **45** (12), 569–81.

HETHERINGTON, M. M., ALTEMUS, M., NELSON, M. L., BERNAT, A. S. and GOLD, P. W. (1994), Eating behavior in bulimia-nervosa – multiple meal analyses. *American Journal of Clinical Nutrition* **60** (6), 864–73.

HILL, A. J. and BLUNDELL, J. E. (1989), Comparison of the action of macronutrients on the expression of appetite in lean and obese human-subjects. *Annals of the New York Academy of Sciences* **575**, 529–31.

HILL, A. J., MAGSON, L. D. and BLUNDELL, J. E. (1984), Hunger and palatability – tracking ratings of subjective experience before, during and after the consumption of preferred and less preferred food. *Appetite* **5** (4), 361–71.

HOLLAND, B., WELCH, A. A., UNWIN, I. D., BUSS, D. H., PAUL, A. A. and SOUTHGATE, D. A. T. (1991), *The Composition of Foods*. Cambridge, The Royal Society of Chemistry and Ministry of Agriculture, Fisheries and Food.

HOLT, S. H., MILLER, J. C., PETOCZ, P. and FARMAKALIDIS, E. (1995), A satiety index of common foods. *European Journal of Clinical Nutrition* **49**, 675–90.

HOWARTH, N. C., SALTZMAN, E. and ROBERTS, S. B. (2001), Dietary fiber and weight regulation. *Nutrition Reviews* **59** (5), 129–39.

JOHNSON, R. K. and FRARY, C. (2001), Choose beverages and foods to moderate your intake of sugars: the 2000 Dietary Guidelines for Americans – what's all the fuss about? *Journal of Nutrition* **131** (10), 2766S–71S.

JOHNSON, S. L., MCPHEE, L. and BIRCH, L. L. (1991), Conditioned preferences – young-children prefer flavors associated with high dietary-fat. *Physiology and Behavior* **50** (6), 1245–51.

JOHNSTONE, A. M., SHANNON, E. L., WHYBROW, S., REID, C. A. and STUBBS, R. J. (2000), Altering the temporal distribution of energy intake with isoenergetically dense foods given as snacks does not affect total daily energy intake in normal weight men. *British Journal of Nutrition* **83** (1), 7–14.

KANT, A. K., GRAUBARD, B. I., SCHATZKIN, A. and BALLARD BARBASH, R. (1995), Proportion of energy intake from fat and subsequent weight change in the NHANES I Epidemiologic Follow-up Study. *American Journal of Clinical Nutrition* **61**, 11–17.

KERN, D. L., MCPHEE, L., FISHER, J., JOHNSON, S. and BIRCH, L. L. (1993), The postingestive consequences of fat condition preferences for flavors associated with high dietary-fat. *Physiology and Behavior* **54** (1), 71–6.

KEYS, A., BREZEK, J., HENSCHEL, A., MICKELSEN, O. and TAYLOR, H. L. (1950), *The Biology of Human Starvation*. Minneapolis, University of Minnesota Press.

KISSILEFF, H. R. (1990), Some suggestions in dealing with palatability – response to Ramirez. *Appetite* **14**, 162–6.

LAPPALAINEN, R., MENNEN, L., VAN WEERT, L. and MYKKANEN, H. (1993), Drinking water with a meal: a simple method of coping with feelings of hunger, satiety and desire to eat. *European Journal of Clinical Nutrition* **47**, 815–19.

LAWTON, G. L., DELARGY, H. J., BROCKMAN, J., SMITH, F. C. and BLUNDELL, J. E. (2000), The degree of saturation of fatty acids influences post-ingestive satiety. *British Journal of Nutrition* **83** (5), 473–82.

LE MAGNEN, J. (1971), Advances in studies on the physiological control and regulation of food intake. *Progress in Physiological Psychology*. E. Stellar and J. M. Sprague. New York, Academic Press. **4**, 203–61.

LEVEILLE, G. A. and FINLAY, J. W. (1997), Macronutrient substitutes: description and uses. *Annals of the New York Academy of Sciences* **819**, 11–21.

LEVINE, A. S. and BILLINGTON, C. J. (1994), Dietary fiber: does it affect food intake and body weight? *Appetite and Body Weight Regulation: Sugar, Fat and Macronutrient Substitutes*. J. D. Fernstrom and G. D. Miller. Boca Raton, FL, CRC Press Inc: 191–200.

LISSNER, L. and HEITMANN, B. L. (1995), Dietary-fat and obesity – evidence from epidemiology. *European Journal of Clinical Nutrition* **49** (2), 79–90.

MAYER, J. (1955), Regulation of energy intake and the body weight – the glucostatic theory and the lipostatic hypothesis. *Annals of the New York Academy of Sciences* **63** (1), 15–43.

MAZLAN, N., HORGAN, G. and STUBBS, R. J. (2001), Mandatory snacks rich in sugar, starch or fat; effect on energy and nutrient intake. *International Journal of Obesity* **25** (Suppl. 2), S54.

MCCRORY, M. A., FUSS, P. J., MCCALLUM, J. E. *et al.* (1999), Dietary variety within food groups: association with energy intake and body fatness in men and women. *American Journal of Clinical Nutrition* **69** (3), 440–7.

MCCRORY, M. A., FUSS, P. J., SALTZMAN, E. and ROBERTS, S. B. (2000), Dietary determinants of energy intake and weight regulation in healthy adults. *Journal of Nutrition* **130** (2S Suppl.), 276S–9S.

MEISELMAN, H. L., WATERMAN, D. and SYMINGTON, L. E. (1974), Armed forces food preferences, US Armt Natrick Development Center Technical Report.

MELA, D. and ROGERS, P. (1998), *Food Eating and Obesity: The Psychobiological Basis of Appetite and Weight Control*. London, Chapman & Hall.

MELA, D. J. and SACCHETTI, D. A. (1991), Sensory Preferences For Fats – Relationships With Diet and Body-Composition. *American Journal of Clinical Nutrition* **53** (4), 908–15.

MILLER, D. L., CASTELLANOS, V. H., SHIDE, D. J., PETERS, J. C. and ROLLS, B. J. (1998), Effect of fat-free potato chips with and without nutrition labels on fat and energy intakes. *American Journal of Clinical Nutrition* **68**, 282–90.

O'DOHERTY, J., ROLLS, E. T., FRANCIS, S. *et al.* (2000), Sensory-specific satiety-related olfactory activation of the human orbitofrontal cortex. *Neuroreport* **11** (4), 893–7.

PRENTICE, A. M. and JEBB, S. A. (2003), Fast foods, energy density and obesity: a possible mechanistic link. *Obesity Reviews* **4**, 187–94.

PRENTICE, A. M. and POPPITT, S. D. (1996), Importance of energy density and macronutrients in the regulation of energy intake. *International Journal of Obesity* **20**: S18–23.

RAMIREZ, I. (1990), What do we mean when we say palatable food? *Appetite* **14** (3), 159–61.

REED, D. R., TORDOFF, M. G. and FRIEDMAN, M. I. (1990), Sham-feeding of corn-oil by rats – sensory and postingestive factors. *Physiology and Behavior* **47** (4), 779–81.

ROGERS, P. J. (1990), Why a palatability construct is needed – comment. *Appetite* **14** (3), 167–70.

ROLLS, B. J. and BELL, E. A. (1999), Intake of fat and carbohydrate: role of energy density. *European Journal of Clinical Nutrition* **53**, S166–73.

ROLLS, B. J. and BELL, E. A. (2000), Dietary approaches to the treatment of obesity. *Medical Clinics of North America* **84** (2), 401-18.

ROLLS, B. J., BELL, E. A. and THORWART, M. L. (1999), Water incorporated into a food but not served with a food decreases energy intake in lean women. *American Journal of Clinical Nutrition* **70** (4), 448–55.

ROLLS, B. J., CASTELLANOS, V. H., HALFORD, J. C. *et al.* (1998), Volume of food consumed affects satiety in men. *American Journal of Clinical Nutrition* **67**, 1170–7.

ROLLS, B. J., ROLLS, E. T., ROWE, E. A. and SWEENEY, K. (1981), Sensory-specific satiety in man. *Physiology and Behavior* **27** (1), 137–42.

SCHOELLER, D. A. (1990), How accurate is self-reported dietary energy-intake. *Nutrition Reviews* **48** (10), 373–9.

SHERWOOD, N. E., JEFFERY, R. W., FRENCH, S. A., HANNAN, P. J. and MURRAY, D. M. (2000), Predictors of weight gain in the Pound of Prevention study. *International Journal of Obesity* **24** (4), 395–403.

SHIDE, D. J. and ROLLS, B. J. (1995), Information about the fat content of preloads influences energy intake in healthy women. *Journal of the American Dietetic Association* **95**, 993–8.

SPITZER, L. and RODIN, J. (1981), Human eating behaviour: a critical review of studies in normal weight and overweight individuals. *Journal for Intake Research* **2**, 293–9.

STEPHEN, A. M. and SIEBER, G. M. (1994), Trends in individual fat consumption in the UK 1900–1985. *British Journal of Nutrition* **71**, 775–88.

STOOKEY, J. D. (2001), Energy density, energy intake and weight status in a large free-living sample of Chinese adults: exploring the underlying roles of fat, protein, carbohydrate, fiber and water intakes. *European Journal of Clinical Nutrition* **55** (5), 349–59.

STUBBS, J., FERRES, S. and HORGAN, G. (2000), Energy density of foods: Effects on energy intake. *Critical Reviews in Food Science and Nutrition* **40** (6), 481–515.

STUBBS, R. J. (1998), Appetite, feeding behaviour and energy balance in human subjects. *Proceedings of the Nutrition Society* **57** (3), 341–56.

STUBBS, R. J. (2001), The effect of ingesting olestra-based foods on feeding behavior and energy balance in humans. *Critical Reviews in Food Science and Nutrition* **41** (5), 363–86.

STUBBS, R. J. and HARBRON, C. G. (1996), Covert manipulation of the ratio of medium- to long-chain triglycerides in isoenergetically dense diets: effect on food intake in *ad libitum* feeding men. *International Journal of Obesity* **20**, 435–44.

STUBBS, R. J., JOHNSTONE, A. M., HARBRON, C. G. and REID, C. (1998a), Covert manipulation of energy density of high carbohydrate diets in 'pseudo free-living' humans. *International Journal of Obesity* **22** (9), 885–92.

STUBBS, R. J., JOHNSTONE, A. M., O'REILLY, L. M., BARTON, K. and REID, C. (1998b), The effect of covertly manipulating the energy density of mixed diets on *ad libitum* food intake in 'pseudo free-living' humans. *International Journal of Obesity* **22** (10), 980–7.

STUBBS, R. J., JOHNSTONE, A. M., O'REILLY, L. M. and POPPITT, S. D. (1998c), Methodological issues relating to the measurement of food, energy and nutrient intake in human laboratory-based studies. *Proceedings of the Nutrition Society* **57**, 357–72.

STUBBS, R. J., MAZLAN, N. and WHYBROW, S. (2001), Carbohydrates, appetite and feeding behavior in humans. *Journal of Nutrition* **131** (10), 2775S–81S.

TORDOFF, M. G. and REED, D. R. (1991), Sham-feeding sucrose or corn-oil stimulates food-intake in rats. *Appetite* **17** (2), 97–103.

WESTERTERP-PLANTENGA, M. S. (2001), Analysis of energy density of food in relation to energy intake regulation in human subjects. *British Journal of Nutrition* **85** (3), 351–61.

WESTERTERP-PLANTENGA, M. S., WIJCKMANS-DUIJSENS, N. E., VERBOEKET-VAN DE VENNE, W. P., DE GRAAF, K. and VAN HET HOF, K. H. (1998), Energy intake and body weight effects of six months reduced or full fat diets, as a function of dietary restraint. *International Journal of Obesity* **22**, 14–22.

WESTSTRATE, J. A. (1992), Effects of nutrients on the regulation of food intake. *Unilever Research*.

WHYBROW, S., MAYER, C., KIRK, T. R. and STUBBS, R. J. (2004), The effect of snack composition on energy intake and body weight. *Proceedings of the Nutrition Society*.

YAO, M. J. and ROBERTS, S. B. (2001), Dietary energy density and weight regulation. *Nutrition Reviews* **59** (8), 247–58.

YEOMANS, M. R. (1996), Palatability and the micro-structure of feeding in humans. The appetizer effect. *Appetite* **27** (2), 119–33.

YEOMANS, M. R. (1998), Taste, palatability and the control of appetite. *Proceedings of the Nutrition Society* **57** (4), 609–15.

YEOMANS, M. R., GRAY, R. W., MITCHELL, C. J. and TRUE, S. (1997), Independent effects of palatability and within-meal pauses on intake and appetite ratings in human volunteers. *Appetite* **29**, 61–76.

ZIZZA, C., SIEGA-RIZ, A. M. and POPKIN, B. M. (2001), Significant increase in young adults' snacking between 1977–1978 and 1994–1996 represents a cause for concern! *Preventive Medicine* **32** (4), 303–10.

10

Dietary fat and weight control

M. Noakes, CSIRO Health Sciences and Nutrition, Australia

10.1 Introduction

It has been argued that the dramatic increase in the prevalence of obesity around the world is primarily due to environmental factors, in particular sedentary lifestyles and consumption of high-fat and energy-dense diets (WHO, 1998). Fat is high in energy and high-fat foods are high in energy density, reducing this macronutrient would appear to be a logical strategy for weight management. However, some (Drewnowski *et al.*, 2004) but not all studies (Crowe *et al.*, 2004) argue that the energy density of foods is not necessarily related to fat content but is inversely related to the water content of foods.

Although some cross-sectional epidemiological studies have linked dietary energy density with higher body mass index (BMI) values, the data are not consistent. At this time, there are no longitudinal cohort data linking dietary energy density with higher obesity risk.

Furthermore, the weight loss observed on *ad libitum* very low carbohydrate high-fat diets (Foster *et al.*, 2003) suggests that reduction of fat and energy density alone may not provide the exclusive strategy for weight management as other dietary factors are clearly involved.

Hence, although dietary fat reduction has been recommended as a useful weight management strategy (Bray and Popkin, 1998; WHO, 1998), the causal link between dietary fat and obesity has been challenged (Shah and Garg, 1996; Willett, 1998).

This chapter is based on a revised and updated version of the Australian National Heart Foundation's Review Paper 'A review of the relationship between dietary fat and overweight/obesity (Sept. 2003)' http://www.heartfoundation.com.au/

The specific research questions of this review were:

- to determine whether dietary fat as a proportion of energy intake is a risk factor for the development and progression of overweight and obesity;
- to assess the effectiveness of fat reduction strategies relative to other dietary strategies for achieving weight loss in overweight and obese individuals and weight maintenance in normal weight, overweight and obese individuals.

10.2 Dietary fat and obesity: epidemiological studies

10.2.1 Ecological studies

Between-population studies have used aggregate level population data (usually national food balance data) and found a positive association between consumption of dietary fat (percent energy from fat) and BMI (Bray and Popkin, 1998). However, it is generally acknowledged that the suggestion that this is a causal relationship is confounded due to differences in physical activity levels, smoking, availability and variety of food, affluence as well as the variable quality of the data (Willett, 1999; Bray and Popkin, 1998; Lissner and Heitmann, 1995).

10.2.2 Cross-sectional studies

Many cross-sectional studies have been conducted in individuals within the same population to examine the correlation between intake of dietary fat (mainly percent energy from fat) and body fatness (mainly BMI). Most cross-sectional studies provide statistical evidence of an association (correlation coefficients ranging from 0.17 to 0.38) between percent energy from fat and body fat in free-living populations. However, a number of studies have reported no association (Lissner and Heitmann, 1995). Similarly, results from cross-sectional studies in children are inconsistent (Davies, 1997; Gazzaniga and Burns, 1993; Guillaume *et al.*, 1998; Lissner and Heitmann, 1995). Shah identified four cross-sectional studies which had controlled for all potential confounders. Two studies reported an inverse and no relationship between obesity and energy or fat intake, whereas the other two found obese individuals consumed more energy and more dietary fat (independent of energy intake) than lean individuals (Shah and Garg, 1996). However, percent energy from fat explained only 1.6% of the total variation in body fat (Shah and Garg, 1996).

Larson *et al.* (1996) examined the relation between fat intake (3-D food records) and intraabdominal adipose tissue in 349 white middle-aged subjects by computed tomography. After adjustment for fat-free mass, sex, age, physical activity, and nonfat energy intake, fat intake was weakly correlated with fat mass, explaining only 2% of the variance (partial $R_2 = 0.018$, $P <$

0.01). In a separate model that evaluated type of fat, saturated fat was positively related (partial $R_2 = 0.025$, $P < 0.01$) to fat mass after adjustment for fat-free mass, sex, age, physical activity, and nonfat energy intake whereas polyunsaturated fat intake was negatively related (partial $R_2 = 0.007$, $P = 0.056$). The authors conclude that this cross-sectional analysis suggests that dietary fat independently plays a very minor role in increasing overall fat mass and does not specifically influence intraabdominal fat.

Since indices of obesity and dietary fat intake are measured simultaneously, cross-sectional studies are not considered sufficient to establish causation (Sempos *et al.*, 1999).

10.3 Dietary fat and obesity: cohort studies

10.3.1 Adults

Participants were selected from health surveys (Rissanen *et al.*, 1991; Paeratakul *et al.*, 1998; Klesges *et al.*, 1992; Jorgensen *et al.*, 1995), on-going cohorts (Colditz *et al.*, 1990; Lissner *et al.*, 1997; Heitmann *et al.*, 1995; Jorgensen *et al.*, 1995) or recruited via advertisements (Kant *et al.*, 1995). Follow-up varied from around 70 to 90%. Baseline dietary fat intake was measured using a range of methodologies and averaged approximately 37% energy from fat in most studies, except for one study conducted in China (about 20% energy from fat). Only one study measured dietary fat intake more than once (Klesges *et al.*, 1992). Most studies analysed the association between weight change and dietary fat as continuous variables. Lissner *et al.* (1997) compared weight change in high fat consumers (>38.5% energy from fat) with low fat consumers (<38.5% energy from fat). Only one study stratified dietary intake according to quartiles of % energy from fat but found that there were no clear trends between quartiles of % energy from fat and weight change in men or women (Kant *et al.*, 1995). Although all studies controlled for total energy intake, not all possible confounding factors were controlled making it difficult to compare study results.

Two studies have reported no association between dietary fat and weight change (Jorgensen *et al.*, 1995; Parker *et al.*, 1997). Another study reported a positive association between dietary fat and weight change (Klesges *et al.*, 1992). The positive association between dietary fat and weight change reported in other studies was dependent on age (Kant *et al.*, 1995), gender (Rissanen *et al.*, 1991; Paeratakul *et al.*, 1998; Kant *et al.*, 1995), health status (Kant *et al.*, 1995), activity levels (Lissner *et al.*, 1997), and genetic predisposition (Heitmann *et al.*, 1995).

The National Health and Nutrition Examination Survey (NHANES) I Epidemiologic Follow-up Study showed no significant association of percent fat energy with weight change in men but was inversely related in women aged <50 y. The association between % energy from dietary fat and weight change in both men and women appears to be stronger in younger people (Kant *et al.*, 1995).

Several studies reported differences in the association between % energy from fat and weight change according to gender. In Finland, neither the intake of energy nor that of any of the macronutrients predicted weight gain in men. In Finnish women, the risk of gaining five or more kilograms in 5.7 years in the highest quintile of intake of energy (*RR* = 2.0 (95% CI,1.2–3.3)), fat (*RR* = 1.7 (95% CI,1.1–2.7)), carbohydrate (*RR* = 1.7 (95% CI,1.0–2.6)), and protein (*RR* = 2.0 (95% CI,1.2–3.3)), was almost twice that of the lowest quintile, after adjusting for potential confounders (Rissanen *et al.*, 1991). In contrast, studies in China and the USA suggest that the association is positive in men but not in women (Kant *et al.*, 1995; Paeratakul *et al.*, 1998).

The Nurses' Health Study suggests dietary intake changes as a result of weight gain (Colditz *et al.*, 1990). Prior to weight gain, there was a positive relationship between weight gain and intakes (grams per day) of total and type of dietary fat as well as sucrose. After subsequent weight gain, an inverse relationship was found between weight gain and total fat, vegetable fat, trans fatty acid, oleic acid, linoleic acid and sucrose.

Physical activity and genetic predisposition was shown to modify the effect of dietary fat on weight gain in women (Lissner *et al.*, 1997; Heitmann *et al.*, 1995). Dietary fat intake was associated with weight gain in sedentary women but not in active women (Lissner *et al.*, 1997). Sedentary women consuming a high fat diet (42.3% energy from fat and 100.2 g fat/day) gained 2.6 kg over 6 years whereas those on a low fat diet (34.1% energy from fat and 73.2 g fat/day) lost 0.6 kg.

Genetically predisposed women, with one or more obese parents, were more susceptible to weight gain when exposed to high dietary fat intakes (Heitmann *et al.*, 1995). Women predisposed to obesity who consumed a diet consisting of 40–45% energy from fat gained 3.5–5.2 kg over 6 years.

The effect of diet on weight gain is small when compared to the effect other non dietary factors have on weight gain. Diet was less predictive of body fat or weight than non dietary factors, particularly physical activity, age and prior weight gain (Rissanen *et al.*, 1991; Colditz *et al.*, 1990; Jorgensen *et al.*, 1995). In men, an increase in fat intake of 100 kcal was associated with an increase in BMI of 0.036 kg/m^2. In comparison, an increase in physical activity by one level (physical activity levels were divided into sedentary, moderate and strenuous according to reported physical activity level at occupation) was associated with a decrease in BMI of 0.12 kg/m^2 in women (Paeratakul *et al.*, 1998). For both genders, an average increase in age of about two years was associated with an increase in BMI of about 0.11 kg/m^2 (Paeratakul *et al.*, 1998). Colditz found that age and prior weight gain were much stronger predictors of weight change than dietary intake (Colditz *et al.*, 1990).

The cross-sectional and prospective relationship between fat intake and body weight in the Pound of Prevention study found that the determinants of weight gain are multifactorial and that exercise, fat intake and total energy intake are all important for long term control of body weight (Sherwood *et al.*, 2000).

Mosca *et al.* (2004) investigated whether insulin resistance modifies the rate of weight gain associated with a high proportion of dietary fat in a longitudinal study in 782 non-diabetic Hispanic and non-Hispanic white subjects who were seen up to three times over a 14-y period. Percentage of energy intake from dietary fat was positively associated with weight gain over time ($P = 0.0103$). High intake of dietary fat was more strongly related to weight gain in women than in men, and in those with insulin resistance.

10.3.2 Children

Several cohort studies have been conducted in children. Measurement of obesity in children is problematic due to differences in growth patterns. A simple measure of body fat, such as BMI, is not ideal for assessing obesity in children because it covaries with height (Bellizzi and Dietz, 1999). Until recently, there has not been an internationally acceptable index to assess childhood obesity nor an established cut-off to define overweight in children (Bellizzi and Dietz, 1999). Consequently, obesity has been assessed and defined differently in studies, making it difficult to compare results.

A 3-year study in 146 American preschool children aged 4 years found baseline levels of % energy from fat were positively associated with changes in obesity status based on 1987 Department of Health and Human Services Norms ($P = 0.05$), after adjusting for known risk factors. BMI increased by 0.168 kg/m^2 as % energy from fat increased by 5% over the 3 yrs (Klesges *et al.*, 1995). However, in a cohort of 112 French children, protein intake (% energy from protein) at 2 yrs of age, but not dietary fat intake, was positively correlated with BMI and subscapular skinfold at 8 years after adjustment for energy intake and parental BMI (Rolland-Cachera *et al.*, 1995).

A study in 4-year-old children, selected according to their familial risk of obesity, reported significantly higher dietary fat intakes (34.4% energy from fat; $P = 0.0004$) in the high risk group (defined as having one to two overweight parents) compared to the low risk group (32.1% energy from fat) (Eck *et al.*, 1992). After 1 year, the high risk group gained marginally more weight than the low risk group ($P = 0.05$). However, the difference in weight gain was small (2.5 vs. 2.2 kg) and may have been affected by physical activity, which was marginally lower in the high risk group (Eck *et al.*, 1992).

A 4-year study in 112 children aged an average 8.6 years found that parent's obesity was the main risk factor for obesity and that dietary intake did not significantly affect risk of obesity (defined as relative BMI > 120%) (Maffeis *et al.*, 1998).

A recent analysis of data from an Australian longitudinal study of children (2 to 15 years) over a 13-year-period reported no significant associations between BMI (converted to standard deviation scores) and intake of any macronutrient estimated from 3-day and 4-day weighed food records (Magarey *et al.*, 2000). However, there was a positive association between dietary fat intake (g/day) and tricep ($P < 0.05$) as well as subscapular

($P < 0.01$) skinfolds (converted to standard deviation scores). Dietary fat intake (g/day) at 6 years was a significant predictor of BMI (SD score) at 8 years ($P < 0.01$) and dietary fat intake (g/day) at 2 years was a significant predictor of subscapular skinfolds (SD score) at 15 yrs ($P < 0.01$) (Magarey *et al.*, 2001). Previous body fatness had the greatest effect on subsequent body fatness.

The risk of a high fat mass (defined as percentage of body fat >20% for males and >30% for females and BMI > 25 kg/m^2) estimated from the sum of four skinfolds and body mass, was measured in a Dutch cohort of 13-year-old children who were followed over a period of 20 years until the age of 32 years (Kemper *et al.*, 1999). Lifestyle factors discriminating high- from low-risk participants included physical activity [OR = 0.81 (0.69 to 0.96)] and % energy from protein [OR = 1.5 (1.2 to 1.8)] but not % energy from fat.

10.4 Mechanisms linking dietary fat and weight gain

To confirm whether dietary fat plays a role in the aetiology of overweight and obesity suggested in some cohort studies, biologically plausible mechanisms must be identified which explain how dietary fat might increase the risk of weight gain.

10.4.1 The effect of dietary fat on energy storage

Several experimental studies have shown that protein and carbohydrate promote their own oxidation whereas fat influences its own oxidation only weakly or not at all (Schutz, 1995; Tremblay *et al.*, 1989). An increase in dietary fat intake produces a positive fat balance, whereas an increase in carbohydrate intake results in a negative fat balance (Proserpi *et al.*, 1997; Schutz, 1995). It has therefore been suggested that dietary fat is more efficiently stored than carbohydrate (Proserpi *et al.*, 1997; Schutz, 1995).

The effect of macronutrient composition on fat storage may only be evident when excess energy is available for storage in the adipose tissue. Under conditions of energy balance, the body seems capable of adapting to variations in fat and carbohydrate intake without displacing macronutrient stores (Stubbs *et al.*, 1996). Normal weight subjects can adjust fat oxidation in response to increased fat intake within 7 days, depending on physical activity levels (Schrauwen *et al.*, 1997). A study which provided seven pairs of normal weight identical twins with either a low fat (20% energy from fat) or high fat (40% energy from fat) diet over 18 days reported no differences in fat oxidation rates between the two diets. Instead, post-prandial fat and carbohydrate oxidation rates tended to reflect the diet's macronutrient ratios (Salzman *et al.*, 1997).

Horton *et al.* (1995) calculated energy storage in assessing the effects of carbohydrate and fat in an overfeeding study lasting 14 days. Although carbohydrate overfeeding resulted in 75 to 85% of excess energy being stored compared to 90 to 95% with fat overfeeding, there was no significant difference between diets in body weight or body composition. By the end of the study (14 days), there was no difference in the proportion of total stored energy stored as body fat. More recently, a 96-hour continuous whole-body calorimetry study provided 50% excess energy as either fat or different sources of carbohydrate and reported no differences in macronutrient oxidation or fat balance in lean and obese women (McDevitt *et al.*, 2000). The authors concluded that the effect of diet type on fat balance is not mediated through differences in their metabolic actions with respect to disposal or total energy expenditure.

10.4.2 The effect of dietary fat on energy expenditure

The components of energy expenditure consists of diet-induced thermogenesis, the basal metabolic rate (BMR) and physical activity. The contribution of diet-induced thermogenesis remains constant at about 10% whereas the contribution of BMR varies from 40 to 60%, depending on the level of physical activity (WHO, 1998).

A study comparing energy balance of six normal weight men in a calorimeter with that of free-living conditions found subjects on the medium fat diet (40% energy from fat) in the sedentary condition were in positive energy balance whereas in the free-living condition, they were in negative energy balance (Stubbs *et al.*, 1995). This study demonstrates the critical role physical activity can play in preventing positive energy balance.

In conditions of energy balance, no differences in energy expenditure have been reported over a range of diets containing from 10% to 80% energy from fat (Prentice, 1998).

10.4.3 The effect of dietary fat on energy intake

Since dietary fat is highly correlated with energy density, it has been proposed that together with its palatability, dietary fat creates a 'fat-related hyperphagia', overriding normal signals of satiety and leading to passive overconsumption (Blundell and Stubbs, 1999). Crowe *et al.* (2004) found that, for both individual foods and diets, there was a positive relationship between energy density and percentage energy as fat and negative relationships between energy density and percentage energy as carbohydrate and percentage water by weight.

Several studies suggest that dietary fat exerts relatively weak effects on satiation and satiety compared to carbohydrate and protein (Blundell *et al.*, 1993). Satiety refers to the effects of a specific food or meal on subsequent food intake after eating has ended. Satiation refers to the processes involved in the termination of a meal.

Studies conducted over 2 to 11 weeks in normal weight women and men reported significantly higher energy density and energy intake on high-fat diets (40 to 60% energy from fat) than on low-fat diets (20 to 25% energy from fat) resulting in positive energy balance and weight gain (Stubbs *et al.*, 1995; Lissner *et al.*, 1987; Kendall *et al.*, 1991). However, in these studies, both macronutrient composition and energy density varied, making it difficult to separate the effect of dietary fat from energy density.

Studies in which energy density and palatability were kept constant found no effect of dietary fat content on voluntary energy intake in normal weight women and men (Van Stratum *et al.*, 1978; Stubbs *et al.*, 1996; Salzman *et al.*, 1997).

The independent effect of energy density and dietary fat was determined in a study of 17 lean and 17 obese females over 4 days. Energy density was manipulated by varying the water and fibre content of foods. Both lean and obese women reduced energy intake by 16% in the low (4.4 kJ/g) compared to the high (6.7 kJ/g) energy density condition. In contrast, there was no difference in energy intake when the fat content of foods was manipulated from 16% to 36% energy from fat (Rolls, 1999). A recent study in lean and obese women examined the effect of energy density on energy intake using meals representative of the typical American diet. There were no differences between lean and obese women. Both consumed 20% less energy on the low (5.23 kJ/g) than on the high (7.32 kJ/g) energy density condition, irrespective of the fat content of the meals (Bell and Rolls, 2001). These studies suggest that, when palatability and energy density are controlled, fat and carbohydrates have similar effects on energy intake. Hence, energy density, rather than dietary fat *per se*, is a major determinant of energy intake regardless of macronutrient content (Rolls, 2000).

According to Rolls (2000), the water content of foods is a critical determinant of energy density, having a larger effect than fat or fibre.

LaFontaine *et al.* (2004) have noted that, although a reduced-fat diet may be low in energy density and hence may protect against weight gain, there are some exceptions. A high intake of commercially available products with reduced fat claims which are low in moisture content could lead to an energy-dense diet, yet a high intake of vegetable-based foods, even with substantial added fat, could reduce energy density and hence may be considered protective against weight gain.

Energy density does elevate energy intake, especially in short-term studies where it can account for >40% of the variance in energy intake (Stubbs and Whybrow, 2004). However, in real life, energy density accounts for only approximately 7% of the variance in energy intake because the determinants of energy intake are multifactorial and also because the short-term effects of energy density on energy intake do not translate into the longer term due to learned compensation from postingestive consequences of consuming familiar food that differ in energy density (Stubbs and Whybrow, 2004).

10.4.4 Effects of palatability

Both increases in portion size and energy density have been shown to result in independent and additive increases in energy intake (Kral *et al.*, 2004). Subjects consumed 56% more energy (925 kJ) when served the largest portion of the higher energy-dense meal than when served the smallest portion of the lower energy-dense meal and did not compensate by eating less at the next.

Energy-dense foods are generally palatable but not satiating making it difficult to separate these factors from energy density in real life (Drewnowski, 1998). The influence of energy density on energy intake seems in part direct, and in part indirect and mediated by palatability (McCrory *et al.*, 2000). However, fat is only one factor in determining palatability, with sugar and particularly salt for obese subjects being significant contributors (Cox *et al.*, 1999). A study in 11 normal weight and 9 post-obese subjects over 14 days compared the impact of a high sucrose (29% energy from fat; 23% energy from sucrose; 59% energy from carbohydrate) to a high starch (28% energy from fat; 59% energy from carbohydrate; 2% energy from sucrose) and high fat diet (46% energy from fat; 41% energy from carbohydrate; 2% energy from sucrose) on *ad libitum* energy intake and body weight (Raben *et al.*, 1997). The energy density of the high sucrose diet (6.9 kJ/g) was comparable to the high starch diet (6.4 kJ/g) and significantly lower than the high fat diet (8.2 kJ/g). However, average energy intake was significantly higher on the high-sucrose (10.3 MJ/d) than on the high-starch diets (9.1 MJ/d) and comparable to the high-fat diet (10.2 ± 0.4 MJ/d). Consequently, there was a significant decrease in body weight (0.7 kg; $P < 0.05$) on the high-starch diet compared to the high-sucrose and high-fat diets. Although the high-sugar and high-fat diets differed significantly in terms of energy density, they had similar impacts on energy intake. This study therefore suggests that factors affecting satiety such as the palatability of the diet and the form of food consumed may also affect energy intake. The high-sucrose diet was the most preferred by subjects and contained large amounts of sucrose-containing drinks which may be less efficient at increasing satiety and suppressing food intake compared with solid foods.

McCrory *et al.* (2000) concluded that energy density, palatability and dietary variety are important dietary components and that these dietary variables may play a greater role than dietary fat *per se* in affecting energy intake and adiposity.

10.5 Low-fat diets and weight loss

10.5.1 Isocaloric energy restricted diets

Several studies have investigated the effect on weight loss of varying the fat and carbohydrate content of isocaloric energy restricted diets. The studies were mainly conducted in obese women. Treatment allocation was randomised in some studies (Powell *et al.*, 1994; Golay *et al.*, 1996a; Lean *et al.*, 1997) but not in others (Alford *et al.*, 1990; Golay *et al.*, 1996b). One study was conducted in a controlled environment and included exercise and a behavioural programme (Golay *et al.*, 1996a). Dietary compliance, based on actual intakes, was measured in free-living subjects in some studies (Powell *et al.*, 1994; Golay *et al.*, 1996b). Alford *et al.* (1990) monitored dietary compliance without reporting actual dietary intakes. Lean *et al.* (1997) did not measure dietary compliance and analysis was based on treatment allocation. Only one study controlled for potential confounders, such as physical activity, baseline scores, caloric intake and deficit in caloric intake between baseline and intervention diets (Powell *et al.*, 1994).

A systematic review by Summerbell *et al.* (1998) compared low-energy, low-fat diets (less than or equal to 30% energy from fat) with low-energy diets that were not low in dietary fat. Low-energy, low-fat diets were as effective as a low-energy diet, which is not low in fat, in achieving weight loss in overweight or obese subjects (Summerbell *et al.*, 1998). This was also found in a Cochrane review by Pirozzo *et al.* (2002). Intervention studies therefore confirm that energy intake, rather than macronutrient composition, is the major determinant of weight loss in overweight and obese individuals.

10.5.2 Low-fat *ad libitum* diets

Several *ad libitum* dietary intervention studies have investigated whether dietary fat increases the risk of weight gain by facilitating excess energy intake in free-living individuals. Studies examined were those specifically designed to investigate the effect of low fat or reduced fat dietary advice on *ad libitum* energy intake and body weight compared to usual dietary intake in normal weight and overweight individuals.

A meta-analysis of 37 low fat dietary intervention studies in free-living subjects lasting more than 3 weeks reported a 0.28 kg decrease in body weight for every 1% decrease in energy as total fat (Yu-Poth *et al.*, 1999). A review of 28 short-term trials of the effect of dietary fat reduction on weight loss in obese individuals showed that a reduction of 10% energy from fat was associated with a reduction in weight of 16 g/day (Bray and Popkin, 1998). A more restrictive meta-analysis of weight loss in 16 *ad libitum* low-fat intervention trials lasting more than 2 months showed that, for every 1% reduction in dietary fat, a weight loss of 0.37 kg (95% CI, 0.15 to 0.60 kg/%) was achieved (Astrup *et al.*, 2000). Astrup *et al.* (2000) reported a weighted difference in weight loss between intervention and control groups of 2.55 kg (95% CI, 1.5 to 3.5; $P < 0.001$). Similarly, Yu-Poth *et al.* found that weight loss in the intervention groups was 2.79 kg larger than in the control group (Yu-Poth *et al.*, 1999).

According to Astrup *et al.* (2000), the effect of *ad libitum* dietary fat reduction on weight loss is dose-dependent. However, Knopp *et al.* (1997) compared diets providing 30%, 26%, 22% and 18% energy from fat and found statistically significant mean reductions in body weight of 2 to 3 kg in each group after 12 months. Energy intake decreased statistically in all diets suggesting that the effect of dietary fat restriction on energy intake was not dose dependent within this range. Reducing dietary fat to 23% energy from fat did not achieve greater weight loss in long term (Sheppard *et al.*, 1991). It is possible that the effect of *ad libitum* dietary fat reduction on energy intake and hence weight loss has a threshold effect with little further gain achieved below 27% energy from fat (Hill *et al.*, 2000).

Since most of these studies were short-term studies (<6 months), it is difficult to predict the long term effect of *ad libitum* dietary fat reduction on body weight. Intervention studies assessing the long-term effect of dietary fat reduction on risk of breast cancer in women suggest weight loss occurs in the first 6 months, with no further weight loss (Lee-Han *et al.*, 1988; Kasim *et al.*, 1993).

Westerterp *et al.* (1996) compared the separate effect of dietary fat reduction and found that men were more sensitive to changes in dietary fat intake than women. Restrained eaters were less likely to gain weight on a high-fat diet (40% energy from fat) than unrestrained eaters (Westerterp-Platenga *et al.*, 1998). Yu-Poth *et al.* (1999) reported significantly greater weight loss in diet intervention with exercise compared to those without exercise. Body weight decreased by 5.66 kg in intervention groups with exercise and by 2.79 kg in intervention groups without exercise (Yu-Poth *et al.*, 1999).

It is unclear whether absolute dietary fat intake (grams) or % energy from fat is more predictive of weight change. Sheppard reported that changes in % energy from fat were more predictive of weight change than changes in total energy intake (Sheppard *et al.*, 1991). Fat reduction of 1% energy from fat in the intervention group resulted in weight loss of 0.1 to 0.25 kg. However, Westerterp *et al.* (1996) reported that change in absolute fat intake explained 70% of the variance in fat mass compared to the fat to carbohydrate ratio which explained only 15%.

10.5.3 High-fat low-carbohydrate *ad libitum* diets

Very low-carbohydrate *ad libitum* diets are unrestricted in dietary fat and hence present an analogous educational strategy of limiting one macronutrient as per low fat *ad libitum* diets. There are surprisingly few studies that have directly compared these two approaches within the same study. A review of very low-carbohydrate diets (<60 g carbohydrate/day or less) from 1966 to early 2003 (Bravata *et al.*, 2003) concluded that weight loss was related to the degree of energy restriction rather than carbohydrate content *per se*. Subsequent to this review there have been a number of studies examining the effect of very low-carbohydrate diets using an *ad libitum* approach as per the Atkins diet.

Body composition was assessed following a very low-carbohydrate diet for 6 weeks in 12 normal weight men and 8 controls (Volek *et al.*, 2002).

Carbohydrate intake decreased from 306 g to 46 g/day with an increase in fat intake from 91 to 157 g while saturated fat increased from 31 g to 56 g. Despite this, fat mass decreased 3.3 kg and lean mass increased by 1.1 kg with no changes in the control group.

A number of randomised controlled trials have subsequently been published which demonstrate that *ad libitum* low-carbohydrate high-fat diets in free living subjects are at least or more effective in achieving weight loss over a 6–12 month period (Sondike *et al.*, 2003; Meckling *et al.*, 2004; Brehm *et al.*, 2003; Foster *et al.*, 2003; Samaha *et al.*, 2003; Stern *et al.*, 2004; Yancy *et al.*, 2004; McAuley *et al.*, 2005). These outcomes seem to be independent of energy density which is higher on the very low-carbohydrate high-fat diet compared to the low-fat dietary pattern. The relative palatability of these dietary patterns has not been reported. It is possible that the satiating effects of higher levels of dietary protein associated with the low-carbohydrate high fat patterns may be implicated in these outcomes which seems to be at odds with the reported effects of energy density (Anderson and Moore, 2004). Concerns about adverse effects on plasma lipids have not been substantiated, suggesting that the effects of weight loss may attenuate any adverse effects of increased saturated fat intake (Noakes and Clifton, 2004; Astrup *et al.*, 2004).

These studies suggest that neither low-fat nor low-carbohydrate dietary patterns are adhered to over longer periods of time and that substantial and regular patient support is needed to achieve sustained weight loss (Knowler *et al.*, 2002). It has been suggested that reduced-carbohydrate dietary patterns may be preferable in reducing the cardiovascular risk profile to low fat high carbohydrate patterns in people with the metabolic syndrome phenotype (Samaha, 2003; Noakes and Clifton, 2004; McAuley *et al.*, 2005).

The above *ad libitum* dietary studies have been conducted in free-living subjects and hence represent the combined effects of behavioural and dietary changes such that energy intake was not controlled. Hence, it is not clear whether these results are caused solely by consequent decreased energy intake or increased energy expenditure. A small preliminary study suggests that, when fat was replaced with carbohydrate in isoenergetic diets in controlled conditions, no differences in fat mass loss has been observed (Segal-Isaacson *et al.*, 2004).

10.6 Summary and conclusions

Evidence from epidemiological, metabolic and intervention studies on the relationship between dietary fat and body weight was inconsistent.

The findings of cohort studies were limited due to the quality of the studies, particularly with respect to the measurement of dietary fat intake. Few studies excluded under-reporters and dietary intake was generally measured only at baseline. Since dietary fat is highly correlated with energy, it is difficult to separate the effect of dietary fat from that of energy. Furthermore, few studies controlled for the confounding effect of physical activity.

In many studies, it was not possible to separate the effect of dietary fat from the behavioural aspects of the treatment diet. Furthermore, many studies included behavioural and lifestyle changes as well as dietary fat reduction strategies.

Metabolic and intervention studies suggest that dietary fat does not directly increase the risk of obesity. It is unlikely that the metabolic effect of dietary fat on energy storage and total energy expenditure increases the risk of overweight (McDevitt *et al.*, 2000). Intervention studies confirm that the energy content, rather than the macronutrient composition, is the most important determinant of weight loss in overweight individuals (Pirozzo *et al.*, 2002).

In many studies, the control group did not receive dietary instruction of the same intensity as the intervention group. Only one study treated intervention and control groups equally (Westerterp *et al.*, 1996). Furthermore, many of these studies included other behavioural and lifestyle changes, making it difficult to determine the independent effect of fat reduction on body weight. The Hawthorne effect describes the modest weight loss achieved during interventions, regardless of the dietary manipulation, as a result of the attention, monitoring and recording provided to the treatment group. In order to determine the independent effect of dietary fat manipulations on weight change, it is preferable to provide the control group with a similar level treatment intensity as the treatment group (Willett, 1999).

A Cochrane systematic review concludes that fat-restricted diets are no better than energy-restricted diets in achieving long term weight loss in overweight or obese people (Pirozzo *et al.*, 2002) confirming that energy intake, rather than fat composition, is the most important dietary determinant of weight loss.

Low-fat *ad libitum* intervention studies and high-fat low-carbohydrate *ad libitum* studies appear to be modestly effective but long-term compliance is poor without ongoing support.

Reducing the overall energy density of the diet to around 5 MJ/g seems to facilitate reduced energy intake. The water content of foods more so than fat content is an important determinant of energy density (Rolls *et al.*, 1999). Hence, including more vegetables in the diet decreases the energy density diets.

Low-fat *ad libitum* diets may help to reduce the energy density of the diet and, in this way, reduce energy intake but effectiveness of this strategy may be limited if highly palatable low-fat foods or energy-dense low-fat foods become widely available. Furthermore, the long-term effectiveness diets low in energy density on weight control needs to be demonstrated. A number of studies have demonstrated that low-fat diets which are higher in dietary protein may have some advantages in short-term and long-term weight management (Luscombe *et al.*, 2003; Skov *et al.*, 1999; Westerterp-Plantenga *et al.*, 2004; McAuley *et al.*, 2005).

Dietary factors, other than energy density, may also impact on energy intake and hence body weight. The palatability and form of the food, such as sugar-containing beverages, may also stimulate energy intake (Raben *et al.*, 1997).

Public health strategies for the prevention of overweight and obesity have encouraged strategies for reducing dietary fat (NHMRC, 1997). However, according to the NIH (1998), and the evidence presented in this review, reducing dietary fat alone without reducing energy intake, is not sufficient for weight loss in overweight and obese individuals. A low-fat diet in addition to portion control and lowering the energy density of foods may assist in the prevention of weight gain but a low-fat diet *per se* represents a small contributor to achieving this goal.

10.7 References

ALFORD B. B., BLANKENSHIP A. C. and HAGEN R. D. (1990), The effects of variations in carbohydrate, protein, and fat content of the diet upon weight loss, blood values, and nutrient intake of adult obese women. *J. Am. Diet. Assoc.*, **90** (4), 534–40.

ANDERSON G. H. and MOORE S. E. (2004 Apr), Dietary proteins in the regulation of food intake and body weight in humans. *J. Nutr.*, **134** (4), 974S–9S.

ASTRUP A., RYAN L. and GRUNWALD G. K. *et al.* (2000), The role of dietary fat in body fatness: evidence from a preliminary meta-analysis of *ad libitum* low-fat dietary intervention studies. *Br. J. Nutr.*, **83** (Suppl 1), S25–32.

ASTRUP A., MEINERT LARSEN T. and HARPER A. (2004 Sep 4), Atkins and other low-carbohydrate diets: hoax or an effective tool for weight loss? *Lancet*, **364** (9437), 897–9.

BELL E. A. and ROLLS B. J. (2001 Jun), Energy density of foods affects energy intake across multiple levels of fat content in lean and obese women. *Am. J. Clin. Nutr.*, **73** (6), 1010–8.

BELLIZZI M. C. and DIETZ W. H. (1999), Workshop on childhood obesity: summary of the discussion. *Am. J. Clin. Nutr.*, **70**, 173S–5S.

BLUNDELL J. E. and STUBBS R. J. (1999), High and low carbohydrate and fat intakes: limits imposed by appetite and palatability and their implications for energy balance. *Eur. J. Clin. Nutr.*, **53** (Suppl 1), S148–65.

BLUNDELL J. E., BURLEY V. J., COTTON J. R. and LAWTON C. L. (1993), Dietary fat and the control of energy intake: evaluating the effects of fat on meal size and postmeal satiety. *Am. J. Clin. Nutr.*, **57** (Suppl), 772S–8S.

BOYD N. F., COUSINS M. and KRIUKOV V. (1992), A randomized controlled trial of dietary fat reduction: the retention of subjects and characteristics of drop outs. *J. Clin. Epidemiol.*, **45**, 31–8.

BRAVATA D. M., SANDERS L. and HUANG J. *et al.* (2003), Efficacy and safety of low-carbohydrate diets: a systematic review. *JAMA*, **289**, 1837–50.

BRAY G. A. and POPKIN B. M. (1998), Dietary fat intake does affect obesity. *Am. J. Clin. Nutr.*, **68**, 1157–73.

BREHM B. J., SEELEY R. J., DANIELS S. R. and D'ALESSIO D. A. (2003), A randomized trial comparing a very low carbohydrate diet and a calorie-restricted low fat diet on body weight and cardiovascular risk factors in healthy women. *J. Clin. Endocrinol. Metab.*, **88**, 1617–23.

COLDITZ G. A., WILLETT W. C., STAMPFER M. J., LONDON S. J., SEGAL M. R. and SPEIZER F. E. (1990), Patterns of weight change and their relation to diet in a cohort of healthy women. *Am. J. Clin. Nutr.*, **51**, 1100–5.

COX D. N., PERRY L., MOORE P. B., VALLIS L. and MELA D. J. (1999 Apr), Sensory and hedonic associations with macronutrient and energy intakes of lean and obese consumers. *Int. J. Obes. Relat. Metab. Disord.*, **23** (4), 403–10.

CROWE T. C., FONTAINE H. L., GIBBONS C. J., CAMERON-SMITH D. and SWINBURN B. A. (2004 Nov), Energy density of foods and beverages in the Australian food supply: influence of macronutrients and comparison to dietary intake. *Eur. J. Clin. Nutr.*, **58** (11), 1485–91.

DAVIES P. S. (1997), Diet composition and body mass index in pre-school children. *Eur. J. Clin. Nutr.*, **51** (7), 443–8.

DREWNOWSKI A. (1998), Energy density, palatability, and satiety: implications for weight control. *Nutr. Revs.*, **56** (12), 347–535.

DREWNOWSKI A., ALMIRON-ROIG E., MARMONIER C. and LLUCH A. (2004 Nov), Dietary energy density and body weight: is there a relationship? *Nutr. Rev.*, **62** (11), 403–13.

ECK L. H., KLESGES R. C., HANSON C. L. and SLAWSON D. (1992), Children at familial risk of obesity: an examination of dietary intake, physical activity and weight status. *Int. J. Obes. Relat. Metab. Disord.*, **16** (2), 71–8.

FOSTER G. D., WYATT H. R., HILL J. O. *et al.* (2003 May 22), A randomized trial of a low-carbohydrate diet for obesity. *N. Engl. J. Med.*, **348** (21), 2082–90.

GAZZANIGA J. M. and BURNS T. L. (1993), Relationship between diet composition and body fatness, with adjustment for resting energy expenditure and physical activity, in preadolescent children. *Am. J. Clin. Nutr.*, **58** (1), 21–8.

GOLAY A., ALLAZ A. F., MOREL Y., DE TONNAC N., TANKOVA S. and REAVEN G. (1996a), Similar weight loss with low- or high-carbohydrate diets. *Am. J. Clin. Nutr.*, **63** (2), 174–8.

GOLAY A., EIGENHEER C., MOREL Y., KUJAWSKI P., LEHMANN T. and DE TONNAC N. (1996b), Weight-loss with low or high carbohydrate diet? *Int. J. Obes. Relat. Metab. Disord.*, **20** (12), 1067–72.

GUILLAUME M., LAPIDUS L. and LAMBERT A. (1998), Obesity and nutrition in children. The Belgian Luxembourg Child Study IV. *Eur. J. Clin. Nutr.*, **52**, 323–8.

HEITMANN B. L. and LISSNER L. (1995 14), Dietary underreporting by obese individuals – is it specific or non-specific? *BMJ*, **311** (7011), 986–9.

HEITMANN B. L., LISSNER L., SORENSEN T. I. A. and BENGTSSON C. (1995), Dietary fat intake and weight gain in women genetically predisposed for obesity. *Am. J. Clin. Nutr.*, **61**, 1213–17.

HILL J. O., MELANSON E. L. and WYATT H. T. (2000), Dietary fat intake and regulation of energy balance: implications for obesity. *J. Nutr.*, **130** (2S Suppl), 284S–8S.

HORTON T., DROUGAS H., BRACHEY A., REED G. W., PETERS J. C. and HILL J. O. (1995), Fat and carbohydrate overfeeding in humans: different effects on energy storage. *Am. J. Clin. Nutr.*, **62**, 19–29.

JØRGENSEN L. M., SØRENSEN T. I., SCHROLL M. and LARSEN S. (1995), Influence of dietary factors on weight change assessed by multivariate graphical models. *Int. J. Obes. Relat. Metab. Disord.*, **12**, 909–15.

KANT A. K., GRAUBARD B. I., SCHATZKIN A. and BALLARD-BARBASH R. (1995), Proportion of energy intake from fat and subsequent weight change in the NHANES I Epidemiologic Follow-up Study. *Am. J. Clin. Nutr.*, **61** (1), 11–17.

KASIM S. E., MARTINO S., KIM P. N. *et al.* (1993), Dietary and anthropometric determinants of plasma lipoproteins during a long-term low-fat diet in healthy women. *Am. J. Clin. Nutr.*, **57**, 146–53.

KEMPER H. C., POST G. B., TWISK J. W. and VAN MECHELEN W. (1999), Lifestyle and obesity in adolescence and young adulthood: results from the Amsterdam Growth And

Health Longitudinal Study (AGAHLS). *Int. J. Obes. Relat. Metab. Disord.*, **23**, S34–40.

KENDALL A., LEVITSKY D. A., STRUPP B. J. and LISSNER L. (1991), Weight loss on a low-fat diet: consequence of the imprecision of the control of food intake in humans. *Am. J. Clin. Nutr.*, **53**, 1124–9.

KLESGES R. C., KLESGES L. M., ECK L. H. and SHELTON M. L. (1995), A longitudinal analysis of accelerated weight gain in preschool children. *Pediatrics*, **95** (1), 126–30.

KLESGES R. C., KLESGES L. M., HADDOCK C. K. and ECK L. H. (1992), A longitudinal analysis of the impact of dietary intake and physical activity on weight change in adults. *Am. J. Clin. Nutr.*, **55**, 818–22.

KNOPP R. H., WALDEN C. E., RETZLAFF B. M. *et al.* (1997), Long-term cholesterol-lowering effects of 4 fat-restricted diets in hypercholesterolaemic and combined hyperlipidemic men: the Dietary Alternative Study. *JAMA*, **278**, 1509–15.

KNOWLER W. C., BARRETT-CONNOR E. and FOWLER S. E. (2002), Reduction in the incidence of type 2 diabetes with lifestyle intervention or metformin. *N. Engl. J. Med.*, **346**, 393–403.

KRAL T. V., ROE L. S. and ROLLS B. J. (2004 Jun), Combined effects of energy density and portion size on energy intake in women. *Am. J. Clin. Nutr.*, **79** (6), 962–8.

LA FONTAINE H. A., CROWE T. C., SWINBURN B. A. and GIBBONS C. J. (2004 Jun), Two important exceptions to the relationship between energy density and fat content: foods with reduced-fat claims and high-fat vegetable-based dishes. *Public Health Nutr.*, **7** (4), 563–8.

LARSON D. E., HUNTER G. R., WILLIAMS M. J., KEKES-SZABO T., NYIKOS I. and GORAN M. I. (1996 Nov), Dietary fat in relation to body fat and intraabdominal adipose tissue: a cross-sectional analysis. *Am. J. Clin. Nutr.*, **64** (5), 677–84.

LEAN M. E., HAN T. S., PRVAN T., *et al.* (1997), Weight loss with high and low carbohydrate 1200 kcal diets in free living women. *Eur. J. Clin. Nutr.*, **51** (4), 243–8.

LEE-HAN H., COUSINS M., BEATON M. *et al.* (1988), Compliance in a randomized clinical trial of dietary fat reduction in patients with breast dysplasia. *Am. J. Clin. Nutr.*, **48**, 575–86.

LISSNER L., HEITMANN B. L. and BENGTSSON C. (1997), Low-fat diets may prevent weight gain in sedentary women: prospective observations from the population study of women in Gothenburg, Sweden. *Obes. Res.*, **5**, 43–8.

LISSNER L. and HEITMANN B. L. (1995), Dietary fat and obesity: evidence from epidemiology. *Eur. J. Clin. Nur.*, **49**, 79–90.

LISSNER L., LEVITSKY D. A., STRUPP B. J., KALKWARF H. J. and ROE D. A. (1987), Dietary fat and the regulation of energy intake in human subjects. *Am. J. Clin. Nutr.*, **46**, 886–92.

LUSCOMBE N. D., CLIFTON P. M., NOAKES M., FARNSWORTH E. and WITTERT G. (2003 May), Effect of a high-protein, energy-restricted diet on weight loss and energy expenditure after weight stabilization in hyperinsulinemic subjects. *Int. J. Obes. Relat. Metab. Disord.*, **27** (5), 582–90.

MAFFEIS C., TALAMINI G. and TATO L. (1998), Influence of diet, physical activity and parents'obesity on children's adiposity: a four-year longitudinal study. *Int. J. Obes. Relat. Metab. Disord.*, **22** (8), 758–64.

MAGAREY A. M., DANIELS L. A. and BOULTON T. J. C. (2001), Prevalence of overweight and obesity in Australian children and adolescents: reassessment of 1985 and 1995 data against new standard international definitions. *Med. J. Aust.*, **174**, 561–4.

MAGAREY A. M., DANIELS L. A., BOULTON T. J. and COCKINGTON R. A. (2001 Jun), Does fat intake predict adiposity in healthy children and adolescents aged 2–15 y? A longitudinal analysis. *Eur. J. Clin. Nutr.*, **55** (6), 471–81.

MARTIN L. J., SU W., JONES P. J., LOCKWOOD G. A., TRITCHLER D. L. and BOYD N. F. (1996), Comparison of energy intakes determined by food records and doubly labeled water in women participating in a dietary-intervention trial. *Am. J. Clin. Nutr.*, **63**, 483–90.

MCAULEY K. A., HOPKINS C. M., SMITH K. J. *et al.* (2005 Jan), Comparison of high-fat and high-protein diets with a high-carbohydrate diet in insulin-resistant obese women. *Diabetologia.*, **48** (1), 8–16.

MCCRORY M. A., FUSS P. J., MCCALLUM J. E. *et al.* (1999), Dietary variety within food groups: association with energy intake and body fatness in adult men and women. *Am. J. Clin. Nutr.*, **69**, 440–7.

MCCRORY M. A., FUSS P. J., SALZMAN E. and ROBERTS S. B. (2000), Dietary determinants of energy intake and weight regulation in healthy adults. *J. Nutr.*, **130** (2S Suppl), 276S–9S.

MCDEVITT R. M., POPPITT S. D., MURGATROYD P. R. and PRENTICE A. M. (2000 Aug), Macronutrient disposal during controlled overfeeding with glucose, fructose, sucrose, or fat in lean and obese women. *Am. J. Clin. Nutr.*, **72** (2), 369–77.

MECKLING K. A., GAUTHIER M., GRUBB R. and SANFORD J. (2002), Effects of a hypocaloric, low-carbohydrate diet on weight loss, blood lipids, blood pressure, glucose tolerance, and body composition in free-living overweight women. *Can. J. Physiol. Pharmacol.*, **80**, 1095–105.

MOSCA C. L., MARSHALL J. A., GRUNWALD G. K., CORNIER M. A. and BAXTER J. (2004 Jun), Insulin resistance as a modifier of the relationship between dietary fat intake and weight gain. *Int. J. Obes. Relat. Metab. Disord.*, **28** (6), 803–12.

NATIONAL HEALTH AND MEDICAL RESEARCH COUNCIL (NHMRC) (1997), Acting on Australia's weight: a strategic plan for the prevention of overweight and obesity. Canberra: AGPS.

NATIONAL INSTITUTES OF HEALTH (NIH) (1998), Clinical guidelines on the identification, evaluation, and treatment of overweight and obesity in adults, the evidence report. *Obes. Res.*, **6** (Suppl 2), 51S–209S.

NOAKES M. and CLIFTON P. (2004 Feb), Weight loss, diet composition and cardiovascular risk. *Curr. Opin. Lipidol.*, **15** (1), 31–5.

PAERATAKUL S., POPKIN B. M., KEYOU G., ADAIR L. S. and STEVENS J. (1998), Changes in diet and physical activity affect the body mass index of Chinese adults. *Int. J. Obes. Relat. Metab. Disord.*, **22**, 424–31.

PARKER D. R., GONZALEZ S., DERBY C. A., GANS K. M., LASATER T. M. and CARLETON R. A. (1997 Feb), Dietary factors in relation to weight change among men and women from two southeastern New England communities. *Int. J. Obes. Relat. Metab. Disord.*, **21** (2), 103–9.

PASCALE R. W., MULLEN M., WING R. R., BONONI P. and BUTLER B. A. (1995), Effects of a behavioural weight loss programme stressing calorie restriction versus calories plus fat restriction in obese individuals with NIDDM or a family history of diabetes. *Diabetes Care*, **18**, 1241–8.

PIROZZO S., SUMMERBELL C., CAMERON C. and GLASZIOU P. (2002), Advice on low-fat diets for obesity. *Cochrane Database Syst. Rev.*, CD003640.

POWELL J. J., TUCKER L., FISHER A. G. and WILCOX K. (1994 Jul–Aug), The effects of different percentages of dietary fat intake, exercise, and calorie restriction on body composition and body weight in obese females. *Am. J. Health Promot.*, **8** (6), 442–8.

PRENTICE A. M. (1998), Manipulation of dietary fat and energy density and subsequent effects on substrate flux and food intake. *Am. J. Clin. Nutr.*, **67** (Suppl), 535S–41S.

PROSERPI C., SPARTI A., SCHUTZ Y., DI V., V., MILON H. and JEQUIER E. (1997), *Ad libitum* intake of a high-carbohydrate or high-fat diet in young men: effects on nutrient balances. *Am. J. Clin. Nutr.*, **66**, 539–45.

RABEN A., MACDONALD I. and ASTRUP A. (1997 Oct), Replacement of dietary fat by sucrose or starch: effects on 14 d ad libitum energy intake, energy expenditure and body weight in formerly obese and never-obese subjects. *Int. J. Obes. Relat. Metab. Disord.*, **21** (10), 846–59.

RISSANEN A. M., HELIOVAARA M., KNEKT P., REUNANEN A. and AROMAA A. (1991), Determinants of weight gain and overweight in adult Finns. *Eur. J. Clin. Nutr.*, **54**, 419–30.

ROLLAND-CACHERA M. F., DEHEEGER M., AKROUT M. and BELLISLE F. (1995), Influence of macronutrients on adiposity development: a follow up study of nutrition and growth from 10 months to 8 years of age. *Int. J. Obes. Relat. Metab. Disord.*, **19** (8), 573–8.

ROLLS B. J. (1999), Energy density but not fat content of foods affected energy intake in lean and obese women. *Am. J. Clin. Nutr.*, **69**, 863–71.

ROLLS B. J., BELL E. A. and THORWART M. L. (1999), Water incorporated into a food but not served with a food decreases energy intake in lean women. *Am. J. Clin. Nutr.*, **70**, 448–55.

ROLLS B. J. (2000), The role of energy density in the overconsumption of fat. *J. Nutr.*, **130** (2S Suppl), 268S–71S.

SALZMAN E., DALLAL G. E. and ROBERTS S. B. (1997), Effect of high-fat and low-fat diets on voluntary energy intake and substrate oxidation: studies in identical twins consuming diets matched for energy density, fiber, and palatability. *Am. J. Clin. Nutr.*, **66**, 1332–9.

SAMAHA F. F., IQBAL N., SESHADRI P. *et al.* (2003), A low-carbohydrate as compared with a low-fat diet in severe obesity. *N. Engl. J. Med.*, **348**, 2074–81.

SCHRAUWEN P., VAN MARKEN LICHTENBELT W. D., SARIS W. H. and WESTERTERP K. R. (1997), Changes in fat oxidation in response to a high-fat diet. *Am. J. Clin. Nutr.*, **66** (2), 276–82.

SCHUTZ Y. (1995), Macronutrients and energy balance in obesity. *Metabolism*, **44** (9) (Suppl 3), 7–11.

SEGAL-ISAACSON C. J., JOHNSON S., TOMUTA V., COWELL B. and STEIN D. T. (2004 Nov), A randomized trial comparing low-fat and low-carbohydrate diets matched for energy and protein. *Obes. Res.*, **12** (Suppl, 2), 130S–40S.

SEMPOS C. T., LIU K. and ERNST N. D. (1999), Food and nutrient exposures: what to consider when evaluating epidemiologic evidence. *Am. J. Clin. Nutr.*, **69** (Suppl), 1330S–8S.

SHAH M. and GARG A. (1996), High-fat and high-carbohydrate diets and energy balance. *Diabetes Care*, **10**, 1142–52.

SHAH M., BAXTER J. E., MCGOVERN P. G. and GARG A. (1996), Nutrient and food intake in obese women on a low-fat or low-calorie diet. *Am. J. Health Promot.*, **10** (3), 179–82.

SHEPPARD L., KRISTAL A. R. and KUSHI L. H. (1991), Weight loss in women participating in a randomized trial of low-fat diets. *Am. J. Clin. Nutr.*, **54** (5), 821–8.

SHERWOOD N. E., JEFFERY R. W., FRENCH S. A., HANNAN P. J. and MURRAY D. M. (2000 Apr), Predictors of weight gain in the Pound of Prevention study. *Int. J. Obes. Relat. Metab. Disord.*, **24** (4), 395–403.

SIGGAARD R., RABEN A. and ASTRUP A. (1996), Weight loss during 12 week's *ad libitum* carbohydrate-rich diet in overweight and normal-weight subjects at a Danish work site. *Obes. Res.*, **4** (4), 347–56.

SKOV A. R., TOUBRO S., RONN B., HOLM L. and ASTRUP A. (1999), Randomized trial on protein vs. carbohydrate in *ad libitum* fat reduced diet for the treatment of obesity. *Int. J. Obes. Relat. Metab. Disord.*, **23** (5), 528–36.

SONDIKE S. B., COPPERMAN N. and JACOBSON M. S. (2003), Effects of a low-carbohydrate diet on weight loss and cardiovascular risk factor in overweight adolescents. *J. Pediatr.*, **142**, 253–8.

STERN L., IQBAL N., SESHADRI P. *et al.* (2004 May 18), The effects of low-carbohydrate versus conventional weight loss diets in severely obese adults: one-year follow-up of a randomized trial. *Ann. Intern. Med.*, **140** (10), 778–85.

STUBBS R. J. and WHYBROW S. (2004 Jul), Energy density, diet composition and palatability: influences on overall food energy intake in humans. *Physiol. Behav.*, **81** (5), 755–64.

STUBBS R. J., RITZ P., COWARD W. A. and PRENTICE A. M. (1995), Covert manipulation of the ratio of dietary fat to carbohydrate and energy density: effect on food intake and energy balance in free-living men eating *ad libitum. Am. J. Clin.*, **62**, 330–7.

STUBBS R. J., HARBRON C. G. and PRENTICE A. M. (1996), Covert manipulation of the dietary fat to carbohydrate ratio of isoenergetically dense diets: effect on food intake in feeding men *ad libitum. Int. J. Obes.*, **20**, 651–60.

SUMMERBELL C. D., JONES L. V. and GLASZIOU P. P. (1998), The long-term effect of advice on low-fat diets in terms of weight loss: an interim meta-analysis. *J. Hum. Nutr. Diet.*, **11**, 209–17.

TREMBLAY A., PLOURDE G., DESPRES J.-P. and BOUCHARD C. (1989), Impact of dietary fat content and fat oxidation on energy intake in humans. *Am. J. Clin. Nutr.*, **49**, 799–805.

VAN STRATUM P., LUSSENBURG R. N., VAN WEZEL L. A., VERGROESEN A. J. and CREMER H. D. (1978), The effect of dietary carbohydrate: fat ratio on energy intake by adult women. *Am. J. Clin. Nutr.*, **31**, 206–12.

VOLEK J. S., SHARMAN M. J., LOVE D. M. *et al.* (2002), Body composition and hormonal responses to a carbohydrate-restricted diet. *Metabolism*, **51**, 864–70.

WESTERTERP K. R., VERBOEKET-VAN DE VENNE W. P., WESTERTERP-PLANTENGA M. S., VELTHUIS-RE WIERIK E. J., DE GRAAF C. and WESTSTRATE J. A. (1996), Dietary fat and body fat: an intervention study. *Int. J. Obes. Relat. Metab. Disord.*, **20**, 1022–6.

WESTERTERP-PLANTENGA M. S., WIJCKMANS-DUIJSENS N. E., VERBOEKET-VAN DE VENNE W. P., DE GRAAF K., VAN HET HOF K. H. and WESTSTRATE J. A. (1998 Jan), Energy intake and body weight effects of six months reduced or full fat diets, as a function of dietary restraint. *Int. J. Obes. Relat. Metab. Disord.*, **22** (1): 14–22.

WESTERTERP-PLANTENGA M. S., LEJEUNE M. P., NIJS I., VAN OOIJEN M. and KOVACS E. M. (2004 Jan), High protein intake sustains weight maintenance after body weight loss in humans. *Int. J. Obes. Relat. Metab. Disord.*, **28** (1), 57–64.

WILLETT W. C. (1998 Dec), Dietary fat and obesity: an unconvincing relation. *Am. J. Clin. Nutr.*, **68** (6): 1149–50.

WILLETT W. C. (1999 Jul), Reply to JQ Purnell, RH Knopp, and JD Brunzell (letter). *Am. J. Clin. Nutr.*, **70** (1), 108A–109.

WORLD HEALTH ORGANIZATION (1998), *Obesity. Preventing and Managing the Global Epidemic*. Geneva: World Health Organization.

YANCY W. S. JR, OLSEN M. K., GUYTON J. R., BAKST R. P. and WESTMAN E. C. (2004 May 18), A low-carbohydrate, ketogenic diet versus a low-fat diet to treat obesity and hyperlipidemia: a randomized, controlled trial. *Ann. Intern. Med.*, **140** (10), 769–77.

YU-POTH S., ZHAO G., ETHERTON T., NAGLAK M., JONNALAGADDA S. and KRIS-ETHERTON P. M. (1999), Effects of the national Cholesterol Education Programme's Step I and Step II dietary intervention programmes on cardiovascular disease risk factors: a meta-analysis. *Am. J. Clin. Nutr.*, **69**, 632–46.

11

Carbohydrates, glycemic responses and weight control

K. Teff, Monell Chemical Senses Center, USA

11.1 Introduction

The public has a long-standing hate–love relationship with carbohydrates. Depending on the period of history, sucrose has either been sought after and revered or vilified and rejected. Sucrose, a disaccharide composed of one molecule of glucose and one molecule of fructose, is a processed carbohydrate, which has been accused of causing a variety of health problems ranging from hyperactivity to food allergies. To date, these accusations have never been supported scientifically. However, recent epidemiological studies are implicating foods containing high concentrations of processed carbohydrates in the etiology of chronic diseases such as obesity, diabetes and dyslipidemia (Frost *et al.*, 1999; Salmeron *et al.*, 1997a). Thus, there has been renewed concern over the type and amount of carbohydrate in the diet.

The overall objective of this chapter is to explore what is known about the acute and chronic physiological responses to carbohydrate intake and the potential mechanisms by which different types of carbohydrate may contribute to disease outcome, particularly the components of the metabolic syndrome. Specifically, methodological approaches used in the determination of the glycemic responses to a meal and the many factors which modify the glycemic responses will be discussed. In addition, the evidence supporting the proposed mechanisms by which glycemic responses may influence weight and body adiposity will be evaluated. These include the relationship between carbohydrate and hyperinsulinemia as well as the effect of carbohydrates on satiety and subsequent food intake. It is hoped that a better understanding of the complexity of this issue will be reached as well as an acknowledgment of the limitations of current knowledge.

11.2 The glycemic index (GI): definition and methodological issues

The differential effects of various carbohydrates on blood glucose was first brought to light by Jenkins in 1981 when he proposed that the 'glycemic index' of a food could be used as a tool for the dietary management of type 1 diabetes (Jenkins *et al.*, 1981). High glycemic index (HGI) foods were those that resulted in high plasma glucose values in contrast to low glycemic index (LGI) foods which elicit modest increases in plasma glucose. To determine the GI of a food, the early studies compared 50g portions of various carbohydrates with 50g of glucose. Blood samples were taken over a 2-hour period and the area under the curve (AUC) above the fasting level was calculated and expressed as a percentage of the area obtained after ingestion of glucose. More recently, foods have been compared to a 50g portion of white bread, which is now the standard comparison. Because the GI does not take into consideration the total amount of carbohydrate ingested within a meal, the glycemic load (GL) has been proposed to account for total carbohydrate ingested (Salmeron *et al.*, 1997b). The GL is calculated by multiplying the GI by the total carbohydrate in the diet. More specific calculations can be made by calculating the GI of each carbohydrate and multiplying by the quantity of carbohydrate and then summing the total of each food. However, it should be noted that GL can be reduced by either reducing the total amount of carbohydrate consumed or by changing the foods consumed to low glycemic index foods.

Concerns have been raised with regards to the validity of the methodology used in the calculation of the glycemic index. Variability and lack of standardization have been two overarching concerns. One criticism has been the use of white bread, which inherently carries a higher degree of variability both in terms of macronutrient composition and weighing precision than glucose (Pi-Sunyer, 2002). Time of day is also a contributor to the irreproducibility of GI measurements. Greater differences in glycemic responses to different foods are often seen following an overnight fast but these differences are minimized at lunch time (Jenkins *et al.*, 1982).

One critical issue has revolved around the 2h time period as the endpoint calculation of the area under the curve. Following ingestion of mixed nutrient meals, blood glucose levels have not always returned to baseline values by the 2h time point, particularly in diabetics, thereby underestimating the area under the curve (AUC). It has been demonstrated that, by allowing a 4-hour period, differences in GI of foods are substantially minimized (Gannon and Nuttall, 1987). All in all, the variation and lack of reproducibility in the measurement of the glycemic index as a measure of diet quality limits its usefulness as a means of determining the pathophysiological consequences of specific carbohydrates.

Of even greater concern is whether the physiological effects of single test meals used in determining the GI can be extrapolated to long-term dietary intake of a variety of foods. The vast majority of research conducted on GI falls into one of two categories, acute single meal experiments or epidemiological studies with limited physiological parameters. Only a handful of studies have been conducted that coupled chronic dietary intake and detailed physiological responses to the meals. Thus, there are inherent differences between many of the studies, making comparisons very difficult.

11.3 Factors affecting the glycemic index of foods

Many factors influence the rate of appearance and disappearance and magnitude of glucose levels in the blood after a meal. The physical form and the preparation of a food play an important role in determining postprandial blood glucose levels. For example, raw foods are digested more slowly than cooked foods and therefore, even for the same food, elicit lower GI values (Granfeldt *et al.*, 1991). Typically, the more highly processed foods elicit higher GI values. However, this is not always the case, as whole wheat bread and white bread have equivalent GI values. Surprisingly, sucrose has a lower GI value than the white bread standard but potatoes and carrots have higher GIs (Table 11.1). Thus, GI values are not always intuitively obvious and, from a nutritional point of view, consumption of micronutrient-containing potatoes and carrots would be superior to the ingestion of pure sucrose.

11.3.1 Liquid vs. solid forms of carbohydrate

Of primary importance in determining the magnitude and patterning of blood glucose levels following food ingestion is the form of the food ingested. Solids and liquids are emptied from the stomach by different mechanisms and at different rates (Keith, 1980). Liquids are emptied from

Table 11.1 Glycemic index of a variety of common foods

Apple juice	39 ± 5
Coca-Cola®	53 ± 7
French fries	72 ± 0
Gatorade®	78 ± 13
Wheat bread	52 ± 0
Brown rice	55 ± 5
Instant white rice	69 ± 12
Chicken nuggets	46 ± 4
All-Bran cereal	42 ± 5
Coco Pops cereal	77 ± 8

Note: Values taken from Foster-Powell *et al.* (2002).

the stomach and nutrients absorbed from the intestine quickly, resulting in rapid increases in blood glucose and subsequent rapid clearance by insulin. When liquids, typically carbohydrate beverages, are consumed on their own, independent of a meal, the large rapid post-prandial rise in insulin can result in a drop of blood glucose levels below baseline. The same amount of carbohydrate in a solid form will elicit relatively blunted glucose and insulin profiles with no incidence of hypoglycemia. The difference in glucose responses between solid and liquid forms of carbohydrates has implications both in terms of the glycemic index as well as the obesity epidemic. With respect to the glycemic index, many of the hypothesized mechanisms attributed to the effect of high glycemic index foods on chronic disease (Ludwig, 2002) may be applicable to carbohydrate beverages but not mixed nutrient meals. However, in our current dietary culture, high carbohydrate beverages in the form of soft drinks, sweetened coffees, fruit juices and athletic drinks are consumed heavily and often unassociated with a meal. In fact, the consumption of these beverages has increased dramatically over the past 50 years (Putnam *et al.*, 2002). These beverages, which are highly caloric, do not contain any micronutrients or dietary fiber but contribute significantly to daily caloric intake. Thus, it is possible that the correlations reported by epidemiological studies between high GI foods and disease could be due to the ingestion of these beverages. In fact, significant associations between soft drink consumption and obesity have been reported in a number of studies (Ludwig *et al.*, 2001; Schulze *et al.*, 2004; Willett *et al.*, 2002).

An additional factor may be that liquid calories are not physiologically accounted for in the same manner as solids. Thus, in pre-load experiments, subjects given a caloric load in the form of a liquid do not adjust their subsequent food intake in contrast to the caloric compensation exhibited when the pre-load is in the form of a solid. Although some studies do suggest a degree of compensation (Anderson and Woodend, 2003), the fact that preparatory responses such as the vagally mediated cephalic phase hormonal responses which typically occur at the onset of food ingestion, are not evident during the ingestion of sweet, caloric or non-caloric liquids lends a physiological basis to this phenomenon (Teff, 1994; Teff *et al.*, 1995). Activation of the vagus nerve during food ingestion plays an important role in optimizing nutrient metabolism. In the absence of vagal activation, nutrient metabolism tends to be impaired or suboptimal. Pancreatic polypeptide, a hormone released from the pancreas solely in response to stimulation of the vagal nerve provides an indirect measure of vagal activation. Figure 11.1 illustrates the pancreatic polypeptide in response to the sham-feeding of a carbohydrate food compared to the ingestion of a glucose sweetened beverage. The absence of a pancreatic polypeptide response indicates that activation of the vagus nerve did not take place and suggests that optimal metabolism of the incoming nutrients is unlikely to occur. Thus, it is possible that sweetened beverages contribute to obesity directly by contributing

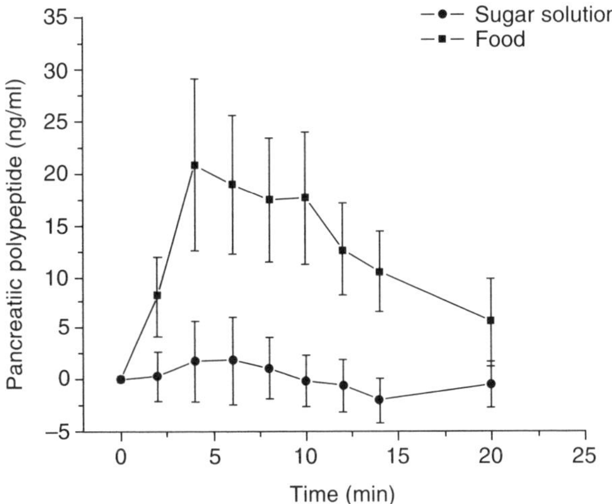

Fig. 11.1 Mean ± S.E. pancreatic polypeptide levels in ten normal weight healthy men following either a 2-minute sham-feed of apple pie (squares) or sipping and spitting a sugar solution (circles).

to daily caloric intake but also indirectly as the calories associated with sweetened liquids bypass the normal regulatory mechanisms such that no dietary compensation takes place.

11.3.2 Type of carbohydrate

The relationship between an ingested carbohydrate and its related GI value is not always intuitively obvious. This is because the rate of digestion and absorption of each type of carbohydrate is dependent on the chemical structure and preparation of the food. Carbohydrates can be divided structurally into two categories: simple and complex. The complex carbohydrate category includes: long polymers of glucose or other monosaccharides, including the branched form, amylopectin and the linear form, amylase as well as soluble and insoluble fibers. Simple carbohydrates include the mono- (glucose, fructose, galactose) and disaccharides (sucrose, maltose and lactose). The segregation of carbohydrates into the two categories can be misleading if, as was the belief a number of years ago, it is assumed that complex carbohydrates are absorbed more slowly than simple carbohydrates. In fact, some forms of starch are actually digested at the same rate as glucose.

Whole grain foods such as whole wheat bread, brown rice or wheat pasta, would typically be considered within the complex carbohydrate category and considered part of a low GI diet. Unexpectedly, minimal differences in GI values between the whole wheat and the processed form of the food are observed. However, whole grain foods often contain various micronutrients, particularly from the B vitamin family. Thus, even though they may elicit similar GIs as processed foods, they have additional nutritional components. Wholegrain foods are associated with lower rates of cardiovascular disease (Hu, 2003; Liu *et al.*, 2001) and type 2 diabetes (Meyer *et al.*, 2000). Conversely, foods containing sugars do not necessarily elicit high GI values. Brand-Miller *et al.* (1995) compared 39 foods and examined glycemic and insulin responses in healthy adults. A wide range of foods were tested including those with naturally occurring sugars such as fruit and dairy products as well as those with added sugars including confectioneries, sweetened cereals and cookies. The authors concluded that the foods with added sugars did not produce higher glucose or insulin responses than starchy foods. However, many highly processed foods, particularly those with added sugars, rarely contain the essential micronutrients and are primarily conveyors of calories and taste quality such as sweetness.

The most common simple carbohydrates found in the diet, glucose and fructose, can result in vastly different GI values and patterns of metabolic fuels and hormones. Ingestion of glucose results in rapid increases in plasma glucose, resulting in high GI values. In contrast, fructose ingestion has minimal effects on blood glucose and insulin and is associated with a low GI. Thus, the GIs of the two sweeteners are very different and because of this, fructose has been touted as a better sweetener both for the healthy non-diabetic population and diabetics. However, fructose ingestion elicits other unexpected differences in hormones compared with glucose ingestion. Teff *et al.* compared the effects of fructose-sweetened and glucose-sweetened beverages, each ingested with equicaloric mixed nutrient meals, in normal weight healthy women (Teff *et al.*, 2004). As expected, fructose ingestion resulted in lower levels of insulin and glucose levels compared to glucose ingestion. In addition, fructose decreased circulating levels of leptin, a satiety hormone and resulted in significantly elevated triglycerides compared to the glucose challenge. Furthermore, the orexigenic hormone ghrelin was not as fully suppressed following fructose as occurred during glucose ingestion. This metabolic profile consisting of a decrease in two hormones mediating satiety (leptin and insulin) and unsuppressed levels of a hormone stimulating food intake (ghrelin) is one that could potentially promote food intake.

In addition, elevation of triglycerides is a known marker of cardiovascular disease. Thus, the fructose found in sweetened beverages may contribute to the elevations in lipids associated with ingestion of high-glycemic index foods (see below). It should be noted, however, that high fructose corn syrup, the sweetener typically used in soft drinks, contains both fructose and glucose and that the ingestion of high fructose corn syrup would probably result in intermediary effects on triglycerides compared to the effect of fructose alone. However, taking into account the large quantity of ingested sweetened beverages, the enormous amount of calories associated with them as well as the potential metabolic consequences on lipids and satiety hormones, it is not surprising that ingestion of sweetened beverages has been found to be associated with weight gain and incidence of type 2 diabetes (Schulze *et al.*, 2004).

11.3.3 Macronutrient effects on the glycemic index and insulin secretion

Meals are almost always composed of combinations of protein, fat and carbohydrate. Even snacks such as potato chips, doughnuts and chocolate bars are combinations of fat and carbohydrate, although some, such as hard candy and popcorn are primarily composed of carbohydrate. Combinations of macronutrients elicit very different hormonal and glucose patterns in response to meal ingestion, depending on the quantity and combination of the macronutrients and, therefore, evaluation of single foods can be misleading with regards to the overall effect of meal ingestion on glucose and insulin (Ercan *et al.*, 1994).

The macronutrients have differential potencies with regards to their ability to act as insulin secretagogues. The magnitude of insulin secreted is dependent on a direct effect of the macronutrient on the beta-cell of the pancreas and an indirect effect on gut hormone release, which unto themselves modulate insulin secretion. Glucose, for example, is the most potent insulin secretagogue, both because of its direct effect on insulin secretion as well as its effect on glucagon-like peptide (GLP) and glucose-dependent insulinotropic protein (GIP) release. Protein when added to a carbohydrate meal also enhances insulin secretion, increases GLP release but has no effect on GIP (Elliott *et al.*, 1993). In contrast, fat, which has no direct effect on insulin secretion, does stimulate GLP (Meier and Nauck, 2005) and GIP (Elliott *et al.*, 1993) release. Ghrelin, the orexigenic hormone released from the stomach, is more potently suppressed by glucose and protein but relatively insensitive to fat (Overduin *et al.*, 2005), suggesting one potential mechanism mediating the lower satiating value of fat. Thus, varying the macronutrient composition of a meal has profound effects on insulin and gut hormone secretion, which are not adequately represented by looking at the glucose responses alone. Furthermore, as the gut peptides play a role in the regulation of food intake, the differential effects of the macronutrients on gut peptide release may be one of the mechanisms mediating the differential degrees of satiety and energy regulation provided by the various diets under evaluation (Choi and Anderson, 2001).

11.4 Glucose response and chronic disease

The underlying assumption with regards to use of the GI as a marker for the development of chronic disease is that low glycemic responses are optimal while high peak glucose levels are potentially detrimental. This idea, however, originates from the perspective of limiting glycemic excursions in the treatment of diabetics, the original purpose of the glycemic index. For type 1 diabetes, minimizing glycemic excursions is an important dietary objective due to the vascular complications associated with hyperglycemia. In addition, a decrease in glycemic excursions will decrease insulin requirements and the potential of hypoglycemic events. However, for non-diabetics, the same objectives are not necessarily relevant. In non-diabetics, a large rapid increase in plasma glucose is usually followed by a rapid return of glucose to baseline. Therefore, the question is whether an acute high glucose response, without a sustained return to baseline is potentially of concern from the viewpoint of optimal health.

An interesting physiological illustration is the comparison of a pure carbohydrate meal and a carbohydrate plus fat meal on blood glucose levels. Figure 11.2 illustrates the plasma glucose response to a high carbohydrate drink (left) compared with a high carbohydrate, high fat food (right). In the figure on the left, the glucose levels rise quickly and return to baseline rapidly. In the figure on the right, the addition of fat to a meal significantly delays gastric emptying. The peak glucose response is lower but the return to baseline is delayed and at the 2h time point, plasma glucose has not returned to baseline. The blunted peak response would contribute to a lower GI value than the carbohydrate alone while the delayed return to baseline would not be accounted for by the 2h endpoint included in the methodology of the glycemic index. If we consider the question of optimal temporal patterning, one must decide whether acute high glucose excursions (carbohydrate alone) are more perturbing from a physiological point of view than prolonged mildly elevated plasma glucose levels (carbohydrate and fat) leading to sustained stimulation of the beta-cell and insulin release. There is evidence that early rapid, large responses are metabolically more

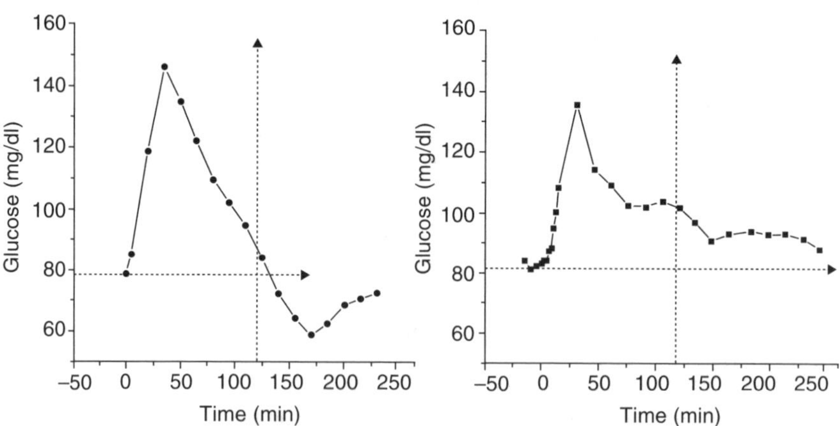

Fig. 11.2 Mean ± S.E. glucose levels (mg/dl) in ten normal weight healthy men following ingestion of 50g of a glucose solution (left graph) or ingestion of carbohydrate and fat snack (200kcal; 35% fat) (right graph).

efficient that delayed blunted responses, insulin being the prime example. Delayed early insulin release is associated with impaired glucose tolerance. Supplementation of insulin during the very early period at the onset of food ingestion improves post-prandial glucose responses in obese individuals (Teff and Townsend, 1999). An absent first phase insulin response is highly predictive of type 2 diabetes (Kahn *et al.*, 2001) and, in fact, is associated with a marked impairment in the inhibition of hepatic gluconeogenesis (Luzi and DeFronzo, 1989). Thus, rapid and large insulin responses are critical to achieving glucose homeostasis. Of perhaps greater concern are sustained post-prandial glucose and insulin levels, typically observed following ingestion of hypercaloric, high fat diets. Chronic post-prandial elevations in both glucose and insulin are each independent risk factors for the macrovascular complications of diabetes and cardiovascular disease (Gin and Rigalleau, 2000). The likelihood of post-prandial hyperglycemia and hyperinsulinemia will be greater following consumption of a hypercaloric, high fat meal and particularly so, in an insulin-resistant population.

11.4.1 Insulin as the mediator of chronic disease

A number of large epidemiological studies designed to evaluate the influence of dietary intake and dietary patterns on the development of chronic diseases such as obesity and diabetes have found positive correlations between the ingestion of high GI foods and outcome variables such as BMI, indices of insulin resistance and diabetes (Hodge *et al.*, 2004; Salmeron *et al.*, 1997a; Schulze *et al.*, 2004). While a variety of mechanisms have been postulated, by and large, insulin has been suggested as the most likely mitigating factor in the relationship between HGI foods and chronic disease. Ironically, insulin levels are not measured or taken into consideration in the calculation of the GI. Despite this, the overarching hypothesis is that high glycemic index foods stimulate excessive and prolonged insulin secretion which increases deposition of nutrients, resulting in increased fat mass. The increased fat mass associated with obesity leads to an increase in non-esterified free fatty acids (NEFA) delivery to the circulation, which as described below contributes to insulin resistance.

11.4.2 The glycemic index, insulin resistance and diabetes

Insulin resistance, a decline in the efficacy of insulin to stimulate glucose uptake has been proposed in the etiology of chronic diseases such as type 2 diabetes, hypertension and cardiovascular disease (Reaven, 1988). Thus, preventing the development of insulin resistance is of significant clinical importance. The prevailing construct with regards to the development of insulin resistance, from the simplistic point of view necessary within the confines of this chapter, is that sustained increases in NEFA contribute to the development of differential tissue sensitivity to insulin, such that insulin is unable to stimulate glucose uptake from the muscle and inhibit free fatty acid release from the adipose tissue. However, these effects are tissue and mechanism dependent because, while there is hepatic insulin resistance with respect to the inhibition of gluconeogenesis, insulin is still capable of stimulating triglyceride synthesis. The increase in both NEFA and triglycerides further decreases insulin sensitivity, in a cyclical worsening of the insulin resistant state. In addition, to compensate for the increase in insulin resistance, the pancreatic beta-cell secretes more insulin. Thus, individuals with insulin resistance typically exhibit elevated fasting insulin levels and compensatory hyperinsulinemia. In some individuals, insulin secretion becomes inadequate to maintain euglycemia and at this point, frank type 2 diabetes develops (Frayn, 2001).

Determination of insulin resistance, particularly with the objective of assessing differential tissue sensitivity, is difficult even within the laboratory setting. The gold standard for the measurement of insulin resistance is the euglycemic, hyperinsulinemic clamp which when paired with a tracer allows determination of whole body versus hepatic insulin resistance (Felber *et al.*, 1993). The frequently sampled intravenous glucose tolerance test (FSIGT) is also used to measure insulin sensitivity and is highly correlated to the clamp (Bergman *et al.*, 1987). Occasionally, one of these more sensitive methods has been used to determine the effect of diet on insulin sensitivity. However, neither method is feasible for either large clinical trials or epidemiological studies and the majority of large studies have used either fasting insulin and glucose levels or a mathematical combination of both such as the HOMA or QUICKI (Kanauchi *et al.*, 2003). While these approaches are moderately correlated to the clamp and may give some indirect measure of insulin resistance, they provide no information on individual tissue sensitivity, nor are they reliable for individuals who have any degree of beta-cell failure. Therefore, bearing these limitations in mind, it is difficult to draw definitive conclusions with regards to the effect of various diets on insulin resistance.

The evidence supporting a causative relationship between high glycemic index diets and insulin resistance in humans is in fact, very weak. While a couple of studies suggest that low glycemic index diets increase insulin sensitivity (Frost *et al.*, 1998; Ludwig *et al.*, 1999) or conversely that relatively short-term (4 days) high GI diets increase insulin resistance (Brynes *et al.*, 2003), most studies showed either no association between GI and insulin resistance (Jenkins and Jenkins, 1987; Kiens, 1996) or a positive association (Kiens, 1996). Bessesen (2001) reviewed the literature on the role of carbohydrates in insulin resistance and pointed out that despite evidence in animals, simple sugars such as fructose and glucose do not appear to contribute to insulin resistance in humans. Similarly, Daly concluded that, to date, there have been no major studies showing a negative effect of sucrose *per se* on insulin sensitivity. Furthermore, he pointed out that some of the negative effects of sugars may occur only in the context of a high-fat diet (Daly, 2003).

If, instead of insulin resistance, one uses the incidence of diabetes as an end point, the data are inconsistent. A number of studies found positive associations between GI and the incidence of diabetes (Hodge *et al.*, 2004; Salmeron *et al.*, 1997a, b; Schulze *et al.*, 2004) while three found no association (Marshall *et al.*, 1997; Meyer *et al.*, 2000; Stevens *et al.*, 2002). However, if one examines the association between total carbohydrate intake and onset of diabetes, neither the San Luis Valley study (Marshall *et al.*, 1997), the Health Professionals Follow-up study (Salmeron *et al.*, 1997a), the Nurses Health Study (Salmeron *et al.*, 1997b) or the IOWA Women's health study (Meyer *et al.*, 2000) found a significant relationship.

Willett *et al.* (2002) discussed his re-analysis of a number of studies in which they found that those individuals falling within the highest quintile of glycemic load had a significantly greater risk of diabetes. He also examined individual food predictors of type 2 diabetes, comparing the Nurses Health Study at two different periods (1980–1986; 1986–1992) and the Health Professionals Follow-up study. Some foods were consistent positive predictors in all three studies, including French fried potatoes, white bread, cola beverages and white rice. The consistency of these foods as predictors of type 2 diabetes may be more indicative of poor diet quality as opposed to providing implications for the relevancy of high GI diets in promoting disease.

11.4.3 The glycemic index: hypoglycemia and its consequences

It has been suggested that the large increase in insulin following high GI foods leads to hypoglycemia and subsequent counter-regulatory responses including the release of glucagon, free fatty acids and catecholamines. As increases in circulating free fatty acids and sympathetic activation are associated with decreases in insulin sensitivity, the counter-regulatory responses could potentially exacerbate the development of insulin resistance (Ludwig, 2002). In addition, insulin and the resultant hypoglycemia are both thought to stimulate food intake.

Despite citations of hypoglycemia following high GI foods (Roberts, 2000), comparison of plasma glucose levels in subjects following ingestion of high and low GI diets provides little evidence of postprandial hypoglycemia. To some extent, the available data for comparison are rather limited. GI values by themselves do not provide the required information to determine the presence or absence of hypoglycemia and in many of the larger studies, blood sampling was not part of the protocol. Conversely, in those studies which did provide post-prandial glucose data sampled at a rate adequate to document a hypoglycemic episode, individual foods were compared as opposed to high and low-glycemic meals. For example, one study reported a significant drop below baseline in plasma glucose following ingestion of an extruded chickpea bread breakfast compared to breakfasts composed of white bread or chickpea flour bread (Johnson *et al.*, 2005). In contrast, Brand-Miller *et al.* (1995) tested a wide variety of foods containing both natural and added sugars and reported no incidence of rebound hypoglycemia.

Most meals are composed of a mixture of macronutrients and usually the presence of fat in a meal will slow gastric emptying (see discussion above) and prevent the occurrence of hypoglycemia (Ercan *et al.*, 1994). However, when simple sugars are added artificially to meals with the objective of altering the GI, hypoglycemia has been reported. There is one study demonstrating a modest hypoglycemic and epinephrine response following ingestion of a high GI index meal composed of mixed nutrients (Ludwig *et al.*, 1999). In this study, obese teenage boys were given high, medium and low GI breakfasts and blood samples were taken for 5 hours after the meal. The medium and high GI breakfast challenges contained half the amount of protein as the low GI group and were supplemented with fructose and dextrose respectively. The glucose levels after the high GI breakfast were significantly lower compared with the other two groups at 4.5 and 5 hours post-prandially. Plasma epinephrine was also shown to be significantly higher during the last hour of the study. Surprisingly, glucagon, which one would expect to be elevated in the context of a counter-regulatory response to hypoglycemia, was actually decreased following the medium and high GI meals and elevated following the low GI meals. This argues against the occurrence of a counter-regulatory response occurring to hypoglycemia and suggests that the reported increase in epinephrine was due to stress.

Only a limited number of studies have examined the effect of ingestion of high and low glycemic diets on plasma glucose over 24 h periods or following long-term ingestion of the meals and at the same time, monitored blood glucose responses. Daly compared a high sucrose to a high starch diet and took blood samples over a 24 h period. Even within the context of this non-physiological diet, blood glucose levels did not drop below 65 mg/dl (Daly 2003; Daly *et al.*, 1998). In one of the few studies, comparing the effect of high and low GI meals on metabolic fuels and hormones at 3 and then 30 days on the diets, Kiens and Richter (Kiens, 1996) found that, while the LGI diet was initially associated with lower levels of plasma insulin and glucose, by 30 days, no significant differences due to diet were found. No evidence of hypoglycemia was found at any time point on either diet. Even rats placed on high and low glycemic index diets, did not exhibit post-prandial hypoglycemia during an oral glucose tolerance test administered 14 weeks after diet initiation (Pawlak *et al.*, 2004). All in all, while individual foods may potentially result in low blood glucose levels, there appears to be little data demonstrating that high glycemic index meals elicit hypoglycemia on a consistent basis.

11.4.4 The glycemic index, lipids and cardiovascular disease

A number of studies suggest that high glycemic index diets may be associated with increased free fatty acids, triglycerides or increased LDL-cholesterol (Ford & Liu, 2001; Frost *et al.*, 1999; Liu *et al.*, 2001). However, like much of the work in this area, the results are complex and difficult to interpret due to differences in diet composition, study design and the duration of the test diet. For example, Wolever and Mehling (2003) tested the effect of four isocaloric breakfasts followed by a standardized lunch and measured plasma glucose, insulin, free fatty acids (FFAs) and triglycerides. The breakfasts were composed of 80% carbohydrate (either high or low GI foods), 20% protein and 10% fat or 41% carbohydrate (either high or low GI foods), 20% protein and 30% fat. The study demonstrated significantly different levels of FFAs during the rebound phase prior to lunch. The low-carbohydrate, low GI breakfast resulted in significantly elevated FFA levels and impaired second-meal carbohydrate tolerance. However, the high carbohydrate, low GI breakfast, resulted in lower FFAs and improved second meal tolerance. This study demonstrates the importance of meal context and how interactions between macronutrient quantity and composition can result in very different physiological responses.

Kiens and Richter (Kiens and Richrer, 1996), in an elegantly designed protocol, compared long-term ingestion (30 days) of high and low GI diets and conducted a euglycemic, hyperinsulinemic clamp at 3 and 30 days post ingestion. They found that while initially plasma glucose and insulin levels were lower on the low GI diet, by 30 days no differences were evident. In addition, they found that the low GI diet resulted in higher FFA levels during part of the day, a possible explanation for the reduction in insulin sensitivity also observed with the low GI diet. Wolever and Mehling (2003) examined the effect of high and low GI diets in subjects with impaired glucose tolerance and found that after 4 months on the assigned diets, triglycerides were elevated following the low GI diet. Frost *et al.* (1999) conducted a retrospective analysis of a survey of British adults and found that the glycemic index was the only dietary variable significantly related to serum HDL-cholesterol. More recently, the same author undertook a prospective, randomized trial in patients with coronary heart disease, comparing a low glycemic index diet to a control group who received healthy eating dietary advice. No significant differences in lipid levels between the two groups were found, although the authors attributed this to the masking of an effect by concurrent drug therapy (Frost *et al.*, 2004). In another randomized, intervention trial in overweight, healthy subjects, low glycemic index diets lowered LDL cholesterol compared to those on a high GI diet (Brynes *et al.*, 2003). Liu *et al.* (2001) found a very significant correlation between quintiles of glycemic load and fasting triglycerides, particularly in women with a BMI over 25. In addition to these effects on circulating lipid levels, a number of studies also show a significant positive correlation between glycemic index and cardiovascular disease. Thus, there appears to be some limited data demonstrating a relationship between GI and dyslipidemia, although based on the available physiological evidence it is difficult to ascertain the mechanism for this effect.

11.5 GI foods, food intake and weight control

In the 1950s, Mayer (1953) proposed the glucostatic theory of food intake regulation, postulating that low levels of blood glucose stimulate eating while high levels are inhibitory. Based on this theory, foods that elicit large postprandial increases in blood glucose would be more satiating than those resulting in lower post-prandial levels. While there are many studies both refuting and supporting this theory, over the last few years, the idea emerged that the North American diet, composed of highly processed foods and easily digested carbohydrate, contributed to a decrease in satiety, leading to an increase in food intake and obesity. High GI foods were proposed as the prototypic culprits due to their rapid rate of digestion and absorption. Furthermore, it was suggested that the high levels of insulin consecutive to ingestion of high GI foods could promote food intake (Rodin, 1991) and elicit hypoglycemia, which unto itself was recognized as a mechanism for the stimulation of hunger (Ludwig *et al.*, 1999; Roberts, 2000).

Short-term studies investigating the effect of high and low GI foods (or meals) on satiety and food intake typically use one of two designs: ingestion of a single meal coupled with measurements of glucose, insulin and indices of satiety and hunger, or a pre-load design in which subjects ingest a fixed amount of a test food and then at the subsequent meal, are permitted to eat *ad libitum* while hunger and satiety are monitored. A number of studies report an inverse relationship between the glycemic and insulin index of single foods and satiety such that low GI foods had higher satiety ratings in healthy volunteers (Holt *et al.*, 1992; Holt and Miller, 1995). Similarly, in obese teenage boys who consumed low, medium and high GI foods at breakfast, a significant decrease in food intake was observed following the low GI pre-load breakfast (Ludwig *et al.*, 1999). Lavin and Read (1995) compared the effects of a glucose drink, without and with guar gum, to examine the effect of glucose absorption on gastric emptying, satiety and hunger. Similar effects of the two treatments on plasma glucose were observed but insulin was significant higher after glucose alone. The addition of guar gum to the glucose decreased hunger and increased fullness although no differences in gastric emptying were observed. The authors concluded that the addition of the guar gum delayed the absorption of glucose from the small intestine.

Conversely, another study tested 38 common foods, grouped into six categories, and found no relationship between the glycemic score and satiety. However, a negative correlation was found between insulin area under the curve responses and *ad libitum* food intake at 120 min, suggesting that those foods with high post-prandial insulin levels were associated with decreased satiety 2 hours later (Holt *et al.*, 1996). Anderson *et al.* (2002) have also shown an inverse association between the area under the curve for blood glucose and food intake. These authors have demonstrated that, while high GI foods reduce appetite and food intake within an hour after ingestion, low GI foods appear to have a delayed effect, exhibiting satiating effects at 3 hours post ingestion (Anderson and Woodend, 2003). Synthesizing the results of the short-term studies, there is no underlying consistent pattern of relationships among blood glucose levels, satiety and food intake. This is not surprising. Glucose and insulin are just two of many factors involved in the short-term (i.e. meal-to-meal regulation) and long-term regulation of energy balance. It is unlikely that the measurement of insulin and glucose would be predictive of such a complex and vital behavior.

In a compelling article, Raben (2002) reviewed all the literature, both short-term and longer-term studies, that investigated the relationship between GI, satiety and weight loss in humans up until 2002. In 31 short-term studies of less than 1 day, low GI foods were associated with increased satiety in 15 studies, while the remaining 16 either found no significant differences or reduced satiety. When *ad libitum* food intake was monitored, low GI foods reduced food intake in seven studies but not in eight others. Longer-term studies, of which there were 20, showed a similar distribution of results, with 14 reporting no significant difference between high and low GI foods with respect to weigh loss. Of the remaining six, low GI diets promoted weight loss in four studies while the high GI diet promoted weight loss in two. Thus, the author concluded that it was premature to recommend low glycemic index diets as the ideal weight loss regimen. Furthermore, a recent study showed that the additional education of patients on the GI of foods coupled to a recognized behavioral weight loss programme, does not improve weight loss compared to the weight loss programme alone. These data suggest that, from a practical point of view, knowledge of GI composition is not a particularly good tool for diet selection (Carels *et al.*, 2005). In conclusion, as noted by a number of authors (Raben, 2002; Bessesen, 2001), a definitive study comparing diets varying solely in GI, in which subjects are permitted to eat a*d libitum* and weight fluctuate, has not been conducted.

11.5.1 Implications and recommendations

To date, there is insufficient evidence to recommend a low glycemic diet for the prevention of chronic disease, including obesity and weight loss. The literature on the glycemic index reveals startling inconsistencies at every level, ranging from the acute studies investigating satiety and the hypothesized mechanisms mediating the pathophysiological consequences, to the epidemiological studies examining the relationship between GI and chronic disease. The inconsistencies in the literature are a reflection of both the limitations of the GI index as an indicator of optimal dietary intake and of the inherent complexity of the relationship between diet and health. Categorization of foods into those that elicit high and low glycemic responses not only falsely 'villainizes' glucose and insulin, two molecules essential for life, but oversimplifies the importance of dietary context and the interplay of total calories, macro- and micro-nutrients in determining the overall 'healthfulness' of a diet.

The reported associations between GI values and disease may indicate that the GI is a marker, not for diets that elicit high or low blood glucose values, but instead for diet quality. As discussed by Willett *et al.* (2002), certain foods (cola beverages, white bread, cereals) consistently appear as markers of chronic disease across studies. It seems obvious from a nutritional standpoint that these highly caloric foods containing few macronutrients reflect poor diet quality when compared to many of the foods falling into the low GI category, i.e. high fiber vegetables, unprocessed, raw, whole grain foods and dairy products. Consumption of these high GI foods would most likely be less detrimental if they were not ingested within the context of a hypercaloric diet, containing high levels of fat as well as carbohydrate.

Specific concerns should be raised with regards to the consumption of caloric beverages (with the exception of dairy products). This statement is based on two facts: (i) the highly caloric nature of these beverages and (ii) the physiological consequences of liquid sugar ingestion, both with regards to the role liquid sugars may play in energy homeostasis (or lack thereof) as well as their direct metabolic consequences. Fructose is particularly troubling because of the observed effect on triglyceride levels and its potential contribution to a metabolic profile associated with a decrease in satiety. Individuals attempting to lose or maintain weight should be discouraged from consumption of any caloric beverage except low-fat milk.

In conclusion, the equation for weight maintenance is very simple: the amount of calories ingested must equal the amount expended. As a society, our activity level has dropped tremendously over the last few decades. This suggests that the number of calories we ingest must decrease proportionately. Ironically, we cook less and eat more frequently in restaurants where, since the 1950s, the portion sizes of foods have more than doubled and, in some cases, have quadrupled. The bitter but simple fact is that, as a society we must eat less and exercise more. Instead of polarizing itself over issues that are relatively minor, the scientific community should educate the public to negotiate an environment, which is conducive to good health by simplifying approaches and helping individuals adhere to dietary regimens.

11.6 References

ANDERSON, G. H., CATHERINE, N. L. A. and WOLEVER, T. M. S. (2002), 'Inverse association between the effect of carbohydrate on food intake and blood glucose in young men.' *Am. J. Clin. Nutr.*, **76**, 547–52.

ANDERSON, G. H. and WOODEND, D. (2003), 'Effect of glycemic carbohydrates on short-term satiety and food intake.' *Nutr. Rev.*, S17–26.

BERGMAN, R., PRAGER, R., VOLUND, A. and OLEFSKY, J. (1987), 'Equivalence of the insulin sensitivity index in man derived by the minimal model method and the euglycemic glucose clamp.' *J. Clin. Invest.*, **79**, 790–800.

BESSESEN, D. H. (2001), 'The role of carbohydrates in insulin resistance.' *J. Nutr.*, **131**, 2782S–6S.

BRAND-MILLER, J., PANG, E. and BROOMHEAD, L. (1995), 'The glycaemic index of foods containing sugars: comparison of foods with naturally-occurring vs. added sugars.' *Br. J. Nutr.*, **73**, 613–23.

BRYNES, A. E., MARK EDWARDS, C., GHATEI, M. A. *et al.* (2003), 'A randomized four-intervention crossover study investigation the effect of carbohydrates on daytime profiles of insulin, glucose, non-esterified fatty acids and triacylglycerols in middle-aged men.' *Br. J. Nutr.*, **89**, 207–18.

CARELS, R. A., DARBY, L. A., DOUGLASS, O. M., CACCIAPAGLIA, H. M. and RYDIN, S. (2005), 'Education on the glycemic index of foods fails to improve treatment outcomes in a behavioral weight loss programme.' *Eating Behaviors*, **6**, 145–50.

CHOI, Y. H. and ANDERSON, G. H. (2001), 'An interaction between hypothalamic glucagon-like peptide-1 and macronutrient composition determines food intake in rats.' *J. Nutr.*, **131**, 1819–25.

DALY, M. (2003), 'Sugars, insulin sensitivity and the postprandial state.' *Am. J. Clin. Nutr.*, **78**, 865S–72S.

DALY, M. E., VALE, C., WALKER, M. *et al.* (1998), 'Acute effects on insulin sensitivity and diurnal metabolic profiles of a high-sucrose compared with a high-starch diet.' *Am. J. Clin. Nutr.*, **67**, 1186–96.

ELLIOTT, R. M., MORGAN, L. M., TREDGER, J. A., DEACON, S., WRIGHT, J. and MARKS, V. (1993), 'Glucagon-like peptide-1 (7–36) amide and glucose-dependent insulinotropic polypeptide secretion in response to nutrient ingestion in man: acute post-prandial and 24-h secretion pattern.' *J. Endocr.*, **138**, 159–66.

ERCAN, N., NUTALL, F. Q. and GANNON, M. C. (1994), 'Effect of added fat on the plasma glucose and insulin response to ingested potato given in various combinations as two meals in normal individuals.' *Diabetes Care*, **17**, 1453–9.

FELBER, J. P., ACHESON, K. J. and TAY, L. (1993), *From Obesity to Diabetes.* John Wiley, Chichester, UK.

FORD, E. and LIU, S. (2001), 'Glycemic index and serum high-density lipoprotein cholesterol concentration among US adults.' *Arch. Intern. Med.*, **161**, 572–6.

FOSTER-POWELL, K., HOLT, S. H. A. and BRAND-MILLER, J. C. (2002), 'International table of glycemic index and glycemic load values: 2002.' *Am. J. Clin. Nutr.*, **76**, 5–56.

FRAYN, K. N. (2001), 'Adipose tissue and the insulin resistance syndrome.' *Proc. Nutr. Soc.*, **60**, 375–80.

FROST, G., LEEDS, A., MARGARA, R. and DORNHOOST, A. (1998), 'Insulin sensitivity in women at risk of coronary heart disease and the effect of a low glycaemic index diet.' *Metabolism*, **47**, 1245–51.

FROST, G., LEEDS, A. A., DORE, C. J., MADEIROS, S., BRADING, S. and DOMHORST, A. (1999), 'Glycaemic index as a determinant of serum HDL-cholesterol concentration.' *Lancet*, **353**, 1045–48.

FROST, G., BRYNES, A. E., BOVILL-TAYLOR, C. and DORNHORST, A. (2004), 'A prospective randomized trial to determine the efficacy of a low glycaemic index diet given in addition to healthy eating and weight loss advice in patients with coronary heart disease.' *Eur. J. Clin. Nutr.*, **58**, 121–7.

GANNON, M. C. and NUTTALL, F. Q. (1987), 'Factors affecting interpretation of post-prandial glucose and insulin areas.' *Diabetes Care*, **10**, 759–63.

GIN, H. and RIGALLEAU, H. (2000), 'Post-prandial hyperglycemia. Post-prandial hyperglycemia and diabetes.' *Diabet. Metab.*, **26**, 265–72.

GRANFELDT, Y., BJORK, I. and HAGANDER, B. (1991), 'On the importance of processing conditions, product thickness and egg addition for the glycaemic and hormonal responses to pasta: a comparison with bread made with past ingredients.' *Eur. J. Clin. Nutr.*, **45**, 489–99.

HODGE, A. M., ENGLISH, D. R., O'DEA, K. and GILES, G. G. (2004), 'Glycemic index and dietary fiber and the risk of type 2 diabetes.' *Diabetes Care*, **27**, 2701–6.

HOLT, S., BRAND, J., SOVENY, C. and HANSKY, J. (1992), 'Relationship of satiety to post-prandial glycaemic, insulin and cholecystokinin responses.' *Appetite*, **18**, 129–41.

HOLT, S. H., BRAND-MILLER, J. and PETROCZ, P. (1996), 'Interrelationships among post-prandial satiety, glucose and insulin responses and changes in subsequent food intake.' *Eur. J. Clin. Nutr.*, **50**, 788–97.

HOLT, S. H. and MILLER, J. B. (1995), 'Increased insulin responses to ingested foods are associated with lessened satiety.' *Appetite*, **24**, 43–54.

HU, F. B. (2003), 'Plant-based foods and prevention of cardiovascular disease: an overview.' *Am. J. Clin. Nutr.*, **78**, 544S–51S.

JENKINS, D. J. and JENKINS, A. L. (1987), 'The glycemic index, fiber, and the dietary treatment of hypertriglyceridemia and diabetes.' *J. Am. Coll. Nutr.*, **6**, 11–17.

JENKINS, D. J., WOLEVER, T. M. and TALYOR, R. H. (1981), 'Glycemic index of food: a physiological basis for carbohydrate exchange.' *Am. J. Clin. Nutr.*, **34**, 362–4.

JENKINS, D. J. A., WOLEVER, T. M. S. and TAYLOR, R. H. *et al.* (1982), 'Slow release carbohydrate improves second meal tolerance.' *Am. J. Clin. Nutr.*, **35**, 1339–46.

JOHNSON, S. K., THOMAS, S. J. and HALL, W. H. (2005), 'Palatability and glucose, insulin and satiety responses of chickpea flour and extruded chickpea flour bread eaten as part of a breakfast.' *Eur. J. Clin. Nutr.*, **59**, 169–76.

KAHN, S. E., MONTGOMERY, B., HOWELL, W. *et al.* (2001), 'Importance of early phase insulin secretion to intravenous glucose tolerance in subjects with type 2 diabetes mellitus.' *J. Clin. Endocrinol. Metab.*, **86**, 5824–9.

KANAUCHI, M., YAMANO, S., KANAUCHI, K. and SAITO, Y. (2003), 'Homeostasis model assessment of insulin resistance, quantitative insulin sensitivity check index, and oral glucose insulin sensitivity index in nonobese, nondiabetic subjects with high-normal blood pressure.' *J. Clin. Endocrinol. Metab.*, **88**, 3444–6.

KEITH, K. A. (1980), 'Gastric emptying of liquids and solids: roles of proximal and distal stomach.' *Am. J. Physiol.*, **239**, G71–6.

KIENS, B. and RICHTER, E. A. (1996), 'Types of carbohydrate in an ordinary diet affect insulin action and muscle substrates in humans.' *Am. J. Clin. Nutr.*, **63**, 47–53.

LAVIN, J. H. and READ, N. W. (1995), 'The effect on hunger and satiety of slowing the absorption of glucose: relationship with gastric emptying and postprandial blood glucose and insulin responses.' *Appetite*, **25**, 89–96.

LIU, S., MANSON, J. E., STAMPFER, M. J. *et al.* (2001), 'Dietary glycemic load assessed by food-frequency questionnaire in relation to plasma high-density-lipoprotein cholesterol and fasting plasma triacylglycerols in postmenopausal women.' *Am. J. Clin. Nutr.*, **73**, 560–6.

LUDWIG, D. S., MAJZOUB, J. A., AL-ZAHRANI, A., DALLAL, G. E., BLANCO, I. and ROBERTS, S. B. (1999), 'High glycemic index foods, overeating, and obesity.' *Pediatrics*, **103**, E23–7.

LUDWIG, D. (2002), 'The glycemic index: physiologic mechanisms relating to obesity, diabetes, and cardiovascular disease.' *JAMA*, **287**, 2414–23.

LUDWIG, D., PETERSON, K. and GORTMAKER, S. (2001), 'Relation between consumption of sugar-sweetened drinks and childhood obesity: a prospective, observational analysis.' *Lancet*, **357**, 505–8.

LUZI, L. and DEFRONZO, R. A. (1989), 'Effect of loss of first-phase insulin secretion on hepatic glucose production and tissue glucose disposal in humans.' *Am. J. Physiol.*, **257**, E241–6.

MARSHALL, J. A., HOAG, S., SHETTERLY, S. and HAMMAN, R. F. (1997), 'Dietary fat predicts conversion from impaired glucose tolerance to NIDDM.' *Diabetes Care*, **17**, 50–6.

MAYER, J. (1953), 'Glucostatic mechanism of the regulation of food intake.' *N. Engl. J. Med.*, **249**, 13–16.

MEIER, J. J. and NAUCK, M. A. (2005), 'Glucagon-like peptide 1 (GLP-1) in biology and pathology.' *Diabetes Metab. Res. Rev.*, **21**, 91–117.

MEYER, K. A., KUSHI, L. H., JACOBS, D. R., STAVIN, J., SELLERS, T. A. and FOLSOM, A. R. (2000), 'Carbohydrates, dietary fiber, and incident type 2 diabetes in older women.' *Am. J. Clin. Nutr.*, **71**, 921–30.

OVERDUIN, J., FRAYO, R. S., GRILL, H. J., KAPLAN, J. M. and CUMMINGS, D. E. (2005), 'Role of the duodenum and macronutrient type in ghrelin regulation.' *Endocrinology*, **146**, 845–50.

PAWLAK, D. B., KUSHNER, J. A. and LUDWIG, D. S. (2004), 'Effects of dietary glycemic index on adiposity, glucose homeostasis, and plasma lipids in animals.' *Lancet*, **364**, 778–85.

PI-SUNYER, X. (2002), 'Glycemic index and disease.' *Am. J. Clin. Nutr.*, **76**, 290S–8S.

PUTNAM, J., ALLSHOUSE, J. and KANTOR, L. S. (2002), 'U.S. per capita food trends: increased calories, refined carbohydrates and fats.' *Food Rev.*, **25**, 2–15.

RABEN, A. (2002), 'Should obese patients be counseled to follow a low-glycemic index diet? No.' *Obes. Rev.*, **3**, 245–56.

REAVEN, G. M. (1988), 'Banting lecture 1988. Role of insulin resistance in human disease.' *Diabetes*, **37** (12), 1595–607.

ROBERTS, S. B. (2000), 'High-glycemic index foods, hunger, and obesity: is there a connection?' *Nutr. Rev.*, **58**, 163–9.

RODIN, J. (1991), 'Effects of pure sugar vs. mixed starch fructose loads on food intake.' *Appetite*, **17**, 213–19.

SALMERON, J., ASHERIO, M., RIMM, E. B., COLDITZ, G. A., WING, A. L. and WILLETT, W. C. (1997a), 'Dietary fiber, glycemic load, and risk of NIDDM in men.' *Diabetes Care*, **20**, 545–50.

SALMERON, J., MANSON, J. E., STAMPLER, M. J., COLDITZ, G., WING, A. L. and WILLETT, W. C. (1997b), 'Dietary fiber, glycemic load and risk of non-insulin dependent diabetes mellitus in women.' *JAMA*, **277**, 472–7.

SCHULZE, M. B., MANSON, J. E., LUDWIG, D. *et al.* (2004), 'Sugar-sweetened beverages, weight gain, and incidence of type 2 diabetes in young and middle-aged women.' *JAMA*, **292**, 927–34.

STEVENS, J., AHN, K., JUHAERI, H. D., STEFFAN, L. and COUPER, D. (2002), 'Dietary fiber intake and glcyemic index and incidence of diabetes in African-American and white adults: the ARIC study.' *Diabetes Care*, **25**, 1715–21.

TEFF, K. L. (1994), 'Cephalic phase insulin release in humans: mechanism and function', in *Appetite and Body Weight Regulation: Sugar, Fat and Macronutrient Substitutes*, J. D. Fernstrom and G. D. Miller, eds., CRC Press, Boca Raton, 37–50.

TEFF, K. L., DEVINE, J. and ENGELMAN, K. (1995), 'Sweet taste: effect on cephalic phase insulin release in men.' *Physiol. Behav.*, **57** (6), 1089–95.

TEFF, K. L., ELLIOTT, S. S., TSCHOP, M. *et al.* (2004), 'Dietary fructose reduces circulating insulin and leptin, attenuates postprandial supression of ghrelin, and increases triglycerides in women.' *J. Clin. Endocrinol. Metab.*, **89**, 2963–72.

TEFF, K. L. and TOWNSEND, R. R. (1999), 'Early phase insulin infusion and muscarinic blockade in obese and lean subjects.' *Am. J. Physiol.*, **277**, R198–208.

WILLETT, W., MANSSON, J. and LIU, S. (2002), 'Glycemic index, glycemic load, and risk of type 2 diabetes.' *Am. J. Clin. Nutr.*, **76**, 274S–80S.

WOLEVER, T. M. S. and MEHLING, C. (2003), 'Long-term effect of varying the source or amount of dietary carbohydrate on postprandial plasma glucose, insulin, triacylglycerol, and free fatty acids concentrations in subjects with impaired glucose tolerance.' *Am. J. Clin. Nutr.*, **77**, 612–21.

12

Protein intake and weight control

P. Clifton, CSIRO Health Sciences and Nutrition, Australia

12.1 Introduction

This chapter will examine the role protein may have in maintaining weight, enhancing weight loss and maintaining that weight loss long term. There are three proposed mechanisms of action for this effect: enhanced satiety, enhanced thermogenesis and sparing of lean tissue and each of these will be examined in detail both in acute studies and in the fewer long-term studies available. The postulated mechanism for the enhanced satiety will also be explored, although there is very little consistent evidence on this point. The role of higher protein diets in the control of lipids, glucose, insulin and blood pressure will be described. A major issue with high protein diets is long-term safety and this particular aspect will be closely examined. A confounding factor in the examination of high protein diets is that the distribution of the two other macronutrients may vary widely, from very high fat to moderate fat, and this may influence the results observed as well as public and professional response to the diet and the results.

12.2 Protein intake and satiety

Protein in many studies appears to be more satiating than either fat or carbohydrate. This area has been continually examined over the last 50 years. Fryer (1959) found examining 12 male students with 9-week dietary periods that feelings of hunger were greatest on the low protein diet while satiety was greatest on the low carbohydrate/high protein diet. Other studies using similar satiety scales found that high protein meals were more satisfying

(Hill and Blundell, 1986; Vandewater and Vickers, 1995; Westerterp-Plantenga *et al.*, 1999). Stubbs *et al.* (1996, 1999) found protein-rich meals more satiating but energy intake after the test meal was not different. Johnstone *et al.* (1996) found that overfeeding protein in six men over 1 day led to greater feelings of satiety compared with both fat and carbohydrate but this did not influence energy intake on the subsequent 2 days.

12.2.1 Positive findings

Using a more objective measure, although one easily confounded by observation and dietary restraint of participants – the measured amount of food eaten at a subsequent meal after a full test meal or a preload, Booth *et al.* (1970) found that the majority of subjects consumed more food after a low protein test meal than a high protein test meal. Barkeling *et al.* (1990) showed a 12% decrease in energy intake ($P < 0.05$) at the subsequent meal 4 hours after a meat casserole compared with a low protein vegetarian casserole while Porrini *et al.* (1994) showed similar effects with meatballs compared with pasta. Johnson and Vickers (1993) found a high protein preload decreased the weight of food eaten compared with the high fat and high carbohydrate preloads, but caloric intake was reduced only compared to the high fat ($N = 14$ students). Positive effects of protein were also found by de Castro and Elmore (1988), de Castro (1987) and Araya *et al.* (2000). Huon and Wootton (1991) also found *ad libitum* intake was higher 4 hours after a low protein meal. Poppitt *et al.* (1998) found that a protein preload reduced food intake 90 minutes later by about 400 kJ (about 16%). Westerterp-Plantenga *et al.* (1999) showed a mixed high protein (31%), high carbohydrate fixed energy diet (61%) had greater satiating effects over a 36-hour period compared with a low protein (9%), high fat meal (61%) in eight lean, female students. Marmonier *et al.* (2000) found that a high protein meal delayed the request for dinner by 60 minutes compared with 25 for fat and 34 for carbohydrate but food intake was not affected.

However, these test meals differed widely in physical and sensory properties so it cannot be concluded that it was the protein conferring these effects. Lattner designed a study so that the sensory properties of the meals were exactly the same. In 12 lean female students 31% more calories were eaten at a subsequent dinner with high CHO liquid lunch (450 kcal, 99% carbohydrate from polycose) than high protein liquid (71% protein) meal or a 50% protein, 50% carbohydrate lunch (Latner and Schwartz, 1999). The protein was a dried powder mix derived from whey.

As all of these studies used subjects of normal weight, it is difficult to generalise to those who are overweight or who have weight concerns such as restrained eaters. There is some evidence for reduced sensory-specific satiety in the obese. In this study obese women were found to have a significantly slower decline in salivation due to repeated food cues. The effects of meal composition on subsequent craving and binge eating in women with reported frequent episodes of craving was assessed by Gendall (1999). Three isocaloric meals (chicken salad, fruit and cream or a mixture of both) were provided on 3 separate days. Appetite and mood ratings were taken before and at four intervals up to 150 min after meal consumption. Subsequent *ad libitum* food intake was recorded in diaries. Premeal hunger, appetite and mood ratings were similar across meal type. After the protein-rich meal, craving for sweet, carbohydrate-rich foods was significantly higher than after the carbohydrate and mixed meals. The first *ad libitum* eating episodes after the protein meal contained significantly higher absolute and proportional amounts of total carbohydrate and sucrose and were more likely to be categorised as a binge than were those after the carbohydrate and mixed meals. This is in contrast to the results of Barkeling suggesting that either the form of protein meal (i.e. chicken vs. meat or salad vs. casserole) or nature of subjects was responsible for the divergent outcomes.

12.2.2 Negative findings

Negative findings (i.e. no differences in food intake) were seen by Geliebter (1979), Rolls *et al.* (1988), Rolls and McDermott (1991), De Graaf *et al.* (1992), Driver (1988), Stubbs *et al.* (1996, 1999), Johnstone *et al.* (1996), Vozzo *et al.* (2003) and Raben *et al.* (2003). In the latter study a breakfast containing 32% protein, 31% fat and 37% carbohydrate was compared to one containing 65% carbohydrate and 12% protein or 65% fat and 12% protein. The meals were normal whole foods, had the same amount of energy and energy density was the same. The 20% protein increase is well within normal meal variations. The energy supplied was adequate (2500 kJ for women and 3000 kJ for men) although the participant numbers were not great (n = 19). The *ad libitum* test meal was a fixed meal (pasta and meat sauce and vegetables) and probably did not allow for wide differences in intake, although intake was 4.2 (protein-rich meal) to 5 MJ (fat and carbohydrate-rich meals). Dietary restraint in the women was probably marked in this study. No difference was seen with satiety scales either. This difference of 16% has been found to be significant in other studies and is probably typical of normal meal studies and is clearly of significance long term even if not statistically significant in this study. Vozzo found that a 3 MJ protein preload suppressed food intake by 29% over the next 7 hours compared with no preload while a high carbohydrate preload suppressed it by 17%. However, with 16 lean men and five treatments, the study was not powered to show significance for this level of difference.

12.2.3 Conclusion

On an energy basis, protein is probably more satiating than the other macronutrients especially when the interval to the next meal is short (e.g.

90 minutes) but, with normal meals taken at normal intervals, sometimes this difference is not observed. Protein-enriched snacks may delay the interval, to the next meal, while protein-rich meals may prevent later snacking although the latter has not been tested.

12.2.4 Sensory-specific satiety

One of the problems faced in trying to rate sensations of hunger and satiety is the existence of sensory-specific satiety. This occurs when foods that have been eaten decrease more in liking than foods that have not been eaten. Sensory-specific satiety has been studied by Rolls (1986), Rolls *et al.* (1988) who demonstrated that, if several foods which differed in taste, appearance and texture, are offered in succession, the consumption of the meal will be higher than when only one food is given. Thus, overeating may occur when a wide variety of foods is readily available (Birch and Deysher, 1986). Johnson and Vickers (1992) showed a trend for high-protein foods to decrease more in liking than low-protein foods concluding that protein foods showed greater sensory-specific satiety. Sensory-specific satiety is more dependent on the taste, texture and color than macronutrient or energy content of food (Rolls *et al.*, 1988). Sensory-specific satiety is pronounced in adolescents and diminished in elderly people (Rolls and McDermott, 1991; Rolls, 1994). Sensory-specific satiety does not depend on food ingestion as olfactory sensory-specific satiety can be induced by smelling the food (Rolls and Rolls, 1997). Odor variety in a meal could be expected to enhance intake.

12.2.5 Protein type

Very little attention has been paid to protein type and its role in satiation. Uhe *et al.* (1992) tested fish, beef and chicken meals in six lean men. Fish was the most satiating (by visual analogue scale, VAS) and this was related to the slow appearance of amino acids and a higher tryptophan/neutral amino acid ratio. However, the numbers are too small to make any firm conclusions. Essential plasma amino acid levels were related to dietary intake (other than lysine and tryptophan). Lang *et al.* (1998, 1999) tested a variety of protein sources (egg albumin, casein, gelatin, soy protein, pea protein, and wheat gluten) and found no differences in satiety for 8 hours or subsequent intake for 24 hours in 9–12 subjects with meals containing 22–23% protein. Hall *et al.* (2003) found a 1700 kJ liquid preload containing 48 g of whey reduced *ad libitum* intake at a buffet 90 minutes later by 829 kJ or 18% compared with an equivalent casein preload in 16 subjects. There were no measured differences in hunger, desire to eat or fullness after the first study with an *ad libitum* meal. In a second study ($n = 9$) a fixed meal was offered at 42 g/kg 90 minutes after the same preloads. However, the composition of the buffet meal was individually determined, based on the subjects preferences and was not reported in the paper. Fullness was increased and desire to eat was reduced more by the whey preload (plus lunch) over 180 minutes. The whey led to higher total amino acid levels at 70 and 90 minutes after the preload, which surprisingly persisted after the lunch. These results are the opposite of Uhe's results. Although there are quite significant differences in amino acid composition between whey and casein this was not reflected in amino acid profile for some of the amino acids. Five of 13 amino acids were higher with whey, while the rest except for proline were no different. Proline was higher with casein, reflecting its higher level in casein. Arginine, phenylalanine, methionine and tyrosine, although higher in casein, were not different in plasma, suggesting that whey may somehow induce slower clearance of amino acids. Gastric emptying as measured by paracetamol levels was faster with casein. In addition GLP1, GIP and CCK were 28–65% higher over the 180 minutes following the whey meal plus lunch. With GIP this difference was mostly before the 90-minute meal while with GLP1 the majority of the difference occurred after 90 minutes.

Amino acids

A relationship between fluctuations in plasma amino acids was suggested by Mellinkoff *et al.* in 1956 and revived by George Bray in 1997. Administration of 400 mg of the dipeptide aspartame inhibited food intake at lunch by 15% but 200 mg of either of the constituent phenylalanine or aspartic acid had no effects (Rogers *et al.*, 1991).

Habituation

Long *et al.* (2000) showed that the response to a high protein meal is dependent on the habitual protein intake. Fourteen subjects were divided into two groups depending on their habitual protein intake – either 1 g/kg/d or 1.4 g/kg/d. An acute high protein (2.2 g/kg/d) test was performed with the protein consumed across the day as breakfast, lunch and dinner with satiety tested by VAS. The protein intake was then lowered in the low protein group to 0.75 g/kg and increased to 1.96 g/kg in the high protein group for a 14-day period and then the test was repeated. Finally, in the high protein group the protein intake was lowered to 0.85 g/kg for 2 days and the test repeated. Overall, the high protein test meal was more satiating (by VAS) on the low protein diet than the high protein, although the differences were not marked. Lowering the protein intake in the high protein group for 2 days had no effect on satiety ratings.

12.3 Protein intake and energy intake

Most studies have shown that protein has a higher thermic effect than either fat or carbohydrate. Dauncey and Bingham (1983) had six subjects live in a calorimeter for 28 hours on 12 occasions and showed that a high protein diet led to 12% greater total energy production ($P < 0.001$) compared with a high glucose diet. Karst *et al.* (1984) examined this issue in 12 healthy males with indirect calorimetry for 6 hours after 1, 2 and 4 MJ meals of three protein types (egg white, gelatin and casein), two carbohydrates (starch and hydrolysed starch) and two fats (sunflower oil and butter). The thermic effect of protein was three times greater than carbohydrate, while fat produced no thermic effect. An increased meal size was associated with an increased thermic effect. Satiety was not assessed. Crovetti *et al.* (1998) showed that the thermic effect of a 2333 kJ meal containing 68% protein was three times greater than a meal of similar total and percentage energy of fat or carbohydrate. Feelings of fullness were greater with the high protein meal and were related to the thermic effect of the meal. Westerterp-Plantenga *et al.* (1999) showed with a mixed high protein (31%), high carbohydrate (61%) fixed energy diet had greater satiating effects over a 36-hour period compared with a low protein (9%), high fat meal (61%) in 8 lean, female students. The thermic effect of the high protein meal was greater (14% of meal energy) compared with the high fat meal (10.5% of meal energy) and the satiety assessed by VAS was related to the thermogenic effect both within one diet and between diets. In a review of this area Westerterp (2004) calculated that, for each 1% change in energy from protein, the thermic effect of the meal increased by 0.22%, but this was based on a regression analysis of 19 individual studies in which only two studies had interventions with differing protein levels. Raben *et al.* (2003) has offered a contrary view. She studied a larger number of subjects (19) and tested four meals rich in either protein (32% of energy), carbohydrate (65% of energy), fat (65% of energy), or alcohol (23% of energy) for 5 hours with indirect calorimetry. Although the thermic effect of alcohol was greater than the other meals (27% of meal energy), it had no effect on either satiety or energy consumed at a subsequent meal. Leptin was profoundly suppressed by alcohol (−1 ng/ml or about 25%), which may have nullified the enhanced thermic effect.

The relationship between the thermic effect of a meal and its satiating effects still need to be clarified, although there is little doubt that protein meals have an enhanced thermic effect.

12.4 Short- and long-term studies of protein intake and its effects

The studies are essentially designed to test the metabolic effects of a high protein intake, especially on lipids and lean mass and do not allow the effect of enhanced satiety to be demonstrated as energy intake is controlled.

The role of protein levels in very low calorie diets (400–800 kcal/day) in sparing lean body mass is still controversial. Earlier studies from Hoffer found that high protein, low carbohydrate diets were optimal while later studies from Vazquez suggested that moderate protein (50–70 g/day) but high carbohydrate (>75 g/day) diets were optimal.

There is no consensus that macronutrient composition influences insulin sensitivity. Earlier studies suggested that high carbohydrate/high fibre weight stable diets enhanced insulin sensitivity compared with high fat diets (Riccardi *et al.*, 1984), but subsequent studies have suggested either no difference (Borkman *et al.*, 1991) or the opposite effect (Garg *et al.*, 1988); the latter study only used plasma insulin and glucose as indices of insulin resistance. There has been little work examining the effect of protein, but zero or low protein isocaloric diets have been shown to lower blood glucose and increase insulin sensitivity in normals and diabetics (Hoffer *et al.*, 1998; Lariviere *et al.*, 1994).

O'Dea *et al.* (1989) found that a high protein (62% of calories for 2 weeks) diet was as effective at improving glucose control in type 2 diabetics as a high carbohydrate, high fibre diet. Lariviere *et al.* (1994) found a severely protein restricted diet lowered average daily blood glucose by 30% despite a lowering of daily insulin doses by 25% in type 1 diabetics. Pomerleau *et al.* (1993) found that a moderate protein diet (0.8 g/kg) improved renal function in type 2 diabetics and normal subjects compared with a high protein diet (2.0 g/kg) and both had similar effects on glycemic control.

Piatti *et al.* (1994) investigated the effects of two hypocaloric (800 kcal) diets on body composition and insulin sensitivity in 25 normal glucose-tolerant obese women. The two diets had the following composition, 45% protein, 35% carbohydrate (CHO), and 20% fat (10 subjects), and 60% CHO, 20% protein, and 20% fat (15 subjects), both lasted 21 days. Both diets induced a similar decrease in body weight and fat mass whereas fat-free mass decreased only after the high carbohydrate diet. 3-methylhistidine excretion (an index of muscle breakdown) was reduced by 48% after the high protein diet and remained unchanged after the high carbohydrate diet ($P < 0.05$). Insulin sensitivity, as assessed by clamp studies, increased in the high protein group and decreased in the high carbohydrate group. This effect may be related to the loss of lean mass in the high carbohydrate group.

One small study of 13 men has examined the effect of moderate caloric restriction and increased dietary protein in obese subjects with insulin resistance (Baba *et al.*, 1999). In this study, an energy restricted (80% of resting energy expenditure or 1760 kcal/day) high protein (45%), low carbohydrate (25%) diet led to greater weight loss over a 4 week period (8.6 kg vs. 6.0 kg) compared with a normal protein (12%) diet. Much of the difference in weight loss between diets was due to water rather than fat loss. With the high protein diet, however, the fall in resting energy expenditure with weight loss was reduced to –132 kcal/day (5%) compared to –384 kcal/day (or 16%) on the low protein diet. This could potentially lead to a difference between diets of up to 0.8 kg of fat loss over the subsequent month.

In two studies in overweight men and women, one group with insulin resistance (Farnsworth *et al.*, 2003) and one group with diabetes (Parker *et al.*, 2002), we have demonstrated that a high protein weight loss diet (28–30% of energy from protein diet) from mixed sources enhances fat loss by 1–2 kg over 12 weeks, particularly in women, in comparison with a normal protein weight loss diet (14–15% of energy from protein) and spared lean mass. In the diabetic women the difference in fat loss was 5.3 vs. 2.8 kg with an abdominal fat loss of 1.3 vs. 0.7 kg. In the hyperinsulinemic group of women, lean loss was reduced by 1.4 kg with a high protein diet. No effect was seen in men in either study, perhaps related to the lower intake of protein on a g/kg basis. There was no effect of an increased protein intake on blunting the fall in resting energy expenditure.

In another weight loss study in 50 overweight subjects (40 women and 10 men) with mildly elevated plasma triglyceride or glucose levels or with hypertension, we contrasted a 6 MJ weight loss diet containing 30% protein, 30% fat and 40% carbohydrate with one containing 15% protein, 30% fat and 55% carbohydrate over a 12-week period. Although there was a 1.1 kg greater loss on the high protein diet (9.8 kg vs. 8.7 kg), this difference was not statistically significant ($P = 0.4$). There were also no differences in fasting lipids, free fatty acids, glucose or insulin at 12 weeks. With weight loss, there was a larger decrease in insulin levels during the oral glucose tolerance test on the high protein (40–45 mIU/l) as compared to the high carbohydrate diet (24 mIU/l), suggesting an increase in insulin sensitivity, possibly due to preservation of lean body mass. This effect, however, was seen in men only and the study has significant limitations as fasting insulin levels were not matched in the two groups.

We have studied the effect of a high protein, high red meat diet in 12-week randomised parallel design of two 5600 kJ diets, high meat (HM) 34% protein 46% carbohydrate 20% fat or low meat (LM) 17% protein 64% carbohydrate 20% fat (Noakes *et al.*, 2005, in press). One hundred women with a mean BMI of 32.6 and mean age of 49.3 years completed the study with a weight loss of -7.6 ± 3.3 (HM, Mean ± SD) and -6.9 ± 3.5 kg (LM) and fat (-5.7 ± 4.0, -4.6 ± 3.7) and a lean mass loss of (-1.6 ± 1.9, -1.8 ± 1.8 kg) These changes were different from baseline but not between diets. There was a significant interaction between diet and baseline triglyceride ($P < 0.05$). Subjects with a high TG (>1.5 mmol/l) had greater loss of weight on the HM diet 7.9 ± 0.7 vs. 5.9 ± 0.4 kg ($P = 0.02$) and a greater loss of fat (6.3 vs. 3.6 kg) and abdominal fat (1.0 vs. 0.05 kg).

12.4.1 Lipids

In weight stable studies Wolfe and Giovannetti (1991) demonstrated that replacement of carbohydrate with protein in mildly hyperlipidemic subjects lowered LDL cholesterol by 6.4%, lowered triglyceride by 23% and increased HDL cholesterol by 12%. Similar effects were seen in normolipidemic volunteers (Wolfe and Piche, 1999). There are no other studies to confirm or refute this. In the studies of Skov *et al.* (1999a) plasma triglyceride and free fatty acid levels were significantly lowered only on the high protein, low carbohydrate diet. However, this may not be a specific function of the protein as similar changes in plasma triglyceride are seen with fat/carbohydrate exchanges in both weight stable (4) and weight loss studies (5). LDL cholesterol was not different between diets in this study, unlike the Wolfe studies above.

We have also shown that replacing dietary carbohydrate with protein, while keeping fat constant at <28% energy during weight loss, has been effective in preserving HDL and achieving a greater LDL cholesterol reduction in obese subjects with type 2 diabetes. In this study women on the high protein (low glycemic load) diet lost significantly more total (5.3 vs. 2.8 kg, $P = 0.009$) and abdominal (1.3 vs. 0.7 kg, $P = 0.006$) fat compared with the women on the low protein diet (high glycemic load). These observations suggest that a high protein and therefore low glycemic load diet is a valid diet choice for reducing CVD risk in type 2 diabetes (Parker *et al.*, 2002).

In the high red meat study (Noakes, 2005, in press), TG fell by 8% in the low meat diet and 22% in the high meat diet (ns). HDL cholesterol fell 5–8% and LDL cholesterol and glucose fell by 7% and 4%, respectively, with no differences between diets. Fasting insulin fell by 16–27% with no significant differences between diets. Vitamin B12 increased by 9% on HM and fell by 13% on LM ($P < 0.01$) but fasting plasma homocysteine did not change. Plasma folate was unchanged. Urine markers of bone turnover increased by 8–12% and calcium excretion decreased by 1 mmol/day with no differences between diets. Bone density did not change.

12.4.2 *Ad libitum*

There are two *ad libitum* studies. Dumesnil and colleagues (2001), in a short-term (6-day), *ad libitum* study, in 12 overweight men, investigated the effects of a low fat high-protein diet compared with a low fat diet. The *ad libitum* low fat diet induced a 28% increase in plasma TAG levels and a 10% reduction in plasma HDL-C. In contrast, the high protein diet resulted in a spontaneous decrease (25%) in total energy intake, a significant decrease in plasma TAG (35%) and plasma insulin levels. The study also had a pair-fed aspect, in which subjects ate a high carbohydrate diet but with the same reduced energy intake as during the high protein diet. There was a trend for a decrease in plasma HDL-C, a significant increase in hunger ($P < 0.0002$) and decrease in satiety ($P < 0.007$) on the energy-restricted diet. The results of this study suggest that a high protein diet may offer some protection against the over-consumption of energy.

Skov *et al.* (1999) demonstrated that *ad libitum* choice of a high protein (25% of calories) diet from a clinic shop leads to greater weight loss compared with a normal protein (12%) diet with losses of 8.9 and 5.1 kg, respectively, over a 6-month period. Dietary fat intake was maintained at 30% of calories in both diets. Body fat loss was greater on the high protein diet (7.6 vs. 4.3 kg) but there was no difference between the diets in loss of lean body mass. There were no changes in the control group. More subjects lost >10 kg in the HP group (35%) than in the HC group (9%).

Layman fed 24 overweight and obese women either a high protein diet (125 g protein/day) or a low protein diet (68 g/day) with 50 g of fat and 7100 kJ. After 10 weeks weight loss was 7.53 and 6.96 kg, respectively, with a fat/lean ratio loss of 6.3 vs. 3.8. Neither fat nor lean loss separately were different between diets. Triglyceride fell by 21% in the high protein group and the high protein group reported higher satiety. Layman has hypothesised that leucine stimulates muscle protein synthesis and enhances uptake of glucose by muscle (Layman, 2003).

12.4.3 Longer-term studies (12 months or longer)

In a 12-month follow-up of 43 hyperinsulinemic subjects on high and low protein diets, weight loss was 4.1 and 2.9%, respectively, (ns) but long-term compliance to the diet as assessed by urea/creatinine ratio was poor and there was no difference between protein intakes at 12 months (Brinkworth *et al.*, 2004). In a second study, 38 diabetic subjects were followed for 12 months after an 8-week weight loss study on either a high protein or low protein diet. Although compliance to the protein level was good (as assessed by urea/creatinine ratio), there was no difference in outcomes and all of the fat lost in the short-term study was regained. Despite fat regain, there was continuing loss of lean tissue over the whole 12-month follow-up period. In spite of this fat regain, HDL cholesterol rose by over 10% in both groups and CRP continued to fall (G.D. Brinkworth unpublished data). The high protein diet group had a significantly lower blood pressure level at the end of 12 months compared with the normal protein group.

In a third 12-month study, 78 women completed a 12-month weight loss programme comparing a dietary allocation to a higher protein, high meat diet (HM) with a low meat, high carbohydrate diet (HC). At 12 months, overall weight loss was not different at 4.7 and 4.4 kg, HM and HC, respectively. However, when protein intake, calculated from dietary records, at 12 months was used as a criterion, then weight loss was greater in the group who consumed more than 88 g/day of protein, 6.5 kg vs. 3.1 kg ($P = 0.03$). The dietary records were validated with urinary urea/creatinine ratios. However, this weight difference did not translate into a difference in central fat loss between the two groups. Lipids, glucose, insulin, C-reactive protein (CRP) and homocysteine were all improved by weight loss with no differences between groups. A higher serum B12 was seen in the higher protein group and folate levels were not different between groups.

12.5 Very low carbohydrate, high protein diets

Low carbohydrate and high protein diets have recently re-emerged as a popular weight loss strategy. Four recent studies have reported on the use of low carbohydrate diets in the treatment of obesity (Foster *et al.*, 2003). In the first of these studies 63 subjects were randomised to either low-carbohydrate, high-protein, high-fat diets (low GL) or low-calorie, high-carbohydrate, low-fat diets (high GL). Subjects on the low-carbohydrate diet lost more weight than subjects on the conventional diet at 3 months (–6.8 ± 5.0 vs. –2.7 ± 3.7 percent of body weight, $P = 0.001$) and 6 months (–7.0 ± 6.5 vs. –3.2 ± 5.6 percent of body weight, $P = 0.02$). However, the difference was not maintained at 12 months (–4.4 ± 6.7 vs. –2.5 ± 6.3 percent of body weight, $P = 0.26$) (Foster *et al.*, 2003). Samaha *et al.* (2003) randomly assigned 132 severely obese subjects to a low carbohydrate (<30 g/day) diet or an energy restricted (500 calories off usual diet) and fat-restricted (<30% of calories) diet for 6 months. Subjects on the low-carbohydrate diet lost more weight than those on the low-fat diet (–5.8 ± 8.6 kg vs. –1.9 ± 4.2 kg, $P = 0.002$) and had greater decreases in triglyceride levels. Differences in energy intake, assessed by a 24 hr recall method, did not reach significance. Whether the results seen in these studies are related more to the low carbohydrate diet, the ketogenic nature of the diet or the higher protein level is not clear. After 12 months, there was no difference in weight loss between the two groups but triglyceride decreased more and HDL cholesterol less in the low carbohydrate group. In the 54 subjects with diabetes HbA1c decreased more on the low carbohydrate diet. Brehm *et al.* (2003) found a low carbohydrate diet lowered weight by 8.5 kg compared with 3.9 kg on a conventional diet at 6 months in 42 women. In none of the above studies was LDL different on the low carbohydrate, high fat diet, although Sondike *et al.* (2003) found a fall in LDL cholesterol only on the low fat diet.

In another study from our group (unpublished) very low fat (10%) (VLF), high unsaturated fat (30%) (HUF) and very low carbohydrate (4%) (VLC) diets were compared. The VLC diet, resulted in a greater weight loss of 9.2% compared to the VLF (7.3%) and HUF (7.0%) ($P = 0.034$). However, loss of lean mass was significantly greater on the VLC and VLF (31–32% of weight loss) compared to the HUF diet (21%). LDL-C increased on the ketogenic diet but decreased 0.40 ± 0.11 mmol/l on the VLF diet and 0.34 ± 0.14 mmol/l on the HUF diet ($P = 0.009$). The VLC diet had the greatest triglyceride reduction (–0.73 ± 0.12 mmol/l) followed by the HUF diet (–0.15 ± 0.07 mmol/l) and lastly the VLF (–0.06 ± 0.13 mmol/l). Similarly, diet composition significantly affected the change in HDL-C with an increase on the ketogenic diet (0.06 ± 0.03 mmol/l) whereas the other two diets resulted in similar net decreases of 0.06 ± 0.03 mmol/l. Plasma homocysteine increased 6.6% on the ketogenic diet, decreased 6.8% on the VLF and remained unchanged on the HUF diet ($P = 0.026$ for diet effect). The ketogenic diet lowered fasting insulin significantly more than the other diets with a 33% reduction compared to the 19% fall on the HUF diet and no change on the VLF diet ($P < 0.001$). All diets resulted in a significant decrease in fasting glucose, blood pressure and CRP with weight loss ($P < 0.05$). These results suggest that, under isocaloric conditions, the ketogenic diet results in some improvements but also some deterioration in cardiovascular risk factors compared to conventional weight loss patterns. It is unclear what the net effect on CVD risk is imparted by the ketogenic diet. Both these studies have as yet uncompleted 1 year follow-up phases.

12.5.1 Protein intake, insulin release and plasma insulin levels

It has been demonstrated on many occasions that protein meals provoke the release of insulin leading to higher plasma insulin levels postprandially and increased excretion of C-peptide when compared with fat in both normals and diabetics. Whether protein is as potent as glucose at releasing insulin is not clear.

Using normal volunteers, Hoogwerf *et al.* (1986) found that, gram for gram, protein was twice as potent as carbohydrate in releasing insulin (as assessed by 24h urinary C-peptide) while Krezowski *et al.* (1986) demonstrated that protein produced an insulin response that was only 28% of that of the same amount of glucose (as assessed by area under the plasma insulin curve over 4 hours). The combination of insulin and glucose was not synergistic.

Spiller *et al.* (1987) found that the addition of 16g protein to 58g glucose doubled the area under the insulin curve in normals and that the level at 2 hours was directly related to the amount of protein ingested when protein was increased. Glucose area was decreased by increasing amounts of protein.

In diabetics and normals there are significant differences between protein types, with cottage cheese being most potent and egg white being least potent at raising plasma insulin with meat, fish and soy protein being intermediate (Gannon *et al.*, 1988; Westphal *et al.*, 1990). In diabetics, protein was 4–8 times more potent per gram than glucose but it was much weaker in normals. Howe (1990) demonstrated that beef was less potent than both soy isolate and cottage cheese.

Thus substitution of protein for dietary carbohydrate would be expected to reduce the post-prandial glucose response with a maintained or augmented insulin response. Whether this would lead to better glucose control or less risk of long-term complications in diabetics or insulin-resistant subjects is not clear.

12.6 Safety of high protein diets

12.6.1 Cardiovascular disease

Concern has been expressed over the safety of high protein diets. Ecological studies show that countries consuming relatively low protein (and low fat) diets have lower rates of cardiovascular disease. However, there are many potentially confounding factors with large differences between countries in social and cultural factors. One cohort study, The Honolulu Heart Study (McGee *et al.*, 1984), showed that higher protein intakes were associated with more cardiovascular disease after adjustment for plasma cholesterol and other conventional risk factors, while saturated fat ceased to be significant after adjustment. Opposite results have been demonstrated recently in the Nurses Health Study (Hu *et al.*, 1999) where women in the highest quintile of protein consumption (24% of energy) had a 28% lower rate of ischaemic heart disease compared with the lowest quintile (14.7% of energy) after adjustment for conventional risk factors. Adjustment for the intakes of specific fats did not alter this relationship. As the Nurses Health Study is a much larger study, with several estimates of dietary intake over the period of observation, it is likely to be more reliable than the earlier study. Increased dietary protein is also related to lower blood pressure in many studies (Obarzanek *et al.*, 1996).

12.6.2 Bone turnover and calcium metabolism

Cross-cultural studies have shown a positive relationship between hip fracture rate and animal protein intake (Abelow *et al.*, 1992) and this has been confirmed in some within-country studies, especially for non-dairy animal protein combined with a low calcium intake (Meyer *et al.*, 1992). Feskanich *et al.* (1996) showed a 23% higher fracture rate in women in the highest quintile of animal protein intake. Sellmeyer *et al.* (2001) demonstrated that elderly women with a high ratio of animal to vegetable protein had greater loss of bone from the femoral neck and a higher rate of hip fractures. Other studies have demonstrated opposite effects (Munger *et al.*, 1999; Promislow *et al.*, 2002; Hannan *et al.*, 2000; Dawson-Hughes and Harris, 2002; Rapuri *et al.*, 2003; Shapses *et al.*, 1995). There are equally contradictory studies on calcium balance and protein intake. Hegsted and Linkswiler (1981), Schuette and Linkswiler (1982) and Kerstetter *et al.* (1999) have found increased calcium excretion, a negative calcium balance and increased bone turnover when calcium and phosphate were fixed and protein (especially non-dairy) was increased. Spencer *et al.* (1978, 1983) and Roughhead *et al.* (2003) with meat feeding studies and Pannemans *et al.* (1997) with a variety of protein sources in young and elderly people found no or minimal effects.

Protein increases glomerular filtration rate but sulphur-rich protein and phosphorus may decrease reabsorption from the tubule while the acid load from the protein may increase calcium mobilisation from bone, so overall there is no effect on calcium balance. Skov *et al.* (2002) found that bone loss was less on the high protein diet compared with a normal protein diet after 6 months of weight loss.

In all weight loss studies that we have performed, calcium excretion has fallen with no differences between high and low protein diets. In a study contrasting two high protein diets, one based on dairy and rich in calcium and one based on meat and low in calcium, we found a reduced excretion of collagen crosslinks on the high calcium diet but in both diets calcium excretion decreased. Only on a ketogenic diet did we find that calcium excretion was enhanced, probably due to metabolic acidosis.

12.6.3 Renal disease

Although high protein intakes increase renal plasma flow and glomerular filtration rate and renal size, there is no evidence that this has a negative effect on renal function long term. Skov *et al.* (1999) found no changes in albuminuria. Lentine and Wrone (2004) suggested in a review of this area that population-level data indicate graded risk for progressive renal functional decline with increasing protein intake among women with mild renal insufficiency, and support a possible association of higher protein consumption with the risk of microalbuminuria in people with concomitant diabetes and hypertension. In one study we performed in diabetic subjects we found weight decreased albumin excretion with no differences between high and low protein diets. Clearly, more work needs to be done in this area. Knight *et al.* (2003) found that protein intake was associated with a borderline significant decline in renal function in women with glomerular filtration rates of between 55 and 80 ml/min per 1.73 m^2 and this was mostly associated with animal protein rather than dairy protein.

12.7 Future trends

A major issue with high protein diets is maintaining long-term compliance. Once outside the trial framework, the percentage of calories from protein tends to drift downwards towards 20%. Although a reduced absolute amount of protein is a factor, there tends to be an increase in calories from fat and carbohydrate, suggesting the satiating effect may weaken with time. Clearly, there needs to be the development of a wide variety of protein-enriched products so that protein can be derived from wider sources than meat and dairy, especially for women. Both wheat and soy protein can be used to enrich a wide variety of products. Once this occurs then it will be easier to maintain higher protein intakes long term and assess the impact on bone health and renal function. There needs to be a lot more work on understanding the factors that aid and hinder compliance to both a high protein diet and a calorie-reduced diet. I would certainly like to see a wide variety of high protein, low fat foods available in the marketplace as I believe they have the potential to contribute significantly to a reduction in food intake. In addition, the availability of a wide variety of protein sources, especially vegetable and low fat protein-enriched dairy sources, would allay concerns about relying heavily on red meat as a source of protein.

People with type 2 diabetes are frequently overweight and have renal disease and it is imperative that this population group be closely studied. Another perceived, but controversial, side effect of one commonly consumed form of protein, red meat, is an increase in the risk of colon cancer. This can only be addressed by invasive studies in humans with colonic biopsies being examined for genomic and epigenomic damage and changes in key enzymes such as cyclo-oxygenase 2 and the apoptosis pathway.

A further issue is the maintenance of a high protein intake after a gastric bypass, stapling or other forms of gastric reduction. Although these are initially very successful, there is a significant relapse rate. An increase in protein at this point may be beneficial, although this has not yet been tested in clinical trials. Meat is not useful in this situation so other forms of protein-enriched foods are required.

Another potential area of research is the use of high protein meal replacements for moderate caloric reduction weight loss (as opposed to low calorie diets) in contrast to the current high carbohydrate meal replacements. A novel area that requires exploration is the use of personalised web-based or mobile phone-based diet plans, advice and reinforcement in contrast to face-to-face group or individualised care.

The current widespread use in the USA of a low and very low carbohydrate diet needs to be managed with industry to reduce the fat content of the diet and increase the protein, fibre and water content to maximise the satiety and minimise any adverse health effects of this dietary strategy. Fats need to be as unsaturated as possible. Consumers clearly need guidance from health professionals in this area.

12.8 Sources of information and advice

Reputable American government and health organisation sites:

www.cdc.gov/nccdphp/dnpa/obesity/; www.nlm.nih.gov/medlineplus/obesity.html; www.pslgroup.com/obesity.htm; www.naaso.org/information/;

European links: www.obesity-diet.com/
www.who.int/dietphysicalactivity/publications/facts/obesity/en/

12.9 References

ABELOW, B. J., HOLFORD, T. R. and INSOGNA, K. L. (1992), 'Cross-cultural association between dietary animal protein and hip fracture: a hypothesis,' *Calcif. Tissue Int.*, **50** (1), 14–18.

AGUS, M. S., SWAIN, J. F., LARSON, C. L., ECKERT, E. A. and LUDWIG, D. S. (2000), 'Dietary composition and physiologic adaptations to energy restriction,' *Am. J. Clin. Nutr.*, **71** (4), 901–7.

ARAYA, H., HILLS, J., ALVINA, M. and VERA, G. (2000), 'Short-term satiety in preschool children, a comparison between high protein meal and a high complex carbohydrate meal,' *Int. J. Food Sci. Nutr.*, **51** (2), 119–24.

BABA, N. H., SAWAYA, S., TORBAY, N., HABBAL, Z., AZAR, S. and HASHIM, S. A. (1999), 'High protein vs. high carbohydrate hypoenergetic diet for the treatment of obese hyperinsulinemic subjects,' *Int. J. Obes. Relat. Metab. Disord.*, **23** (11), 1202–6.

BARKELING, B., RÖSSNER, S. and BJÖRVELL, H. (1990), 'Effect of a high-protein meal (meat) and a high-carbohydrate meal (vegetarian) on satiety measured by automatic computerized monitoring of subsequent food intake,' *Int. J. Obes.*, **14** (9), 743–51.

BASDEVANT, A., CRAPLET, C. and GUY-GRAND, B. (1993), 'Snacking patterns in obese French women,' *Appetite*, **21** (1), 17–23.

BELL, E. A. and ROLLS, B. J. (2001), 'Energy density of foods affects energy intake across multiple levels of fat content in lean and obese women,' *Am. J. Clin. Nutr.*, **73** (6), 1010–8.

BIRCH, L. L. and DEYSHER, M. (1986), 'Caloric compensation and sensory-specific satiety, evidence for self regulation of food intake by young children,' *Appetite*, **7**, 323–31.

BLUNDELL, J. E. and BURLEY, V. J. (1987), 'Satiation, satiety and the action of fibre on food intake,' *Int. J. Obes.*, **11** Suppl 1, 9–25.

BLUNDELL, J. E. and MACDIARMID, J. I. (1997), 'Fat as a risk factor for overconsumption, satiation, satiety, and patterns of eating,' *J. Am. Diet. Assoc.*, **97** (Suppl), S63–9.

BOBBIONI-HARSCH, E., HABICHT, F., LEHMANN, R., JAMES, R. W., ROHNER-JEANRENAUD, F. and GOLAY, A. (1997), 'Energy expenditure and substrates oxidative patterns after glucose, fat or mixed load in normal-weight subjects,' *Eur. J. Clin. Nutr.*, **51**, 370–4.

BOOTH, D. A., CHASE, A. and CAMPBELL, A. T. (1970), 'Relative effectiveness of protein in the late stages of appetite suppression in man,' *Physiol. Behav.*, **5**, 1299–302.

BORKMAN, M., CAMPBELL, L. V., CHISHOLM, D. J. and STORLIEN, L. H. (1991), 'Comparison of the effects on insulin sensitivity of high carbohydrate and high fat diets in normal subjects,' *J. Clin. Endocrinol. Metab.*, **72** (2), 432–7.

BRAY, G. A. (1997), 'Amino acids, protein, and body weight,' *Obes. Res.*, **5** (4), 373–6.

BREHM, B. J. SEELEY, R. J. DANIELS, S. R. and D'ALESSIO, D. A. (2003), 'A randomized trial comparing a very low carbohydrate diet and a calorie-restricted low fat diet on body weight and cardiovascular risk factors in healthy women,' *J. Clin. Endocrinol. Metab.*, **88** (4), 1617–23.

BRINKWORTH, G. D., NOAKES, M., KEOGH, J. B., LUSCOMBE, N. D., WITTERT, G. A. and CLIFTON, P. M. (2004), 'Long-term effects of a high-protein, low-carbohydrate diet on weight control and cardiovascular risk markers in obese hyperinsulinemic subjects,' *Int. J. Obes. Relat. Metab. Disord.*, **28** (5), 661–70.

CROVETTI, R., PORRINI, M., SANTANGELO, A. and TESTOLIN (1998), 'The influence of thermic effect of food on satiety,' *Eur. J. Clin. Nutr.*, **52** (7), 482–8.

DAUNCEY, M. J. and BINGHAM, S. (1983), 'Dependence of 24 h energy expenditure in man on the composition of the nutrient intake,' *Br. J. Nutr.*, **50** (1), 1–13.

DAWSON-HUGHES, B. and HARRIS, S. S. (2002), 'Calcium intake influences the association of protein intake with rates of bone loss in elderly men and women,' *Am. J. Clin. Nutr.*, **75**, 773–9.

DE CASTRO, J. M. (1987), 'Circadian rhythms of the spontaneous meal pattern, macronutrient intake, and mood of humans,' *Physiol. Behav.*, **40** (4), 437–46.

DE CASTRO, J. M. (1996), 'How can eating behavior be regulated in the complex environments of free-living humans?' *Neurosci. Biobehav. Rev.*, 20, 119–23.

DE CASTRO, J. M. (2000), 'Eating behavior, lessons from the real world of humans,' *Nutrition* **16**, 800–13.

DE CASTRO, J. M. and ELMORE, D. K. (1988), 'Subjective hunger relationships with meal patterns in the spontaneous feeding behavior of humans, evidence for a causal connection,' *Physiol. Behav.*, **43**, 159–65.

DEGRAAF, C., HULSHOF, T., WESTSTRATE, J. A. and JAS, P. (1992), 'Short-term effects of different amounts of protein fats and carbohydrates on satiety,' *Am. J. Clin. Nutr.*, **55**, 33–8.

DE GRAAF, C., DE JONG, L., S. and LAMBERS, A. C. (1999), 'Palatability affects satiation but not satiety,' *Physiol. Behav.*, **66**, 681–8.

DRIVER, C. J. I. (1988), 'The effect of meal composition on the degree of satiation following a test meal and possible mechanisms involved,' *Br. J. Nutr.*, **60**, 441–9.

DUMESNIL, J. G., TURGEON, J., TREMBLAY, A. *et al.* (2001), 'Effect of a low-glycaemic index–low-fat–high protein diet on the atherogenic metabolic risk profile of abdominally obese men,' *Br. J. Nutr.*, **86** (5), 557–68.

FARNSWORTH, E., LUSCOMBE, N. D., NOAKES, M., WITTERT, G., ARGYIOU, E. and CLIFTON, P. M. (2003), 'Effect of a high-protein, energy-restricted diet on body composition, glycemic control, and lipid concentrations in overweight and obese hyperinsulinemic men and women,' *Am. J. Clin. Nutr.*, **78** (1), 31–9.

FESKANICH, D., WILLETT, W. C., STAMPFER, M. J. and COLDITZ, G. A. (1996), 'Protein consumption and bone fractures in women,' *Am. J. Epidemiol.*, **143**, 472–9.

FLINT, A., RABEN, A., BLUNDELL, J. E. and ASTRUP, A. (2000), 'Reproducibility, power and validity of visual analogue scales in assessment of appetite sensations in single meal test studies,' *Int. J. Obes. Relat. Metab. Disord.*, **24**, 38–48.

FOSTER, G. D., WYATT, H. R., HILL, J. O. *et al.* (2003), 'A randomized trial of a low-carbohydrate diet for obesity,' *N. Engl. J. Med.*, **348** (21), 2082–90.

FRENCH, S. J. and CECIL, J. E. (2001), 'Oral, gastric and intestinal influences on human feeding,' *Physiol. Behav.*, **74** (4–5), 729–34.

FRYER, J. H. (1959), 'Physiology of appetite and hunger,' *NY State J. Med.*, **59**, 4418–21.

FRYER, J. H., MOORE, N. S., WILLIAMS, H. H. and YOUNG, C. M. (1955), 'A study of the interrelationship of the energy-yielding nutrients, blood glucose levels, and subjective appetite in man,' *J. Lab. Clin. Med.*, **45**, 684–96.

GANNON, M. C., NUTTALL, F. Q., NEIL, B. J. and WESTPHAL, S. A. (1988), 'The insulin and glucose responses to meals of glucose plus various proteins in type 2 diabetic subjects,' *Metabolism*, **37** (11), 1081–8.

GANNON, M. C., NUTTALL, F. Q., LANE, J. T. and BURMEISTER, L. A. (1992), 'Metabolic response to cottage cheese or egg white protein, with or without glucose, in type 2 diabetic subjects,' *Metabolism*, **41** (10), 1137–45.

GARG, A., BONANOME, A., GRUNDY, S. M., ZHANG, Z. J. and UNGER, R. H. (1988), 'Comparison of a high-carbohydrate diet with a high-monounsaturated-fat diet in patients with non-insulin-dependent diabetes mellitus,' *N. Engl. J. Med.*, **319** (13), 829–34.

GELIEBTER, A. A. (1979), 'Effects of equicaloric loads of protein, fat, and carbohydrate on food intake in the rat and man,' *Physiol. Behav.*, **22**, 267–73.

GENDALL, K. A., JOYCE, P. R. and ABBOTT, R. M. (1999), 'The effects of meal composition on subsequent craving and binge eating,' *Addict. Behav.*, **24** (3), 305–15.

HALL, W. L., MILLWARD, D. J., LONG, S. J. and MORGAN, L. M. (2003), 'Casein and whey exert different effects on plasma amino acid profiles, gastrointestinal hormone secretion and appetite,' *Br. J. Nutr.*, **89** (2), 239–48.

HANNAN, M. T., TUCKER, K. L., DAWSON-HUGHES, B., CUPPLES, L. A., FELSON, D. T. and KIEL, D. P. (2000), 'Effect of dietary protein on bone loss in elderly men and women, the Framingham Osteoporosis Study,' *J. Bone. Miner. Res.*, **15**, 2504–12.

HEANEY, R. P. (1998), 'Excess dietary protein may not adversely affect bone', *J. Nutr.*, **128**, 1054–7.

HEGSTED M. and LINKSWILER, H. M. (1981), 'Long-term effects of level of protein intake on calcium metabolism in young adult women,' *J. Nutr.*, **111** (2), 244–51.

HEINI, A. F., KIRK, K. A., LARA-CASTRO, C., WEINSIER, R. L. (1998), 'Relationship between hunger-satiety feelings and various metabolic parameters in women with obesity during controlled weight loss,' *Obes. Res.*, **6** (3), 225–30.

HETHERINGTON, M., ROLLS, B. J. and BURLEY, V. J. (1989), 'The time course of sensory-specific satiety,' *Appetite*, **12**, 57–68.

HILL, A. J. and BLUNDELL, J. E. (1982), 'Nutrients and behaviour, research strategies for the investigation of taste characteristics, food preferences, hunger sensations and eating patterns in man,' *J. Psychiatr. Res.*, **17**, 203–12.

HILL, A. J. and BLUNDELL, J. E. (1986), 'Macronutrients and satiety, the effects of a high-protein or high-carbohydrate meal on subjective motivation to eat and food preferences,' *Nutrit. Behav.*, **3**, 133–44.

HILL, A. J. and BLUNDELL, J. E. (1990), 'Comparison of the action of macronutrients on the expression of appetite in lean and obese humans,' *Ann. NY Acad. Sci.*, **597**, 529–31.

HILL, A. J., MAGSON, L. D. and BLUNDELL, J. E. (1984), 'Hunger and palatability, tracking ratings of subjective experience before, during and after the consumption of preferred and less preferred food,' *Appetite*, **5**, 361–71.

HOFFER, L. J., BISTRIAN, B. R., YOUNG, V. R., BLACKBURN, G. L. and WANNEMACHER, R. W. (1984), 'Metabolic effects of carbohydrate in low-calorie diets,' *Metabolism*, **33** (9), 820–5.

HOFFER, L. J., TAVEROFF, A. and HAMADEH, M. J. (1998), 'Dietary protein restriction alters glucose but not protein metabolism in non-insulin-dependent diabetes mellitus,' *Metabolism*, **47** (9), 1145–51.

HOLBROOK, T. L. and BARRETT-CONNOR, E. (1991), 'Calcium intake, covariates and confounders,' *Am. J. Clin. Nutr.*, **53**, 741–4.

HOOGWERF, B. J., LAINE, D. C. and GREENE, E. (1986), 'Urine C-peptide and creatinine (Jaffe method) excretion in healthy young adults on varied diets, sustained effects of varied carbohydrate, protein, and meat content,' *Am. J. Clin. Nutr.*, **43** (3), 350–60.

HOWE, J. C. (1990), 'Postprandial response of calcium metabolism in postmenopausal women to meals varying in protein level/source,' *Metabolism*, **39** (12), 1246–52.

HU, F. B., STAMPFER, M. J., MANSON, J. E. *et al.* (1999), 'Dietary protein and risk of ischemic heart disease in women,' *Am. J. Clin. Nutr.*, **70**, 221–7.

HULSHOF, T., DE GRAAF, C. and WESTSTRATE, J. A. (1993), 'The effects of preloads varying in physical state and fat content on satiety and energy intake,' *Appetite*, **21** (3), 273–86.

HUON, G. F. and WOOTTON, M. (1991), 'The role of dietary carbohydrate and of knowledge of having eaten it in the urge to eat more,' *Int. J. Eating Disord.*, **10**, 31–42.

JOHNSON, J. and VICKERS, Z. (1992), 'Factors influencing sensory-specific satiety,' *Appetite*, **19**, 15–31.

JOHNSON, J. and VICKERS, Z. (1993), 'Effects of flavor and macronutrient composition of food servings on liking, hunger and subsequent intake,' *Appetite*, **21**, 25–39.

JOHNSTONE, A. M., STUBBS, R. J. and HARBRON, C. G. (1996), 'Effect of overfeeding macronutrients on day-to-day food intake in man,' *Eur. J. Clin. Nutr.*, **50**, 418–30.

KARST, H., STEINIGER, J., NOACK, R. and STEGLICH H.-D. (1984), 'Diet-induced thermogenesis in man, thermic effects of single proteins, carbohydrates and fats depending on their energy amount,' *Ann. Nutr. Metab.*, **28**, 245–52.

KERSTETTER, J. E., MITNICK, M. E., GUNDBERG, C. M. *et al.* (1999), 'Changes in bone turnover in young women consuming different levels of dietary protein,' *J. Clin. Endocrinol. Metab.*, **84** (3), 1052–5.

KNIGHT, E. L., STAMPFER, M. J., HANKINSON, S. E., SPIEGELMAN, D. and CURHAN, G. C. (2003), 'The impact of protein intake on renal function decline in women with normal renal function or mild renal insufficiency,' *Ann. Intern. Med.*, **138** (6), 460–7.

KREZOWSKI, P. A., NUTTALL, F. Q., GANNON, M. C. and BARTOSH, N. H. (1986), 'The effect of protein ingestion on the metabolic response to oral glucose in normal individuals,' *Am. J. Clin. Nutr.*, **44** (6), 847–56.

KRISTENSEN, S. T., HOLM, L., RABEN, A. and ASTRUP, A. (2002), 'Achieving "proper" satiety in different social contexts – qualitative interpretations from a cross-disciplinary project, sociomaet,' *Appetite*, **39**, 207–15.

LANG, V., BELLISLE, F., OPPERT, J. M. *et al.* (1998), 'Satiating effect of proteins in healthy subjects, a comparison of egg albumin, casein, gelatin, soy protein, pea protein, and wheat gluten,' *Am. J. Clin. Nutr.*, **67** (6), 1197–204.

LANG, V., BELLISLE, F., ALAMOWITCH, C. *et al.* (1999), 'Varying the protein source in mixed meal modifies glucose, insulin and glucagon kinetics in healthy men, has weak effects on subjective satiety and fails to affect food intake,' *Eur. J. Clin. Nutr.*, **53** (12), 959–65.

LARIVIERE, F., CHIASSON, J. L., SCHIFFRIN, A. *et al.* (1994), 'Effects of dietary protein restriction on glucose and insulin metabolism in normal and diabetic humans,' *Metabolism*, **43**, 462–7.

LATNER, J. D. and SCHWARTZ, M. (1999), 'The effects of a high-carbohydrate, high-protein or balanced lunch on later food intake and hunger ratings,' *Appetite*, **33**, 119–28.

LAYMAN, D. K. (2003), 'The role of leucine in weight loss diets and glucose homeostasis,' *J. Nutr.*, **133** (1), 261S–7S.

LAYMAN, D. K. and BAUM, J. I. (2004), 'Dietary protein impact on glycemic control during weight loss,' *J. Nutr.*, **134** (4), 968S–73S.

LAYMAN, D. K., BOILEAU, R. A., ERICKSON, D. J. *et al.* (2003), 'A reduced ratio of dietary carbohydrate to protein improves body composition and blood lipid profiles during weight loss in adult women,' *J. Nutr.*, **133** (2), 411–17.

LE BLANC, J., DIAMOND, P. and NADEAU, A. (1991), 'Thermogenic response to palatable protein- and carbohydrate-rich food,' *Horm. Metab. Res.*, **23**, 336–40.

LENTINE, K. and WRONE, E. M. (2004), 'New insights into protein intake and progression of renal disease,' *Curr. Opin. Nephrol. Hypertens.*, **13** (3), 333–6.

LINN, T., GEYER, R., PRASSEK, S. and LAUBE, H. (1996), 'Effect of dietary protein intake on insulin secretion and glucose metabolism in insulin dependent diabetes,' *J. Clin. Endocrinol. Metab.*, **81**, 3938–43.

LONG, S. J., JEFFCOAT, A. R. and MILLWARD, D. J. (2000), 'Effect of habitual dietary-protein intake on appetite and satiety,' *Appetite*, **35** (1), 79–88.

MARMONIER, C., CHAPELOT, D. and LOUIS-SYLVESTRE, J. (2000), 'Effects of macronutrient content and energy density of snacks consumed in a satiety state on the onset of the next meal,' *Appetite*, **34**, 161–8.

MARMONIER, C., CHAPELOT, D., FANTINO, M. and LOUIS-SYLVESTRE, J. (2002), 'Snacks consumed in a nonhungry state have poor satiating efficiency, influence of snack composition on substrate utilization and hunger,' *Am. J. Clin. Nutr.*, **76** (3), 518–28.

MCGEE, D. L., REED, D. M., YANO, K., KAGAN, A. and TILLOTSON, J. (1984), 'Ten-year incidence of coronary heart disease in the Honolulu Heart Programme. Relationship to nutrient intake,' *Am. J. Epidemiol.*, **119** (5), 667–76.

MELLINKOFF, S. M., FRANKLAND, M., BOYLED and GREIPEL, M. (1956), 'Relationship between serum amino acid concentration and fluctuations in appetite,' *J. Appl. Physiol.*, **8** (5), 535–8.

MEYER, H. E., PEDERSEN, J. I., LOKEN, E. B. and TVERDAL, A. (1997), 'Dietary factors and the incidence of hip fracture in middle-aged Norwegians. A prospective study,' *Am. J. Epidemiol.*, **145**, 117–23.

MUNGER, R. G., CERHAN, J. R. and CHIU, B. C. (1999), 'Prospective study of dietary protein intake and risk of hip fracture in postmenopausal women,' *Am. J. Clin. Nutr.*, **69**, 147–52.

NOAKES, M., KEOGH, J. B., FOSTER, P. R. and CLIFTON, P. M. (in press), 'Effect of an energy restricted high protein low fat diet relative to a conventional high carbohydrate low fat diet on weight loss, body composition, nutritional status and markers of cardiovascular health in obese women,' *Am. J. Clin. Nutr.*, 2005 (in press).

NUTTALL, F. Q. and GANNON, M. C. (1990), 'Metabolic response to egg white and cottage cheese protein in normal subjects,' *Metabolism*, **39** (7), 749–55.

NUTTALL, F. Q., MOORADIAN, A. D., GANNON, M. C., BILLINGTON, C. and KREZOWSKI, P. (1984), 'Effect of protein ingestion on the glucose and insulin response to a standardized oral glucose load,' *Diabetes Care*, **7** (5), 465–70.

OBARZANEK, E., VELLETRI, P. A. and CUTLER, J. A. (1996), 'Dietary protein and blood pressure,' *JAMA*, **275**, 1598–603.

O'DEA, K., TRAIANEDES, K., IRELAND, P. *et al.* (1989), 'The effects of diet differing in fat, carbohydrate, and fiber on carbohydrate and lipid metabolism in type II diabetes,' *J. Am. Diet. Assoc.*, **89** (8), 1076–86.

PALLOTTA, J. A. and KENNEDY P. J. (1968), 'Response of plasma insulin and growth hormone to carbohydrate and protein feeding,' *Metabolism*, **17**, 901–8.

PANNEMANS, D. L., SCHAAFSMA, G. and WESTERTERP, K. R. (1997), 'Calcium excretion, apparent calcium absorption and calcium balance in young and elderly subjects, influence of protein intake,' *Br. J. Nutr.*, **77**, 721–9.

PARKER, B., NOAKES, M., LUSCOMBE, N. and CLIFTON, P. (2002), 'Effect of a high-protein, high-monounsaturated fat weight loss diet on glycemic control and lipid levels in type 2 diabetes,' *Diabetes Care*, **25** (3), 425–30.

PIATTI, P. M., MONTI, F., FERMO, I. *et al.* (1994), 'Hypocaloric high-protein diet improves glucose oxidation and spares lean body mass: comparison to hypocaloric high-carbohydrate diet,' *Metabolism*, **43** (12), 1481–7.

PLATA-SALAMAN, C. R. (2000), 'Ingestive behavior and obesity,' *Nutrition*, **16**, 797–9.

POMERLEAU, J., VERDY, M., GARREL, D. R. and NADEAU, M. H. (1993), 'Effect of protein intake on glycaemic control and renal function in type 2 (non-insulin-dependent) diabetes mellitus,' *Diabetologia*, **36** (9), 829–34.

POPPITT, S. D., MCCORMACK, D. and BUFFENSTEIN, R. (1998), 'Short-term effects of macronutrient preloads on appetite and energy intake in lean women,' *Physiol. Behav.*, **64**, 279–85.

PORRINI, M., CORVETTI, R., RISO, P., SANTANGELO, A. and TESTOLIN, G. (1994), 'Effects of physical and chemical characteristics of food on specific and general satiety,' *Physiol. Behav.*, **57**, 461–8.

PRENTICE, A. M., BLACK, A. E., MURGATROYD, P. R., GOLDBERG, G. R. and COWARD, W. A. (1989), 'Metabolism or appetite, questions of energy balance with particular reference to obesity,' *J. Hum. Nutr. Diet.*, **2**, 95–104.

PROMISLOW, J. H., GOODMAN-GRUEN, D., SLYMEN, D. J. and BARRETT-CONNOR, E. (2002), 'Protein consumption and bone mineral density in the elderly, the Rancho Bernardo Study,' *Am. J. Epidemiol.*, **155**, 636–44.

RABEN, A., HOLST, J. J., CHRISTENSEN, N. J. and ASTRUP, A. (1996), 'Determinants of postprandial appetite sensations, macronutrient intake and glucose metabolism,' *Int. J. Obes. Relat. Metab. Disord.*, **20** (2), 161–9.

RABEN, A., AGERHOLM-LARSEN, L., FLINT, A., HOLST, J. J. and ASTRUP, A. (2003), 'Meals with similar energy densities but rich in protein, fat, carbohydrate, or alcohol have different effects on energy expenditure and substrate metabolism but not on appetite and energy intake,' *Am. J. Clin. Nutr.*, **77** (1), 91–100.

RABINOWITZ, D., MERIMEE, T. J., MAFFEZZOLI, R. and BURGESS, J. A. (1966), 'Patterns of hormonal release after glucose, protein, and glucose plus protein,' *Lancet*, **2**, 454–6.

RAPURI, P. B., GALLAGHER, J. C. and HAYNATZKA, V. (2003), 'Protein intake, effects on bone mineral density and the rate of bone loss in elderly women,' *Am. J. Clin. Nutr.*, 77, 1517–25.

RICCARDI, G., RIVELLESE, A., PACIONI, D., GENOVESE, S., MASTRANZO, P. and MANCINI, M. (1984), 'Separate influence of dietary carbohydrate and fibre on the metabolic control in diabetes,' *Diabetologia*, **26** (2), 116–21.

ROGERS, P. J., KEEDWELL, P. and BLUNDELL, J. E. (1991), 'Further analysis of the short-term inhibition of food intake in humans by the dipeptide L-aspartyl-L-phenylalanine methyl ester (aspartame),' *Physiol. Behav.*, **49** (4), 739–43.

ROLLS, B. J. (1986), 'Sensory-specific satiety,' *Nutr. Rev.*, **44**, 93–101.

ROLLS, B. J. (1994), 'Appetite and satiety in the elderly,' *Nutr. Rev.*, **52**, S9–10.

ROLLS, B. J. and MCDERMOTT, T. M. (1991), 'Effects of age on sensory-specific satiety,' *Am. J. Clin. Nutr.*, **54**, 988–96.

ROLLS, E. T. and ROLLS, J. H. (1997), 'Olfactory sensory-specific satiety in humans,' *Physiol. Behav.*, **61**, 461–73.

ROLLS, B. J. and ROE, L. S. (2002), 'Effect of the volume of liquid food infused intragastrically on satiety in women,' *Physiol. Behav.*, **76** (4–5), 623–31.

ROLLS, B. J., HETHERINGTON, M. and BURLEY, V. J. (1988), 'The specificity of satiety, the influence of foods of different macronutrient content on the development of satiety,' *Physiol. Behav.*, **43**, 145–53.

ROLLS, B. J., BELL, E. A. and THORWART M. L. (1999), 'Water incorporated into a food but not served with a food decreases energy intake in lean women,' *Am. J. Clin. Nutr.*, **70** (4), 448–55.

ROLLS, B. J., BELL, E. A. and WAUGH, B. A. (2000), 'Increasing the volume of a food by incorporating air affects satiety in men,' *Am. J. Clin. Nutr.*, **72** (2), 361–8.

ROUGHHEAD, Z. K., JOHNSON, L. K., LYKKEN, G. I. and HUNT, J. R. (2003), 'Controlled high meat diets do not affect calcium retention or indices of bone status in healthy postmenopausal women,' *J. Nutr.*, **133**, 1020–6.

SAMAHA, F. F., IQBAL, N., SESHADRI, P. *et al.* (2003), 'A low-carbohydrate as compared with a low-fat diet in severe obesity,' *N. Engl. J. Med.*, **348** (21), 2074–81.

SCHUETTE, S. A. and LINKSWILER, H. M. (1982), 'Effects on Ca and P metabolism in humans by adding meat, meat plus milk, or purified proteins, plus Ca and P to a low protein diet,' *J. Nutr.*, **112** (2), 338–49.

SELLMEYER, D. E., STONE, K. L., SEBASTIAN, A. and CUMMINGS, S. R. (2001), 'A high ratio of dietary animal to vegetable protein increases the rate of bone loss and the risk of fracture in postmenopausal women. Study of Osteoporotic Fractures Research Group,' *Am. J. Clin. Nutr.*, **73**, 118–22.

SHAPSES, S. A., ROBINS, S. P., SCHWARTZ, E. I. and CHOWDHURY, H. (1995), 'Short-term changes in calcium but not protein intake alter the rate of bone resorption in healthy subjects as assessed by urinary pyridinium cross-link excretion,' *J. Nutr.*, **125**, 2814–21.

SKOV, A. R., TOUBRO, S., RØNN, B., HOLM, L. and ASTRUP, A. (1999a), 'Randomized trial on protein versus carbohydrate in *ad libitum* fat-reduced diets for the treatment of obesity,' *Int. J. Obes. Relat. Metab. Disord.*, **23**, 528–36.

SKOV, A. R., TOUBRO, S., BULOW, J., KRABBE, K., PARVING, H. H. and ASTRUP, A. (1999b), 'Changes in renal function during weight loss induced by high vs. low-protein low-fat diets in overweight subjects,' *Int. J. Obes. Relat. Metab. Disord.*, **23** (11), 1170–7.

SKOV, A. R., HAULRIK, N., TOUBRO, S., MOLGAARD, C. and ASTRUP, A. (2002), 'Effect of protein intake on bone mineralization during weight loss, a 6-month trial,' *Obes. Res.*, **10** (6), 432–8.

SONDIKE, S. B., COPPERMAN, N. and JACOBSON, M. S. (2003), 'Effects of a low-carbohydrate diet on weight loss and cardiovascular risk factor in overweight adolescents,' *J. Pediatr.*, **142** (3), 253–8.

SPENCER, H., KRAMER, L., OSIS, D. and NORRIS, C. (1978), 'Effect of a high protein (meat) intake on calcium metabolism in man,' *Am. J. Clin. Nutr.*, **31** (12), 2167–80.

SPENCER, H., KRAMER, L., DEBARTOLO, M., NORRIS, C. and OSIS, D. (1983), 'Further studies of the effect of a high protein diet as meat on calcium metabolism,' *Am. J. Clin. Nutr.*, **37** (6), 924–9.

SPILLER, G. A., JENSEN, C. D., PATTISON, T. S., CHUCK, C. S., WHITTAM, J. H. and SCALA, J. (1987), 'Effect of protein dose on serum glucose and insulin response to sugars,' *Am. J. Clin. Nutr.*, **46** (3), 474–80.

STEIN, K. (2000), 'High protein, low-carbohydrate diets. Do they work?' *J. Am. Dietet. Assoc.*, **100** (7), 760–1.

STUBBS, R. J., VAN, WYK, M. C. W., JOHNSTONE, A. M. and HARBRON, C. G. (1996), 'Breakfast high in protein, fat or carbohydrate, effect on within-day appetite and energy balance,' *Eur. J. Clin. Nutr.*, **50**, 409–17.

STUBBS, J., RABEN, A. and WESTERTERP-PLANTENGA, M. S. (1999), 'Substrate metabolism and appetite in humans,' In Westerterp-Plantenga, M. S., Steffens, A. B., Tremblay, A., eds. *Regulation of Food Intake and Energy Expenditure*. Milan, Edra, 59–83.

STUBBS, J., FERRES, S. and HORGAN, G. (2000), 'Energy density of foods, effects on energy intake,' *Crit. Rev. Food. Sci. Nutr.*, **40** (6), 481–515.

SWAMINATHAN, R., KING, R. F. G. J., HOMFIELD, J., SIWEK, R. A., BAKER, M. and WALES, J. K. (1985), 'Thermic effect of feeding carbohydrate, fat, protein and mixed meal in lean and obese subjects,' *Am. J. Clin. Nutr.*, **42**, 177–81.

TAPPY, L. (1996), 'Thermic effect of food and sympathetic nervous system activity in humans,' *Reprod. Nutr. Dev.*, **36**, 391–7.

TEFF, K. L., YOUNG, S. N. and BLUNDELL, J. E. (1989), 'The effect of protein or carbohydrate breakfasts on subsequent plasma amino acid levels, satiety and nutrient selection in normal males,' *Pharmacol. Biochemi. Behav.*, **34**, 829–37.

UHE, A. M., COLLIER, G. R. and O'DEA, K. (1992), 'A comparison of the effects of beef, chicken and fish protein on satiety and amino acid profiles in lean male subjects,' *J. Nutr.*, **122** (3), 467–72.

VAN LOON, L. J. C., SARIS, W. H., VERHAGEN, H. and WAGENMAKERS, J. M. (2000), 'Plasma insulin responses after ingestion of different amino acid or protein mixtures with carbohydrate,' *Am. J. Clin. Nutr.*, **72**, 96–105.

VANDEWATER, K. and VICKERS, Z. (1995), 'Higher-protein foods produce greater sensory-specific satiety,' *Physiol. Behav.*, **59**, 579–83.

VAZQUEZ, J. A., KAZI, U. and MADANI, N. (1995), 'Protein metabolism during weight reduction with very-low-energy diets: evaluation of the independent effects of protein and carbohydrate on protein sparing,' *Am. J. Clin. Nutr.*, **62** (1), 93–103.

VOZZO, R., WITTERT, G., COCCHIARO, C. *et al.* (2003), 'Similar effects of foods high in protein, carbohydrate and fat on subsequent spontaneous food intake in healthy individuals,' *Appetite*, **40** (2), 101–7.

WESTERTERP-PLANTENGA, M., ROLLand, V., WILSON, S. and WESTERTERP, K. (1999), 'Satiety related to 24-h diet-induced thermogenesis during high protein/carbohydrate versus high fat diets measured in a respiration chamber,' *Eur. J. Clin. Nutr.*, **53**, 495–502.

WESTERTERP, K. R. (2004), 'Diet induced thermogenesis' http://www.nutritionandmetabolism.com/content/1/1/5 Review.

WESTPHAL, S. A., GANNON, M. C. and NUTTALL, F. Q. (1990), 'Metabolic response to glucose ingested with various amounts of protein,' *Am. J. Clin. Nutr.*, **52** (2), 267–72.

WOLFE, B. M. and GIOVANNETTI P. M. (1991), 'Short term effects of substituting protein for carbohydrate in the diets of moderately hypercholesterolemic human subjects,' *Metabolism*, **40**, 338–43.

WOLFE, B. M. and PICHE, L. (1994), 'Exchanging dietary protein for carbohydrate in normolipidemic human subjects lowers LDLC,' *Atherosclerosis*, **109**, 71 (abstr).

YANOVSKI, S. Z., LEET, M., YANOVSKI, J. A. *et al.* (1992), 'Food selection and intake of obese women with and without binge-eating disorder,' *Am. J. Clin. Nutr.*, **56**, 975–80.

WOLFE, B. M. and PICHE, L. A. (1999), 'Replacement of carbohydrate by protein in a conventional-fat diet reduces cholesterol and triglyceride concentrations in healthy normolipidemic subject,' *Clin. Invest. Med.*, **22** (4), 140–8.

13

Alcohol, energy balance and obesity

R. D. Mattes, Purdue University, USA

13.1 Introduction

While the adverse consequences of alcohol abuse are well established, accumulating evidence that moderate consumption may hold beneficial effects for heart disease[1,2] has prompted increased interest in additional positive and negative roles of alcohol in the diet. A key concern relates to the contribution of energy from alcohol since overweight/obesity is prevalent globally. The relative importance of genetic, metabolic and behavioral factors in the etiology and maintenance of these conditions is not well characterized. However, recent marked increases in population body weight and body fat suggest an important contribution of behavior.[3,4] This, in turn, underscores the importance of understanding the role of alcohol in the diet since, relative to all energy-yielding macronutrients, its ingestion is under the greatest volitional control.

13.2 Drinking patterns

There is wide diversity in the level and patterns of alcohol ingestion across and within nations. Intake is lowest in the Eastern Mediterranean region with an annual per capita intake of about 0.6 liters of absolute alcohol for the population 15 years of age and older.[5] The highest intake of about 13.9 liters occurs in Eastern European countries. Per capita intake levels in Western Europe are roughly 12.9 liters and in the Americas 9.0–9.3 liters are consumed annually. All estimates of intake must be interpreted cautiously because of difficulty in obtaining reliable data. Self-reported intake levels represent only 40–60% of reported alcohol sales[6] and sales figures do not include home-made beverages or untaxed products. Further, data collected via household surveys clearly miss segments of the population that are not homeowners and this can be a sub-group of higher alcohol consumers than the general population. Another important qualification for consumption data is that it is expressed as a per capita average and the distribution of intake within nations is highly skewed. For example, in the United States, the upper 2.5% of the drinking population consumes 25% of the national total, the top 5% of drinkers account for 40% of the total, the upper 10% of the population ingests 60% of the total and the top 25% consume 90% of the total.[7] It should be emphasized that these figures represent percentages of any-time drinkers who constitute two-thirds of the population.

Given the wide range of consumption levels internationally, the contribution of alcohol to total national daily energy intakes also varies markedly. Clearly, it is of most concern, from an energy balance perspective, in countries with higher absolute levels of intake. Again, using the USA as an example, alcohol contributes about 4.5% of energy to the US diet, but accounts for approximately 10% of total energy intake among those who drink.[8] However, this ranges up to 50% in the heaviest consumers.

Heavy drinkers may be defined as males who consume greater than 40 g of alcohol per day (equivalent to about four drinks per day) and females who ingest greater than 20 g of alcohol per day. The proportion of heavy drinkers in a population roughly parallels the absolute level of intake (e.g. higher in industrialized nations, highest in Eastern Europe). The percentage ranges from 0.1% in the Eastern Mediterranean nations to 18.6% in Eastern Europe.[5] The effects of this high level of intake on body weight are not uniform and probably reflect the impact it has on total lifestyle and physiological processes. A number of studies report a positive association between energy intake from alcohol and body weight or BMI[9–12] in heavy users. This is reportedly due to high levels of energy contributed by alcohol as well as shifts in diet resulting in higher intakes of animal products and fat with reduced consumption of fruits and vegetables.[9] Because alcohol ingestion impairs lipid oxidation, such a dietary shift would be expected to promote adipose tissue and weight gain. However, many researchers note body weight is not increased in this sub-group.[13] The latter is often attributed to a generalized decrease in diet quality and total energy intake from other sources.[14] Increased fat oxidation and energy expenditure have also been observed in this group.[13,15,16] Other work documents weight loss and malnutrition in the heaviest drinkers.[17] As alcohol abuse progressively disrupts healthful behaviors and physiological processes, weight and fitness decline. Because of the complexity of the issues related to energy balance in alcoholics and the fact that they represent only a minority of drinkers, the balance of this review will focus on the larger group of moderate consumers.

Definitions of moderate consumption vary somewhat across nations, but generally fall in the range of no more than two standard drinks per day for males and one standard drink per day for females. Current knowledge of the energetics of alcohol metabolism in this group is open to considerable debate. Nearly all studies indicate moderate alcohol consumption elicits little or no compensatory dietary response so total energy intake increases in approximate proportion to the energy contributed by the alcohol. Clinical studies suggest that the energy from alcohol is available to the body and, because it both increases total intake and spares fat for storage, it poses a threat for positive energy balance and weight gain. However, a substantial epidemiological literature, as well as some clinical data, indicates the increment in energy contributed by alcohol does not result in increased body weight. This paradox has been highlighted repeatedly,[8,18,19] but not resulted in systematic studies to definitively resolve the matter. Such work is warranted not only to clarify the role of alcohol itself in energy balance, but potentially to yield new insights on basic energy metabolism that may lend themselves to more effective weight management practices. Current knowledge on the topic is reviewed below.

13.3 Links between moderate alcohol ingestion and body weight

There are large bodies of conflicting epidemiological data on the association between alcohol ingestion and body weight.[20] The number of prospective studies of alcohol consumption and weight gain is limited. Data from Finland and Switzerland indicate there is a significant positive association.[10,20] No association was observed in Denmark[21] and prospective studies in the USA have yielded inconsistent findings.[22,23] Recent analyses of the Health Professionals Follow-up study, a prospective trial of 16587 males, revealed no association between alcohol intake and change of waist circumference over a 10-year period.[24]

Numerous cross-sectional studies report positive associations between alcohol consumption and indices of body weight and fat mass. Findings from the French centers of the World Health Organization (WHO) MONICA study reveal significant positive associations between alcohol consumption and waist-to-hip ratio and waist girth in both sexes,[25] confirming similar findings from prior studies involving individuals of varying nationalities (e.g. French, Italian and US), races (African American, Caucasian), age groups and genders.[20,26–29] Univariate and multivariate, cross-sectional analyses have also revealed positive associations between alcohol ingestion and body weight or body mass index.[20,29–33] These data often reveal gender differences with stronger associations noted in males. This has been replicated in surveys from different nations (e.g. France, UK, Finland).[22,34–36] While alcohol ingestion may be especially problematic among individuals consuming high fat diets,[37] this is not a necessary condition. Data from the Oxford Vegetarian Study reveal alcohol intake is independently associated with BMI in male vegetarians with low fat intakes.[36]

In contrast to the positive findings from these trials, there is a very substantive body of epidemiological evidence that either does not support an association between alcohol ingestion and body weight or BMI or reveals an inverse relationship. The NHANES I study demonstrated no association between body mass index (BMI) and alcohol intake in 2614 men and an inverse association among 4616 women.[37] This was replicated in NHANES II with 5265 men and 5664 women[38] as well as the Nurses Health Study and Health Professionals Follow-up Study which included 89538 females and 48493 males.[39] A non-gender specific negative association was also reported in the Lung Health Study with 3618 males and 2141 females.[40] Similar results have been noted in various European trials as well.[41,42] The Kaiser Permanente Women Twins Study ($N = 352$ pairs) found drinkers had lower BMI than abstainers[43] and a study of 1911 male monozygotic twin pairs observed no association between alcohol ingestion and body weight.[44] In the latter study, clear differences were observed in comparisons of smokers vs. non-smokers indicating the assessment methods were sensitive.

Drinking pattern may also influence regional adiposity. Alcohol ingestion is associated with central fat deposition,[45] especially among binge drinkers.[40] A recent study reports that frequent moderate drinkers have the lowest and binge drinkers have highest abdominal height.[46] Whether this is correlational or causal is not known. Stress, smoking and high dietary fat ingestion are associated with both alcohol use and central adiposity. A more causal role could be attributable to an alcohol effect on endocrine (e.g. cortisol, glucocorticoid) status.[26,30]

Taken together, the epidemiological literature provides strong evidence both supporting and negating an association between alcohol consumption and body weight. To help resolve such conflicting survey data, insights may be sought from tightly controlled, intervention trials to determine which view is best supported mechanistically. Evidence is available from studies exploring the effects of alcohol on appetite, food choice, metabolic efficiency and energy expenditure.

13.3.1 Alcohol and appetite

The data on alcohol's influence on appetite indicate it either enhances hunger or has little effect, thereby permitting positive energy balance where food is available and palatable. Several different laboratories have published data in the past few years documenting an appetite stimulating effect of alcohol. Heatherington *et al.*[47] observed decreased fullness ratings after a meal preceded by a 24 g serving of alcohol as compared to a non-alcoholic beverage. Total energy intake was higher when alcohol was consumed. Yeomans *et al.*[48] reported increased hunger during the early part of a meal following an 18 g alcohol beverage and greater energy intake among unrestrained males. Westerterp-Plantenga and Verwegen[49] noted that provision of a 37 g alcohol aperitif led to an increased eating rate, longer meal duration, later satiation and longer eating post-maximal satiation compared to isocaloric drinks containing protein, fat or carbohydrate. Energy intake was also higher with alcohol consumption in that study. Poppitt *et al.*[50] noted no change of hunger, but higher energy intake with alcohol consumption. Thus, the available evidence indicates alcohol is an acute appetite stimulant and may facilitate positive energy balance. Whether this is attributable to alcohol's psychoactive properties, learned behavior or influence on metabolic processes involved with energy regulation is not known.

13.3.2 Alcohol and food choice

There is compelling evidence that alcohol elicits a weak compensatory dietary response (i.e. spontaneous reduced intake of other energy-yielding foods and beverages to offset the extra energy from alcohol). Dietary intake studies overwhelmingly indicate total energy consumption is higher in alcohol users than non-users by an amount roughly comparable to the calories added by the alcohol.[39,50–54] HANES I data reveal partial dietary compensation in direct proportion to alcohol intake, but the maximum was 42% in males and 16% in females and this often occurred through skipped meals reflecting an effect of high alcohol use on lifestyle rather than one only on dietary habits. Another study involving heavy drinking, but nutritionally replete men, observed no dietary compensation.[55] Poor compensation has been reported by light and heavy, young and elderly as well as male and female consumers.[51,53,55,56] One study, conducted in a metabolic unit, noted modest compensation, 37% of the energy added as alcohol.[57] Collectively, these data strongly indicate that alcohol poses a risk for positive energy balance.

Incomplete compensation may be attributable to a blunted release of satiety hormones. Alcohol administration to rats with a high fat diet suppresses cholecystokinin (CCK) release.[58] Further, obese rats chronically consuming alcohol are less sensitive to higher concentrations of CCK (e.g. 2 µg/kg) than lean controls.[59] Evidence that CCK plays an important role in food intake of rats and piglets on a liquid diet indicates these findings may be alcohol, rather than fluid-specific.[60,61] CCK promotes satiety in humans[62,63] so its reduction could facilitate increased total energy intake.

Leptin, also holds satiety properties.[64–66] Given its strong association with body fat mass,[67] which changes slowly, its effects were, and are, believed to contribute to long-term regulation. However, accumulating evidence also supports an acute influence on appetite, feeding and energy balance (e.g.[66,68,69]). Although there are exceptions,[70] an association between leptin concentration and hunger/satiety has been reported in obese females,[66] post-obese and control females[71] and in females on prolonged energy restriction.[72] Several groups have documented a postprandial rise of plasma leptin[68,71] and, where it was assessed,[68] leptin concentration was a strong predictor of the inter-meal interval ($r = 0.91$). Further, levels at one meal were strongly negatively correlated with intake at the next meal ($r = -0.85 - r = -0.95$). The shift in leptin levels was related to an increased free fatty acid concentration – a change that occurs with alcohol consumption. In rats, recent evidence indicates alcohol ingestion reduces serum leptin levels,[73] thereby facilitating food intake. Whether this occurs in humans, either acutely after a meal or after chronic alcohol ingestion, is not known. Leptin may also modify food preferences and the macronutrient composition of the diet.[74,75] Another mechanism by which leptin may express its satiety effect is through inhibition of gastric emptying.[76] Given the rapid transit of fluids through the gut, it is hypothesized alcohol may escape this control on feeding, thereby accounting for its less than expected satiety effect.

An inverse association between GI transit time and hunger has long been recognized.[77–79] The effects of alcohol on GI transit are complex. Acute dosing studies with healthy subjects indicate alcohol increases,[80] decreases[81] or does not alter[82,83] gastric emptying. Effects are modified by the form of alcohol delivery (e.g. alone or as beer or wine) as well as the nature of the meal being tracked (liquid versus solid). Mouth to cecum transit appears to be accelerated, at least for fluids.[84] This may be due to an insensitivity of the duodenal osmoreceptors to alcohol.[80,83] While evidence suggests these measures of transit are slowed in alcoholics,[82] the influence of chronic moderate alcohol consumption in healthy adults remains poorly characterized.

Alcohol intake may also modify ingestion of other macronutrients which variously influence energy balance. The liking for sweetness is linked to genetic risk for alcoholism as measured by family history[85] and chronic alcohol consumption has been associated with a heightened preference for sweetness.[86] However, an inverse association between alcohol and carbohydrate intake has generally been reported.[32,43] An inverse association has also been reported between alcohol and fat intake based on survey data.[87] This could account for the failure to observe an increment in body weight with alcohol use even when total energy intake is elevated. Dietary fat may exert an energy independent influence on body weight.[88,89] However, there are other reports of a positive association between alcohol and fat intake.[20,51]

13.3.3 Alcohol and energy balance

Because weight gain would be expected if the energy from alcohol is biologically available, this scenario does not require elaboration. The case where body weight is not increased despite higher reported energy intake, the alcohol energy paradox, does warrant further consideration. Based on a model that body weight is a function of energy consumed, energy stored and energy expended, this seeming energy paradox must be due to (a) insensitivity of dietary measurements (e.g. dietary compensation occurs but has been undetected in dietary surveys), (b) offsetting shifts of body composition (e.g. fluid reduction and fat gain) that result in no net change of body weight, (c) excretory energy loss and/or (d) increased energy expenditure via resting metabolic rate (REE), postprandial thermogenesis (TEF), non-exercise activity thermogenesis (NEAT) and/or physical activity (PA).

13.3.4 Insensitivity of dietary intake measurement

The apparent paradox between reported energy intake and body weight among moderate drinkers could be due to inaccurate self reports of alcohol and total energy consumption. However, because alcohol is consumed in discrete episodes by light to moderate drinkers, frequency of use is reasonably well recalled (correlation coefficient with diet records = 0.7–0.85).[90–92] If errors are made, they tend to be underestimates[93] which would make the discrepancy between intake and body weight more pronounced. Dietary intake is also notoriously difficult to quantify in free-living individuals. However, the consistency of the dietary data from multiple studies involving thousands of participants and the greater tendency to under-report intake suggests insensitivity of dietary intake data is an unlikely explanation for an alcohol intake-body weight discrepancy.

13.4 Alcohol and energy intake

Controlled studies conducted in metabolic wards have yielded mixed findings on the efficiency of alcohol metabolism. However, the preponderance of evidence demonstrates the energy yield from alcohol is comparable to that from carbohydrate (which clearly supports weight gain if consumed in excess of energy need). Seventy-five per cent of the energy from alcohol is available for ATP synthesis when metabolized through the alcohol dehydrogenase pathway.[94] The value drops to 50% with the microsomal ethanol oxidizing system (MEOS), but the contribution of this pathway is unclear under conditions of moderate intake. Individual variability in the activity of this system has been proposed as an explanation for variance in energy balance and body weight.[94] Several short-term studies monitoring energy expenditure by indirect calorimetry have documented that alcohol and carbohydrate are used with comparable efficiency.[95,96] This has also been reported in more comprehensive, longer term (i.e. 7-day;[97] 4–5 week[98] and 3 month[99]) trials involving moderate levels of alcohol ingestion. These data demonstrate that alcohol is a utilizable energy source, albeit at a level comparable to carbohydrate rather than 7.1 kcal/g as suggested by bomb calorimetry. However, alcohol may be especially problematic because it spares lipid metabolism, thereby promoting lipid storage and weight gain.[37,95,96,100]

While the evidence noted above supports the bioavailability of energy from alcohol, this is an issue that remains open to debate. In several seminal metabolic studies, Leiber *et al.*[101] demonstrated that replacement of up to 50% of energy derived from carbohydrate with alcohol led to weight loss and the addition of alcohol (1400 kcal) to an energy sufficient diet did not lead to weight gain. These data challenge the view that energy from alcohol is available. However, their relevance to conditions of moderate intake is uncertain. At high doses, the efficiency of alcohol metabolism is reduced. A more recent free-feeding study provided about 8% of energy as alcohol to 14 normal weight males.[102] No changes in body weight, resting metabolic rate or respiratory quotient were noted over the 6-week diet and control (abstinence) periods. The authors interpreted their findings as evidence that the energy from alcohol is not used efficiently. However, the study had low statistical power, did not accurately measure non-resting energy expenditure and used lean subjects on low fat diets (conditions less likely to show effects). Thus, the conclusion must be interpreted cautiously.

Even if true, the hypothesis that alcohol energy is not efficiently used may require qualification. Several studies indicate obese individuals derive more energy from alcohol than lean individuals. In one controlled feeding study, the addition of 20–30% of energy as alcohol to the basal diet did not result in an increase of body weight in six lean subjects, but three of six obese participants gained weight.[103] Another study provided participants diets with and without 30 g/d alcohol that were adjusted to maintain body weight over 3-month periods.[99] Obese subjects required about 135 kcal less dietary energy during alcohol ingestion whereas the leaner participants required about 210 kcal more dietary energy to maintain body weight. While suggestive of a difference in efficiency of alcohol metabolism, these data require further verification. The former study defined obesity as body weight ≥120% of ideal and two of the three weight gainers had values of 120% and 123%. In the second study, the lean and obese had mean BMI values of 22.6 and 25.2 kg/m^2. Thus, in neither case were patients markedly obese. More recently, alcohol consumers were observed to have higher central abdominal fat than abstainers, but the association was attributable to higher levels among individuals at elevated genetic risk of abdominal obesity.[104] This supports a possible genetic basis for differential responses to energy derived from alcohol.

13.4.1 Alcohol and energy losses/expenditure

Alcohol may be lost directly via breath, urine and feces. With high doses, this may account for 10–15% of a load.[105] However, under conditions of moderate use, where blood alcohol levels remain low, these routes of alcohol excretion are minor.[98,106] Estimates in humans are in the range of 2–5%.[107,108] Still, over time, these routes may contribute to the loss of energy and less than expected influence of alcohol on body weight.

A lack of dietary response or weight gain to alcohol ingestion may be due to alcohol-induced increased energy expenditure. This may occur through increased resting energy expenditure (REE), the thermogenic effect of feeding (TEF), physical activity (PA) and/or non-exercise activity thermogenesis (NEAT). Chronic high levels of alcohol ingestion are associated with elevated REE.[106,109,110] The relevance of this shift to chronic moderate drinkers is uncertain, but, in one study, acute administration of 29 ml of pure alcohol to moderately drinking women led to an increase in energy expenditure that exceeded the energy content of the alcohol.[111] This is suggestive of an elevation of REE. Indirect calorimetry indicates 15–25% of alcohol energy is lost as heat.[8,112,113] In that TEF typically accounts for only 8–10% of ingested energy from mixed meals, alcohol appears to have an especially high TEF. As noted above, some evidence indicates energy from alcohol and carbohydrate are used equally efficiently,[8,97,99,112] but other data show the former yields only 80% of the latter.[114] In contrast, it is also well known that alcohol spares fat oxidation acutely and this would favor fat storage.

Physical activity is the second largest component of total daily energy expenditure. It is highly variable and, for logistical reasons, difficult to measure. Observational data in rats indicate locomotion increases during alcohol infusion.[114] Findings from unvalidated questionnaires generally do not support an association between activity and alcohol ingestion in humans.[102,115–117] However, data from the Kaiser Permenante Women Twins study revealed a significantly lower proportion of drinkers among participants with low activity levels compared to non-drinkers.[44] Further, the Copenhagen City Heart study data indicate there are a higher percentage of abstainers who are inactive during leisure time and a lower percentage that are active during work relative to individuals consuming 1–27 drinks per week.[118] Recently, a positive association was observed between the habitual level of physical activity and alcohol ingestion ($r = 0.41$) in a group of older (mean age 61 ± 5 years) males ($n = 24$) and females ($n = 20$), but no increment was observed on days when alcohol was consumed compared to days of abstinence.[119] Physical activity was unaffected by alcohol ingestion in a metabolic ward study, but this environment limits normal behavior and constraints were placed on activity.[113]

A potentially important source of energy expenditure under conditions of energy surplus is NEAT, the energy used for activities such as sitting, standing, body posture transitions and fidgeting. It is a source of energy expenditure that has not been routinely assessed. However, when 16 adults were supplied with 1000 kcal over requirements for 8 weeks, up to two-thirds of increased energy expenditure was attributable to NEAT.[120] It appears to be a mechanism for resisting weight gain when excess energy is consumed. Based on the epidemiological and dietary literature, it appears that the alcohol adds to the diet rather than replace other energy sources so the role of NEAT is potentially important.

Taken together, these data on energy loss/expenditure provide plausible explanations for the view that alcohol does not promote positive energy balance and weight gain. Whether the underlying assumption that alcohol does not promote positive energy balance is valid and which mechanism may account for such a finding warrants further consideration.

13.5 Alcohol and body composition

Assuming moderate drinkers do ingest more total energy, the failure to note expected changes in body weight may be due to unmeasured shifts of body composition. If body fat increases consistent with the increment in energy intake, but water decreases, there could be no net change of body weight. Alcohol has diuretic properties after acute administration.[121] In a study involving nasogastric alcohol or carbohydrate formula infusion, weight reduction observed with the former treatment over a 7-day period was attributable primarily to fluid loss.[105] Whether this could account for the inconsistency between energy intake and body weight in drinkers is unclear since the diuretic effect subsides with chronic use.[122] However, in a national survey of alcohol consumption in women, there was an inverse association between drinking frequency and body water.[123]

13.6 Summary and research needs

The role of moderate alcohol consumption in energy balance remains largely unresolved. The one facet of this issue where there is consensus is that moderate drinking elicits a weak compensatory dietary response. Thus, the energy from alcohol largely adds to the diet rather than replacing other energy sources. In light of this, the widespread use of alcohol, its lack of essentiality, and the increasing prevalence of overweight/obesity, it is vital that the role of alcohol in energy balance be clarified. The epidemiological data on this point are mixed. Some work indicates that moderate consumption is associated with higher body weight, BMI and/or girth whereas an equally substantive body of evidence reveals no association between alcohol consumption and these indices. Explanations for this seeming inconsistency may lie in a failure to fully account for differences in the genetics of the populations assessed as well as drinking patterns and types of beverages consumed. Further work exploring these issues would be a considerable contribution to understanding the health effects of alcohol intake. Clarification of the correlational data will also help to better focus intervention trials aimed at establishing mechanisms for noted associations. The existing literature is mixed on the bioavailability of alcohol. Some work suggests the true energy value to drinkers is roughly comparable to that of carbohydrate whereas others report inefficient conversion of energy from alcohol resulting in a very limited impact on body weight. Whether this is attributable to metabolic inefficiency, insensitivity of measures of body composition, and/or influences of energy expenditure is not known. Application of the most sensitive tools (e.g. underwater weighing or DEXA for body composition, indirect calorimetry and doubly labeled water for energy expenditure) should make it possible to resolve the contributions of each of these factors. Work in this area may provide insights not only on the role of alcohol in the diet, but also on novel approaches for preventative or therapeutic weight management more generally.

13.7 References

1 HANNA, E. Z., CHOU, S. P. and GRANT, B. F. (1997), The relationship between drinking and heart disease morbidity in the United States: results from the national health interview survey. *Alc. Clin. Exp. Res.* **21**, 111–18.

2 KLATSKY, A. L., ARMSTRONG, M. A. and FRIEDMAN, G. D. (1997), Red wine, white wine, liquor, beer, and risk for coronary artery disease hospitalization. *Am. J. Cardiol.* **80**, 416–20.

3 RAVUSSIN, E. and BOGARDUS, C. (2000), Energy balance and weight regulation: genetics versus environment. *Br. J. Nutr.* **83** (Suppl 1), S17–20.

4 HILL, J. O. and PETERS, J. C. (1998), Environmental contributions to the obesity epidemic. *Science* **280**, 1371–7.

5 REHM, J., REHN, N., ROOM, R. *et al.* (2003), The global distribution of average volume of alcohol consumption and patterns of drinking. *Eur. Addict. Res.* **9**, 147–56.

6 DUFOUR, M. C. (2001), If you drink alcoholic beverages do so in moderation: what does this mean? *J. Nutr.* **131**, 552S–61S.

7 STOCKWELL, T. (1998), Towards guidelines for low-risk drinking: quantifying the short- and long-term costs of hazardous alcohol consumption. *Alc. Clin. Exp. Res.* **22**, 63S–9S.

8 LANDS, W. E. M. (1993), A summary of the workshop 'alcohol and calories: a matter of balance'. *J. Nutr.* **123**, 1338–41.

9 KESSE, E., CLAVEL-CHAPELON, F., SLIMANI, N. and VAN LIERE M. (2001), E3N Group. Do eating habits differ according to alcohol consumption? Results of a study of the French cohort of the European prospective investigation into cancer and nutrition (E3N-EPIC)[1–4]. *Am. J. Clin. Nutr.* **74**, 322–7.

10 RISSANEN, A. M., HELIOVAARA, M., KNEKT, P., REUNANEN, A. and AROMAA, A. (1991), Determinants of weight gain and overweight in adult Finns. *Eur. J. Clin. Nutr.* **45**, 419–30.

11 WEATERALL, R. and SHAPER, A. G. (1988), Overweight and obesity in middle-aged British men. *Eur. J. Clin. Nutr.* **42**, 221–31.

12 WANNAMETHEE, S. G. and SHAPER, A. G. (2003), Alcohol, body weight, and weight gain in middle-aged men. *Am. J. Clin.* **77**, 1312–7.

13 ADDOLORATO, G., CAPRISTO, E., GRECO, A. V., STEFANINI, G. F. and GASBARRINI, G. (1998), Influence of chronic alcohol abuse on body weight and energy metabolism: is excess alcohol consumption a risk factor for obesity or malnutrition? *J. Intern. Med.* **244**, 387–95.

14 HILLERS, V. N. and MASSEY, L. K. (1985), Interrelationships of moderate and high alcohol consumption with diet and health status. *Am. J. Clin. Nutr.* **41**, 356–65.

15 ADDOLORATO, G., CAPRISTO, E., GRECO, A. V., CAPUTO, F., STEFANINI, G. F. and GASBARRINI, G. (1998), Three months of abstinence from alcohol normalizes energy expenditure and substrate oxidation in alcoholics: a longitudinal study. *Am. J. Gastroenterol.* **93**, 2476–81.

16 LEVINE, J. A., HARRIS, M. M. and MORGAN, M. Y. (2000), Energy expenditure in chronic alcohol abuse. *Eur. J. Clin. Invest.* **30**, 779–86.

17 FALCK-YTTERM, Y. and MCCULLOUGH, A. J. (2000), The effect of alcohol on body composition. *Am. J. Gastroenterol.* **95**, 2156–9.

18 LEIBEL, R. L., DUFOUR, M., HUBBARD, V. S. and LANDS, W. E. M. (1993), Alcohol and calories: A matter of balance. *Alcohol.* **10**, 429–34.

19 LIEBER, C. S. (1991), Perspectives: do alcohol calories count. *Am. J. Clin. Nutr.* **54**, 976–82.

20 SUTER, P. M., MAIRE, R. and VETTER, W. (1995), Is an increased waist:hip ratio the cause of alcohol-induced hypertension? The AIR 94 study. *J. Hypertens.* **13**, 1857–62.

21 VADSTRUP, E. S., PETERSEN, L., SORENSEN, T. I. A. and GRONBAEK, M. (2003), Waist circumference in relation to history of amount and type of alcohol; results from the Copenhagen City Heart Study. *Int. J. Obes.* **27**, 238–46.

22 GORDON, T. and KANNEL, W. B. (1983), Drinking and its relation to smoking, BP, blood lipids, and uric acid. *Arch. Intern. Med.* **143**, 1366–74.

23 LIU, S., SERDULA, M. K., WILLIAMSON, D. F., MOKDAD, A. H. and BYERS, T. (1994), A prospective study of alcohol intake and change in body weight among US adults. *Am. J. Epidemiol.* **140**, 912–20.

24 KOH-BANERJEE, P., CHU, N. F., SPIEGELMAN, D. *et al.* (2003), Prospective study of the association of changes in dietary intake, physical activity, alcohol consumption, and smoking with 9 year gain in waist circumference among 16 587 US men. *Am. J. Clin. Nutr.* **78**, 719–27.

25 DALLONGEVILLE, J., MARECAUX, N., DUCIMETIERE, P. *et al.* (1998), Influence of alcohol consumption and various beverages on waist girth and waist-to-hip ratio in a sample of French men and women. *Int. J. Obes.* **22**, 1178–83.

26 RANDRIANJOHANY, A., BALKAU, B., CUBEAU, J., DUCIMETIÈRE, P., WARNET, J-M. and ESCHWÈGE, E. (1993), The relationship between behavioural pattern, overall and central adiposity in a population of healthy French men. *Int. J. Obes.* **17**, 651–5.

27 SLATTERY, M. L., MCDONALD, A., BILD, D. E. *et al.* (1992), Associations of body fat and its distribution with dietary intake, physical activity, alcohol, and smoking in blacks and whites. *Am. J. Clin. Nutr.* **55**, 943–9.

28 ARMELLINI, F., ZAMBONI, M., FRIGO, L. *et al.* (1993), Alcohol consumption, smoking habits and body fat distribution in Italian men and women aged 20–60 years. *Eur. J. Clin. Nutr.* **47**, 52–60.

29 LAWS, A., TERRY, R. B. and BARRETT-CONNOR, E. (1990), Behavioral covariates of waist-to-hip ratio in Racho Bernardo. *Am. J. Pub. Hlth.* **80**, 1358–62.

30 SUTER, P. M., HASLER, E. and VETTER, W. (1997), Effects of alcohol on energy metabolism and body weight regulations; is alcohol a risk factor for obesity? *Nutr. Rev.* **55**, 157–71.

31 TROISI, R. J., WEISS, S. T., SEGAL, H. R., CASSANO, P. A., VOKONAS, P. S. and LANDSBERG, L. (1990), The relationship of body fat distribution to blood pressure in normotensive men: the normative aging study. *Int. J. Obes.* **14**, 515–25.

32 HELLERSTEDT, W. L., JEFFERY, R. W. and MURRAY, D. M. (1990), The association between alcohol intake and adiposity in the general population. *Am. J. Epidemiol.* **132**, 594–611.

33 SEPPÄ, K., SILLANAUKEE, P., PITKÄJÄRVI, T., NIKKILÄ, M. and KOIVULA, T. (1992), Moderate and heavy alcohol consumption have no favorable effect on lipid values. *Arch. Intern. Med.* **152**, 297–300.

34 MARQUES-VIDAL, P., MONTAYE, M. and HAAS, B. *et al.* (2001), Relationships between alcoholic beverages and cardiovascular risk factor levels in middle-aged men, the PRIME study. *Atherosclerosis* **157**, 431–40.

35 GREGORY, J., FOSTER, K., TYLER, H. and WISEMAN, M. (1990), *The Dietary and Nutritional Survey of British Adults.* HMSO: London.

36 APPLEBY, P. N., THOROGOOD, M., MANN, J. I. and KEY, T. J. (1998), Low body mass index in non-meat eaters: the possible roles of animal fat, dietary fiber and alcohol. *Int. J. Obes.* **22**, 454–60.

37 SUTER, P. M., SCHUTZ, Y. and JEQUIER, E. (1992), The effect of alcohol on fat storage in healthy subjects. *N. Engl. J. Med.* **326**, 983–7.

38 WILLIAMSON, D., FORMAN, M., BINKIN, N., GENTRY, E., REMINGTON, P. and TROWBRIDGE, F. (1987), Alcohol and body weight in United States adults. *Am. J. Pub. Hlth.* **77**, 1324–30.

39 COLDITZ, G. A., GIOVANNUCCI, E., RIMM, E. B., STAMPFER, M. J., ROSNER, B., SPEIZER, F. E., GORDIS, E. and WILLET, W. C. (1991), Alcohol intake in relation to diet and obesity in women and men. *Am. J. Clin. Nutr.* **54**, 49–55.

40 ISTVAN, J., MURRAY, R. and VOLLKER, H. (1995), The relationship between patterns of alcohol consumption and body weight. *Int. J. Epidemiol.* **24**, 543–6.

41 LAHMANN, P. H., LISSNER, L., GULLBERG, B. and BERGLUND, G. (2000), Sociodemographic factors associated with long-term weight gain, current body fatness and central adiposity in Swedish women. *Int. J. Obes.* **24**, 685–94.

42 POMERLEAU, J., MCKEIGUE, P. M. and CHATURVEDI, N. (1999), Factors associated with obesity in South Asian, Afro-Caribbean and European women. *Int. J. Obes.* **23**, 25–33.

43 MAYER, E. J., NEWMAN, B., QUESENBERRY, JR. C. P., FRIEDMAN, G. D. and SELBY, J. V. (1993), Alcohol consumption and insulin concentrations: role of insulin in associations of alcohol intake with high-density lipoprotein cholesterol and triglycerides. *Circulation* **88**, 2190–7.

44 EISEN, S. A., LYONS, M. J., GOLDBERG, J. and TRUE, W. R. (1993), The impact of cigarette and alcohol consumption on weight and obesity: an analysis of 1911 monozygotic male twin pairs. *Arch. Intern. Med.* **153**, 2457–63.

45 SUTER, P. M., HÄSLER, E. and VETTER, W. (1997), Effects of alcohol on energy metabolism and body weight regulation: is alcohol a risk factor for obesity? *Nutr. Rev.* **55**, 157–71.

46 DORN, J. M., HOVEY, K., MUTI, P., FREUDENHEIM, J. L., RUSSEL, NOCHAJSKI, T. H. and TREVISAN, M. (2003), Alcohol drinking patterns differentially affect central adiposity as measured by abdominal height in women and men. *J. Nutr.* **133**, 2655–62.

47 HEATHERINGTON, M. M., CAMERON, F., WALLIS, D. J. and PIRIE, L. M. (2001), Stimulation of appetite by alcohol. *Physiol. Behav.* **74**, 283–9.

48 YEOMANS, M. R., HAILS, N. J. and NESIC, J. S. (1999), Alcohol and the appetizer effect. *Behav. Pharmacol.* **10**, 151–61.

49 WESTERTERP-PLANTENGA, M. S. and VERWEGEN, C. R. T. (1999), The appetizing effect of an aperitif in overweight and normal-weight humans. *Am. J. Clin. Nutr.* **69**, 205–12.

50 POPPITT, S. D., ECKHARDT, J. W., MCGONAGLE, J., MURGATROYD, P. R. and PRENTICE, A. M. (1996), Short-term effects of alcohol consumption on appetite and energy intake. *Physiol. Behav.* **60**, 1063–70.

51 JACQUES, P. F., SULSKY, S., HARTZ, S. C. and RUSSELL, R. M. (1989), Moderate alcohol intake and nutritional status in nonalcoholic elderly subjects. *Am. J. Clin. Nutr.* **50**, 875–83.

52 DE CASTRO, J. M. and OROZCO, S. (1989), Moderate alcohol intake and spontaneous eating patterns of humans: evidence of unregulated supplementation. *Am. J. Clin. Nutr.* **50**, 875–83.

53 ROSE, D., MURPHY, S. P., HUDES, M. and VITERI, F. E. (1995), Food energy remains constant with increasing alcohol intake. *J. Am. Diet. Assoc.* **95**, 698–700.

54 TREMBLAY, A., WOUTERS, E., WENKER, M., ST-PIERRE, S., BOUCHARD, C. and DESPRES, J. P. (1995), Alcohol and a high fat diet: a combination favoring overfeeding. *Am. J. Clin. Nutr.* **62**, 639–44.

55 RISSANEN, A., SARLIO-LAHTEENKORVA, S., ALFTHAN, G., GREF, C-G. and SALASPURO, M. (1987), Employed problem drinkers; a nutritional risk group? *Am. J. Clin. Nutr.* **45**, 456–61.

56 OROZCO, S. and DE CASTRO, J. M. (1991), Effects of alcohol abstinence on spontaneous feeding patterns in moderate alcohol consuming humans. *Pharmacol. Biochem. Behav.* **40**, 867–73.

57 FOLTIN, R. W., KELLY, T. H. and FISCHMAN, M. W. (1993), Alcohol as an energy source in humans: comparison with dextrose-containing beverages. *Appetite* **20**, 95–110.

58 HORNE, W. I. and TSUKAMATO, H. (1993), Dietary modulation of alcohol-induced pancreatic injury. *Alcohol* **10**, 481–4.

59 WEATHERFORD, S. C., FIGLEWICZ, D. P., PARK, C. R. and WOODS, S. C. (1993), Chronic alcohol consumption increases sensitivity to the anorexic effect of cholescytokinin. *Am. J. Physiol.* **265**, R211–5.

60 BARANYIOVA, E. and HULLINGER, R. L. (1999), Effects of cholecystokinin on liquid diet intake of early weaned piglets. *Physiol. Behav.* **68**, 163–8.

61 KONTUREK, P. C., KONTUREK, S. J., BRZOZOWSKI, T. and HAHN, E. G. (1999), Gastroprotection and control of food intake by leptin. Comparison with cholecystokinin and prostaglandins. *J. Physiol. Pharmacol.* **50**, 39–48.

62 PI-SUNYER, X., KISSILEFF, H. R., THORNTON, J. and SMITH, G. P. (1982), C-Terminal octapeptide of cholecystokinin decreases food intake in obese men. *Physiol. Behav.* **29**, 627–30.

63 LIEVERSE, R. J., JANSEN, L. B. M. J., MASCLEE, A. A. M. and LAMERS, C. B. H. W. (1982), Satiety effects of a physiological dose of cholecystokinin in humans. *Gut.* **36**, 176–9.

64 MANTZOROS, C. S. (1999), The role of leptin in human obesity and disease: a review of the current evidence. *Ann. Intern. Med.* **130**, 671–80.

65 TRAYHURN, P., HOGGARD, N., MERECER, J. G. and RAYNER, D. V. (1999), Leptin: fundamental aspects. *Int. J. Obes.* **23** (Suppl 1), 22–8.

66 HEINI, A. F., LARA-CASTRO, C., KIRK, K. A., CONSIDINE, R. V., CARO, J. F. and WEINSER, R. L. (1998), Association of leptin and hunger-satiety ratings in obese women. *Int. J. Obes.* **22**, 1084–7.

67 CAMPOSTANO, A., GRILLO, G., BESSARIONE, D., DE GRANDI, R. and ADAMI, G. F. (1998), Relationship of serum leptin to body composition and resting energy expenditure. *Horm. Metab. Res.* **30**, 646–7.

68 CHAPELOT, D., AUBERT, R., MARMONIER, C., CHABERT, M. and LOUIS-SYLVESTRE, J. (2000), An endocrine and metabolic definition of the intermeal interval in humans; evidence for a role of leptin on the prandial pattern through fatty acid disposal. *Am. J. Clin. Nutr.* **72**, 421–31.

69 WISSE, B. E., CAMPFIELD, L. A., MARLISS, E. B., MORAIS, J. A., TENEBAUM, R. and GOUGEON, R. (1999), Effect of prolonged moderate and severe energy restriction and refeeding on plasma leptin concentrations in obese women. *Am. J. Clin. Nutr.* **70**, 321–30.

70 ROMON, M., LEBEL, P., VELLY, C., MARECAUX, N., FRUCHART, J. C. and DALLONGEVILLE, J. (1999), Leptin response to carbohydrate or fat meal and association with subsequent satiety and energy intake. *Am. J. Physiol.* **277**, E855–61.

71 RABEN, A. and ASTRUP, A. (2000), Leptin is influenced both by predisposition to obesity and diet composition. *Intl. J. Obes.* **24**, 450–9.

72 KEIM, N. L., STERN, J. S. and HAVEL, P. J. (1998), Relation between circulating leptin concentrations and appetite during a prolonged, moderate energy deficit in women. *Am. J. Clin. Nutr.* **68**, 794–801.

73 HINEY, J. K., DEARTH, R. K., LARA, F., SRIVASTAVA, S. and LESDEES, W. (1999), Effects of alcohol on leptin secretion and the leptin-induced luteinizing hormone (LH) release from last juvenile female rats. *Alc. Clin. Exp. Res.* **23**, 1785–92.

74 LARSSON, H., ELMSTAHL, S., BERGLUND, G. and AHREN, B. O. (1998), Evidence for leptin regulation of food intake in humans. *J. Clin. Endocrinol. Metab.* **83**, 4382–5.

75 KARHUNEN, L. J., LAPPALAINEN, R. I., HAFFNER, S. M. *et al.* (1998), Serum leptin, food intake and preferences for sugar and fat in obese women. *Int. J. Obes.* **22**, 819–21.

76 MATRINEZ, V. (1999), Intracerebroventricular leptin inhibits gastric emptying of a solid nutrient meal in rats. *NeuroReport* **10**, 3217–21.

77 ROSENZWIG, M. R. The mechanisms of hunger and thirst. In: Fredrick M, Toate S (eds), *Biological Foundation of Behavior*, Open U. Press: Phil, 1986. Pp. 73–143.

78 RABEN, A., TAGLIABUE, A., CHRISTENSEN, N. J., MADSEN, J., HOLST, J. J. and ASTRUP, A. (1994), Resistant starch: the effect on postprandial glycemia, hormonal response, and satiety. *Am. J. Clin. Nutr.* **60**, 544–51.

79 COUNCIL ON SCIENTIFIC AFFAIRS. (1989), Dietary Fiber and Health. *J. Am. Med. Assoc.* **262**, 542–6.

80 KAUFMAN, S. E. and KAYE, M. D. (1979), Effect of alcohol upon gastric emptying. *Gut.* **20**, 688–92.

81 JIAN, R., DUCROT, F., NAJEAN, Y., CORTOT, A. and MODIGLIANI, R. (1983), Effect of alcohol on gastric-emptying of an ordinary meal in man. *Gut.* **24** (4), A363.

82 WEGENER, M., SCHAFFSTEIN, J., DILGER, U., COENEN, C., WEDMANN, B. and SCHMIDT, G. (1991), Gastrointestinal transit of solid-liquid meal in chronic alcoholics. *Dig. Dis. Sci.* **35**, 917–23.

83 MOORE, J. G., CHRISTIAN, P. E., DATZ, F. L. and COLEMAN, R. E. (1981), Effect of wine on gastric emptying in humans. *Gastroenterology* **81**, 1072–5.

84 PFEIFFER, A., HOGL, B. and KAESS, H. (1992), Effect of alcohol and commonly ingested alcoholic beverages on gastric emptying and gastrointestinal transit. *Clin. Invest.* **70**, 487–91.

85 KAMPOV-POLEVOY, A. B., GARBUTT, J. C. and KHALITOV, E. (2003), Family history of alcoholism and response to sweets. *Alcohol. Clin. Exp. Res.* **27**, 1743–9.

86 KAMPOV-POLEVOY, A. B., GARBUTT, J. C., DAVIS, C. E. and JANOWSKY, D. S. (1998), Preference for higher sugar concentrations and tridimensional personality questionnaire scores in alcoholic and nonalcoholic men. *Alcoholism: Clin. Exp. Res.* **22**, 610–4.

87 SUBAR, A. F., ZIEGLER, R. G., PATTERSON, B. H., URSIN, G. and GRAUBARD, B. (1994), US dietary patterns associated with fat intake; the 1987 national health interview survey. *Am. J. Pub. Hlth.* **84**, 359–6.

88 TURNER, L. A. and KANO, M. J. (1992), Dietary fat and body fat: a multivariate study of 205 adult females. *Am. J. Clin. Nutr.* **56**, 616–22.

89 ASTRUP, A. (1993), Dietary composition, substrate balances, and body fat in subjects with a predisposition to obesity. *Int. J. Obes.* **17**, S32–6.

90 FERRARONI, M., DECARLI, A., FRANCESCHI, S. *et al.* (1996), Validity and reproducibility of alcohol consumption in Italy. *Int. J. Epidemiol.* **25**, 775–82.

91 LIU, S., SERDULA, M. K., BYERS, T., WILLIAMSON, D. F., MOKDAD, A. H. and FLANDERS, D. (1996), Reliability of alcohol intake as recalled from 10 years in the past. *Am. J. Epidemiol.* **143**, 177–86.

92 KAAKS, R., SLIMANI, N. and RIBOLI, E. (1997), Pilot phase studies on the accuracy of dietary intake measurements in the EPIC project: overall evaluation of results. *Int. J. Epidemiol.* **26** (Suppl 1), S26–36.

93 GIOVANNUCCI, E., COLDITZ, G., STAMPFER, M. J. *et al.* (1991), The assessment of alcohol consumption by a simple self-administered questionnaire. *Am. J. Epidemiol.* **133**, 810–7.

94 SUTER, P. M. (2000), The paradox of the alcohol-paradox – another step towards the resolution of the 'alcohol energy wastage' controversy. *Eur. J. Clin. Invest.* **30**, 749–50.

95 SONKO, B. J., PRENTICE, A. M., MURGATROYD, P. R., GOLDBERG, G. R., VAN DE VEN, M. L. H. M. and COWARD, W. A. (1994), Effect of alcohol on postmeal fat storage. *Am. J. Clin. Nutr.* **59**, 619–25.

96 MURGATROYD, P. R., VAN DE VEN, M. L. H. M., GOLDBERG, G. R. and PRENTICE, A. M. (1996), Alcohol and the regulation of energy balance: overnight effects on diet-induced thermogenesis and fuel storage. *Br. J. Nutr.* **75**, 33–45.

97 RUMPLER, W. V., RHODES, D. G., BAER, D. J., CONWAY, J. M. and SEALE, J. L. (1996), Energy value of moderate alcohol consumption by humans. *Am. J. Clin. Nutr.* **64**, 108–14.

98 REINUS, J. F., HEYMSFIELD, S. B., WISKIND, R., CASPER, K. and GALAMBOS, J. T. (1989), Alcohol: relative fuel value and metabolic effects in vivo. *Metabolism* **38**, 125–35.

99 CLEVIDENCE, B. A., TAYLOR, P. R., CAMPBELL, W. S. and JUDD, J. T. (1995), Lean and heavy women may not use energy from alcohol with equal efficiency. *J. Nutr.* **125**, 2536–40.

100 TREMBLAY, A. (1999), The effects of exercise and alcohol intake on energy balance and food intake. *Progress in Obesity Research*: 8, Eds. Guy-Grand B., Ailhaud G., London, John Libbey & Co.

101 PIROLA, R. C. and LIEBER, C. S. (1972), The energy cost of the metabolism of drugs, including alcohol. *Pharmacology* **7**, 185–96.

102 CORDAIN, L., BRYAN, E. D., MELBY, C. L. and SMITH, M. J. (1997), Influence of moderate daily wine consumption on body weight regulation and metabolism in healthy free-living males. *J. Am. Coll. Nutr.* **16**, 134–9.

103 CROUSE, J. R. and GRUNDY, S. M. (1984), Effects of alcohol on plasma lipoproteins and cholesterol and triglyceride metabolism in man. *J. Lipid. Res.* **25**, 486–96.

104 GREENFIELD, J. R., SAMARAS, K., JENKINS, A. B., KELLY, P. J., SPECTOR, T. D. and CAMPBELL, L. V. (2003), Moderate alcohol consumption, dietary fat composition, and abdominal obesity in women: evidence for gene-environment interaction. *J. Clin. Endocrinol. Metab.* **88**, 5381–6.

105 KALANT, H. (1971), Absorption, diffusion, distribution, and elimination of alcohol: effects of biological membranes. In: Begleiter KB (ed), *The Biology of Alcoholism*. New York: Plenum, pp. 1–62.

106 ADDOLORATO, G., CAPRISTO, E., GRECO, A. V., STEFANINI, G. F. and GASBARRINI, G. (1997), Energy expenditure, substrate oxidation, and body composition in subjects with chronic alcoholism: new findings from metabolic assessment. *Alcoholism: Clin. Exp. Res.* **21**, 962–7.

107 LEAKE, C. D. and SILVERMAN, M. (1996), *Alcoholic Beverages in Clinical Medicine*. Chicago: Yearbook Medical Pub, Inc. Pp. 54.

108 NORBERG, A., GABRIELSSON, J., JONES, A. W. and HAHN, R. G. (2000), Within- and between-subject variations in pharmacokinetic parameters of alcohol by analysis of breath, venous blood and urine. *Br. J. Clin. Pharmacol.* **49**, 399–408.

109 ADDOLORATO, G., CAPRISTO, E., GRECO, A. V., CAPUTO, F., STEFANINI, G. F. and GASBARRINI, G. (1998), Three months of abstinence from alcohol normalizes

energy expenditure and substrate oxidation in alcoholics: a longitudinal study. *Am. J. Gastroenterol.* **93**, 2476–81.

110 JHANGIANI, S. S., AGARWAL, N., HOLMES, R., CAYTEN, C. G. and PITCHUMONI, C. S. (1986), Energy expenditure in chronic alcoholics with and without liver disease. *Am. J. Clin. Nutr.* **44**, 323–9.

111 KLESGES, R. C., MEALER, C. Z. and KLESGES, L. M. (1994), Effects of alcohol intake on resting energy expenditure in young women social drinkers. *Am. J. Clin. Nutr.* **59**, 805–9.

112 BLOCK, G., DRESSER, C. M., HARTMAN, A. M. and CARROLL, M. D. (1985), Nutrient sources in the American diet: quantitative data from the NHANES II survey. *Am. J. Epidemiol.* **122**, 27–40.

113 SUTER, P. M., JEQUIER, E. and SCHUTZ, Y. (1994), Effect of alcohol on energy expenditure. *Am. Physiol. Soc.* **35**, R1204–12.

114 KIEFER, S. W. and DOPP, J. M. (1989), Taste reactivity to alcohol in rats. *Behav. Neurosci.* **103**, 1318–26.

115 GRUCHOW, H. W., SOBOCINSKI, K. A., BARBORIAK, J. J. and SCHELLER, J. G. (1985), Alcohol consumption, nutrient intake and relative body weight among US adults. *Am. J. Clin. Nutr.* **42**, 289–95.

116 JONES, B. R., BARRETT-CONNER, E., CRIQUI, M. H. and HOLDBROK, M. J. (1982), A community study of calorie and nutrient intake in drinkers and non-drinkers and non-drinkers of alcohol. *Am. J. Clin. Nutr.* **35**, 135–9.

117 TOFLER, O. B., SAKER, B. M., ROLLO, K. A., BURVILL, M. J. and STENHOUSE, N. (1969), Electrocardiogram of the social drinker in Perth, Western Australia. *Br. Heart J.* **31**, 306–13.

118 FAGRELL, B., DEFAIRE, U., BONDY, S., CRIQUI, M., GASIANO, M., GRONBAEK, M., JACKSON, R., KLATSKY, A., SALONEN, J. and SHAPER, A. G. (1999), The effects of light to moderate drinking on cardiovascular diseases. *J. Intern. Med.* **246**, 331–40.

119 WESTERTERP, K. R., MEIJER, E. P., GORIS, A. H. C. and KESTER, A. D. M. (2004), Alcohol energy intake and habitual physical activity in older adults. *Br. J. Nutr.* **91**, 149–52.

120 LEVINE, J. A., EBERHARDT, N. L. and JENSEN, M. D. (1999), Role of nonexcercise activity thermogenesis in resistance to fat gain in humans. *Science* **283**, 212–4.

121 LINKOLA, J., YLIKARHRI, R. and FYHRQUIST, F. (1978), Plasma vasopressin in alcohol intoxication and hangover. *Acta. Physiol. Scand.* **104**, 180–7.

122 VANDYKE, H. B. and AMES, E. G. (1951), Alcohol diuresis. *Acta. Endocrinol.* **7**, 110–21.

123 WILSNACK, S. C. and WILSNACK, R. W. (1995), Drinking and problem drinking in US women: patterns and recent trends, in Galanter M (ed): *Recent Developments in Alcoholism*, vol 12. *Alcoholism and Women.* New York, Plenum, pp. 29–60.

14

The use of fat replacers for weight loss and control

J. Miller Jones, College of St Catherine, USA and S. Jonnalagadda, Novartis Medical Nutrition, USA

14.1 Introduction

Obesity rates for both children and adults have increased dramatically in the USA, the UK and Western Europe (WHO, 1998; Centers for Disease Control and Prevention, 2002; Nielsen *et al.*, 2002). The obesity epidemic is fueled by readily available, inexpensive food, especially energy dense, high fat foods and increased portion size coupled, which both lead to the over-consumption of calories (Young and Nestle, 2003; Smiciklas-Wright *et al.*, 2003; Swinburn and Egger, 2002; Nielsen and Popkin, 2003; Rolls *et al.*, 2002; Roe and Rolls, 2004). Since increases in the energy density of foods have also been shown to increase energy intake (Kral *et al.*, 2004; Devitt and Mattes, 2004; DeCastro, 2004), it is reasonable to assume that ingestion of foods, which lower energy density by any means including the use of fat replacers, would result in lower overall food energy intake. Thus manipulation of the energy density of the diet can lower energy consumption by 20% to 25% and can lead to modest changes in body weight (Kral *et al.*, 2002; Bell and Rolls, 2001). These data indicate that a reduction in the proportion of fat in the diet by 10% can result in a corresponding reduction of 238 kcal/day of total energy intake and can produce a weight loss of ~3.2 kg. Therefore, lowering the fat content of foods, by using fat replacers, has potential for lowering the energy density of foods, which can be helpful in the struggle to maintain a healthy weight (Astrup *et al.*, 2000).

14.2 Types of fat replacers

Fat replacers are called by many synonyms with various nuances in their usage. The various names are distinguished in Box 14.1. Fat replacers in food must do two things if they are to help consumers with weight loss. First, they must replicate all or some of the functional properties of fat and, in so doing, impart the sensory properties attributed to fat such as a rich, creamy mouth feel and a tender texture. No one fat replacer is likely to provide all the functions of fat such as flavor, texture, lubrication, keeping quality, volume or heat transfer. Second, they must lower the fat and calorie content of the food. They do this either by enabling the holding of air and water or by being less well absorbed. Fat replacers are most frequently used to replace fat in products with a high fat content and are used in a variety of food products, including frozen desserts, processed meats, cheese, sour cream,

Box 14.1 Fat replacer terms

Fat replacers – can provide some or all of the functions of fat
usually yield fewer calories than fat
may or may not provide the same nutrients as the fat they replace

Fat substitutes – resemble conventional fats and oils and provide all food functions of fat
replace fat on a gram-for-gram basis
are usually stable at cooking and frying temperatures
yield less than 9 kcal/g
in some cases are not absorbed at all, so yield no calories

Fat analogs – provide food with many of the characteristics of fat
provide lower digestibility than common dietary fats
alter nutritional value

Fat extenders – optimize the functionality of fat
allow a decrease in the usual amount of fat in the product

Fat mimetics – mimic one or more of the sensory and physical functions of fat in the food
are either carbohydrate, protein, or fat components alone or in combination
provide from 0–9 kcal/g
provide lubricity, mouth feel and other characteristics of fat by holding water
are unsuitable for fat functions such as frying due to additional water
may be used for baking and at retort temperatures
may be subject to excessive browning at high heat

salad dressings, snack chips and baked goods. At the height of the interest in low fat foods, more than 1000 fat-modified foods were introduced, with fat modified snacks being the fastest growing category of products in supermarkets at the time (Schwenk and Guthrie, 1997; Calorie Control Council, 2004).

There are three broad categories of fat replacers on the market. Since fat replacers may contain calories, food manufacturers using these products should ensure that the final product is not only reduced in fat, but also reduced in calories. In the end, the food with fat replacers will be of little value for weight reduction if it fails to cause a significant reduction in calories.

Carbohydrate-based fat replacers use carbohydrate polymers and dietary fibers, such as cellulose, dextrins, maltodextrins, polydextrose, gums, fiber, and modified starch, to replace fat. Carbohydrate-based fat replacers can provide up to 4 kcal/g if the carbohydrate is fully digestible. Often the calories are lower than this since the fat replacers are either dietary fibers, which are not digested or only fermented to some degree, or digestible carbohydrates mixed with water so they provide 0–2 kcal/g. In some cases fibers, such as cellulose, are ground into micro particles that can form gels for use as fat substitutes, e.g. Oatrim® and Z-trim®. Carbohydrate-based fat replacers used in a variety of foods including dairy-type products, frozen desserts, sauces, salad dressings, processed meats, baked goods, spreads, chewing gums and sweets, but cannot replace fats in frying.

Protein-based fat replacers are made from many different types of protein but soy, egg, milk or whey proteins are common. Microparticulation of protein into tiny, spherical particles that provide a creamy mouth feel similar to fats helps protein to function as a fat replacer. Blending protein with carbohydrates is another way to create fat replacers. Several studies have shown that combinations of ingredients in fat replacer formulations create synergy that helps lower fat and helps retain desirable product texture (Ordonez *et al.*, 2001; Ruthig *et al.*, 2001; El-Nager *et al.*, 2002; Conforti *et al.*, 2001; Conforti and Archilla, 2001). Fat replacers from protein and protein blends do provide 4 kcal/g, but they may provide only 1 to 4 kcal/g either because they hold water or are used in lesser amounts than fat. For example, 1 g of Simplesse® can replace 3 g of fat in cream.

Protein-based fat replacers have been used in fat-free ice cream, low-fat cheese, low-fat baked goods and reduced fat versions of butter, sour cream, cheese, yogurt, salad dressing, margarine, mayonnaise, baked goods, coffee creamers, soups and sauces. Often, a combination of these fat replacers can have tremendous potential in the development of fat modified foods with greater acceptability while lowering the total energy and fat intake.

Fat-based fat replacers include common fats that have had chemical alterations of fatty acids so that they deliver less than 9 calories per gram. Some fat-based fat replacers pass through the body partially or totally unabsorbed. Thus they provide less than 9 kcal/g or no calories at all. For example, Olestra (Olean®) is a sucrose polyester consisting of a mixture of hexa, hepta and octa esters of sucrose, esterified with long chain fatty acids. It has the organoleptic and thermal properties of fat, but cannot be hydrolyzed by gastric or pancreatic lipase. The unhydrolyzed molecule is too large to be absorbed in the gastrointestinal tract and, therefore, cannot be metabolized for energy with a net effect of yielding no calories. Other fat-based fat replacers such as SALATRIM (short and long chain triglyceride molecule) and Caprenin, a substitute for cocoa butter in candy bars, are only partially digested and absorbed and provide 5 kcal/g. Some fat replacers such as Enova™ oil are structured diglycerides and are metabolized differently than triglycerides, so that some of the energy is lost as heat rather than stored as adipose.

Emulsifiers can be another type of fat-based substance that can be used as a fat replacer. They may be used with water to replace all or part of the shortening content in cake mixes, cookies, icings, vegetable and dairy products. They provide the same number of calories as fat, but since less is used in the formulation the resultant product has less total fat and energy. Mono- and diglycerides are currently used in foods as fat replacers and other substances such as dialkyl dihexadecylmalonate, esterified propoxylated glycerol, and trialkoxytriartallate are in various stages of development.

14.3 The role of fat replacers in weight loss

Fat replacers can potentially impact overall diet quality and help with weight loss and maintenance. For example, salad dressings and spreads made with fat replacers can help enhance appeal of other nutritious foods such as vegetables and fruit. Thus, fat replacers may help increase the intake of satiety producing low calorie, high fiber, nutrient-dense foods while adding few calories. In meat and other food items, fat replacers such as prunes, raisins or cherry paste or wild rice replace some of the fat and increase the antioxidant value of foods while lowering calories.

14.3.1 Impact of protein-based fat replacers

Since protein-based fat replacers are from milk powder, whey, soy or legumes, they not only have potential to lower calories, but can also increase protein in the diet or offer some nutritional advantages of the individual protein. Some preliminary data indicate that protein may have an impact on satiety and food consumption in the short term (Anderson and Moore, 2004; Layman and Baum, 2004). Furthermore, protein-based fat replacers have the potential to increase the protein in the diet and a high protein to carbohydrate ratio has been associated in studies with greater weight loss than diets with a lower ratio (Layman, 2004). Dairy-based proteins may add calcium, which has been shown in some studies to be related to weight loss

(Zemel, 2004). Thus protein-based fat replacers might offer two benefits to the calorie conscious eater.

14.3.2 Impact of fiber-based fat replacers

Fiber-based fat replacers may offer calorie savings while increasing fiber in the diet (Inglett, 2002). Some types of fiber have been shown to regulate food intake, to aid in both preventing weight gain and helping with weight maintenance (Archer *et al.*, 2004; Toeller *et al.*, 2001; Laitinen *et al.*, 2004; Howarth *et al.*, 2001). One study with male diabetics shows the utility of a fiber-based-fat replacer in dealing with obesity and complications associated with it. In this study those who chose diets rich in fiber-based fat replacers along with sugar replacers and other lifestyle changes reduced body weight and body mass index more than those eating the standard treatment plan. In addition, there were greater decreases in HbA1C[1] and increases in HDL cholesterol (Reyna *et al.* 2003). In like manner, inclusion of foods made with fat replacers such as Mimex or Oatrim® (a powdered soluble oat fiber containing beta-glucans) has been observed to not only lower blood lipids, systolic blood pressure, improve glucose tolerance and antioxidant status but also lower body weight (Inglett, 2002; Larion *et al.*, 2003). Liu *et al.* (2003) noted that those in the Harvard Nurses' Health Study cohort who had the highest fiber intakes were least likely to gain weight.

14.3.3 Impact of fat-based fat replacers

Fat-based fat replacers have also been associated with caloric dilution (Glueck *et al.*, 1982), decreased caloric intake and changes in appetite (Burley *et al.*, 1994). In a study with lean and overweight subjects eating foods prepared with a fat emulsion of palm oil and oat oil (Olibra®) as a fat replacer, there was decreased total energy intake for up to 36 hours post-consumption. Use of Olibra® as a fat substitute in yogurt significantly reduced the energy and macronutrient intakes relative to use of milk fat (Burns *et al.*, 2000, 2001, 2002).

14.3.4 Impact of fat replacers

Use of fat replacers in foods such as mayonnaise, hotdogs and chips has been shown to decrease the energy and fat in products by as much as 50%. In a study where subjects were offered either full fat or fat-free Olestra containing chops, total fat intake was reduced from 32 to 43% on regular chips to 27–30% with Olestra chips (Miller *et al.*, 1998). In one study the use of fat-free chips did not have a positive impact on diets if consumers were

[1] Hemogloblin A1C is the best measure of glucose control because it will be high only if glucose has been elevated for a sustained period of time.

regarded as moderate or high Olestra consumers. This subset of consumers increased total energy intake by 209 kcal/d and carbohydrate intake by 37 g/d, compared to a reduction of 87 kcal/d and 14 g/d, respectively, among those not moderate or heavy consumers ($P = 0.01$) (Satia-Bouta *et al.*, 2003). While the changes in percent energy from carbohydrate and total fat were not significant in this study, the small changes in the energy intake over time may lead to increases in body weight, emphasizing the importance of reduced fat products being low in energy and not consumed in excessive quantities.

Some studies showed greater weight loss with the use of fat replacers. Bray *et al.* (2002) and Lovejoy *et al.* (2000) observed weight loss of 6.3 kg over 6 months with fat-substituted diets, wherein Olestra substituted a portion of the full-fat diet, while decreasing digestible fat to 25% but retaining palatability comparable to a diet with 33% of energy from fat. Significant reductions were also observed in body fat (–5.9 kg), total cholesterol (–10 mg/dl), and LDL-cholesterol (–12 mg/dl) compared to the regular (33% in fat) group. Likewise, Weststrate *et al.* (1998) noted that providing free access to reduced fat products resulted in a reduction in energy intake and percent energy from fat, while it was associated with an increase in percentage energy from carbohydrate, especially among individuals classified as high fat consumers. Body weight remained stable in the reduced fat group, while it increased significantly by about 1 kg in the full-fat group. In addition, cardiovascular disease risk factors such as blood lipids, and hemostatic factors, were lower in the reduced fat group compared to the full fat group.

Kennedy and colleagues (1999, 2001, 2003) showed that the selection of low-fat grain mixtures, cakes, cookies and pies not only lowered fat and saturated fat, it resulted in a less energy-dense diet. The individuals consuming lower fat foods were more likely to meet nutrient requirements than those consuming higher fat foods even though they were eating 400–500 kcal less (Kennedy *et al.*, 2003).

Thus one strategy for combating the obesity epidemic may involve the switch from consumption of full-fat products to lower calorie, reduced fat alternatives. Lyle *et al.* (1992) estimated that a 30% reduction in fat calories and a total calorie reduction of 800 kcal can be achieved per week if fat free products from food categories such as cheese, sour cream, frozen desserts, commercial sweets, and baked goods were substituted for their regular versions. The Olestra Post-Market Surveillance Study (Patterson *et al.*, 2000) showed that an intake of 2 g/d of Olestra replaced 18 kcal of fat/d (6570 kcal/y), equivalent to a 0.85 kg decrease in body weight.

Existing evidence suggests that reduced-fat diets and foods are an important strategy that can help lower energy density of foods and limit total fat and energy intake in fighting the obesity epidemic (Sigman-Grant *et al.*, 2003). Fat replacers, thus, can play a useful role in maintaining the palatability of reduced fat foods without sacrificing the hedonic qualities of the food or putting the population at a safety risk (Box 14.2) (Swanson *et al.*,

Box 14.2 Safety of fat replacers

Consumer safety concerns over ingredients added to compensate for fat removal highlight the need for educating the general population about fat replacers and their proper use. Safety of most fat replacers is not an issue as the majority of fat replacers are widely used as food additives and have 'generally recognized as safe' (GRAS) status.

Fat replacers that are approved food additives have raised health concerns. Polydextrose can have a laxative effect, while Olestra may cause leaky and fatty stools and loss of fat-soluble vitamins. Olestra was approved in 1996 for use in savory snacks such as potato chips, crackers and tortilla chips. Manufacturers were required to add vitamins A, D, E and K to Olestra-containing foods to compensate for Olestra's effects on these vitamins, and to place a warning label informing consumers that Olestra may cause abdominal cramping, loose stools, inhibit absorption of fat-soluble vitamins and other nutrients. Subsequent, scientific review has led the FDA to conclude that the warning is no longer warranted (US Food and Drug Administration, 2003). There is limited evidence at the present time to suggest any long-term adverse consequences associated with the consumption of these or any other reduced fat foods developed using the approved fat replacers.

2002). Therefore, on a population level, replacing only 1–2 g of fat/day, by using fat replacers and fat modified foods can prevent excess weight gain and associated chronic diseases and help in promoting health (WHO, 1998; Eldridge *et al.*, 2002). On the other hand, foods prepared with fat replacers that neither lower calories nor encourage the consumption of foods that are central to the dietary recommendations may do little to improve the quality of the diet or to help with obesity. Excessive consumption of brownies, cookies, snack cakes and crisps (chips) and other such foods made with fat replacers may do little to help in the battle against obesity. This may be especially problematic if the consumer erroneously believes that fat-free means calorie free and takes this as a license to consume unlimited amounts.

14.4 Conclusions

Fat replacers have facilitated the development of reduced fat and fat-free foods that have the taste and texture of high fat foods with less fat and fewer calories. The food industry provided a variety of low-fat products and a segment of the public responded by consuming these products. The actual use of reduced fat foods by the general population is influenced by dietary advice and recommendations, individual health concerns, sensory characteristics of products, usefulness in the dietary pattern and willingness to accept the fat substitute. A US survey done in 2000 revealed that the top three reasons for using reduced fat products were to stay in better overall health, to eat or drink healthier foods and beverages, and to reduce intake of fat and calories (American Dietetic Association, ADA, 2003; Calorie Control Council, 2004). Thus, when fat replacers enable the provision of palatable, lower calorie foods, they can be one strategy in the battle to lose or maintain desirable weight. On the other hand, fat replacers that neither lower calories nor enable consumption of foods which are useful in weight reduction and maintenance plans may be of little use. In like manner, the over consumption of foods containing fat replacers by consumers who are either misled by irresponsible manufacturers or misconstrue package claims and equate fat-free or reduced fat with a license to ingest unlimited amounts obviates any potential benefits of fat replacers in the diet. No food or fat replacer supplants the need for practicing moderation and good nutrition.

14.5 References

AMERICAN DIETETIC ASSOCIATION, ADA (2004), 'Nutrition and You: Trends 2002. Final Report'. Available at: www.eatright.org. Accessed 12/06/2003.

ANDERSON G. H. and MOORE S. E. (2004), 'Dietary proteins in the regulation of food intake and body weight in humans', *J. Nutr.*, **134**, 974S–9S.

ARCHER, B. J., JOHNSON, S. K., DEVEREUX, H. M., and BAXTER, A. L. (2004), 'Effect of fat replacement by inulin or lupin-kernel fibre on sausage patty acceptability, post-meal perceptions of satiety and food intake in men', *Br. J. Nutr.*, **91**, 591–9.

ASTRUP, A., GRUNWALD, G. K., MELANSON, E. L., SARIS, W. H. and HILL, J. O. (2000), 'The role of low-fat diets in body weight control: a meta-analysis of *ad libitum* dietary intervention studies', *Int. J. Obes. Relat. Metab. Disord.*, **24**, 1545–52.

BELL, E. A. and ROLLS B. J. (2001), 'Energy density of foods affects energy intake across multiple levels of fat content in lean and obese women', *Am. J. Clin. Nutr.*, **73**, 1010–8.

BRAY G. A., LOVEJOY J. C., MOST-WINDHAUSER M. *et al.* (2002), 'A nine-month randomized clinical trial comparing a fat-substituted and fat-reduced diet in healthy obese men: the Ole Study', *Am. J. Clin. Nutr.*, **76**, 928–34.

BURLEY V. J., COTTON J. R., WESTSTRATE J. A. and BLUNDELL J. E. (1994), 'Effect on appetite of replacing natural fat with sucrose polyester in meals or snacks across one whole day', In Ditschuneit H, Gries FA, Hauner H, Schusdziarra V, Wechsler JG (eds). *Obesity in Europe.*, Libbey, London, 227–33.

BURNS A. A., LIVINGSTONE M. B. E., WELCH R. W., DUNNE A. and ROWLAND I. R. (2002), 'Dose-response effects of a novel fat emulsion (Olibra™) on energy and macronutrient intakes up to 36 h post-consumption', *Eur. J. Clin. Nutr.*, **56**, 368–77.

BURNS A. A., LIVINGSTONE M. B. E., WELCH R. W., DUNNE A., REID A. and ROWLAND I. R. (2001), 'The effects of yoghurt containing a novel fat emulsion on energy and macronutrient intake in lean, overweight and obese subjects', *Int. J. Obes. Relat. Metab. Disord.*, **25**, 1487–96.

BURNS A. A., LIVINGSTONE M. B. E., WELCH R. W. *et al.* (2000), 'Short-term effects of yoghurt containing a novel fat emulsion on energy and macronutrient intakes in non-obese subjects', *Int. J. Obes. Relat. Metab. Disord.*, **24**, 1419–25.

CALORIE CONTROL COUNCIL (2004), 'Fat replacers: Food ingredients for healthy eating', available at: http://www.caloriecontrol.org/fatreprint.html. Accessed 5/6/2004.

CAPRENIN http://www.chiroweb.com/archives/15/13/07.html.

CENTERS FOR DISEASE CONTROL AND PREVENTION: MONITORING THE NATION'S HEALTH (2002), 'Dietary intake of macronutrients, micronutrients, and other dietary constituents: United States, 1988–94', *Vital and Health Statistic*, **11**, 9–85.

CONFORTI F. D. and ARCHILLA L. (2001), 'Evaluation of a maltodextrin gel as a partial replacement for fat in a high-ratio white-layer cake', *Int. J. Consumer. Sci.*, **25**, 238–45.

CONFORTI F. D., NEE P. and ARCHILLA L. (2001), 'The synergistic effects of maltodextrin and high-fructose corn sweetener 90 in a fat-reduced muffin', *Int. J. Consumer Sci.*, **25**, 3–8.

DE CASTRO J. M. (2004), 'Dietary energy density is associated with increased intake in free-living humans', *J. Nutr.*, **134**, 335–41.

DEVITT A. A. and MATTES R. D. (2004), 'Effects of food unit size and energy density on intake in humans', *Appetite*, **42**, 213–20.

ELDRIDGE A. L., COOPER D. A. and PETERS J. C. (2002), 'A role for olestra in body weight management', *Obes. Rev.*, **3**, 17–25.

EL-NAGER G., CLOWES G., TUDORICA C. M., KURI V. and BRENNAN C. S. (2002), 'Rheological quality and stability of yog-ice cream with added inulin', *Int. J. Dairy. Tech.*, **55**, 89–93.

ENOVA http://lowfatcooking.about.com/od/healthandfitness/p/enovaoil.htm.

GLUECK C. J., HASTINGS M. M., ALLEN C. *et al.* (1982), 'Sucrose polyester and covert caloric dilution', *Am. J. Clin. Nutr.*, **35**, 1352–9.

HILL D. S., KNOX B., HAMILTON J., PARR H. and STRINGER M. (2002), 'Reduced-fat foods: the shopper's viewpoint', *Int. J. Consumer. Studies*, **26**, 44–57.

HOWARTH N. C., SALTZMAN E. and ROBERTS S. B. (2001), 'Dietary fiber and weight regulation', *Nutr. Rev.*, **59**, 129–39.

INGLETT G. Development of beta-glucan compositions and their health benefits. Annual Meeting Of The Institute Of Food Technologists June 19, 2002. Available at: http://www.ars.usda.gov/research/publications/publications.htm Accessed 6/14/2004.

KENNEDY E. T., BOWMAN S. A. and POWELL R. (1999), 'Dietary-fat intake in the US population', *J. Am. Coll. Nutr.*, **18**, 207–12.

KENNEDY E., BOWMAN S. and POWELL R. (2001), 'Assessment of the effect of fat-modified foods on diet quality in adults, 19–50 years, using data from the Continuing Survey of Food Intake by Individuals', *J. Am. Diet. Assoc.*, **101**, 455–60.

KRAL T. V., ROE L. S. and ROLLS B. J. (2002), 'Does nutrition information about the energy density of meals affect food intake in normal-weight women?', *Appetite*, **39**, 137–45.

KRAL T. V., ROE L. S. and ROLLS B. J. (2004), 'Combined effects of energy density and portion size on energy intake in women', *Am. J. Clin. Nutr.*, **79**, 962–8.

LAIRON D., BERTRAIS S., VINCENT S. *et al.* (2003), 'Dietary fibre intake and clinical indices in the French Supplementation en Vitamines et Mineraux AntioXydants (SU.VI.MAX) adult cohort', *Proc. Nutr. Soc.*, **6**, 11–5.

LAITINEN J., PIETILAINEN K., WADSWORTH M., SOVIO U. and JARVELIN M. R. (2004), 'Predictors of abdominal obesity among 31-y-old men and women born in Northern Finland in 1966', *Eur. J. Clin. Nutr.*, **58**, 180–90.

LAYMAN, D. K. (2004), Dietary protein and weight. IFT 2004. Annual meeting Las Vegas.

LAYMAN D. K. and BAUM J. I. (2004), 'Dietary protein impact on glycemic control during weight loss', *J. Nutr.*, **34**, 968S–73S.

LIU S., WILLETT W. C., MANSON J. E., HU F. B., ROSNER B. and COLDITZ G. (2003), 'Relation between changes in intakes of dietary fiber and grain products and changes in weight and development of obesity among middle-aged women', *Am. J. Clin. Nutr.*, **78**, 920–7.

LOVEJOY J. C., LEFEVRE M., BRAY G. A. *et al.* (2000), 'Beneficial effects of a low-fat diet on health risk factors is mediated by weight-loss in middle age men', *North American Association for the Study of Obesity (NAASO)*, Long Beach, CA.

LYLE B. J., MCMAHON K. E. and KREUTLER P. A. (1992), 'Assessing the potential dietary impact of replacing dietary fat with other macronutrients', *J. Nutr.*, **122**, 211–6.

MILLER D. L., CASTELLANOS V. H., SHIDE D. J., PETERS J. C. and ROLLS B. J. (1998) Effect of fat-free potato chips with and without nutrition labels on fat and energy intakes. *Am. J. Clin. Nutr.*, **68**, 2, 282–90.

NIELSEN S. J, and POPKIN B. M. (2003), 'Patterns and trends in food portion sizes, 1977–1998', *JAMA*, **289**, 450–3.

NIELSEN S. J., SIEGA-RIZ A. M. and POPKIN B. M. (2002), 'Trends in energy intake in U.S. between 1977 and 1996: similar shifts seen across age groups', *Obes. Res.*, **10**, 370–8.

OATRIM http://www.ars.usda.gov/is/AR/archive/dec98/nutrim1298.pdf Visited 02/05.

OLESTRA http://www.olean.com Visited 02/05.

OLIBRA http://www.lipid.se/olibra/main.html Visited 02/05.

ORDONEZ M., ROVIRA J. and JAIME I. (2001), 'The relationship between the composition and texture of conventional and low-fat frankfurters', *Int. J. Fd. Sci. Tech.*, **36**, 749–58.

PATTERSON R. E., KRISTAL A. R., PETERS J. C. *et al.* (2000), 'Changes in diet, weight, and serum lipid levels associated with olestra consumption', *Arch. Intern. Med.*, **160**, 2600–4.

REYNA N. Y., CANO C., BERMUDEZ V. J. *et al.* (2003), 'Sweeteners and beta-glucans improve metabolic and anthropometrics variables in well controlled type 2 diabetic patients', *Am. J. Ther.*, **10**, 438–43.

ROE L. S. and ROLLS B. J. (2004). 'Combined effects of energy density and portion size on energy intake in women', *Am. J. Clin. Nutr.*, **79**, 962–8.

ROLLS B. J., MORRIS E. L. and ROE L. S. (2002), 'Portion size of food affects energy intake in normal-weight and overweight men and women', *Am. J. Clin. Nutr.*, **76**, 1207–13.

RUTHIG D. J., SIDER D. and MECKLING-GILL K. A. (2001), 'Health benefits of dietary fat reduction by a novel fat replacer: Mimix', *Int. J. Fd. Sci. Nutr.*, **52**, 61–9.

SALATRIM (Benefat) http://www.danisco.com/emulsifiers/productrange/benefat.asp.

SATIA-BOUTA J., KRISTAL A. R., PATTERSON R. E. *et al.* (2003), 'Is olestra consumption associated with changes in dietary intake, serum lipids, and body weight?', *Nutrition*, **19**, 754–79.

SCHWENK N. E. and GUTHRIE J. F. (1997), 'Trends in marketing and usage of fat-modified foods: implications for dietary status and nutrition promotion', *Fam. Eco. Nutr. Rev.*, **10**, 16–32.

SIGMAN-GRANT M., WARLAND R. and HSIEH G. (2003), 'Selected lower-fat foods positively impact nutrient quality in diets of free-living Americans', *J. Am. Diet. Assoc.*, **103**, 570–6.

SIMPLESSE http://www.cpkelco.com/simplesse/ Visited 02/05.

SMICIKLAS-WRIGHT H., MITCHELL D. C., MICKLE S. J. and GOLDMAN J. D. (2003), 'Cook A. Foods commonly eaten in the United States, 1989–1991 and 1994–1996: are portion sizes changing?', *J. Am. Diet. Assoc.*, **103**, 41–7.

SWANSON R. B., PERRY J. M. and CARDEN L. A. (2002), 'Acceptability of reduced-fat brownies by school-aged children', *J. Am. Diet. Assoc.*, **102**, 856–9.

SWINBURN B. and EGGER G. (2002), 'Preventive strategies against weight gain and obesity', *Obes. Rev.*, **3**, 289–301.

TOELLER M., BUYKEN A. E., HEITKAMP G., CATHELINEAU G., FERRISS B., MICHEL G. and EURODIAB IDDM complications study group (2001), 'Nutrient intakes as predictors of body weight in European people with type 1 diabetes', *Int. J. Obes. Relat. Metab. Disord.*, **25**, 1815–22.

WESTSTRATE J. A., VAN HET HOF K. H., VAN DEN BERG H. *et al.* (1998), 'A comparison of the effect of free access to reduced fat products or their full fat equivalents on food intake, body weight, blood lipids and fat-soluble antioxidants levels and haemostasis variables', *Eur. J. Clin. Nutr.*, **52**, 389–95.

WHO, WORLD HEALTH ORGANIZATION CONSULTATION ON OBESITY (1998), *Obesity: Preventing and Managing the Global Epidemic*, World Health Organization: Geneva.

YOUNG L. R. and NESTLE M. (2003), 'Expanding portion sizes in the US marketplace: Implications for nutrition counseling', *J. Am. Diet. Assoc.*, **103**, 231–4.

ZEMEL M. (2004), 'Calcium and weight', IFT Annual Meeting, Las Vegas.

Z-TRIM http://www.ars.usda.gov/is/pr/1996/z-trim896.htm. Visited 02/05.

15

Intense sweeteners and sugar replacers in the regulation of food intake and body weight

R. Abou Samra and G. Harvey Anderson, University of Toronto, Canada

15.1 Introduction

The role of non-caloric (intense) compared with caloric sweeteners in influencing appetite and food intake has received considerable attention over the past 60 years, but to date there has been little agreement on their impact on food intake and body weight. Intense sweeteners provide sweetness without calories and have been used primarily in beverages or as tabletop sweeteners. However, this role is broadening with the availability of heat stable intense sweeteners like sucralose. Sucrose and other sugars, particularly high-fructose corn syrups, have been the primary caloric sweetener. However, in recent years a new group of caloric sweeteners, identified as sugar replacers, has emerged. Sugar replacers are carbohydrates but are not sugars. They have bulk and texture similar to sugars, but have fewer calories. Because sugar replacers are less sweet than sucrose, high intensity sweeteners are often added to them in food preparations.

It is perhaps not surprising that it has been difficult to derive a definitive understanding of the role of sweeteners on the regulation of food intake and body weight. Sweetness alone is a factor influencing food choice and intake but the energy consumed from the diet or food is also subject to regulation by physiological mechanisms that strive to maintain body weight. Despite numerous experimental studies of the role of sugars and high-intensity sweeteners in weight control, it cannot be concluded that they have contributed to either the prevention of body weight gain or to the achievement of weight loss goals. There is some evidence, however, that they influence dietary intake patterns. Replacing the carbohydrate content of the diet contributed to by sugars with high intensity sweeteners contributes to net increases in fat and protein intakes and a partial decrease in carbohydrate intake (Beaton *et al.*, 1992), which might increase energy intake and body weight over the long term (Lissner *et al.*, 1987; Saris *et al.*, 2000). Sugar replacers have received little investigation.

This review has two objectives. First is to examine the effect of replacing sweetness from sugars with that from high-intensity sweeteners or from sugar replacers on intake regulation and body weight. A second objective is to provide suggestions for approaches that might lead to a better understanding of the effect of sweeteners on food intake and body weight.

15.2 Intense sweeteners, sugar replacers and weight control

Major sources of high intensity sweeteners are beverages and tabletop powder (Toledo and Ioshi, 1995; Leclercq *et al.*, 1999). Currently in the United States five have been approved (Table 15.1) (2004c). The first intense sweeteners, primarily saccharin or sodium cyclamate, were marketed to people who, for medical reasons, were advised to follow dietary restrictions. Initially, the goal of providing sweetness without calories from sugars was motivated by the mistaken view that sucrose was unsuitable for consumption by individuals with diabetes. Thus it was thought that sweeteners providing sweetness without calories would help diabetics reduce carbohydrate intake, achieve better control of blood glucose and body weight and have a more varied diet.

Since that time, there has been a steady and significant change in consumer perception of energy-free or energy-reduced sweeteners: they are no longer for the few, but for the majority. Increased health consciousness has brought a strong demand for a wide variety of good tasting, light foods and beverages. Nine in 10 consumers in the USA use sweeteners other than sugars (Bright, 1999). In European countries, as well as in developing countries, demand for reduced energy sweeteners has increased due to the growing interest in health, an ageing population and in recognition of their role in making limited diets more palatable (Bright, 1999).

Although people with diabetes generally consume less sugars than other groups in the population (Duffy and Anderson, 1998; Renwick, 1999; Butchko and Stargel, 2001), this may change. In the past 10 years, guidelines for the dietary treatment of diabetes have changed from avoiding 'simple' sugars to monitoring the total amount of carbohydrate consumed (1994). In the current recommendations, sugars are acceptable as a carbohydrate in the diet of those with diabetes (2003; Franz *et al.*, 2003). This change in dietary guidance has come about because of the recognition that caloric sweeteners increase blood glucose less than many commonly consumed foods such as bread and potatoes. Thus avoidance of sugars is not the solution to glycemic control for those who have insulin resistance or diabetes.

Table 15.1 High-intensity sweeteners

Type	Energy value (kcal/g)	Sweetness (compared with sucrose)
Saccharin	0	200–700×
Aspartame	4[a]	160–220×
Acesulfame-K	0	200×
Sucralose	0	600×
Neotame	0	8000×

[a] This sweetener does provide energy; however, because of the intense sweetness, the amount of energy derived from it is negligible.

15.2.1 Sweeteners and their role in managing obesity

The prevalence of obesity is increasing and it is a significant public health problem in many countries (James *et al.*, 2001). Technologically, the use of intense sweeteners to develop 'diet' beverages has been a success. However, the growing epidemic of obesity does little to support the effectiveness of calorie-reduced or -free sweeteners in the prevention of obesity.

The food supply offers consumers a wide range of choice in sweet foods and beverages. One distinguishing characteristic among sweeteners is the energy that they provide. Nutritive or caloric sugar replacers provide a sweet taste and a source of energy; non-nutritive sugar replacers are sweet without energy.

15.3 Caloric sugar replacers: sugar alcohols

Products sweetened with sugar alcohols (also known as polyols) are appearing on the market more frequently and are promoted for weight management because they have the potential to reduce the energy content contributed by sugars in confectionery and other foods. Sugar alcohols are chemically defined as saccharide derivatives in which a ketone or aldehyde group is replaced by a hydroxyl group (Zumbe *et al.*, 2001). They are classified according to the number of saccharide units present in the molecule (see Table 15.2). They are naturally present in small amounts in some fruits and vegetables and are commercially produced by hydrogenation of mono-, di- or polysaccharides (Dills, 1989). Sugar alcohols have been considered an ideal substitute for sugar because they possess similar physical and chemical properties but less energy than sugar. Most sugar alcohols have an energy content 1.0 to 2.5 kcal/g less than sucrose or other carbohydrates because they are absorbed slowly and incompletely from the intestine leading to fermentative degradation by intestinal flora. However, intakes >10 to 20 g/day of certain sugar alcohols may cause flatulence, diarrhea, and other gastrointestinal symptoms. Since tolerance for sugar alco-

Table 15.2 Sugar alcohols

Type	Energy value (kcal/g)	Description
Monosaccharide polyols:		
Sorbitol	2.6	50–70% as sweet as sucrose; 50–80% absorbed from the human small intestine
Mannitol	1.6	50–70% as sweet as sucrose; 50% absorbed from the human small intestine
Xylitol	2.4	As sweet as sucrose; 50% absorbed from the human small intestine
Erythritol	0.2	60–80% as sweet as sucrose
D-Tagatose	1.5	75–92% as sweet as sucrose
Disaccharide polyols:		
Isomalt	2	45–65% as sweet as sucrose; 50–60% absorbed from the small intestine
Lactitol	2	30–40% as sweet as sucrose; 0% absorbed from the small intestine
Maltitol	2.1	90% as sweet as sucrose; ≈50–75% absorbed from the small intestine
Trehalose	4	45% as sweet as sucrose
Polysaccharide polyols:		
HSH[a]	3	25–50% as sweet as sucrose

[a] hydrogenated starch hydrolysate.

hols may be limited by their laxative effects, their impact on overall energy balance has been judged to be small, at most, approximately 20–40 kcal/day (Wolever *et al.*, 2002).

Until recently, the use of sugar alcohols in manufactured foods was limited mainly to their presence in small amounts in candy and chewing gum, foods that also have few calories. However, high-calorie products sweetened with sugar alcohols and labeled as 'low carbohydrate' or 'carbohydrate free' such as chocolates, cookies, ice cream, breakfast cereals and breads have come onto the market (2004e).

15.3.1 Sugar alcohols and weight control

The effect of foods sweetened with sugar alcohols on food intake and satiety has received little examination. Ingestion of 25 g of xylitol or lactitol in place of 25 g of glucose did not lead to a change in thermogenesis and net energy balance (Natah *et al.*, 1997). Because many sugar alcohol-sweetened foods are high in fat, are energy dense and are labeled 'sugar-free' in the USA (2004a), it is possible that their use will alter the composition or nutritional adequacy of the diet and lead to excess energy intake (Wolever *et al.*, 2002). For example, subjects not informed about the composition of yogurt consumed less energy while eating low-fat yogurt than when given regular yogurt (Shide and Rolls, 1995). Conversely, when they were given products that were identified as regular or low in fat, they consumed more energy on the day they were given the low-fat yogurt. Excessive energy intake in any form relative to expenditure leads to weight gain, and ingestion of energy-dense foods, whether high in fat or carbohydrate, promotes over-consumption (Stubbs *et al.*, 1996).

Further research is required to define the effects of sugar alcohols on food intake and energy balance. It has been proposed that sugar replacers have an advantage because, in addition to being somewhat lower in energy content than sugars, they have less effect on blood glucose (Natah *et al.*, 1997), and therefore reduce the glycemic load of the diet. However, there is no evidence that the glycemic index of a food and diet is related to weight control (2004b). Furthermore, it is unlikely that the small amount of sugar alcohols that can be added to the diet could have a detectable effect on energy balance because the caloric reduction achieved by their substitution for sugars is small.

It would perhaps be informative to examine the effect of sugar replacers on short-term appetite and food intake after being consumed in a beverage or food. Sugars raise blood glucose and insulin, simulate the release of gut peptide hormones involved in satiety mechanisms and suppress ghrelin, the hunger hormone, from the stomach (Woods, 2004). In short-term studies the meal size after sugars is inversely related to blood glucose (Anderson *et al.*, 2002). It might, therefore, be that sugar alcohols fail to suppress food intake in proportion to the calories that they contain, because they fail to stimulate these satiety signals. Their putative benefit might, therefore, be better evaluated by measuring physiological biomarkers of satiety than by food intake preloads. It is difficult to detect the effect of differences among preload treatments on later food intake if they differ by less than 100 kcal (Anderson and Woodend, 2003).

15.4 Non-caloric sugar replacers: high-intensity sweeteners

Intense sweeteners are many times sweeter than sucrose and deliver sweet taste with few calories (see Table 15.1). Depending on the carrier used to deliver the high intensity sweetener, the energy from adding sweetness from sugars (approximately 4 kcal/g) can be almost completely eliminated. High intensity sweeteners are mostly used in diet beverages and 'light' semi-solid foods, such as yogurts, puddings and frozen desserts.

Sweetness is a taste that is innate and is fully expressed in newborn infants. It is a property of foods that has been vigorously examined for its role in food selection and appetite control. Unfortunately, a mixture of excessive expectations of the public for simple solutions combined with research reports that often feed these expectations and are later proved to be wrong contributes to confusion about its role among consumers and public health authorities. For example, the current widespread demand among the public for high intensity sweeteners has been created by the simplistic assumption that substitution of sugars with high intensity sweeteners providing very few or no calories will prevent weight gain. Indeed, it has been suggested that, by replacing intake of added sugars with non-caloric sweeteners, a reduction of energy intake of 380 kcal/day would occur (2004c). However, this assumes that energy intake regulatory systems will not detect the deficit and will lead to increased intake of energy from other sources (Beaton *et al.*, 1992).

At the present time the role of sweetness mediated by high intensity sweeteners in the regulation of energy intake and energy balance is uncertain. Many experimental approaches have been used. Most often the studies are short term and include measuring subjective appetite or food intake after subjects consume food or beverages that are either unsweetened, or are sweetened with a non-caloric or a caloric sweetener. The results are influenced by many factors, including the form of treatment (liquid vs. solid), the amount (volume and calories), the knowledge of the subjects (that is what they are told about the treatments), the time at which subjective appetite and food intake is measured, and age and gender of the subjects. Often, both the design and the interpretation of the study results are based on physiological mechanisms of intake control, yet it is rare that physiological measures are made and associated with the food intake behavior.

Associations based on epidemiological data are often problematic because food intake usually measures the current diet and anthropometric characteristics of the individual at the time of the survey. However, body fat accumulates over a significant duration of time and present diet may not reflect the diet that led to the current body weight status.

15.4.1 High-intensity sweeteners and short-term appetite and food intake

A considerable increase in research on the effect of sweetness and caloric substitution came about with the introduction of aspartame to the food supply and its wide spread use in beverages and as a table-top sweetener. A thorough review of studies reported to 1991 was published by Rolls (1991) and led to the conclusion that aspartame has not been found to increase food intake and that the consumption of aspartame sweetened foods or drinks is associated with either no change or a reduction in food intake. It was also concluded that data from long-term studies are very limited. The addition of new and the more widespread uses of high intensity sweeteners and now sugar replacers provides additional motivation to determine their impact on food intake and body weight, but to date the conclusion put forth by Rolls seems equally sound. The following is therefore not a comprehensive summary of all publications, but is aimed at informing the reader of the issues that have been raised.

The notion that high intensity sweeteners would increase appetite and food intake arose in the 1980s. The appealing rationale was that high intensity sweeteners increase appetite through cephalic stimulation (e.g. the taste, smell and sight of food) (Blundell and Hill, 1986; Rogers and Blundell, 1989; Tordoff and Alleva, 1990b). Conversely, it has been proposed that intense sweeteners have post-ingestive consequences that can lead to stimulation of physiologic systems that either suppress (Black *et al.*, 1993) or increase (Rogers and Blundell, 1989) energy intake and subsequent eating occasions.

Intense sweeteners in beverages and intake control

Blundell and Hill (Blundell and Hill, 1986) originally popularized the notion that sweetness and therefore aspartame-sweetened beverages led to an increase in subjective appetite and possibly food intake (Rogers *et al.*, 1988). They rationalized that, because sweetness is most often associated with calories, it would be expected to lead to subtle changes in metabolism aimed at preparing the body for incoming calories. But, when these calories are not forthcoming, the person experiences an increase in appetite. Many attempts to replicate the report of Blundell and Hill (Blundell and Hill, 1986) have failed (Rolls, 1991), except in one study where 340 mg of aspartame was added to water at twice the normal concentration found in familiar beverages, creating a very sweet drink (Black *et al.*, 1993). An increase in appetite compared to an unsweetened control was reported that lasted for 20–30 min (see Fig. 15.1). However, the aspartame drink had no impact on energy intake or on food selection measured 60 min later.

When studies have used a familiar drink (Canty and Chan, 1991; Black *et al.*, 1991a,b; Rolls, 1991; Holt *et al.*, 2000) they have been unable to detect an effect of aspartame on appetite. The effect of aspartame-sweetened diet soft drinks on short-term subjective appetite and food intake of young adult males is similar to that of carbonated mineral water and is associated with volume, not sweetness (Black *et al.*, 1991a,b). Compared with 280 ml, 560 ml of a diet soda decreased appetite more for the next 30–45 min, but there were no effects on food intake at the meal 60 min later. Furthermore, the suppression in appetite that was observed after the consumption of 560 ml of a diet soda (containing 340 mg aspartame) was not due to the aspartame content of the drink but was due to the volume, because 560 ml of carbonated mineral water suppressed appetite to the same extent and for the same duration (Black *et al.*, 1993).

Because the subjective appeal of most foods decrease following ingestion of aspartame drinks (Black *et al.*, 1993), sweetness alone in beverages

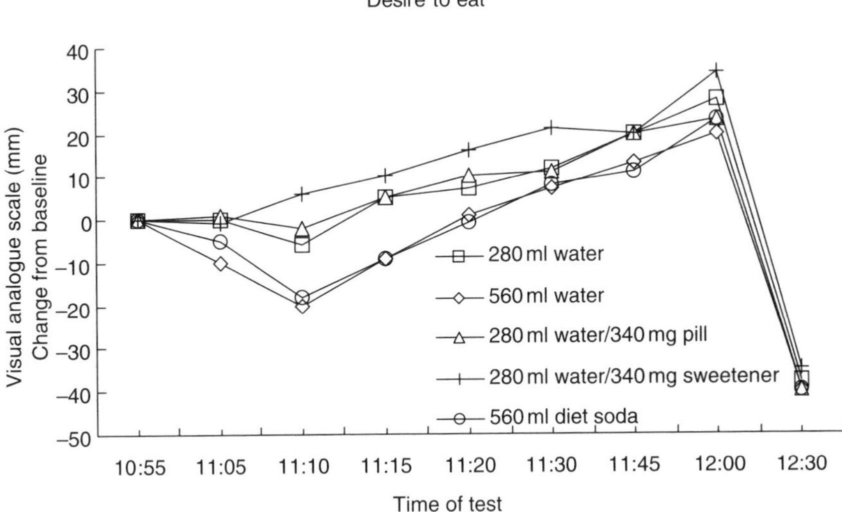

Fig. 15.1 Subjective measures of Desire to Eat for subjects following consumption of preloads as indicated. Note that consuming 340 mg of aspartame as a sweetener in mineral water increases subjective appetite, while consuming the same amount in two gelatin capsules (labeled 'pill' in figure) does not. Also 560 ml of mineral water reduces subjective appetite to the same extent as 560 ml of aspartame sweetener diet soda.

is more likely to suppress than to stimulate food intake. Indeed, several studies indicate that sweetness without calories in drinks suppresses appetite and food intake in both adults (Rodin, 1990; Canty and Chan, 1991; Anderson and Woodend, 2003) and children (Birch *et al.*, 1989). In the studies reported by Woodend and Anderson (Anderson and Woodend, 2003), the effect on food intake 1 hour later was similar among sweet drinks containing either a non-caloric sweetener (sucralose) or containing 25 g and 50 g of sucrose. However, compared with the unsweetened water control, food intake was lower after the sucrose drinks. Similarly, an earlier report found that non-caloric drinks sweetened with either aspartame or saccharin reduced hunger ratings to an amount intermediate between the equally sweet sucrose (20 g) drink and the water control (Canty and Chan, 1991). Although food intake 60 min later was not different among the treatments, it may have been if measured earlier at the times that appetite was suppressed. Young children respond to sweetness by decreasing food intake. Two to 5-year-old children reduced their food intake up to 60 min after consuming an aspartame-sweetened beverage compared to the effects of a water control, but not as much as when they consumed sweetened energy-containing (200 kcal) drinks (Birch *et al.*, 1989).

At the same time that sweetness from aspartame in beverages was proposed to increase food intake, the same group (Rogers *et al.*, 1990, 1991) reported that ingesting aspartame in the usual amounts in familiar soft-drinks, but without taste (in a gelatin capsule), led to a decrease in appetite and food intake, but once again their results could not be reproduced by others (Black *et al.*, 1993). They suggested that the decrease might be due to the post-ingestive effects of the phenylalanine component of aspartame; but they were unable to show an effect of phenylalanine alone when given in the amount found in aspartame (200 mg) (Rogers *et al.*, 1991). In contrast, adults who consumed much larger quantities, that is 5 or 10 g of aspartame, compared to an equivalent quantity of alanine, showed no statistically significant decrease in appetite or food intake (Ryan-Harshman *et al.*, 1987). Rogers and Blundell (Rogers and Blundell, 1994) subjected the same data to re-analysis by applying retrospective statistics and by pooling data from two separate experiments and concluded that the results supported their view that aspartame and phenylalanine decreased food intake. Unfortunately, their re-analysis did not capture the physiological mechanisms of intake regulation that provided the underpinnings for the design of the original study by Ryan-Harshman *et al.* (1987). The original study used equal weight nitrogen loads with alanine as the control for the phenylalanine and aspartame treatments. This was done in order to determine if taking a large quantity of phenylalanine or aspartame in pill form suppressed food intake through the food intake regulatory mechanisms associated with phenylalanine (Ryan-Harshman *et al.*, 1987). Phenylalanine when given in large amounts to monkeys (500 mg/kg) (Gibbs *et al.*, 1976) suppressed food intake in association with an increase in plasma cholecystokinin (CCK), a known satiety hormone (Woods, 2004). Phenylalanine is also a precursor for tyrosine and catecholamine synthesis in the brain, and catecholamines are regulators of food intake (Anderson *et al.*, 1988). Alanine was selected as the placebo for three reasons. First, carbohydrate would not be appropriate because even 10 g would raise blood glucose and insulin. Second, no intake regulatory mechanism has been associated with its ingestion, and third, it provided similar amounts of nitrogen and energy to the aspartame and phenylalanine test treatments. The results of the original study showed clearly that alanine, phenylalanine and aspartame when given in amounts of either 5 or 10 g (about 75 and 150 mg/kg, respectively) resulted in the same food intake from a buffet lunch 1 hour later. Although CCK was not measured, plasma amino acid concentrations were over ten times higher after the phenylalanine treatment than after the alanine control, suggesting that a central effect of phenylalanine on catecholaminergic regulation of food intake response did not occur. Therefore, it can be concluded that there is neither a physiological rationale nor experimental data supporting the hypothesis that aspartame has unique effects on intake regulatory mechanisms or on food intake when consumed in either large amounts or in amounts contained in familiar foods and beverages.

The situation described in the above shows that not only study design elements are key to the outcomes of studies, but also that the perspective of the investigator is more likely geared to the interpretation of results within the context of his or her expertise and familiar concepts. In future investigations, it might be more enlightening if physiological and behavioral scientists undertook joint studies, and biomarkers of intake regulation were measured to associate these with hypothesized mechanisms and intake behavior. Co-operation in research designs would be a more useful application of energy and intellect rather than wasting it on acrimonious debate such as that arising (Rogers and Blundell, 1993) after the review by Rolls (Rolls, 1991).

Intense sweeteners and solid or semi-solid foods in intake control

Adding high intensity sweeteners to solid and semi-solid foods have also produced mixed results with both increased (Rogers and Blundell, 1989) and decreased (Mattes, 1990) energy intake reported, suggesting that, at best, the results are reproducible and applicable only to the specific situation described by the experiment. Again, the results are highly dependent on the choice of subjects (age, gender), time of measurements, the physical characteristics of the foods used, their volume and the caloric difference between the treatments. Certain studies compare the effects of adding high intensity sweeteners to foods with the unsweetened food and others make the comparison with a similar food to which a caloric sweetener has been added.

The same investigators reporting sweetness in beverages increases appetite have provided evidence that sweetness added to semi-solid food increases later food intake. For example, saccharin-sweetened yogurt fed to young men and women was reported to stimulate appetite and lead to greater cumulative (preload plus meals) food intake at lunch 1 hour later and throughout the remainder of the day, when compared to unsweetened equicaloric yogurt (Rogers and Blundell, 1989). Similarly, when 50 g glucose and maltodextrin were added to the unsweetened yogurt, the sweet (glucose) yogurt resulted in greater cumulative food intake than after the maltodextrin containing yogurt, suggesting that the consequence of sweetness lasts throughout the day and is independent of source. It is curious that, in this study, saccharin is proposed to have post-ingestional effects beyond its sweetness to account for its continued stimulation of food intake over the rest of the day but the similar effect of glucose was ignored. Again, this type of study would be improved by physiological measures to support the hypothesized mechanisms.

In contrast, an increase in intake due to sweetness was not found in a number of studies. In a comparison of the effects of equicaloric breakfasts based on cereals either unsweetened or sweetened with aspartame or sucrose, subsequent food intakes at lunch, dinner or snacks were not affected by sweetness (Mattes, 1990). Another breakfast study also found that it was the energy value (300 vs. 700 kcal) of the breakfast and not the presence of sweetness, whether from aspartame or sucrose, that determined later food intake of normal weight non-dieting men and women (Drewnowski *et al.*, 1994a,b). In this study, the yogurt-like creamy white cheese treatments were plain, sweetened with aspartame or with sucrose, or sweetened with aspartame and supplemented with maltodextrin. Complete energy compensation was also observed in a longer-term residential study, conducted with six normal-weight, non-dieting males (Foltin *et al.*, 1990). The carbohydrate content of lunch was reduced by 400 kcal, mostly by substituting aspartame for sugar. When subjects were informed about which sweetener was in the lunch, they made up for the energy deficit by dinner-time on every day of the experiment by consuming additional foods rather than increased amount of the modified food. On the other hand, if food volume is maintained, intense sweeteners replacing sucrose might reduce energy intake, thereby aiding weight loss. Normal-weight men and women given low- or high-calorie versions of a pudding or gelatin dessert in the same volume consumed similar amounts of food at a buffet lunch presented 2 h later (Rolls *et al.*, 1989). Similarly, while food intake after an aspartame-sweetened drink was not found to be different from water alone, the aspartame-sweetened water drink resulted in lower cumulative caloric consumption (the sum of the calories in the drink and those consumed at the test meal) compared to the glucose-containing preload beverage (Rodin, 1990).

Taken together, these studies suggest that caloric content and volume of the test meals are factors exerting stronger effects than sweetness on later food intake and possibly energy balance. However, this remains to be determined. It might be informative if some of the new intense sweeteners such as sucralose, which as yet has no physiological link other than its sweetness to intake regulation (Mezitis *et al.*, 1996), was utilized and more comparisons made among sweeteners in future studies.

15.4.2 High-intensity sweeteners and weight control

The worldwide increase in the prevalence of obesity has been associated with increased caloric sweetener availability and the assumption has been made that a reduction is in order (1998). It seems unlikely, however, that intense sweeteners and sugar replacers are the solution; because in countries where obesity and overweight are characteristic of over 50% of the population, the use of intense sweeteners has also increased many-fold in 30 years. In the USA diet soft drinks have accounted for 25% of total soft drinks available for consumption over the past 15 years (2004d), but this has not slowed the continued rise in obesity. As pointed out in two recent reviews, data from epidemiological studies and from short-term intervention trials are insufficient to lead to the conclusion that replacing added sugars with intense sweeteners in the diet is beneficial to body weight control (St-Onge and Heymsfield, 2003; Vermunt *et al.*, 2003).

It is very difficult to determine cause and effect in the associations found between sweetener consumption and body weight. Epidemiological studies have associated self-reported high intensity sweetener consumption with weight gain in women (Colditz *et al.*, 1990), and high intensity sweetened soft drinks with obesity in children (Giammattei *et al.*, 2003). In a prospective cohort study, a positive association was found between increased use of saccharin and body-weight both at the start of the study and after a 4-year follow-up (Parker *et al.*, 1997). On the other hand, in a cross-sectional study with 2450 Spanish men and women, intake of cyclamate, a high intensity sweetener, was negatively correlated with BMI (Serra-Majem *et al.*, 1996). Because increased body fat accrues over an extended duration of time, and food records measure present diet, it is impossible to make any conclusions from epidemiological studies. It is possible that, at the time of the survey, subjects who are concerned about their body weight have already switched to low-energy sweeteners to prevent further weight gain (Colditz *et al.*, 1990).

A number of intervention trials have investigated the effects of replacing sugars with intense sweeteners on body-weight. Most are of a very short duration, making it difficult to detect reliable changes in body weight. However, one recent study was conducted for a duration of 10 weeks and provided some indication of a benefit to consuming high intensity sweetened foods and beverages rather than their energy-containing equivalents (Raben *et al.*, 2002). Overweight male and female subjects were asked to consume a minimum amount of sucrose sweetened or artificially sweetened foods and beverages each day. The artificial sweeteners included aspartame, acesulfame K, sucralose and saccharin. In the sucrose group 70% of sucrose came from beverages and 30% from solid foods. About 80% of the artificial sweeteners were in beverages and 20% in solid food. Beverages were soft drinks or flavored fruit juices and foods were yogurt, marmalade, ice cream and stewed fruits (Raben *et al.*, 2002). The amount provided by these foods and drinks was equalized on a weight basis. The group consuming sweetened food and beverages gained an average of 1.6 kg, while those consuming the artificially sweetened foods lost 1.0 kg. Their energy intake at week 10 was 28% lower than those on the sucrose diet. The high intensity sweetener-supplemented group already had a lower sucrose intake prior to the start of the study and daily energy intakes decreased by approximately 105 kcal, an amount that would produce a 0.9 kg weight loss over a 10-week period. The differences observed between the sucrose-supplemented group and the high intensity sweetener-supplemented group was due to the fact that subjects consuming the sucrose-containing supplements did not decrease their carbohydrate intakes to compensate for the added calories provided by the supplements; thus resulting in significant increases in carbohydrate consumption. On the other hand, subjects in the high intensity sweetener-supplemented group did not modify their carbohydrate consumption but consumed significantly higher amounts of fat and protein as a percentage of energy as predicted by Beaton *et al.* (1992). Because protein suppresses appetite more than carbohydrate (Anderson and Moore, 2004), the increase in food intake may have been due to the increase in carbohydrate and decrease in protein intake but not due to sugar *per se*. Furthermore, in considering the results, however, it is important to note that subjects who consumed the sucrose-sweetened products consumed 28% of their energy as sucrose. This amount was nearly three times their baseline intakes and approximately twice the average intake of added sugars in the US population and therefore may not be relevant to their usual diets and their relationship to obesity.

The ecological validity of this study is also in doubt because it does little to elucidate whether obese persons consuming their usual diet will benefit from switching from sugar-based foods and beverages to reduced energy sweetened foods. In order to bring about the differences observed, the sucrose group was on a very high added sugar diet and were required to consume the equivalent in fluid of three to four 360 ml soft drinks per day. Furthermore, it does little to answer the role of sucrose or sweetness *per se* in the weight gain. What would have been the outcome if the beverages and foods contained a carbohydrate source other than sucrose, but with and without an added high intensity sweetener? Sweetness alone does not lead to overeating as has been proposed, and these results cannot be used to suggest that sucrose is different from any other sweetened carbohydrate.

Another short-term 3-week study showed similar results. Substituting aspartame-containing beverages for high-fructose corn syrup beverages decreased caloric intake in men and women and led to significant reduction in body weight in men (Tordoff and Alleva, 1990a) but again the subjects were required to consume large amounts of beverages compared with their usual intakes. In this study they supplemented their regular diets with either four 300-ml bottles of soda sweetened with aspartame (i.e. diet soda), four 300-ml bottles of soda sweetened with high fructose corn syrup (i.e. regular soda), or no soda for 3 weeks, with each treatment being administered in random order. Energy intakes during both soda periods were equally decreased (i.e. excluding the soda calories) relative to during the no soda period. Because regular soda provided an energy source, however, these results show that compensation did not occur during regular soda consumption compared with diet soda consumption.

Another approach to studying the effect of replacing energy from sugar with high intensity sweeteners is shown in the studies by Porikos and colleagues (Porikos *et al.*, 1977, 1982; Porikos and Pi-Sunyer, 1984). Energy intakes of volunteer subjects were measured before, during, and after the covert substitution of aspartame for sugar, which made up 25% of the total dietary calories. However, several alternative explanations for the reduced energy intake during the aspartame phase have been proposed (Porikos *et al.*, 1977, 1982; Porikos and Pi-Sunyer, 1984). First, in these studies the subjects were gaining weight during the baseline period on sugar. When aspartame was used in the diet, the reduction in caloric intake stabilized weight but did not result in weight loss. When sugar was re-introduced, once again weight began to increase. This observation suggests that the subjects were probably overeating during baseline, possibly because of the wide array of food presented to them on an *ad libitum* basis, and that the caloric dilution may have reduced intake by making it difficult (if not impossible) to consume sufficient bulk to maintain the previously elevated intake. Second, all subjects experienced a sugar/aspartame/sugar rotation in the diet, and so there is no data on subjects exposed to an aspartame/sugar/aspartame rotation. This makes it difficult to distinguish between the impact of familiarity with the diet and the role of the sweetener in the diet. For example, it could be argued that there was significant over-consumption, even hyperphagia, during the first 3 to 6 days of the study (the duration of the initial sugar period) due to the novelty of the diet. What might the intake have been if aspartame were used as the sweetener during the first 6 days? Might intake have been elevated during this time?

Many studies report that replacing the caloric sweeteners in a diet with a non-caloric sweetener results in little if any change in energy intake and body weight (Van Itallie *et al.*, 1988; Mattes, 1990; Mattes *et al.*, 1988; Gatenby *et al.*, 1997). Subjects consumed a larger volume of food when the caloric density is reduced and so maintained energy intake (Foltin *et al.*, 1988, 1990).

Non-caloric sweetener may, however, play a role in facilitating compliance to a weight maintenance programme even though they do not assist in weight loss, but at present this association is based on only one study. Groups of obese men and women on an energy-restricted diet for 12 weeks (Kanders *et al.*, 1988), either required to or prohibited from use of aspartame-sweetened products, had a similar weight loss. Similarly, a later clinical trial of obese women showed weight loss to be similar on weight-reducing diets containing sucrose or aspartame, but found that women who were assigned to the aspartame-containing diet maintained better weight loss over the 3 years than women who were assigned to the high-sucrose diet (Blackburn *et al.*, 1997).

15.5 Implications and recommendations

After 30 years of intensive research to identify the role of sweeteners in the etiology of obesity, we remain unable to provide consistent and useful advice to the industry, public health authorities, regulators and consumers. One wonders if we are asking the wrong questions. In a recent editorial Jenkins *et al.* ask the question 'Too much sugar, too much carbohydrate or just too much?' (Jenkins *et al.*, 2004). Although their discussion is aimed at carbohydrates, it applies more broadly and suggests that attempts to solve the obesity conundrum by sweeteners alone is an attempt at micromanaging a complex problem.

In a food environment that is plentiful, varied and increasing in its appeal (Briefel and Johnson, 2004), is it realistic to believe that by replacing sugars with high intensity sweeteners in our foods and diets we will prevent obesity? The majority of high intensity sweeteners have been around in beverages for many years and as a result may just replace water or other non-caloric beverages. Will new sweeteners that are heat stable and low in energy help? Perhaps we can fool people by reducing energy density of foods, but such foods are already available and people are free to choose what they want to eat. They simply eat too much and we do not know why, although a plethora of explanations have been offered.

High intensity sweeteners and sugar replacers in foods and beverages cannot replace the consumers' responsibility for moderation and wise food selection. However, they can provide palatable alternatives to caloric sweeteners and give consumers choice. It seems unlikely that this will do much to stem the obesity tide unless the individual consumer understands the concept of too much food and too little exercise in determining energy balance.

In order to stop the current trends in obesity, a great deal more research should be directed to understanding the etiology and to terminating the continued rise in overweight and obesity in children. Almost all of the published research on intake regulation has been conducted in adults who are a product of their health behavior and food-based experiences over many years. Children need to be empowered to have better health behaviors than their parents but we have little understanding of how children learn healthy behaviors around food and exercise. The school and public health systems should be more involved in the formation of positive health behaviors in children and in helping parents understand the adverse effects of obesity in childhood and what to do to prevent it. Academics, the food industry and government should be co-operating in stopping childhood obesity, or as has been recently predicted, this may be the first time in history that children will not live as long as their parents (Olshansky *et al.*, 2005).

Finally, as with the many areas of nutrition research that do not produce unequivocal results, it would be of value to both industry and public health and regulatory authorities to have consensus and to communicate consistent messages. However, they must also contribute to consensus and advancement of the research by encouraging and supporting the application of evidence-based decision-making processes to areas of controversy (Anderson *et al.*, 2003).

15.6 References

(1994), 'Nutrition recommendations and principles for people with diabetes mellitus', *J. Am. Diet. Assoc.*, **94**, 504–6.

(1998), In *Report of a WHO consultation on Obesity* Geneva.
(2003), 'Clinical Practice Guidelines for the Prevention and Management of Diabetes in Canada', *Canadian Journal of Diabetes*, **27** (suppl 2), S27–31.
(2004a), United States Food and Drug Administration, Center for Food Safety and Applied Nutrition, Maryland.
(2004b), American Dietetics Association.
(2004c), 'Position of the American Dietetic Association: use of nutritive and non-nutritive sweeteners', *J. Am. Diet. Assoc.*, **104**, 255–75.
(2004d), United States Department of Agriculture – Economic Research Service.
(2004e), International Food Information Council, Washington DC.
ANDERSON, G. H. and MOORE, S. E. (2004), 'Dietary proteins in the regulation of food intake and body weight in humans', *J. Nutr.*, **134**, 974S–9S.
ANDERSON, G. H. and WOODEND, D. (2003), 'Consumption of sugars and the regulation of short-term satiety and food intake', *Am. J. Clin. Nutr.*, **78**, 843S–9S.
ANDERSON, G. H., BIALIK, R. J. and LI, E. T. S. (1988), In *NATO Workshops on Amino Acids Availability and Brain Functions in Health and Disease* (Ed, Heuther, G.) Max-Planck-Institute, Gottingen, FRG.
ANDERSON, G. H., CATHERINE, N. L. WOODEND, D. M. and WOLEVER, T. M. (2002), 'Inverse association between the effect of carbohydrates on blood glucose and subsequent short-term food intake in young men', *Am. J. Clin. Nutr.*, **76**, 1023–30.
ANDERSON, G. H., BLACK, R. M. and HARRIS, S. (2003), 'Preface: Dietary Guidelines: Past Experience and New Approaches', *J. Am. Diet. Assoc.*, **103** (Suppl 2), S3–7.
BEATON, G. H., TARASUK, V. and ANDERSON, G. H. (1992), 'Estimation of possible impact of non-caloric fat and carbohydrate substitutes on macronutrient intake in the human', *Appetite*, **19**, 87–103.
BIRCH, L. L., MCPHEE, L. and SULLIVAN, S. (1989), 'Children's food intake following drinks sweetened with sucrose or aspartame: time course effects', *Physiol. Behav.*, **45**, 387–95.
BLACK, R. M., LEITER, L. A. and ANDERSON, G. H. (1993), 'Consuming aspartame with and without taste: differential effects on appetite and food intake of young adult males', *Physiol. Behav.*, **53**, 459–66.
BLACKBURN, G. L., KANDERS, B. S., LAVIN, P. T., KELLER, S. D. and WHATLEY, J. (1997), 'The effect of aspartame as part of a multidisciplinary weight-control programme on short- and long-term control of body weight', *Am. J. Clin. Nutr.*, **65**, 409–18.
BLUNDELL, J. E. and HILL, A. J. (1986), 'Paradoxical effects of an intense sweetener (aspartame) on appetite', *Lancet*, **1**, 1092–3.
BRIEFEL, R. R. and JOHNSON, C. L. (2004), 'Secular trends in dietary intake in the United States', *Annu. Rev. Nutr.*, **24**, 401–31.
BRIGHT, G. (1999), In *Low-calorie Sweeteners: Present and Future*, Vol. 85 (Ed, A. Corti) S. Karger AG, Basel, Switzerland, pp. 3–8.
BUTCHKO, H. H. and STARGEL, W. W. (2001), 'Aspartame: scientific evaluation in the postmarketing period', *Regul. Toxicol. Pharmacol.*, **34**, 221–33.
CANTY, D. J. and CHAN, M. M. (1991), 'Effects of consumption of caloric vs. noncaloric sweet drinks on indices of hunger and food consumption in normal adults', *Am. J. Clin. Nutr.*, **53**, 1159–64.
COLDITZ, G. A., WILLETT, W. C., STAMPFER, M. J., LONDON, S. J., SEGAL, M. R. and SPEIZER, F. E. (1990), 'Patterns of weight change and their relation to diet in a cohort of healthy women', *Am. J. Clin. Nutr.*, **51**, 1100–5.
DILLS, W. L. JR. (1989), 'Sugar alcohols as bulk sweeteners', *Annu. Rev. Nutr.*, **9**, 161–86.
DREWNOWSKI, A., MASSIEN, C., LOUIS-SYLVESTRE, J., FRICKER, J., CHAPELOT, D. and APFELBAUM, M. (1994a), 'Comparing the effects of aspartame and sucrose on motivational ratings, taste preferences, and energy intakes in humans', *Am. J. Clin. Nutr.*, **59**, 338–45.

DREWNOWSKI, A., MASSIEN, C., LOUIS-SYLVESTRE, J., FRICKER, J., CHAPELOT, D. and APFELBAUM, M. (1994b), 'The effects of aspartame versus sucrose on motivational ratings, taste preferences, and energy intakes in obese and lean women', *Int. J. Obes. Relat. Metab. Disord.*, **18**, 570–8.

DUFFY, V. B. and ANDERSON, G. H. (1998), 'Position of the American Dietetic Association: use of nutritive and nonnutritive sweeteners', *J. Am. Diet. Assoc.*, **98**, 580–7.

FOLTIN, R. W., FISCHMAN, M. W., EMURIAN, C. S. and RACHLINSKI, J. J. (1988), 'Compensation for caloric dilution in humans given unrestricted access to food in a residential laboratory', *Appetite*, **10**, 13–24.

FOLTIN, R. W., FISCHMAN, M. W., MORAN, T. H., ROLLS, B. J. and KELLY, T. H. (1990), 'Caloric compensation for lunches varying in fat and carbohydrate content by humans in a residential laboratory', *Am. J. Clin. Nutr.*, **52**, 969–80.

FRANZ, M. J., BANTLE, J. P., BEEBE, C. A. *et al.* (2003), 'Evidence-based nutrition principles and recommendations for the treatment and prevention of diabetes and related complications', *Diabetes Care*, **26**, S51–61.

GATENBY, S. J., AARON, J. I., JACK, V. A. and MELA, D. J. (1997), 'Extended use of foods modified in fat and sugar content: nutritional implications in a free-living female population', *Am. J. Clin. Nutr.*, **65**, 1867–73.

GIAMMATTEI, J., BLIX, G., MARSHAK, H. H., WOLLITZER, A. O. and PETTITT, D. J. (2003), 'Television watching and soft drink consumption: associations with obesity in 11- to 13-year-old schoolchildren', *Arch. Pediatr. Adolesc. Med.*, **157**, 882–6.

GIBBS, J., FALASCO, J. D. and MCHUGH, P. R. (1976), 'Cholecystokinin-decreased food intake in rhesus monkeys', *Am. J. Physiol.*, **230**, 15–18.

HOLT, S. H., SANDONA, N. and BRAND-MILLER, J. C. (2000), 'The effects of sugar-free vs. sugar-rich beverages on feelings of fullness and subsequent food intake', *Int. J. Food. Sci. Nutr.*, **51**, 59–71.

JAMES, P. T., LEACH, R., KALAMARA, E. and SHAYEGHI, M. (2001), 'The worldwide obesity epidemic', *Obes. Res.*, **9**, 228S–33S.

JENKINS, D. J., KENDALL, C. W., MARCHIE, A. and AUGUSTIN, L. S. (2004), 'Too much sugar, too much carbohydrate, or just too much?', *Am. J. Clin. Nutr.*, **79**, 711–2.

KANDERS, B. S., LAVIN, P. T., KOWALCHUK, M. B., GREENBERG, I. and BLACKBURN, G. L. (1988), 'An evaluation of the effect of aspartame on weight loss', *Appetite*, **11**, 73–84.

LECLERCQ, C., BERARDI, D., SORBILLO, M. R. and LAMBE, J. (1999), 'Intake of saccharin, aspartame, acesulfame K and cyclamate in Italian teenagers: present levels and projections', *Food Addit. Contam.*, **16**, 99–109.

LISSNER, L., LEVITSKY, D. A., STRUPP, B. J., KALKWARF, H. J. and ROE, D. A. (1987), 'Dietary fat and the regulation of energy intake in human subjects', *Am. J. Clin. Nutr.*, **46**, 886–92.

MATTES, R. (1990), 'Effects of aspartame and sucrose on hunger and energy intake in humans', *Physiol. Behav.*, **47**, 1037–44.

MATTES, R. D., PIERCE, C. B. and FRIEDMAN, M. I. (1988), 'Daily caloric intake of normal-weight adults: response to changes in dietary energy density of a luncheon meal', *Am. J. Clin. Nutr.*, **48**, 214–9.

MEZITIS, N. H., MAGGIO, C. A., KOCH, P., QUDDOOS, A., ALLISON, D. B. and PI-SUNYER, F. X. (1996), 'Glycemic effect of a single high oral dose of the novel sweetener sucralose in patients with diabetes', *Diabetes Care*, **19**, 1004–5.

NATAH, S. S., HUSSIEN, K. R., TUOMINEN, J. A. and KOIVISTO, V. A. (1997), 'Metabolic response to lactitol and xylitol in healthy men', *Am. J. Clin. Nutr.*, **65**, 947–50.

OLSHANSKY, S. J., PASSARO, D. J., HERSHOW, R. C. *et al.* (2005), *N. Engl. J. Med.*, **352**, 1138–45.

PARKER, D. R., GONZALEZ, S., DERBY, C. A., GANS, K. M., LASATER, T. M. and CARLETON, R. A. (1997), 'Dietary factors in relation to weight change among men and women from two southeastern New England communities', *Int. J. Obes. Relat. Metab. Disord.*, **21**, 103–9.

PORIKOS, K. P. and PI-SUNYER, F. X. (1984), 'Regulation of food intake in human obesity: studies with caloric dilution and exercise', *Clin. Endocrinol. Metab.*, **13**, 547–61.

PORIKOS, K. P., BOOTH, G. and VAN ITALLIE, T. B. (1977), 'Effect of covert nutritive dilution on the spontaneous food intake of obese individuals: a pilot study', *Am. J. Clin. Nutr.*, **30**, 1638–44.

PORIKOS, K. P., HESSER, M. F. and VAN ITALLIE, T. B. (1982), 'Caloric regulation in normal-weight men maintained on a palatable diet of conventional foods', *Physiol. Behav.*, **29**, 293–300.

RABEN, A., VASILARAS, T. H., MOLLER, A. C. and ASTRUP, A. (2002), 'Sucrose compared with artificial sweeteners: different effects on *ad libitum* food intake and body weight after 10 wk of supplementation in overweight subjects', *Am. J. Clin. Nutr.*, **76**, 721–9.

RENWICK, A. G. (1999), 'Intake of intense sweeteners', *World Rev. Nutr. Diet.*, **85**, 178–200.

RODIN, J. (1990), 'Comparative effects of fructose, aspartame, glucose, and water preloads on calorie and macronutrient intake', *Am. J. Clin. Nutr.*, **51**, 428–35.

ROGERS, P. J. and BLUNDELL, J. E. (1989), 'Separating the actions of sweetness and calories: effects of saccharin and carbohydrates on hunger and food intake in human subjects', *Physiol. Behav.*, **45**, 1093–9.

ROGERS, P. J. and BLUNDELL, J. E. (1993), 'Intense sweeteners and appetite', *Am. J. Clin. Nutr.*, **58**, 120–2.

ROGERS, P. J. and BLUNDELL, J. E. (1994), 'Reanalysis of the effects of phenylalanine, alanine, and aspartame on food intake in human subjects', *Physiol. Behav.*, **56**, 247–50.

ROGERS, P. J., CARLYLE, J. A., HILL, A. J. and BLUNDELL, J. E. (1988), 'Uncoupling sweet taste and calories: comparison of the effects of glucose and three intense sweeteners on hunger and food intake', *Physiol. Behav.*, **43**, 547–52.

ROGERS, P. J., PLEMING, H. C. and BLUNDELL, J. E. (1990), 'Aspartame ingested without tasting inhibits hunger and food intake', *Physiol. Behav.*, **47**, 1239–43.

ROGERS, P. J., KEEDWELL, P. and BLUNDELL, J. E. (1991), 'Further analysis of the short-term inhibition of food intake in humans by the dipeptide L-aspartyl-L-phenylalanine methyl ester (aspartame)', *Physiol. Behav.*, **49**, 739–43.

ROLLS, B. J. (1991), 'Effects of intense sweeteners on hunger, food intake, and body weight: a review', *Am. J. Clin. Nutr.*, **53**, 872–8.

ROLLS, B. J., LASTER, L. J. and SUMMERFELT, A. (1989), 'Hunger and food intake following consumption of low-calorie foods', *Appetite*, **13**, 115–27.

RYAN-HARSHMAN, M., LEITER, L. A. and ANDERSON, G. H. (1987), 'Phenylalanine and aspartame fail to alter feeding behavior, mood and arousal in men', *Physiol. Behav.*, **39**, 247–53.

SARIS, W. H., ASTRUP, A., PRENTICE, A. M. *et al.* (2000), 'Randomized controlled trial of changes in dietary carbohydrate/fat ratio and simple vs. complex carbohydrates on body weight and blood lipids: the CARMEN study. The Carbohydrate Ratio Management in European National diets', *Int. J. Obes. Relat. Metab. Disord.*, **24**, 1310–8.

SERRA-MAJEM, L., RIBAS, L., INGLES, C., FUENTES, M., LLOVERAS, G. and SALLERAS, L. (1996), 'Cyclamate consumption in Catalonia, Spain (1992): relationship with the body mass index', *Food Addit. Contam.*, **13**, 695–703.

SHIDE, D. J. and ROLLS, B. J. (1995), 'Information about the fat content of preloads influences energy intake in healthy women', *J. Am. Diet. Assoc.*, **95**, 993–8.

ST-ONGE, M. P. and HEYMSFIELD, S. B. (2003), 'Usefulness of artificial sweeteners for body weight control', *Nutr. Rev.*, **61**, 219–21.

STUBBS, R. J., HARBRON, C. G. and PRENTICE, A. M. (1996), 'Covert manipulation of the dietary fat to carbohydrate ratio of isoenergetically dense diets: effect on food intake in feeding men *ad libitum*', *Int. J. Obes. Relat. Metab. Disord.*, **20**, 651–60.

TOLEDO, M. C. and IOSHI, S. H. (1995), 'Potential intake of intense sweeteners in Brazil', *Food Addit. Contam.*, **12**, 799–808.

TORDOFF, M. G. and ALLEVA, A. M. (1990a), 'Effect of drinking soda sweetened with aspartame or high-fructose corn syrup on food intake and body weight', *Am. J. Clin. Nutr.*, **51**, 963–9.

TORDOFF, M. G. and ALLEVA, A. M. (1990b), 'Oral stimulation with aspartame increases hunger', *Physiol. Behav.*, **47**, 555–9.

VAN ITALLIE, T. B., YANG, M. U. and PORIKOS, K. P. (1988), 'Use of aspartame to test the "body weight set point" hypothesis', *Appetite*, **11**, 68–72.

VERMUNT, S. H., PASMAN, W. J., SCHAAFSMA, G. and KARDINAAL, A. F. (2003), 'Effects of sugar intake on body weight: a review', *Obes. Rev.*, **4**, 91–9.

WOLEVER, T., PIEKARZ, A., HOLLANDS, M. and YOUNKER, K. (2002), 'Sugar alcohols and diabetes: a review', *Can. J. Diabetes.*, **26**, 356–62.

WOODS, S. C. (2004), 'Gastrointestinal satiety signals I. An overview of gastrointestinal signals that influence food intake', *Am. J. Physiol. Gastrointest. Liver Physiol.*, **286**, G7–13.

ZUMBE, A., LEE, A. and STOREY, D. (2001), 'Polyols in confectionery: the route to sugar-free, reduced sugar and reduced calorie confectionery', *Br. J. Nutr.*, **85**, S31–45.

16

Dietary fibre and weight control

K. Ryttig, Farmaservice Ltd, Denmark

16.1 Introduction

A few perceptive individuals have, throughout history, recognised the importance of dietary fibre in the diet. Hippocrates was already aware of the effect of dietary fibre, or roughage, on the gastrointestinal tract.[1] Throughout history a few researchers have advocated the use of dietary fibre as a tool for obtaining good health, but others were directly against the use of dietary fibre, because they considered the provoked weight reduction to be a side effect in comparison to the alleviation of constipation. This weight reduction was considered a drawback.[1]

Cleave was among the first to make the important observation that many of the most common diseases in highly developed countries, e.g. overweight, hypertension and coronary diseases, were rare or absent in less developed countries.[2] He linked the high intake of refined sugar to the development of those diseases. Trowell and Burkett proposed, based upon Cleave's theory, that the so-called 'westernised disorders' were due not to the high intake of refined sugar, but to the lack of dietary fibre in the diet.[3]

The theory proposed by Trowell and Burkett has been generally accepted for many years. However, several national surveys recently have indicated a fall in dietary fibre intake.[4] Several public health agencies have consequently proposed an increase intake of dietary fibre, up to 30g of dietary fibre per day.[5]

Trowell[6] has stated that fibre-depleted foods appear to be a risk factor in the pathogenesis of overweight and possible hypertension. Despite that, treatment of overweight with high fibre food or dietary fibre supplement has, even recently, been considered with much caution or even scepticism.

In a report on obesity by the Royal College of Physicians of London[7] published in 1983, dietary fibre was mentioned in the chapter 'The management of the overweight and obese'. Dietary fibre was classified under the subsection 'Very low energy containing diets', and the authors stated that dietary fibres 'have been advocated in the treatment of overweight in adults, but there is little satisfactory evidence as yet that they have appreciable advantages in term of weight loss'. The Royal College of Physicians had previously published *Medical Aspects of Dietary Fibre*,[1] where the authors stated that, although epidemiology pointed towards a lower prevalence in societies with high intake of dietary fibre, there was little evidence that dietary fibre *per se* could prevent obesity. However, the report mentioned that slimming diets should contain some dietary fibre in order to avoid constipation, a side effect often experienced by people on low caloric diets. In *Dietary Fibre Perspectives 1*[8] it was stated in the chapter reviewing dietary fibre in obesity that 'the importance of dietary fibre with respect to obesity is still unclear as only a few studies have addressed this issue'. However, the authors indicated that soluble fibre particularly could facilitate weight reduction and prevent weight gain.

In the Fifth and Sixth International Congresses on Obesity in 1986 and 1990 a whole section was devoted to dietary fibre in the management of overweight. At the Fifth Congress it was concluded that there was some evidence that dietary fibre could facilitate weight reduction, but none concerning weight maintenance, which is much more difficult for most overweight subjects to sustain. At the Congress in 1990, the mechanisms of action of dietary fibre in the management of overweight were assessed. In the international authoritative textbook *Obesity* by Björntorp and Brodoff,[9] a chapter by Leeds was devoted to dietary fibre and obesity. The author concludes, after reviewing the different mechanism of action of dietary fibre in overweight and the evidence for efficacy, that dietary fibre does influence some of the variables related to energy intake in the short term, but what happens in the long term is uncertain. The results of the different performed trials have to be scrutinised carefully.

In a Nordic textbook,[10] the authors of the treatment chapter recommend that the amount of dietary fibre in the diet should be increased to 25 to 35 g/day, but no further assessment of the efficacy or lack of efficacy of dietary fibre was mentioned. Pasman concluded in her thesis[11] that supplementation of fibre is mainly effective in the short term studies, but the applicability for long-term studies is still under debate. Furthermore, the number of long-term studies is limited.

16.2 Defining dietary fibre

The term dietary fibre was first used by Hipsley for an agent protecting against toxaemia in pregnancy.[12] Dietary fibre is a heterogeneous mixture of substances predominantly found in the plant cell wall. Trowell first defined dietary fibre as the skeletal remnants of the plant cell that was not hydrolysed by the alimentary enzymes of man.[13] However, the plant cell wall contains other structural components that are not associated with dietary fibre. Consequently Trowell *et al.* expanded the definition to include all plant polysaccharides and lignin resistant to enzyme digestion. This physiological definition has a number of deficiencies such as indigestibility and ignores physiological properties such as influence on digestion and absorption of nutrients, both macro- and micronutrients.

Indigestibility implies that dietary fibre is not broken down by the enzymes in the upper part of the gastrointestinal tract, because this part of the human gastrointestinal tract does not contain an enzyme capable of cleaving β-1–4 bonds. Dietary fibre is, however, degraded to short fatty acids in the large bowel.[14] These short fatty acids are easily absorbed and contribute to energy metabolism.

By processing and cooking food, material such as starch and Maillard polymers are formed. It has been discussed whether such artefact products should not be incorporated into the dietary fibre definition, because this product possesses some of the properties of dietary fibre. For a further discussion concerning definition of dietary fibre and added fibre see Dietary Reference Intake, Standing Committee on the scientific evaluation of dietary reference intake, Food and Nutrition Board 2001.[15] A chemical definition of dietary fibre was consequently proposed to encompass the plant non-starch polysaccharides. Dietary fibre plus associated substances such as waxes, cutins, cell-wall bound protein, cell-wall bound minerals and other cell-wall bound material have been named dietary fibre complexes.[16] Other terminology such as plantix, non-nutritive fibre or biopolymers has been proposed.[17] Only the terminology proposed by Trowell has been generally accepted.

16.2.1 Classifications of dietary fibre

The dietary fibre components are predominantly located in the cell-wall structure. Other indigestible plant material such as cutin, waxes, protein etc. are closely related to dietary fibre.

The structure can be divided chemically into cellulose, hemi-cellulose, pectic substances, other polysaccharides and lignin. Dietary fibre is also normally divided into a water-insoluble fraction, consisting of cellulose and lignin, and water soluble components, encompassing the major part of the hemi-cellulose compounds, gums, β-glucans, mucilages and pectin. The water-insoluble components have predominantly been attributed to properties exerted locally in the gastrointestinal tract in contrast to the water soluble compounds, which have been attributed to influencing carbohydrate and fat metabolism. However, a survey by Leeds has revealed that this distinction may be too categorical.[9] Cellulose is a linear polymer of β-1–4-

linked glucose units. It has a high molecular weight and the compound is held together within the chain and adjacent chains by hydrogen bonds.

Fructans, which contains two molecules of fructose, is now considered dietary fibre. The principal fructan is inulin.

Hemi-cellulose comprises those cell-wall polysaccharides that are solubilised by aqueous alkali after removal of water-soluble and pectic polysaccharides. The hemi-cellulose has main chains of β-1–4-linked pyranoside sugars as in cellulose. Frequently, hemi-cellulose is closely associated with cellulose by hydrogen bonding. The individual classification of hemicellulose is based upon the dominant monomeric sugar component.[18]

The pectic group is a complex of polysaccharides where D-galacturonic acid is the dominant constituent.

Other polysaccharides are a heterogenous group including water-soluble algar polysaccharides, gums and mucilages. These products are used as emulsifiers, stabilisers and thickeners in the food industry. Components of this group have a complex, highly branched structure.[18]

Lignin is a complex of phenyl propane units.[18]

16.3 Defining obesity

Overweight or obesity is defined as an excessive accumulation of body fat in the organism, which eventually will influence the health of the individual.[19] Measurement or estimation of body fat is rarely done, although simple methods have been developed and validated.[20] Studies on obesity normally depend on measuring weight and height only or on calculating a body mass index by dividing the subject's body weight (kg) by the square of the height (m^2). Based upon the BMI, overweight patients can be divided into several classes, e.g. underweight, normal range, pre-obese, obese class I, II and III.[19] The different classes imply increasing risks of co-morbidities. However, to characterise and classify an obese person from a health point of view, not only is the total amount of fat, or a BMI, but also the regional distribution of fat is needed. Excess abdominal fat, measured by a waist circumference or a waist–hip ratio of more than 0.8 in women and 1 in men, carry a bigger risk for developing co-morbidities compared to excess fat accumulation in other locations in the body.[19]

Waist circumference is a convenient measurement unrelated to height but correlated to BMI and waist–hip ratio (WHR).[21] Waist circumference is a measure for the amount of fat located intra-abdominally.[22] Changes in waist circumference seem to reflect changes in risk factors for developing cardiovascular diseases.[23]

16.3.1 Prevalence of overweight

The prevalence of overweight and obesity is increasing at an alarming rate and is now considered an epidemic by the World Health Organization

(WHO).[19] The most comprehensive data on the global prevalence of obesity have emerged from the WHO Monica study.[24] Implying a BMI border of >25 has resulted in prevalence of overweight of more than 50% of the adult population.

In the USA several national surveys such as NHES I,[25] NHANES I, II and III have revealed that obesity is a major problem in USA and, unfortunately, is increasing sharply.[26] Applying a cut-off border of BMI >30 showed that obesity had doubled from 10% in 1960 to 19.7% for females in 1991 and nearly doubled in men from 15% in 1960 to 24.5% in 1991.

Prevalence in Canada shows the same pattern, although with a little lower prevalence, especially for women. The prevalence in European countries shows a pattern of obesity between 5% and 21% for men and between 9% and 45% for women and a sharp increase over the years, with the exception of the Netherlands which has shown a remarkable low increase in obesity for men and women over two decades. The variation in prevalence of overweight in the different countries might be explained by demographic factors, social-cultural differences and behavioural factors.[27]

16.3.2 Epidemiology

Big epidemiological studies (the Multiple Risk Factor Intervention Trial and the Health Professionals' Follow-up Study) have tried to correlate body weight to intake of dietary fibre. In the MRFIT trial[28] it was demonstrated that intake of a low-fat/high fibre diet was correlated to a lower body weight. Increase in dietary fibre was associated with lower weight during the follow-up period.

In the Health Professionals' Study it was demonstrated that a high intake of dietary fibre was correlated to a decrease in coronary heart disease.[29] Wynder *et al.*[30] could demonstrate that people with the highest dietary fibre intake had the lowest BMI and vice versa. This correlation was also demonstrated by Alfieri *et al.* in an observational study.[31] Total dietary fibre intake was found to be significantly higher in normal weight subjects compared to severely obese patients.

16.3.3 Etiology of overweight

The etiology of overweight and obesity is not known, but is most likely multi-factorial. Etiology can be divided into genetic factors and environmental factors. It is a well-known fact that obesity is more frequent in some families. Investigations have clearly demonstrated that, if the subject is obese, the parents are most likely also to be obese.[32,33] Among the environmental factors are changes in the diet and physical activity. In particular, intake of fat has been high and intake is still too high today.[34]

Despite the fact that a reduction in intake of fat has taken place, the prevalence of overweight has increased.[34] A higher intake of highly palatable high fat foods with a low GI and a corresponding lower intake of carbohydrates has been seen since the 1950s and has been suggested as a major reason for the development of obesity.[34] A reduced level of physical activity has also been demonstrated in several studies.[35,36] A lower metabolic rate in some patients has been suggested as a cause for development of overweight.[37] Gain in weight has been seen after pregnancy,[38] after surgery, after certain endocrine disorders and after treatment with steroids, tricyclic antidepressants, and other drugs.[19] It has also been demonstrated that BMI in subjects in highly developed countries increases with age.[39]

16.4 Dietary fibre and the treatment of obesity

Treatment of overweight and obesity is necessary in order to reduce morbidity and mortality. In a Scandinavian population, Waler[40] demonstrated that overweight *per se* was connected with an overall mortality rate of 4%. The mortality rate seems to increase not only with the degree of overweight[19] but also with the length of time of overweight.[19] A weight reduction of 5 to 10% of initial body weight has been documented to reduce the risk factors for developing cardiovascular diseases.[41] Treatment should be started as soon as possible in order to avoid further weight gain.

Management of overweight is a multi-disciplinary task, involving physicians, nutritionists, nurses, physiotherapists, behaviour therapists, psychologists, etc. As pointed out by Rössner,[42] the aim of inducing a sufficient weight reduction to obtain the ideal body weight is not an option in most overweight patients, but obtaining a slightly lower body weight could be the primary goal for most overweight patients and even a slowing down of the weight gain could be a goal *per se* for some patients.

The cornerstone in the management of overweight is changing the subject's behaviour and a well-balanced hypo-caloric diet together with an increase in physical exercise. Dietary fibre as a part of the carbohydrate content in the diet plays an important role in a well-balanced hypo-caloric diet. The hypothesis that dietary fibre could have an impact on body weight originally emerged from epidemiological studies. Investigators working on the African continent in the first half of the last century noticed that body weight in rural living subjects was constant until the age of 30 years after which it actually fell. It was also found that the average weight for Zulu urban men and women were higher compared to rural men and women in the same age group.[43] Unfortunately, no detailed information about the composition of the diet was available, but it was generally known that the diet consisted predominantly of plant material. Trowell[44] pointed out that obesity was rare in a population ingesting a high amount of starchy foods. He also pointed out that high-fibre food induced greater satiety than did low-fibre food of comparable energy content.

A number of clinical trials incorporating dietary fibre in the diet have shown a weight reduction.[45,46] Only few prospective, placebo-controlled trials have been published. The change of diet from low fibre to high fibre inevitably means a simultaneous reduced fat intake and this, together with the high intake of dietary fibre, could be responsible for the weight reduction. The high fibre diet could also result in a longer chewing time, enhanced saliva production and increased gastric filling. The high fibre diet could also have an impact on palatability of the food and consequently on the energy intake.

The availability of dietary fibre supplement paved the way to circumvent some of the above-mentioned inherent obstacles, such as palatability, chewing time and fat content. Several trials using a balanced hypo-caloric diet and a dietary fibre supplement or placebo have been performed in different categories of overweight subjects. In mildly overweight subjects a significant weight reduction in both fibre treated and placebo groups were found. However, the weight reduction in the fibre treated groups with a supplement of approximately 8 g/day were significantly higher compared to placebo. The difference in weight loss in the prospective, placebo-controlled trials occurred after a treatment period of 4 to 6 weeks at a time at which the weight reduction in the placebo groups normally levelled off. However, in the fibre-treated group weight reduction continued after that time.[47]

Treatment of even mildly overweight subjects is in a majority of the cases a long-term process and the subjects could consequently benefit by having a dietary fibre supplement added to the treatment regimen. In mildly overweight subjects a 50% higher weight loss corresponding to a weight loss of approximately 2 kg over a period of 3 months was obtained. One of the reasons for the better result in the fibre-treated group was a better adherence to the treatment regimen.

In prospective, placebo-controlled trials encompassing moderately obese patients a significantly higher weight loss in the fibre treated groups were demonstrated. However, the difference in weight reduction was clinically of minor importance.[47] In order to obtain a clinically significant weight loss in these patients, a sufficiently high dietary fibre supplement has to be provided.[48] A positive effect of a dietary fibre supplementation without simultaneously reduced energy intake has been documented in some, but not all, investigations.[49] The dietary fibre supplement (20 g guar gum) was provided after a diet intervention lasting for 14 months. The diet intervention and the time of administration could have masked the possible positive role of the dietary fibre supplement, because Krotkiewski found a positive effect of the same type and same amount of dietary fibre provided to the patients before lunch and dinner.[50]

In the fibre supplement plus hypo-caloric diet studies, the results are not only dependent upon the fibre supplementation but also on the compliance to the diet. Different amounts of dietary fibre supplement of different origin together with hypo-caloric diet containing different caloric intake have, in most cases, provided a higher weight loss in the fibre-treated group compared to the placebo group. Rössner *et al.* showed, in two studies in moderately overweight patients with an initially body weight of 95 kg to 103 kg (respectively) treated with a hypo-caloric diet of approximately 5 MJ/day and a fibre supplement amounting from 5 g to 7 g/day document, a bigger weight loss in the fibre groups compared to placebo.[51] In a similar study by Rössner *et al.* including 62 moderately overweight patients were provided a hypo-caloric diet amounting to 6.7 MJ/day and a dietary fibre supplement of 6.5 g/day or placebo. The dietary fibre content in the hypo-caloric diet was around 8 g/day. No significant difference in weight loss was found after 2.5 months treatment.[52] One reason for the difference between the obtained results could be the substantially higher content of dietary fibre in the diet in the latter study.

In a 52-week prospective, placebo-controlled study, where 97 patients with a BMI of 27.4 were treated with a hypo-caloric diet of between 5 MJ/day and 6.7 MJ/day and a dietary fibre supplement of 6 g/day or placebo, a significantly higher weight reduction was observed in the fibre-treated group compared to placebo after 27 weeks of treatment. All remaining patients were then provided with an *ad libitum* diet and 6 g/day of dietary fibre for the rest of the period. The adherence to the diet regimen after the first 27-week treatment was significantly higher in the fibre-treated group. A weight reduction continued during the rest of the treatment period.[53] In the treatment of overweight, the following aspects may be considered:

- Early onset of treatment
- Multi-disciplinary nature of task
- There have been a number of clinical trials incorporating dietary fibre in the diet, but not all, have shown a weight reduction
- Only few prospective, placebo-controlled trials have been published
- Very few long-term prospective studies have been published
- The high fibre diet could also have an impact on palatability of the food
- Treatment of overweight subjects is, in a majority of cases, a long-term process

16.4.1 Possible mode of actions of dietary fibre in overweight

According to Heaton,[54] dietary fibre is an obstacle to energy intake. Dietary fibre would reduce energy intake by displacing available nutrients, increasing the chewing time and reducing the absorption efficiency in the gastrointestinal tract. Food rich in dietary fibre has a lower energy density compared to other nutrients. Intake of dietary fibre will consequently provoke a lower energy intake. Together with the lower energy density *per se*, dietary fibre will replace other nutrients with a higher energy density.[55] Increasing the intake of dietary fibre will most likely provoke a reduction in fat intake.[55] When a constant amount of food is consumed, a diet low in energy density will result in a reduced energy intake.[55]

High-fibre food requires increasing chewing time and consequently an increase in saliva production.[48] The higher saliva production after intake of dietary fibre rich food such as the soluble fibre guar gum and pectin could enhance gastric filling thereby increasing satiety.[56] However, the relation between release of CCK, gastric distension and satiety are still debatable.[57] Increasing the intake of dietary fibre will decrease the absorption of energy.[58] Heaton suggested that dietary fibre simply acted as a barrier to hinder the intestinal absorption of energy.[54]

The influence on gastric emptying time of dietary fibre has provided contradictory results. Forty-six patients suffering from irritable bowel syndrome were included in an open, randomised parallel group design study. Half of the patients were treated with dietary fibre tablets containing 8.5 g/day and the remaining patients received a bran product (14 g/day) for 6 weeks. Total transit time decreased significantly in the fibre group only. However, total transit time was initially significantly lower in the bran treated group. Gastric emptying time was initially comparable but significantly shorter in the dietary fibre group after treatment compared to the bran group (Schrijver *et al.*, personal communication).

Leeds *et al.*[59] could document a delay in gastric emptying time with 10 g of pectin added to an oral glucose load. In most cases a dosage above 10 g per day has been necessary to delay gastric emptying time. Rydning *et al.*[60] could, however, not show a change in gastric emptying time with different dosages of both soluble fibre (5 g) and insoluble fibre (10.5 g). The lack of effect in this study could be due to the fact that only eight subjects were assessed.

Gastric emptying time is properly regulated by the composition of the duodenal content. The duodenal mucosa possesses two sets of receptors, one responding to the osmotic effects of the breakdown products, and one responding to the surface tension effect provoked by the breakdown products of lipids.[61] However, the osmolarity effect on gastric emptying time seems to be of minor importance.[62] The mechanisms involved in the control of gastric emptying time involve both neuronal and hormonal interactions.[62] It has been demonstrated that the gastric emptying rate may be correlated to meal energy density and independent of chemical composition and osmolality.[62] Gastric emptying time has been linked to satiety and feeding behaviour.[59]

The post-prandial transit of nutrients commences as a rapid rate, followed by a slower rate. The digested food is absorbed during its transportation in the small intestine. An alteration in small intestinal motility with possible increase in thickness of the unstirred water layer has been proposed by Jenkins.[63] High fibre food may reduce the rate of penetration of digestive enzymes and thereby reduce the rate of supply of substrates for absorption.[64] Supplementation of fibre to glucose tolerance tests results in flattening insulin and gastric inhibitory polypeptide responses.[63] One of the advantages of dietary fibre is a decrease of glucose absorption from the intestinal tract. Anderson *et al.* investigated the influence on glucose absorption with and without different amounts of dietary fibre. The investigation revealed that intake of a high fibre meal provoked a considerable flattening in post-prandial glucose response when fibre was provided both on a short-term period and under long-term period to patients.[58]

As dietary fibre passes the colon, some part of the material is digested by the bacteria.[65] The structure of the fibre is consequently altered. It is also possible that dietary fibre *per se* affects the activities and composition of bacteria in the colon. Supplementation of the diet with dietary fibre has provoked an increased faecal mass containing an increased amount of bacteria, but with no change in the composition of the flora.[66] Cummings reviewed the evidence that non-starch polysaccharides are broken down in the colon.[67] End products are short-chain fatty acids, acetate, propionate and butyrate with acetate as the dominant acid. The different short-chain fatty acids play a very important role in maintaining the integrity of the epithelium in colon.

The hypothesis that butyrate, one of the short-chain fatty acids, protects the colon against developing cancer has been proposed by Kim *et al.*[68]

As well as reducing energy intake, the beneficial effect of dietary fibre on overweight could hypothetically also be due to an influence on energy expenditure. The effect of dietary fibre on energy expenditure has also provided conflicting results. Rössner found a 1% reduction in diet induced thermogenesis when changing from a high-fibre diet to a low-fibre diet.[49] The difference in thermogenesis has been explained by a time-shift in oxidation of the available nutrients.[69]

Raben *et al.* found a lower oxidation of carbohydrates during daytime on a high dietary fibre diet.[70] The 1% changes in diet induced thermogenesis mean a 1 to 2% change in total energy intake. Ryttig *et al.*[71] found no influence of a dietary fibre supplement of 7 g/day on 24-hour energy expenditure in 19 healthy volunteers with an average body weight of 65 kg. Twenty-four hour energy expenditure was measured during a 2-week run-in period. The subjects were then given either fibre or placebo for 2 weeks after which they switched therapy for another 2 weeks. Energy intake, 4.5 MJ/day, and food fibre, 29 g/day, were kept constant during the treatment period. No change in body weight was observed.

Rigaud *et al.*[72] found a significantly higher energy excretion in the faeces in 20 healthy volunteers, who were provided a dietary fibre supplement of 7 g/day in a randomised, double-blind, placebo-controlled trial lasting 6 weeks. Energy intake remained constant during the whole treatment period (2 MJ/day). The mean food fibre intake remained the same during run-in, fibre and placebo treatment (13 g/day). These results indicate that there may be differences in thermogenesis exerted by different carbohydrates and different composition of the diet.[73] The following are aspects of the influence of fibre on overweight worth considering.

Mode of action of dietary fibre in overweight:

- Impact on energy intake
- Some, but not all, trials have shown an impact on gastric emptying time
- Nutrients absorption
- Impact on thermogenesis
- Some, but not all, trials have shown that dietary fibre has an influence on energy excretion.

16.5 Dietary fibre and chronic diseases associated with obesity

16.5.1 Influence of dietary fibre on diabetes mellitus type 1

The high prevalence of diabetes has, in part, been attributed to the low intake of dietary fibre as pointed out by Mann.[74] In the management of diabetes, total energy intake may be the most important issue. Andersson *et al.*[75] reported a beneficial effect of changing the diet to a high fibre/high carbohydrate diet in the management of diabetes. A high fibre/high carbohydrate diet is not an issue for all patients and it was therefore essential that Jenkins *et al.*[76] could demonstrate a hypoglycemic response exerted by guar and viscous gum intake. However, also water-insoluble fibre such as rye bran has been documented as able to reduce insulin requirement significantly in insulin- dependent diabetic patients subjects as shown by Nygren.[77]

Jenkins *et al.* has performed extensive research in order to find out what impact different carbohydrates had on blood glucose.

Carbohydrates can be divided into low glycemic index carbohydrates and high glycemic index carbohydrates.[76] The practical implication of this division originally proposed by Jenkins has been widely discussed, but the glycemic index concept has now been generally accepted.[78] Also, there seems to be a consensus that treatment with high fibre/high carbohydrate diet is now a well-established part of the management of diabetes.

16.5.2 Influence of dietary fibre on diabetes mellitus type 2

Type 2 diabetes is considered a lifestyle disease. There is a direct relationship between the degree of obesity and number of persons with type 2 diabetes. The risk of developing type 2 diabetes can be reduced by lifestyle interventions such as changes in diet, enhanced physical activities and weight reduction.[79] The European Diabetes Association recommends a diet with low glycemic index to patients suffering of type 2 diabetes.[80] This recommendation has further been substantiated by a recently published meta-analysis in which a diet with a low glycemic index was compared with a diet with a high glycemic index and shown to have a better impact on HbA1c.[81] This is in contrast to the recommendations given by the American Diabetes Association, which states that it is the amount and not the type of carbohydrates that has an influence on HbA1c.[82]

16.5.3 Influence of dietary fibre on hypertension

Changes in lifestyle and non-pharmacological therapy approaches have long been considered the first step in the management of hypertension. In the study performed by Rössner *et al.*[52] it was demonstrated that a dietary fibre supplement of between 6 and 7 g/day had a positive influence on both systolic and diastolic blood pressure. The average blood pressure was initially within the normal range (138 mm Hg/86 mm Hg). After 3 months treatment, the blood pressure in both groups was significantly reduced, whereas the diastolic blood pressure was reduced significantly only in the fibre-treated group. The decrease in blood pressure was evident after 2-weeks treatment and before weight reduction was evident. In mild to moderate hypertensive patients a dietary fibre supplement of 7 g/day provoked a significant reduction of 10 mm Hg in systolic blood pressure and 5 mm Hg in diastolic blood pressure.[83] The reduction in blood pressure was independent of a change in weight, because body weight did not change during the treatment (80 kg). Eliasson *et al.*[84] treated 63 patients with a diastolic blood pressure between 90 and 115 mm Hg with a dietary fibre supplement of 7 g/day or matching placebo in a randomised, double-blind parallel group study of 3 months duration. Reduction in systolic blood pressure was the same in both groups, whereas the 5 mm Hg in diastolic blood pressure was evident in the fibre-treated group only. Body weight did not change during treatment. There was no correlation between changes in body weight and blood pressure. Serum insulin decreased significantly only in the fibre-treated group and could have contributed to the blood pressure lowering effect in the fibre group.

16.5.4 Influence of dietary fibre on lipid disorders

Treatment of lipid disorders is first of all dietary intervention with a low intake of saturated fat to 10% of the energy intake and in some cases below. Furthermore, an increase in carbohydrates is required. A weight reduction amounting to 5 to 10% of initial body weight will also have a beneficial effect on the lipid pattern. Anderson *et al.*[85] have demonstrated that water-soluble dietary fibre can reduce blood cholesterol significantly. Some investigators[83,84] could also show that 7 g/day fibre of the water insoluble type had a beneficial effect on s-triglycerides in a placebo-controlled trial. The mechanism of action for that effect is not clear, although weight reduction could play a role. The gastric emptying time, together with the absorptive mechanisms, could also be important for such an effect. Furthermore, a reduction in both cholesterol and triglycerides has been seen in subjects without any concomitant change in body weight.

16.6 Conclusions and future trends

Overweight is today considered one of the biggest health problems. To reduce morbidity and mortality in these patients, an offensive treatment approach has to be imposed. Change of diet to a high fibre/high carbohydrate diet has been shown to provoke a weight reduction in overweight patients. Dietary fibre supplement added to a well-balanced hypo-caloric diet has in prospective, placebo-controlled trials also been shown to result in a significant weight reduction in mild and moderate overweight patients. Dietary fibre seems to be able to influence energy intake, prolong gastric emptying time – although different opinions exist – reduce absorption of nutrients in the small intestine and increase fecal energy excretion.

A weight reduction of 5 to 10% of initial body weight has been demonstrated to result in lowering blood pressure and with a beneficial effect on lipids. Besides the weight reduction effect of the dietary fibre, these supplements have also been shown to exert blood pressure lowering effects independent of the change in body weight. The mechanism of action for those effects are not clear, although an effect on insulin has been suggested. A beneficial effect on some of the lipid parameters has also been seen, probably due to a changed absorption pattern.

Interest for dietary fibre, based upon the number of publications, has been steadily increasing. In particular, the interest for the efficacy of dietary fibre in the management of overweight has been prominent. The effect has been assessed in several publications, reviews and a couple of theses. The effect of dietary fibre in long-term obesity has not been exploited sufficiently to conclude if dietary fibre plays any role here.

The effect of the different water-soluble and water-insoluble fibres on metabolic parameters such as insulin, glucose, lipids, enzymes, etc. has to be further investigated.

Studies on how to increase the amount of dietary fibre in food without negatively influencing the palatability of the food too much should be investigated.

Dietary fibre supplements that could be incorporated into food items should be assessed properly in order to evaluate if such supplements could have an influence on the prevalence of some of the co-morbidities connected to overweight.

The postulated hypothesis that dietary fibre has a beneficial effect on cancer in the gastrointestinal tract, and maybe other forms of cancer should be investigated in detail.

The combination of dietary fibre and the bacterial environment in the colon and the implications need to be investigated further.

16.7 References

1 ROYAL COLLEGE OF PHYSICIANS OF LONDON. (1980), *Medical Aspects of Dietary Fibre.* Tunbridge Wells, Kent: Pitman Medical.

2 CLEAVE, T. L. (1974), *The Saccharine Disease*, Bristol: John Wright & Sons.

3 BURKITT, D. P. and TROWELL, H. C. (1975), *Refined Carbohydrate Food and Disease. Some Implications of Dietary Fibre.* London: Academic Press.

4 HEALTH EDUCATION COUNCIL, A discussion paper on proposal for nutritional guidelines for health education in britain (NACNE 1983).

5 US DEPARTMENT OF AGRICULTURE AND US DEPARTMENT OF HEALTH AND HUMAN SERVICE, 1980.

6 TROWELL, H. C. (1981), Hypertension, obesity, diabetes mellitus and coronary heart disease. In Trowell H. C. and Burkett D. P., eds. *Western Diseases: Their Emergency and Prevention*. London: Edward Arnold, 3–32.

7 ROYAL COLLEGE OF PHYSICIANS OF LONDON (1983), Obesity. *J. R. Coll. Phys. Lond.* **17**, 45–6.

8 KROTKIEWSKY, M. and SMITH, U. (1985), Dietary fibre in obesity. In Leeds A. R. and Avenell A., eds. *Dietary Fibre Perspectives–Reviews and Bibliography 1*, London: John Libbey, 61–7.

9 LEEDS, A. R. (1992), Dietary fibre and obesity. In Björntorp P. and Brodoff B. N., eds. *Obesity*. Philadelphia: J. B. Lippencott, 677–82.

10 HAKALA, P. (1998), Dietary therapy. In Andersen T., Rissanan A. and Rössner S., eds. *A Nordic Text Book in Overweight*, Lund: Studenterlitteratur, 234–48.

11 PASMAN, W. J. (1998), Obesity treatment and weight maintenance. Thesis. Maastricht, 19.

12 HIPSLEY, I. (1953), Dietary 'fibre' and pregnancy toxaemia. *Br. Med. J.* **2**, 420–2.

13 TROWELL, H. (1974), Definition of fibre. *Lancet* **1**, 503.

14 TROWELL, H., SOUTHGATE, D. A. T., WOLEVER, T. M. S., LEEDS, A. R., GASSULL, M. A. and JENKINS, D. J. A. (1976), Dietary fibre redefined. *Lancet* **1**, 65–70.

15 DIETARY REFERENCE INTAKE, STANDING COMMITTEE ON THE EVALUATION ON THE SCIENTIFIC EVALUATION OF DIETARY REFERENCE INTAKE. (2002), Food and Nutrition Board, page 22–25.

16 TROWELL, H. C. (1976), Definition of dietary fibre and hypothesis that it is a protective factor in certain diseases. *Am. J. Clin. Nutr.* **29**, 417–27.

17 SPILLER, G, A., SHIPLEY, E. A. and BLAKE, J. A. (1978), Recent progress in dietary fibre (plantix) in human nutrition, *CRC Crit. Rev. Fd. Sci. Nutr.* **10**, 31–90.

18 THEANDER, O. and ÅMAN, P. (1979), The chemistry, morphology and analysis of dietary fibre components. In Inglett G. E. and Falkeha S. I., eds. *Dietary Fibre Chemistry and Nutrition.* New York: Academic Press, 215–44.

19 OBESITY, PREVENTING AND MANAGING THE GLOBAL EPIDEMIC, REPORT OF A WHO CONSULTATION ON OBESITY. WORLD HEALTH ORGANIZATION, 1998.

20 DURNIN, J. V. G. A. and WORMERSLEY, J. (1974), Body fat assessment from total body density and its estimation from skinfold thickness: measurements on 481 men and women aged from 16–72 years. *Br. J. Nutr.* **32**, 77–97.

21 WHO PHYSICAL STATUS: THE USE AND INTERPRETATION OF ANTHROPOMETRY. Report of a WHO Expert Committee: Geneva, World Health Organization, 1995 (Technical Report Series; No. 854): 368–9.

22 LEAN, M. E, J., HAN, T. S. and MORRISON, C. E. (1995), Waist circumference as a measure for indicating need for weight management. *BMJ* **311**, 158–61.

23 LEAN, M. E. J., HAN, T. S. and DEURENBERG, P. (1996), Predicting body composition by densitometry from simple anthropometric measurements. *Am. J. Clin. Nutr.* **72**, 787–95.

24 LARSSON, B., BENGTSSON, C., BJÖRNTORP, P. *et al.* (1992), Is abdominal fat distribution a major explanation for the sex difference in the incidence of myocardial

infarction? The study of men born in 1913 and the study of women, Göteborg, Sweden. *Am. J. Epidemiol.* **135**, 266–73.

25 WHO MONICA PROJECT: RISK FACTORS. (1989), *Int. J. Epidemiol.* **18** (suppl.1), S46–55.

26 KUCZMARSKI, R. J., FLEGAL, K. M., CAMPELL, S. M. and JOHNSON, C. L. (1994), Increasing prevalence of overweight among US adults. The National Health and Nutrition examination surveys, 1960 to 1991, *JAMA* **272**, 205–11.

27 SEIDELL, J. C. and FLEGAL, K.M. (1997), Assessing obesity: classification and epidemiology. *Br. Med. Bull.* **53**, 238–52.

28 STAMLER, J. and DOLECEK, T. A. (1997), Relation of food and nutrient intakes to body mass in the special intervention and usual care groups in the Multiple Risk Factor Intervention Trial. *Am. J. Clin. Nutr.* **65**, 366–73.

29 RIMM, E. B., ASCHERIO, A., GIOVANNUCI, E., SPIGELMAN, D., STAMPFER, M. J. and WILLET, W. C. (1996), Vegetable, fruit and cereal fiber and risk of coronary heart disease among men. *JAMA* **275**, 447–51.

30 WYNDER, E. L., STELLMAN, S. D. and ZANG, E. A. (1996), High fiber intake. Indicator for a healthy lifestyle. *JAMA* **275**, 486–7.

31 ALFIERI, M. A. H., POMERLEAU, J., GRACE, D. M. and ANDERSSON, L. (1995), Fibre intake of normal weight, moderately and severely obese subjects. *Obes. Res.* **3**, 541–7.

32 HEITMANN, B. L., LISSNER, L., SØRENSEN, T. I. A. and BENGTSSON, C. (1995), Dietary fat intake and weight gain in women genetically predisposed for obesity. *Am. J. Clin. Nutr.* **61**, 1213–7.

33 WHITAKER, R. C., WRIGHT, J. A., PEPE, M. S., SEIDEL, K. D. and DIETZ, W. H. (1997), Predicting obesity in young adulthood from childhood and parental obesity. *N. Engl. J. Med.* **337**, 869–73.

34 LISSNER, L., HEITMANN, B. L. and BENGTSSON, C. (1997), Low fat-diet may prevent weight gain in sedentary women: prospective observations from the population study of women in Gothenburg, Sweden. *Obes. Res.* **5**, 43–8.

35 FOGENHOLM, M., MÄNNISTÖ, S., VARTIAINEN, E. and PIETINEN, P. (1996), Determinants of energy balance and overweight in Finland 1982 and 1992. *Int. J. Obes.* **20**, 1097–104.

36 DIETZ, W. H. and GORTMARKER, S. L. (1985), Do we fatten our children at the television set? Obesity and television viewing in children and adolescents. *Pediatrics.* **75**, 807–12.

37 SHAR, M. and JEFFERY, R. W. (1991), Is obesity due to overeating and inactivity or to a defective metabolic rate? A review. *Ann. Bev. Med.* **13**, 73–81.

38 RÖSSNER, S. and ÖHLIN, A. (1995), Pregnancy as a risk factor for obesity: Lessons from the Stockholm Pregnancy and Weight Development Study. *Obes. Res.* **3** (suppl 2), 267–75.

39 HEITMAN, B. L. (1998), Prevalence, epidemiology, In Andersen T., Rissanan A. and Rössner S., eds. *A Nordic Text Book in Overweight.* Lund: Studenterlitteratur, 44–54.

40 WAALER, H. T. (1984), Height, weight and mortality. The Norwegian experience. *Acta. Med. Scan.* (suppl 679), 1–56.

41 VAN GAAL, L. F., WAUTERS, M. A. and DE LEEUW, I. H. (1997), The beneficial effects of modest weight loss on cardiovascular factors. *Int. J. Obes.* **21** (suppl 1), 5–9.

42 RÖSSNER, S. (1997), Defining success in obesity management. *Int. J. Obes.* **21** (suppl 1), 2–4.

43 HUXLEY, J. (1981), Africa View, 162. London: Chatto & Windus, 1931. Cited in Trowell H. C. and Burkett D. P., eds. *Western Diseases: Their Emergence and Prevention.* London: Edward Arnold.

44 TROWELL, H. (1975), Obesity in the Western world. *Plant Foods Man* **1**, 157–66.

45 EVANS, E. and MILLER, D. S. (1975), Bulking agents in the treatment of obesity. *Nutr. Metab.* **18**, 199–203.

46 MICKELSEN, O., MAKDANI, D. D., COTTON, R. H., TITCOMB, S. T., COMLEY, J. C. and GATTY, R. (1979), Effects of a high fiber bread diet on weight loss in college-age males. *Am. J. Clin. Nutr.* **32**, 1703–9.

47 RYTTIG, K. R. (1990), Clinical effects of dietary fibre supplements in overweight and in hypertension. Thesis. Stockholm.

48 RÖSSNER, S. (1992), Dietary fibre in the prevention and treatment of obesity. In Schweizer T. F. and Edwards C. A., eds. *Dietary Fiber – A Component of Food*, Springer – Verlag, London, 265–77.

49 PASSMAN, W. J., WESTERTERP-PLANTENGA, M. S., MULS, E., VANSANT, G., VAN REE, J. and SARIS, W. H. M. (1997), The effectivness of long-term fiber supplementation on weight maintenance in weight-reduced women. *Int. J. Obes.* **21**, 548–55.

50 KROTKIEWSKI, M. and SMITH, U. (1985), Dietary fibre in obesity. In Leeds A. R. and Avenell A., eds. *Dietary Fibre Perspectives – Reviews and Bibliography 1.* London: John Libbey, 61–7.

51 RÖSSNER, S., VON ZWEIGBERGK, D., ÖHLIN, A. and RYTTIG, K. (1987), Weight reduction with dietary fibre supplements: Results of two double-blind randomized studies. *Acta. Med. Scan* **222**, 83–8.

52 RÖSSNER, S., ANDERSSON, I. L. and RYTTIG, K. (1988), Effects of a dietary fibre supplement to a weight reduction programme on blood pressure. *Acta. Med. Scan.* **223**, 353–7.

53 RYTTIG, K. R., TELLNES, G., HÆGH, L., BØE, E. and FAGERTHUN, H. (1989), A dietary fibre supplement and weight maintenance after weight reduction. *Int. J. Obes.* **13**, 165–71.

54 HEATON, K. W. (1980), Food intake regulation and fiber. In Spiller G. S. and Kay R. M., eds. *Medical Aspects of Dietary Fibre.* New York: Plenum Medical, 223–38.

55 RABEN, A., JENSEN, N. D., MARCKMANN, P., SANDSTRÖM, B. and ASTRUP, A. (1995), Spontaneous weight loss during 11 weeks *ad libitum* intake of low fat/high fiber diet in young, normal weight subjects. *Int. J. Obes.* **19**, 916–23.

56 POPPITT, S. D. (1995), Energy density of diets and obesity. *Int. J. Obes.* **19** (suppl 5), 20–6.

57 READ, N., FRENCH, S. and CUNNINGHAM, K. (1994), The role of the gut in regulating food intake in man. *Nutr. Rev.* **52**, 1–10.

58 ANDERSON, J. W. RANDLES, K. M., KENDELL, C. W. and JENKINS, D. J. (2004), Carbohydrates and fiber recommendations for individuals with diabetes: a quantitative assessment and meta-analysis of the evidence. *J. Am. Coll. Nutr.* **23**, 5–17.

59 LEEDS, A. R., RALPHS, D. N. L., EBEID, F., METZ, G. and DILAWARI, J. B. (1981), Pectin in the dumping syndrome: Reduction of symptoms and plasma volume changes. *Lancet* **1**, 1075–8.

60 RYDNING, A., BERSTAD, A., BERSTAT, T. and HERTZENBERG, L. (1985), The effect of guar gum and the fibre-enriched wheat bran on gastric emptying of a semi solid meal in healthy subjects. *Scand J. Gastroenterol.* **20**, 330–4.

61 HUNT, J. N., CASH, R. and NEWLAND, P. (1978), Energy density of food, gastric emptying and obesity. In Roth H. P. and Mehlman M. A., eds. *Role of Dietary Fiber in Man. Am. J. Clin. Nutr.* **31** (suppl), 259–60.

62 WISEN, O. (1992), Thesis. Studies of digestive functions in human obesity. 12, Stockholm.

63 JENKINS, D. J. A., WOLEVER, T. M. S., JENKINS, A. L. and TAYLOR, R. H. (1984), Dietary fiber, gastrointestinal, endocrine and metabolic effects: Lente carbohydrates. In Vahouny G. V. and Kritchevsky D., eds. *Dietary Fiber: Basic and Clinical Aspects.* New York: Plenum Press, 69–80.

64 JENKINS, D. J. A., JENKINS, A. L., WOLEVER, T. M. S., RAO, A. V. and THOMSON, L. U. (1986), Fiber and starchy foods: gut function and implications in disease. *Am. J. Gastroenterol.* **81**, 920–30.

65 VAN SOEST, P. J. (1978), Dietary fibers: Their definition and nutritional properties. *Am. J. Clin. Nutr.* **31**, 12–20.

66 SALYERS, A. A. (1984), Diet and the colonic environment: Measuring the response of human colonic bacteria to changes in the host's diet. In Vahouny G. V. and Kritchevsky D., eds. *Dietary Fiber: Basic and Clinical Aspects.* New York: Plenum Press, 119–30.

67 CUMMINGS, J. H. (1981), Dietary fibre. *Br. Med. Bull.* **37**, 65.

68 KIM, Y. S., TSAO, D., MORITA, A. and BELLA, A. (1982), Effect of sodium butyrate and three human colorectal edenocarcinoma cell lines in culture. In Malt R. A. and Williamson R. C. N., eds. *Colonic Carcinogenesis*, Falk Symposium 31, M. T. P., Lancaster, England 317.

69 SPARTI, A., SCHUTZ, Y., DI VETTI, V, POLLET, P., MILON, H. and JÉQUIER, E. (1997), Effect of complex carbohydrates on 24 h nutrient oxidation. *Int. J. Obes.* **21** (suppl 2), 18.

70 RABEN, A., CHRISTENSEN, N. J., HOLST, J. J. and ASTRUP, A. (1994), Decreased postprandial thermogenesis and fat oxidation but increased fullness after a high-fiber meal compared with a low-fiber meal. *Am. J. Clin. Nutr.* **59**, 1386–94.

71 RYTTIG, K. R., LAMMERT, O., NIELSEN, E., GARBY, L. and POULSEN, K. (1990), The effect of a soluble dietary fibre supplement on 24-hour energy expenditure during a standardized physical activity programme. *Int. J. Obes.* **14**, 451–5.

72 RIGAUD, D., RYTTIG, K. R., LEEDS, A. R., BARD, D. and APFELBAUM, M. (1987), Effect of a moderate dietary fibre supplement on hunger rating, energy input, and faecal energy output in young healthy volunteers. A randomized, double-blind, cross-over trial. *Int. J. Obes.* **11** (suppl 1), 73–8.

73 LEAN, M. E. J. and JAMES, W. P. T. (1988), Metabolic effects of isoenergetic nutrient exchange over 24 hours in relation to obesity in women. *Int. J. Obes.* **12**, 15–27.

74 MANN, J. I. (1983), in Mann J. L., Pyorala K. and Tescher A., eds. *Diabetes in Epidemiological Perspective.* London. Churchill Livingston, 122–39.

75 ANDERSON, J. W. and CHEN, W.-J. L. (1979), Plant fiber: Carbohydrates and lipid metabolism. *Am. J. Clin. Nutr.* **32**, 346–63.

76 JENKINS, D. J., WOLEVER, T. M., TAYLOR, R. H. *et al.* (1981), Glycemic index of foods: a physiological basis for carbohydrate exchange. *Am. J. Clin. Nutr.* **34** (3), 362–6.

77 NYGREN, C. (1984), Effects of bran in diabetes mellitus. Thesis, Gothenburg and Umeå.

78 JENKINS, D. J., JENKINS, A. L., WOLEVER, T. M., VUKSAN, V., RAO, A. V., THOMSON, L. U. and JOSSE, R. G. (1994), Low glycemic index: lente carbohydrates and physiological effects of altered food frequency. *Am. J. Clin. Nutr.* **59** (suppl), 706–9.

79 NATIONAL BOARD OF HEALTH. (2003), Centre for evaluation and technical assessment. Type 2 diabetes. Medical technology assessment of screening, diagnostic and treatment. Medical technology assessment **5**, 140–5.

80 THE EUROPEAN ASSOCIATION FOR THE STUDY OF DIABETES (the Diabetes and Nutrition Study: Group of the European Association for the Study of Diabetes (EASD). (2000), Recommendations for the nutritional management of patients with diabetes mellitus. *Eur. J. Clin. Nutr.* **54**, 353–5.

81 BRAND-MILLER, J., HAYNE, S., PETOCS, P. and COLAGIURI, S. (2003), Low glycemic index diets in the management of diabetes: a meta-analysis of randomized, controlled trials. *Diabetes Care* **26**, 2261–7.

82 FRANZ, M. J., BANTLE, J. P. BEEBE, C. A. *et al.* (2002), Evidence based nutrition principle and recommendations for the treatment and prevention of diabetes and related complications (technical review). *Diabetes Care* **25**, 148–98.

83 SCHLAMOWITZ, P., HALBERG, T., WARNØE, O., WILSTRUP, F. and RYTTIG, K. (1987), Treatment of mild to moderate hypertension with dietary fibre. Letter to the editor. *Lancet* 622–3.

84 ELIASSON, K., RYTTIG, K. R., HYLANDER, B. and RÖSSNER, S. (1989), A dietary fibre supplement in the treatment of mild hypertension. A randomized, double-blind, placebo-controlled trial. *J. Hypertension*, **13**, 227–32.

85 ANDERSON, J. W., STORY, L., SIELING, B., CHEN, W.-J. L., PETRO, M. S. and STORY, J. (1984), Hypocholesterolemic effects of oat-bran or bean intake for hypercholesterolemic men. *Am. J. Clin. Nutr.* **40**, 1146.

Part III
Commercial strategies, functional targets and agents in weight control

17

Consumer determinants and intervention strategies for obesity prevention

H. C. M. van Trijp, Wageningen University and Unilever Health Institute, The Netherlands, J. Brug, Erasmus University Medical Centre, The Netherlands and R. van der Maas, Unilever Health Institute, The Netherlands

17.1 Introduction

Overweight is an important and growing societal concern. This is probably best exemplified by statistics such as those from the World Health Organization (WHO). Globally, there are now more than 1 billion overweight adults of whom at least 300 million are severely overweight or obese (WHO, 2003, 2004). In the USA, in 1999–2000 approximately 64% of adults aged over 20 yr. were classified as overweight and 30% as obese (Drenowski and Specter, 2004). Childhood overweight is now 13% (*Lancet* Editorial, 2004). Similar prevalence levels have been reported for Australia and the United Kingdom. Slightly lower, but also high and growing, percentages of overweight and obesity are found in most other European countries. Furthermore, the problem of overweight and obesity is not restricted to industrialised countries. Many developing countries now face an obesity epidemic alongside problems related to under-nutrition. Obesity and overweight pose a major public health risk for chronic disease, including type-2 diabetes, cardiovascular disease, hypertension and stroke and certain forms of cancer (WHO, 2004). It is expected that overweight and obesity will soon surpass tobacco as the most important determinant of preventable disease (Peeters *et al.*, 2003). The medical costs associated with the obesity epidemic are staggering and will rise further in the years to come. In the USA alone, medical costs attributable to obesity were US$75 billion and that equates US$175 each year for each USA taxpayer (Finkelstein *et al.*, 2004).

Only very recently has being overweight and obese become a potential health threat for the majority of the population in many countries. Serious overweight and obesity was always the 'exception to the rule'. Interventions to fight overweight and obesity were, therefore, mostly aimed at weight loss treatment. However, with the present epidemic proportions of the problem, and the lack of long-term success of most treatments, population-based weight gain prevention interventions are needed to stop and reverse the epidemic (e.g. Kumanyika *et al.*, 2002). In order to develop, plan and implement effective interventions that promote weight maintenance in the population at large, insight is necessary into the determinants of weight gain. The most proximal determinant of weight gain is clear and simple: a positive energy balance. A positive energy balance means that caloric intake exceeds energy expenditure: eating too much and/or exercising too little. Eating and physical activity behaviours are thus the main cause of weight gain that may eventually result in becoming overweight or obese. Genetic and other biological factors are, of course, also important determinants of being overweight or obese and these factors may, for example, explain why some people seem to put on weight more easily than others do. However, the rapid rise in the worldwide prevalence of obesity cannot be explained by genetic changes (WHO, 1998).

Eating and exercising are not single acts but complex systems of a variety of behaviours. We do not eat calories as such, but many different foods that are combined in meals, prepared and processed in different ways, and consumed at different occasions. Furthermore, knowledge of the behavioural causes of weight gain is not enough. Such knowledge tells us what needs to be changed in order to prevent weight gain, but it does not tell us how we can change such behaviours. For intervention development we need to know why people engage in behaviours that make them gain weight, we need to know the mediators or determinants of the risk behaviours. Only interventions that tackle these mediators will result in behaviour change that may contribute to weight maintenance (Baranowski *et al.*, 1999, 2003; Bartholomew *et al.*, 2001). Each of the specific behaviours that contribute to a too high caloric intake may have its own behaviour specific determinants. For example, the reasons people have for eating energy-dense snacks may be very different from their reasons for choosing high fat instead of leaner milk products.

In line with the scope of this book, the present chapter will focus on the intake side of the energy balance equation: food intake and eating behaviours. We do not argue that energy intake is more important than energy output in promoting weight maintenance. As many others have rightly stated, probably the best strategy to stop and possibly reverse the obesity epidemic is to change food as well as exercise habits. Our focus on just the energy intake side of the equation does illustrate the complexity and multidisciplinarity of the study of the determinants of weight maintenance behaviours, intervention strategies tailored to these determinants, and the fact that this research area is still in its early stages (Crawford, 2002).

Over-consumption of calories, resulting in overweight and obesity is a multiply determined problem with determinants at the individual level of consumers, their direct social environments, as well as at the societal level (Mela, 2001; Swinburn *et al.*, 2004). Over-consumption may be influenced by such different factors as cultural norms about ideal weight and body image, by availability and accessibility of sufficient calories to feed a nation, availability and accessibility of specific foods in local food shops, and the eating behaviours of close relatives and friends.

The most proximal determinants of caloric intake involves a complexity of individual choices and decisions regarding food consumption, including whether to eat, how often to eat, what to eat, and how much to eat (Baranowski *et al.*, 2003). In the end, the societal problem of overweight and obesity finds its origin in the behavioural choices of individual consumers who ingest more calories than they burn. Therefore, prevention of, and solutions to, the problem of over-consumption are to be found in the effectiveness of influencing individual consumers' caloric intakes. As we will argue later in this chapter, this does not imply that interventions to promote weight maintenance should only be targeted at the individual consumers. It is very likely that intervention aiming to change the more distal, environmental determinants of over-consumption are more than necessary in order to make valuable changes in the choices and behaviour of individuals. In this chapter, we review behavioural determinants of caloric over-consumption based on the framework suggested by Rothschild (1999). This framework is particularly appropriate as it covers some of the key categories of determinants also identified in other reviews (e.g. Baranowski *et al.*, 2003) and links them to the most appropriate type of intervention strategy.

Several additional restrictions apply to this chapter. We already mentioned that we would only look at the energy input side of the energy balance equation. We will further aim our arguments at weight maintenance issues, i.e. prevention of weight gain, overweight and obesity, and not at weight loss. Finally, energy intake is the result of the consumption of many specific foods, in different combinations and on different occasions, that differ in their energy content. In this chapter, rather than discussing highly specific determinants of isolated food choices (e.g. determinants of choosing low fat milk or low calorie soft drinks) we address general categories of behavioural determinants of patterns of over-consumption.

Section 17.2 will review some of the most popular health behavioural change models (see also Baranowski *et al.*, 2003) and identify three key categories of behavioural determinants as proposed by Rothschild: motivation, ability and opportunity (MacInnis *et al.*, 1991). Section 17.3 will discuss some of the most important intervention strategies that have been proposed in various recent papers, and these strategies will be linked to the Rothschild framework. Section 17.4 will provide the conclusions.

17.2 Behavioural determinants of obesity

No comprehensive framework for studying and understanding determinants of weight gain inducing behaviours has been developed and agreed upon yet. Many attempts build on more general psychological models of determinants of human behaviour. Such models have been applied and found useful for investigating determinants of eating behaviours (Baranowski *et al.*, 2003; Conner and Armitage, 2002). Rothschild (1999) has suggested dividing behavioural determinants into three broad categories: motivation related, ability related and opportunity related (MacInnis *et al.*, 1991). Motivation involves the perceived self-interest of the consumer to engage in behavioural change. Abilities are the specific resources that are required to translate motivation into behavioural change, and opportunity is the extent to which the environment is supportive or dysfunctional for the behaviour change to occur. Largely based on Baranowski *et al.* (2003), Table 17.1 summarises the most important behavioural theories and some of their core constructs classified by motivation, ability and opportunity.

It is beyond the scope of this chapter to discuss the various models in detail and the reader is referred to Baranowski *et al.* (2003) for a review of these models with their theoretical background. What is important for our purpose is that, despite their differences in focus on theoretical underpinning, Table 17.1 highlights a considerable amount of communality between the models, particularly at the level of motivational constructs and ability.

Most of the models focus on a consumer evaluation of the (expected) positive and negative consequences or attributes of the healthy behaviour vs. the current behaviour as a key determinant of change. The concepts of attitude, cost–benefits, outcome expectancies, positive and negative values of outcomes of the behaviour, pros and cons of behavioural change and perceived self-interest in the behavioural change all address this common theme that we refer to as *decisional balance*. Some models, such as the popular Theory of Planned Behaviour and Social Cognitive Model further posit that *social determination* of behaviour and behavioural change is important.

Most theories further recognise that individual skills and ability should accompany motivation for the behavioural change to occur. *Health and nutrition knowledge* and *self-efficacy/perceived behavioural control* are key consumer resources in translating motivations into actual behaviour. Finally, particularly the (social) ecological models, and to some extent the behavioural learning theory models, work from the underlying assumption that behaviour is largely driven by *external stimuli*, the physical and personal factors in the environment that serve as direct cues for desirable and undesirable behaviour. They reflect the opportunities or lack of opportunities in the cultural, social and physical environment that may shape behaviours, possibly without too much cognitive interference. Other models view the environmental factors as a moderator of the attitude–intention–behaviour links (‘*barriers*’).

Table 17.1 Overview of the most important health behaviour change models and their key components (based on Baranowksi *et al.*, 2003)

Model	Motivation	Ability	Opportunity
Knowledge-Attitude-Behaviour[a]	Change in attitude	(accumulation of) knowledge	
Behaviour Learning Theory[b]	Aversive physiological drive (eg hunger)	Not applicable (stimulus driven)	
Health Belief Model[c] Protection Motivation Theory[d]	Level of perceived threat or the risk of a specific condition (readiness to act) as a combination of perceived seriousness and susceptibility	Self-efficacy	Barriers
Social Cognitive Theory[e]	Outcome expectancies, including social outcome expectancies Self-efficacy expectations	Skills Self-efficacy Self control	
Theory of Planned Behaviour[f]; ASE-model[g]	Positive and negative values of the outcomes of the behaviour Desire to comply with the expectations of the important people in one's life	Perceived behavioural control	
Transtheoretical model[h]	Pros and cons of behavioural change	Self-efficacy Process of change	
(Social) Ecological models[i]	No cognitive motivational concepts	Not clearly delineated. May include cues for action	Ecologies and social ecologies Availability and accessibility of healthy choices
Social Marketing[j]	Perceived self interest	Not well defined; includes self-efficacy	Barriers

Relevant references to each of the behavioural change models.
[a] Baranowski *et al.*, (2003), [b] Birch (1999), [c] Rosenstock (1990), [d] Hodgkin and Orbell (1998), [e] Baranowski *et al.* (2002), [f] Ajzen (1991), [g] Brug *et al.* (1995), [h] Greene *et al.*, (1999); Horvath (1999), [i] Catlin *et al.* (2003), [j] Lefebvre *et al.* (1995).

Because of the many similarities, attempts have been made to integrate the insights from the different theories (see, for example Armitage and Conner, 2000; Bartholomew *et al.*, 2001). These efforts generally support the assumption (e.g. Rothschild, 1999) that behavioural change can be successfully made if people are motivated and able to do so, and when the environment provides sufficient opportunities or even encourages behaviour change. The Rothschild framework thus recognises that motivation to behave is an important but insufficient condition for desired behavioural change. Not only should consumers be willing to act, they should also know what behavioural options they should engage in, and have the specific skills or abilities to act on their intentions. Finally, good intentions often fall short in light of the many seductions or lack of opportunity in the environment. Lack of opportunity refers to the situations in which the individual wants to act, knows what to do, but is unable to do so because there is no environmental mechanism (e.g. behavioural alternatives) at hand. In the next paragraph we will elaborate on these three categories of determinants.

17.2.1 Motivational factors in (over-)consumption

According to the theories discussed, people will only voluntarily restrict their caloric intake in order to promote a neutral energy balance when they are motivated to do so. Motivation is goal-directed arousal. Individuals are motivated to behave when they expect that their self-interest will be served. In the context of overweight, such self-interest may be health related as well as appearance related. Three proximal mediators of intention have been identified: a weighing of pros and cons that are expected from the behaviour, an assessment of how the social environment will react or act related to the behaviour and confidence in one's abilities to engage in the behaviour. We will now discuss the first two, while ability will be discussed later.

Motivation may occur at different levels and under different control mechanism. At the rational conscious *goal-directed level*, consumers may consider being healthy or attractive as an important goal in life (e.g. Satia *et al.*, 2001). Motivation occurs when consumers recognise that their actual situation is different from their ideal situation. Such a discrepancy may provoke goal-directed energy to restore equilibrium, in this particular case to reduce the energy intake. The assumption is that individuals realistically and correctly know their intake levels *vis-à-vis* ideal levels. Motivation may also emerge at the *social level* from a discrepancy between norms imposed by relevant others and the actual behaviour. This includes the social perception of ideal body weight and shape. At the *biological level*, motivation may occur from hard-wired biological mechanisms that favour or disfavour certain consumption patterns. Included are inborn preferences for sweet taste and satiety-conditioned preferences for fat and other energy-dense foods.

Decisional balance
If people perceive or expect a net benefit from a change toward healthy eating, they will be more likely to be motivated to change. On the other hand, motivation to start eating more healthily will be decreased when the unhealthy option is perceived as being less rewarding. This decisional balance, the weighing of expected pros and cons of a behaviour change, is a recurring theme in almost all of the models of human behaviour and behavioural change. Essentially, this defines the consumers' perceived self-interest in the behavioural change. Thus if a person expects more, as well as more important, positive consequences than negative consequences of caloric restriction, he will have a positive attitude and will be more likely to have a positive intention to restrict his dietary intake.

Positive perceived benefits in the desired behaviour reinforce the behavioural change, whereas negative perceived benefits reinforce the existing behaviour. Reinforcement may come from the reduction of aversive physiological drives (e.g. hunger), but also from cognitive mediation (e.g. health-related knowledge and beliefs). In the context of complex eating behaviour, reinforcement can occur in relation to health benefits of dietary habits but also, and more importantly, to the direct rewards of the behaviour in terms of taste, convenience and price. The behavioural learning theory model does assume less conscious cognitive mediation and assumes reinforcement against aversive physiological drives (e.g. hunger reduction). The behavioural economics model as a variant to behavioural learning theory assumes reinforcement more broadly in terms of costs and benefits. The Health Belief Model assumes that the perceived threat of a specific condition is a key motivational construct.

What do people consider to be important pros and cons related to dietary intake? In general, short-term pros and cons are more important than longer-term outcomes. Taste and pleasure are of major importance for most people. People will eat what they like, and disliked foods will not be chosen (Mela, 2001). Certain taste preferences are innate, such as a liking for sweet, a dislike for bitter, and possibly also the tendency to very quickly and easily learn to like the taste of energy dense (i.e. high fat) and thus satiating foods (Birch, 1999; Capaldi, 1996). However, taste preferences can be learned and unlearned (Birch, 1999), and the fact that many people like the taste of coffee, beer or even Brussels sprouts illustrates that we can even unlearn our innate dislike of bitter tastes. Next to taste, the decisional balance of eating fewer calories is also significantly influenced by the need for convenience (e.g. Furst *et al.*, 1996). Many consumers and particularly the 'baby boomers' seem unwilling to choose healthier options if this means compromising in terms of taste and convenience (Backman *et al.*, 2002; Glanz *et al.*, 1998). Similar results are obtained from HealthFocus (2000) studies which indicate that, in the USA and Australia, some 40% of consumers indicated to rarely or never giving up good taste for good health, and in Europe this percentage is as high as 57%. In Europe 42% of consumers indicate to rarely or never giving up convenience for good health compared to 24% in USA and Australia. Also, how well healthy eating is expected to fit with one's lifestyle in general can be a major hindrance to healthier behaviour. Busy lifestyles with little time for food preparation and food consumption tend to stimulate out-of-home consumption and less structured meals (e.g. snacking and grazing). Although neither of these necessarily needs to lead to increased consumption (more eating moments may actually promote energy balance), meals eaten out are often higher in energy than home-made meals and foods eaten in-between meals are mostly energy dense and not negatively compensated by less consumption in regular meals (Swinburn *et al.*, 2004). Not surprisingly 55% of US consumers indicate it is always/usually difficult to eat healthily out of home compared to only 20% who finds it always/usually difficult to eat healthily at home (HealthFocus, 2003).

Health values provide direction to food choices by prioritising the healthy options (Connors *et al.*, 2001). Health beliefs are important in the decisional balance, but most so when the health consequences are expected to be soon, severe and easy to recognise. People may therefore very quickly develop negative attitudes toward foods for which they are allergic or intolerant, i.e. foods that literally make you sick (Capaldi, 1996). However, many energy dense foods provide a comfortable feeling of satiety. The potential negative consequences of overweight, obesity and obesity-related diseases like diabetes or heart disease will present itself only decades later.

Social norms/influences

Much of human behaviour is driven by its social context and this also holds for what to eat, when to eat and in which quantity. Social influences are explicitly incorporated in several of the behavioural models discussed above. Social influence may exert its influence through subjective norms, social support and descriptive norms.

Although the three-meal-per-day pattern, with meals eaten with the family, is certainly not as common as it used to be, eating is still often an overt, public, and thus social behaviour. The ASE-model (Brug *et al.*, 1995; De Vries *et al.*, 1994) recognises three different categories of social influences: subjective norms, social support (or social pressure) and descriptive norms. People tend to do what they think that other people who are important to them want them to do. This is what the construct of subjective norm aims to capture. A person who thinks that his partner and children really want him to restrict his dietary intake in order to lose weight, will be more likely to be motivated to eat less, and thus will be more likely to indeed cut back on food. However, people can also be more directly pressured into participating in certain eating behaviours. We have all experienced that, at a dinner or birthday party, the host asks us in a rather decisive manner if we would like some cake. Social support or social pressure can also be subtler. Every construct can be further subdivided, and different types of social support have been proposed. One distinction is between structural and functional support, where structural support refers to the actual presence of significant others, or social integration, and functional support is the more subjective side, the perceived social support of those significant others. The third social influence is based on example behaviour. People whose significant others eat a low energy diet, will be more likely to do so themselves (e.g. Brug *et al.*, 1994, 1995). This is referred to as descriptive norm, modelling or social learning (Povey *et al.*, 2000). Perceptions of the behaviour of others are also important in self-evaluation by social comparison. People often evaluate their own actions by comparing their behaviour with that of others, especially when more objective evaluation criteria are lacking. For complex behaviours like energy intake, social comparison may be the first and foremost way for people to check their own performance (Oenema and Brug, 2003). Since people do not eat energy, like they smoke a cigarette, but eat different foods with different drinks, in different combinations, prepared in various ways, that all add up to a certain energy intake, it is very difficult for them to check their own behaviour by comparison with an objective recommendation. Social comparison may thus be a likely alternative. Oenema and Brug explored how often, where and with whom people compare themselves in order to evaluate their personal fat intake levels. The results indicated that people make social fat intake comparisons in many everyday situations and are more likely to compare themselves to people in their direct social environment than with famous role models (Oenema and Brug, 2003). Social comparisons are often biased and for everyday health-related behaviours like diet and physical activity, that people believe are under their volitional control, an optimistic bias is most likely (Weinstein, 1984). Many people are, for example, optimistically biased about their fat, fruit and vegetable intake, as well as about their amount of physical activity (Lechner *et al.*, 1998; Ronda *et al.*, 2001). They often think they are doing OK and better than most others, while this is not the case. Different studies also show that people may have a biased perception of their personal weight status. Men tend to be more likely to be optimistically biased about their weight status (they think they are not overweight, while their BMI > 25), while women are more likely to be too pessimistic about their weight status. Men will therefore be unlikely to be motivated to watch their weight while women may be more likely to engage in unnecessary and possibly dysfunctional weight loss attempts (Wardle and Johnson, 2002).

In this paragraph we argued that people tend to do what they want and what they are motivated to do. Motivation or intentions are a fairly good predictor of behaviour (Sheeran, 2002). In their meta-analysis, Godin and Kok (1996) showed intermediate to strong effect sizes for intention-behaviour associations for different health behaviours including diet and physical activities. Sheeran (2002) showed that lack of intention almost guarantees lack of behaviour. However, he also showed that a positive intention is important for behaviour, but certainly no guarantee. Jeffery (2004) showed that interventions tailored to motivation theory were, by and large, ineffective in inducing actual weight loss in obese patients. Simply prescribing dietary or exercise regimens or providing people with exercise equipment is more effective in inducing weight loss (Jeffery, 2004). Lack of abilities and opportunities can prevent good intentions from being turned into effective weight maintenance action.

17.2.2 Ability to change behaviour

People's behavioural choices can be restricted by their abilities. Even if you very much want to change your diet or physical activity pattern, you may just not be capable of actually doing so. Abilities are also related to motivation: people are more likely to intend to do things for which they are confident they will succeed. Rothschild thus recognises 'ability' as a second category of determinants that may promote or restrict energy balance behaviour change. If we want people to volitionally and voluntarily restrict their energy intakes and increase their energy expenditure in order to maintain a healthy weight and prevent weight gain, they should also be able to do so. Since the energy balance behaviours are such complex collections of different acts, people need many skills to maintain their weight. They, for example, need to know and recognise what foods and preparation methods fit better or worse in an energy balanced diet and they should have the skills to resist the urge to eat too much. However, whether a person is able to eat a low-energy diet is not only dependent on personal knowledge and skills, but also on the opportunities the environment offers. One needs fewer personal abilities to eat a low energy diet, when low-energy foods are readily available and prepared by some caretaker (spouse, parent, restaurant chef) than in a situation when one needs to search for, select and prepare such foods oneself. Thus, the opportunities (or lack of opportunities) our environment offers may interact with our personal abilities (see Section 17.2.3).

Knowledge and awareness

To make dietary changes for better bodyweight maintenance, knowledge is necessary about which changes will be effective in weight maintenance. Should one cut back on fat, on carbohydrates, or increase fibre intake? And which foods are high in fat, carbohydrates or fibre? And what are low fat or low-carb alternatives? Furthermore, many interventions to help people to lose weight or prevent weight gain are partly based on 'counting calories' i.e. to self-monitor one's diet to avoid caloric intake above a certain quantity. Knowledge about caloric content of foods is then necessary. However, earlier research has shown (e.g. Patterson *et al.*, 1996) that knowledge is not a direct determinant of healthy eating, but it may be necessary for self-efficacy (see next paragraph and Backman *et al.*, 2002).

The complexity of energy balance behaviour has been mentioned before. Since caloric intake and expenditure are determined by such a complex collection of different specific acts, from choosing foods, portion sizes and preparation methods, to transportation, work and leisure time physical activities, a great deal of knowledge may be necessary to effectively and consciously monitor energy balance behaviours. Not many people have such knowledge, or the arithmetic skills to put such knowledge into daily practice. Many people, therefore, tend to be unaware, and especially overly optimistic of their personal energy balance behaviour (see Social norms/influences in pp 338–40) (Lechner *et al.*, 1997; Ronda *et al.*, 2001) or their personal weight status. For example, in Europe only 20% of consumers self-report to be personally overweight, with as low as 15% in Germany (HealthFocus, 2000). At the same time consumer concern about being overweight seems to be gradually reducing in the USA from 49% being extremely or very concerned in 1994 to 40% in 2002 (HealthFocus, 2003). If people think that they already comply with recommendations for calorie restriction or physical activity, they will not experience a need to change, they will not be motivated to change, and will be much less likely to make actual changes. Also, many people may not be aware of all the possible health consequences of being overweight. In a recent survey in the Netherlands, only 18.3% and 6.3% of a national representative sample of adults aged 25–40 knew that being overweight is associated with higher risks for diabetes and cancer (Wammes *et al.*, 2005). In such instances, educating the public on the serious health consequences may be required to enhance ability. For example, research from HealthFocus (2003) shows that 39% of US consumers agree or strongly agree with the statement that 'it is possible to be overweight and still be healthy'. Similar levels (38%) are found in Australia and even higher (54%) in Europe (HealthFocus, 2000).

Self-efficacy, perceived behaviour control and confidence

Self-efficacy refers to the confidence in one's abilities to perform a desired behaviour in different challenging situations. A large body of research shows that people who have more confidence in their abilities to change are more motivated to change, will put more effort into their attempts to change, and will have a better chance to succeed. Self-efficacy is thus cognition, a perception of one's abilities, and such perceptions may not always be realistic representations of actual skills. Many people have biased perceptions of their own abilities or performance. Unrealistic optimism may result in change attempts that fail, and this will eventually lead to lower self-efficacy and thus a lower likelihood to try again. A pessimistic bias may lead to lack of change attempts.

17.2.3 Opportunities: the obesogenic environment

Childhood and maternal under-nutrition is the number one cause for the global burden of disease (Ezzati *et al.*, 2002) and a large proportion of the world population still live in environments characterised by shortage, rather than abundance, of food. However, for many people in many countries, more calories are available than needed for weight maintenance. In Rothschild's framework, in addition to motivation and ability, weight-maintenance behaviour is also largely determined by the opportunities that the environment presents. Several authors have argued that the present obesity epidemic is primarily the result of a so-called obesogenic environment that increasingly promotes high-energy intakes and sedentary behaviours (e.g. Poston and Foreyt, 1999; Swinburn, this volume; Swinburn *et al.*, 1999, 2004). To paraphrase Battle and Brownell (1996) referring to the US situation it is hard to envision an environment more effective than ours for producing obesity. A number of studies have been published that show associations between different characteristics of the physical or social environment and energy-balance behaviours (Berrigan and Troiano, 2002; Edmonds *et al.*, 2001; Kerr *et al.*, 2004; Sharpe *et al.*, 2004) or weight status indicators (Catlin *et al.*, 2003; Ewing *et al.*, 2003). Environmental restrictions to healthy weight maintenance habits are also perceived by consumers themselves as an important reason for their failure to eat a balanced diet and to be physically active (Bauer *et al.*, 2004). Based on such evidence social-ecological models of health and health behaviour have been proposed to inform prevention of overweight and obesity (Baranowski *et al.*, 2003; Catlin *et al.*, 2003; Green and Kreuter, 1999).

The obesogenic environment has been dissected (e.g. Swinburn *et al.*, 1999) into physical (what is available), economic (cost related to food), political (rules related to food) and socio-cultural (community's or society's attitudes, beliefs and value related to food) environments at the national (macro) or regional/local (micro) level. Some of the more specific, often strongly interrelated, key factors proposed to induce over-consumption include (see e.g. Nicklas *et al.*, 2001; Peters, 2003; Jeffery and Utter, 2003):

- Reduction of meal structures, resulting in more arbitrary and unplanned eating patterns
- An increased per capita availability of food energy
- High accessibility of palatable energy-dense foods
- High exposure to food advertising
- Increased portion sizes

Meals and snacking

Due to more individualised lifestyles within families, the traditional three-meal per day pattern has become less common. Snacking in-between meals has increased as well as out-of-home consumption. Even though distributing energy intake over more eating moments may help to maintain energy balance, most snacks eaten in between meals are energy dense foods that contribute to higher energy intakes (Zizza *et al.*, 2001). Furthermore, eating out has become more common, which may lead to higher energy intakes (French *et al.*, 2001).

An increased per capita availability of food energy and high accessibility of foods

In the USA the per capita food energy availability increased approximately 15% since 1970, and per capita energy availability tracked fairly well with BMI (Jeffery and Utter, 2003). Not only is more than enough food energy available, it has also been made readily accessible in a wide variety of ready-to-eat palatable, energy-dense foods. And in present-day society, such foods are accessible almost everywhere and at anytime, even in schools (Swinburn *et al.*, 2004). Furthermore, most people in industrialised countries have the key resources, e.g. the purchasing power (Peters, 2003), as well as the time, to consume more than enough energy. Also, energy-dense foods and diets tend to be less expensive than foods and diets with lower energy density (Drewnowski and Specter, 2004).

Increased exposure to advertising and other food promotion information sources

In their review, Jeffery and Utter reported that the food industry spends about $50 per person to promote food products, while the USDA spends only approximately $1.50 per person on nutrition education (Jeffery and Utter, 2003). Although the precise effects of food advertising on over-consumption remain unclear, Story and French do show that food advertising aimed at children is mainly for high fat, high sugar, and thus high energy foods, and that such advertising favours over-consumption (Story and French, 2004). The Health Committee of the UK House of Commons in their report on the UK obesity epidemic drew a similar conclusion (Obesity, 2004)

Large portion sizes

Serving size is an important determinant of how much people eat, independent of hunger levels (Capaldi, 1996), and larger serving sizes are associated with higher energy intakes (Matthiessen *et al.*, 2003). Young and Nestle showed that common market place portion sizes exceed the standard serving sizes as defined by the US Department of Agriculture by a factor of 2–8, and that portion sizes have increased significantly, sometimes up to five times the original size (Young and Nestle, 2003). Larger portion sizes are also served in restaurants, with the largest servings in fast food establishments (Nielsen and Popkin, 2003). Soft drink portion sizes have also been increased substantially, and increased soft drink and other sugar containing drinks has been identified as a likely cause for the increased prevalence of being overweight in children and adolescents (Swinburn *et al.*, 2004).

The fact that people in lower socio-economic positions are more likely to be overweight and obese (Van Lenthe and Mackenbach, 2002) may be because their environment may tend to induce a positive energy balance.

Lower socio-economic status neighbourhoods tend to be less safe, have a higher concentration of fast food outlets and fewer opportunities for recreation (Humpel *et al.*, 2004; Van Lenthe *et al.*, 2005). Schools are a micro-environment that has generated substantial interest, particularly for the increasing number of vending machines and fast food outlets in schools and the financial benefits the schools get out of this.

17.3 Intervention strategies

Insight into behavioural determinants of over-consumption is important because these determinants should be changed in order to prevent weight gain. Thus, interventions to prevent weight gain may be as multi-faceted and complex as the behavioural determinants themselves. Rothschild (1999) has suggested differentiating between three general intervention strategies for health issue management and that the appropriateness largely depends on whether unhealthy behaviour finds its basis in lack of motivation, lack of ability and/or lack of opportunity (MacInnis *et al.*, 1991). On the basis of their reward/reinforcement value and degree of voluntary change, Rothschild (1999) differentiates between 'education' (no direct reward and based on voluntary change), 'marketing' (voluntary change but based on reward and self-interest) and 'law' (based on punishment and coercion). *Education*, in the Rothschild terminology, refers *to messages of any type that attempt to inform and/or persuade a target to behave voluntarily in a particular manner but do not provide, on their own, direct and/or immediate reward or punishment.* In other words, education is aimed at providing the basic information on which consumers need to change their behaviour almost altruistically. *Marketing* approaches, on the other hand, try to build in reinforcement and reward and is defined by Rothschild as: *attempts to manage behaviour by offering reinforcing incentives and/or consequences in an environment that invites voluntary exchange.* Finally, *law* differs from the other two strategic tools primarily in its lack of voluntary-ness as this set of tools *involves the use of coercion to achieve behaviour in a non-voluntary manner or to threaten with punishment for non-compliance or inappropriate behaviour.* Others have suggested similar sets of overall strategies although using different terminology such as education, facilitation and regulation (Bartholomew *et al.*, 2001; Brug *et al.*, 2000). Clearly, the three strategic tools are not mutually exclusive and can, and should, be used in combination and in interaction. However, the framework (see Table 17.2) does help to identify in which situation which (combinations of) strategic tools are most appropriate

Intervention strategies to halt the obesity epidemic can focus on each combination of motivation, ability or opportunity to change behaviour. They can be diverse in nature and require specific efforts of various stakeholder groups. In the context of obesity and over-consumption, several

Table 17.2 Type of intervention strategy suggested on key barriers in consumer behaviour

Motivation	Ability	Opportunity	Consumer orientation	Primary tool(s)
Yes	Yes	Yes	Prone to behave	Education
Yes	Yes	No	Unable to behave	Marketing
Yes	No	Yes	Unable to behave	Education Marketing
Yes	No	No	Unable to behave	Education Marketing
No	Yes	Yes	Resistant to behave	Law
No	Yes	No	Resistant to behave	Marketing Law
No	No	Yes	Resistant to behave	Education Marketing Law
No	No	No	Resistant to behave	Education Marketing Law

authors have suggested specific intervention strategies. Rather than listing all the numerous individual attempts, in Table 17.3 we provide a selective overview of the population-based intervention strategies that have been suggested by various obesity taskforces (Swinburn *et al.*, 2004; Kumanyika *et al.*, 2002; WHO, 2003, 2004; IOFT, 2004; New Zealand Health Strategy, 2001; Kelly, 2004; US Department of Health and Human Services, 2001) and recent reviews (Carraro and Garcia Cebrian, 2003; French *et al.*, 2001). We classified these strategies according to the primary stakeholders and the specific category of determinants (motivation, opportunity and ability) they primarily focus on. Many of the intervention strategies require multi-stakeholder approaches, where government (through legislation and community based approaches), food suppliers (marketing) and public health actors (marketing and education) should work together with school and work environments and many others. In our overview of possible intervention strategies, we follow the format suggested by Kumanyika *et al.* (2002) but appreciate that this classification on stakeholders may not be fully accurate and sensitive.

Motivational strategies aim at changing the consumer's decisional balance in favour of the lower calorie alternatives. This can be achieved by making the healthy choice the easy choice in terms of the benefits that consumers derive from the healthier alternative. For example, by giving healthier options and consumption patterns a price advantage (subsidies) or giving unhealthy options and consumption patterns a price disadvantage (taxes, levies). Motivational strategies can also be executed by regulating the marketing and advertising strategies for unhealthy options more

Table 17.3 Examples of population-based intervention strategies as suggested by selective obesity taskforces and recent reviews, classified for their primary focus on motivation, ability or opportunity

Sources		Motivation	Opportunity	Ability
Government				
1,4,9	Price support (subsidies) for healthy foods	X		
2,4,8,9	Economic support for healthy food consumption	X		
4,9	Taxes for unhealthy foods	X		
2	Restrictions on advertisement of calorie dense food	X		
5	Advertisement that promotes healthier eating	X		
1,6,7,9	Ban marketing energy dense foods or drinks in schools, including sponsorship and advertising	X		
1,9	Supply of good fresh water to reduce dependency on sugar soft drinks		X	
1,8,9	Economics (dis)incentives for supply of (un)healthy food		X	
3,6,8	Promoting availability and accessibility of healthy foods		X	
5,6,7,8	Encourage food companies to provide lower energy, more nutritious food marketed at children		X	
4,9	Small levies on unhealthy food for nutritional promotion			X
5,8	Improve maternal nutrition and encouragement of breast feeding			X
5,8	Encourage schools to enact coherent food, nutrition, and physical activities policies			X
2,4,5,6,9	Legislation on correct and readable food labelling and health claims			X
4,6	Nutritional signposting of healthy options through endorsed logos			X
5	Encourage medical and health professionals to participate in the development of public health programmes			X
Food supply				
6	Promote healthy food choices	X		
1,6	Improve nutritional quality of food served in catering outlets		X	
1,6	Improve nutritional quality of general food supply		X	
6	Train catering staff in low fat food preparation and nutritional issues		X	
6	Encourage healthy catering at sports events		X	

1,6	Develop food labelling schemes to help consumers make informed choices		X
6	Encourage labelling info in supermarkets and demonstrations of healthy cooking		X
Media			
1,6,9	Regulate advertising and marketing practices that promote over-consumption of food and drink	X	
1	Ban advertising on television to young children	X	
1,3,6,9	Promote healthy lifestyle culture (incl. Media role models)	X	
2,6,8	Educational campaigns on nutrition and health problems, including weight issues		X
6	Food and nutrition training for media workers to counter misinformation		X
4,6	Communication strategies around key food based messages		X
6,9	Promote the consumption of water over non-alcoholic beverages		X
6,7	Assist parents to assess nutrition information and educate them on food issues		X
NGOs			
1	Promote and support action programmes	X	
Health care			
1,3,6,8	Train doctors and health care workers for preventive action and promotion of healthy diet by patients		X
2,6,7	Develop prenatal, preborn and paediatric care programmes to boost parental awareness of alimentary issues		X
4,7	Community wide intervention programmes to improve dietary patterns		X
4,8	Education and breast feeding support services and health profession training on this issue		X
4,6,7	Individual advice on prevention of weight gain and weight management		X
4	Individual adapted health behaviour change programmes		X
6	Provide nutrition and health information in primary care settings		X
6,7	Family based behaviour modification programmes		X

Table 17.3 *(continued)*

Sources		Motivation	Opportunity	Ability
Health insurance				
6	Link health insurance with health promotion		X	
Education				
1,6,8	Encourage choice of healthy foods (eg reward schemes)	X		
1,4,6,7,8,9	Improve nutritional quality of school meals to expose children to healthy foods and eating patterns		X	
4,6,7,8,9	School food policies/guidelines and standards of food bought and brought to school		X	
1,4,6,7	Empower students to prepare healthy meals; nutritional/cooking skills in curriculum			X
2,8	School based alimentary education and prevention programmes			X
Work places				
1,6	Encourage healthy food choices in staff restaurants through subsidies	X		
1,6,9	Improve nutritional quality of foods available in work places (staff restaurants)		X	
4,8	Food policies in work environments; healthy foods available and promoted		X	
4	Breast feeding-friendly environments		X	
6	Providing obesity and weight control management programmes			X
Direct environment				
1	Increase access of low income groups to healthy foods through community garden programmes and food co-operatives		X	
1,6	Increase access to consumption of F&V through home gardening programmes		X	

Sources: (1) Kumanyika *et al.* (2002), (2) Carraro and Cebrian (2003), (3) WHO (2003, 2004), (4) Swinburn *et al.* (2004), (5) Iotf (2004), (6) New Zealand Health Strategy (2001), (7) Kelly (2004), (8) US Department of Health and Human Services (2001), (9) French *et al.* (2001).

generally and by using social marketing tools to actually enhance and position healthy eating. Media and governmental efforts should go hand in hand with these public health efforts, with the support of non-governmental organisations. Also, such strategies should be extended into the direct environment of the consumer such as in schools and in work places.

Strategies to strengthen abilities need to complement the motivational strategies, to ensure that consumers have accurate and transparent information on the nutrition and health value of food alternatives and dietary habits, as well as the skills to put this knowledge into practice. This is the more conventional educational strategy on nutritional and health problems as well as food-based messages. Governments play a key role in initiating and funding these campaigns, some of which may be funded from small levies on unhealthy products. Also, governments can play a key role in initiating such educational programmes in school environments (school curriculum and education and prevention programmes) and in primary and public health care (community wide intervention programmes). Health insurance companies can play a role here as well, as they also have a vested financial interest. Health care strategies should be based on direct individual contact with the more enduring relationships with the 'patient', allowing for individual advice and tailoring of health behaviour change programmes. However, this would involve training doctors and health care workers for preventive action in the area of overweight and healthy diet. So-called computer-tailored interventions, computer expert systems that provide individually tailored behaviour change advice, may help such health professionals in giving their patients expert advice (Kreuter *et al.*, 2000). Education on, and promotion of, breast-feeding can be one of the complementary strategies. Consumer ability may also be enhanced by correct, clear and simple to understand labelling of food products on the basis of their caloric content, including sign posting through endorsed logos.

In addition to intrinsic motivation and ability to consume healthier diets, availability and accessibility of healthier options (i.e. opportunity to consume) are critical factors in healthier diets. The omnipresence of calorie dense foods in today's societies seriously hampers the translation of motivation, knowledge and skills in actual weight maintenance behaviour. Availability and accessibility of healthier options is largely determined by the food supply (primarily retailers and out-of-home food outlets) on the basis of economic principles. These drivers have an important responsibility in ensuring that the nutritional quality of food in catering outlets and supermarkets is being improved. Schools and work places also share this responsibility in terms of food policies and guidelines on what is being made available, promoted and allowed. If the market does not self-regulate the availability of healthy assortments, on the basis of motivation and purchasing power, governments may have to regulate this on the basis of law, regulations and economic incentives. However, such legislative strategies do assume that consensus exists on what foods promote and what foods prevent weight gain or ill health, in terms of their caloric content, energy-density or nutrient composition. This is far from the case, a situation that probably favours 'promoting good foods' rather than 'penalising bad foods'. Also, the provision of public goods as an alternative (e.g. good quality fresh water) and community-based programmes on fresh produce (e.g. home gardening projects) may further support selection of healthier options.

In summary, Table 17.3 provides support for the three lines of intervention strategies suggested by Rothschild (1999) and provides concrete examples of such intervention strategies. No single driver will be able to redirect current eating patterns, as each of the three lines of intervention strategies requires a joint and collaborative effort of multiple stakeholders. Current public health efforts to halt the obesity epidemic have not been very successful and this may be partly due to the fact that they focus on one category, rather than on all three categories, of behavioural determinants.

17.4 Conclusions

At a conceptual level, this chapter has summarised some of the current thinking on behavioural determinants of over-consumption and how insight into these determinants may help to develop population-based intervention strategies to halt the obesity epidemic.

Most established models on eating behaviour tend to emphasise motivation and skills as key determinants of eating behaviour. More recently, the important role of the environment in shaping energy-balance behaviour has been advocated. However, isolating personal or environmental factors will be insufficient to induce sustainable behaviour change (Baranowski *et al.*, 2003). Peters (2003) recently argued along similar lines, arguing that in our current efforts, the broad spectrum of consumer determinants of eating patterns has been insufficiently taken into account: 'we have attempted to change eating and physical activity patterns, behaviours that are motivated by multiple drivers, not necessarily health, through mediators that are not of primary importance to the individual at the point of decision, given the totality of immediate personal priorities and rewards facing the problem (p 9S–10S)'. We tend to agree with Peters (2003) and Baranowski *et al.* (2003) in that, only if there is a strong consumer motivation based on adequate knowledge on nutrition and health, skills and social facilitation, as well as a supportive physical environment that facilitates rather than hinders healthy energy balance behaviours, will a majority of consumers adopt eating patterns that promote weight maintenance. In current market conditions each of these three conditions is far from satisfied, rendering over consumption almost a 'societal choice' (Peters, 2003). Only with a joint and integrated effort of all key actors in the field (governments, food suppliers, media, health care services, educational systems, NGOs, homes and families and work environments) will we be able to begin to halt and revert obesity as a fact of life (French *et al.*, 2001, Kumanyika *et al.*, 2002). In this chapter we have therefore argued that behavioural change is most likely to occur if motivation, ability and opportunity are all there, which will require education and marketing, as well as legislation (Rothschild, 1999; MacInnis *et al.*, 1991).

Consumer knowledge on diet and health issues and transparency in product supply (in terms of nutritional labelling) are important factors for consumers who are motivated to eat an energy-balanced diet. Also, knowledge on health issues and personal health status can, in itself, underpin the motivation to act. However, when the intrinsic motivation is lacking, more knowledge will not likely materialise in healthier food choices. Although most people are motivated to avoid weight gain in general, the present day environment appears to be too challenging for most people to really avoid weight gain. In line with the Rothschild framework (Rothschild, 1999) more coercion-based approaches (law and regulations) may need to be implemented. As Peters (2003) argued, halting the obesity epidemic will require a number of fundamental changes in the organisation of society. As markets are unlikely to fully self-regulate (in light of limited consumer demand), legislation will be inevitable to 'enforce' motivation and to reduce seduction in the environment. Such legislation should be developed in close collaboration with food suppliers and media to achieve synergy with the activities already going on in the area of health product development and healthy consumption communication. Several multinational food companies have already started to give nutrition and health a more central place in their corporate purposes and are reviewing and adjusting their product portfolios. Legislation should support or enforce this development and further speed it up and help ensure that healthy business can be a profitable business.

However, it is important to realise that the effectiveness of many of the population-based obesity prevention strategies has not yet been established. They are more or less 'common-sense' suggestions, and effective evaluation of such population-wide interventions will be difficult (Rootman *et al.*, 2001). What is, however, clear enough for most well informed experts is that more than health education is needed to halt the obesity epidemic (see Table 17.3). These strategies should be implemented on a trial basis and evaluated for their effectiveness with wide support of the variety of stakeholders. As Nestle and Jacobson (1999) stated: 'without such a national commitment and effective new approaches to making the environment more favourable to maintaining healthy weight, we doubt that the current trend can be reversed'.

17.5 References

AJZEN, I. (1991), 'The theory of planned behavior', *Organ. Behav. Hum. Dec.*, **50**, 179–211.

ARMITAGE, C. J. and CONNER, M. (2000), 'Social cognition models and health behaviour: a structured review', *Psychol. Health*, **15**, 173–89.

BACKMAN, D. R., HADDAD, E. H., LEE, J. W., JOHNSTON, P. K. and HODGKIN, G. E. (2002), 'Psychosocial predictors of healthful dietary behavior in adolescents', *J. Nutr. Educ. Behav.*, **34**, 184–92.

BARANOWSKI, T., CULLEN, K. W. and BARANOWSKI, J. (1999), 'Psychosocial correlates of dietary intake: advancing dietary intervention', *Annu. Rev. Nutr.*, **19**, 17–40.

BARANOWSKI, T., PERRY, C. L. and PARCEL, G. (2002), 'How individuals, environments and health behaviors interact: social cognition theory' in Glanz K, Lewis F M and Rimer B, *Health Behavior and Health Education: Theory, Research and Practice*, 3rd ed., San Fransisco CA, Jossey Bass, 246–79.

BARANOWSKI, T., CULLEN, K. W., NICKLAS, T., THOMPSON, D. and BARANOWSKI, J. (2003), 'Are current health behavioral change models helpful in guiding prevention of weight gain efforts', *Obes. Res.*, 11 (Oct, suppl), 23S–43S.

BARTHOLOMEW, K., PARCEL, G., KOK, G. and GOTTLIEB, N. (2001), *Intervention Mapping; Designing Theory- and Evidence-based Health Education Programs*, Mountain View CA: Mayfield.

BATTLE, E. K. and BROWNELL, K. D. (1996), 'Confronting a rising tide of eating disorders and obesity: treatment vs. prevention and policy', *Addict. Behav.*, **21** (6), 755–65.

BAUER, K. W., YANG, Y. W. and AUSTIN, S. B. (2004), 'How can we stay healthy when you're throwing all of this in front of us? Findings from focus groups and interviews in middle schools on environmental influences on nutrition and physical activity', *Health Educ. Behav.*, **31**, 34–46.

BERRIGAN, D. and TROIANO, R. P. (2002), 'The association between urban form and physical activity in U.S. adults', *Am. J. Prev. Med.*, **23**, 74–9.

BIRCH, L. L. (1999), 'Development of food preferences', *Annu. Rev. Nutr.*, **19**, 41–62.

BRUG, J., LECHNER, L. and DE VRIES, H. (1995), 'Psychosocial determinants of fruit and vegetable consumption', *Appetite.*, **25**, 285–96.

BRUG, J., SCHAALMA, H., KOK, G., MEERTENS, R. and VAN DER MOLEN, H. T. (2000), *Planmatige gezondheidsvoorlichting [planned health education]*, Assen: Van Gorcum.

BRUG, J., VAN ASSEMA, P., LENDERINK, T., GLANZ, K. and KOK, G. J. (1994), 'Self-rated dietary fat intake: association with objective assessment of fat, psychosocial factors and intention to change', *J. Nutr. Educ.*, **26**, 218–23.

CAPALDI, E. D. E. (1996), *Why We Eat What We Eat: The Psychology of Eating*, Washington DC: American Psychological Association.

CARRARO, R. and GARCIA CEBRIAN, M. (2003), 'Role of prevention in the contention of obesity epidemic', *Eur. J. Clin. Nutr.*, **57** (suppl 1), S94–6.

CATLIN, T. K., SIMOES, E. J. and BROWNSON, R. C. (2003), 'Environmental and policy factors associated with overweight among adults in Missouri', *Am. J. Health Promot.*, **17**, 249–58.

CONNER, M. and ARMITAGE, C. J. (2002), *The Social Psychology of Food*, Buckingham, Open University Press.

CONNORS, M., BISOGNI, C. A., SOBAL, J. and DEVINE, C. M. (2001), 'Managing values in personal food systems', *Appetite.*, **36**, 189–200.

CRAWFORD, D. (2002), 'Population strategies to prevent obesity – only few studies attempted so far and with limited success', *Br. Med. J.*, **325** (7367) (Oct 5 2002), 728–9.

DE VRIES, H., BACKBIER, E., DIJKSTRA, M. and VAN-BREUKELEN, G. (1994), 'A Dutch social influence smoking prevention approach for vocational school students', *Health Educ. Res.*, **9**, 365–74.

DREWNOWSKI, A. and SPECTER, S. E. (2004), 'Poverty and obesity: the role of energy density and energy costs', *Am. J. Clin. Nutr.*, **79** (1), 6–16.

EDMONDS, J., BARANOWSKI, T., BARANOWSKI, J., CULLEN, K. W. and MYRES, D. (2001), 'Ecological and socioeconomic correlates of fruit, juice, and vegetable consumption among African-American boys', *Prev. Med.*, **32**, 476–81.

EWING, R., SCHMID, T., KILLINGSWORTH, R., ZLOT, A. and RAUDENBUSH, S. (2003), 'Relationship between urban sprawl and physical activity, obesity, and morbidity', *Am. J. Health Promot.*, **18**, 47–57.

EZZATI, M., LOPEZ, A. D., RODGERS, A., VANDER HOORN, S. and MURRAY, C. J. (2002), 'Selected major risk factors and global and regional burden of disease', *Lancet*, **360**, 1347–60.

FINKELSTEIN, E. A., FIEBELKORN, I. C. and WANG, G. (2004), 'State-level estimates of annual medical expenditures attributable to obesity', *Obes. Res.*, **12** (1), 18–24.

FRENCH, S. A., STORY, M. and JEFFERY, R. W. (2001), 'Environmental influences on eating and physical activity', *Annu. Rev. Publ. Health*, **22**, 309–35.

FRENCH, S. A., STORY, M., NEUMARK-SZTAINER, D., FULKERSON, J. A. and HANNAN, P. J. (2001), 'Fast food restaurant use among adolescents: associations with nutrient intake, food choices and behavioral and psychosocial variables', *Int. J. Obesity*, **25**, 1823–33.

FURST, T., CONNORS, M., BISOGNI, C., SOBAL, J. and FALK, L. (1996), 'Food choice: a conceptual model of the process', *Appetite.*, **26**, 247–56.

GLANZ, K., BASIL, M., MAIBACH, E., GOLDBERG, J. and SNYDER, D. (1998), 'Why Americans eat what they do: taste, nutrition, cost, convenience, and weight control concerns as influences on food consumption', *J. Am. Diet Assoc.*, **98**, 1118–26.

GODIN, G. and KOK, G. (1996), 'The theory of planned behavior: a review of its applications to health-related behaviors', *Am. J. Health Promot.*, **11** (2), 87–98.

GREEN, L. W. and KREUTER, M. W. (1999), *Health Promotion Planning: An Educational and Ecological Approach*, 3rd ed., Mountain View CA: Mayfield.

GREENE, G. W. ROSSI, S. R., ROSSI, J. S., VELICER, W. F., FLAVA, J. L. and PROCHASKA, J. O. (1999), 'Dietary applications of the stages of change model', *J. Am. Diet Assoc.*, **99**, 673–8.

HEALTHFOCUS (2000), 'HealthFocus® Study of Public Attitudes and Actions Toward Shopping and Eating', Europe 2000, St. Petersburg FL, HealthFocus International®.

HEALTHFOCUS (2003), 'The 2003 HealthFocus Trend Report: National Study of Public Attitudes and Actions Towards Shopping and Eating', St. Petersburg FL, HealthFocus International®.

HODGKIN, S. and ORBELL, S. (1998), 'Can Protection Motivation Theory predict behaviour? A longitudinal test exploring the role of previous behavior', *Psychol. Health*, **13**, 237–50.

HORVATH, C. C. (1999), 'Applying the transtheoretical model to eating behavior change: challenges and opportunities', *Nutr. Res. Rev.*, **12**, 281–317.

HUMPEL, N., OWEN, N., LESLIE, E., MARSHALL, A. L., BAUMAN, A. E. and SALLIS, J. F. (2004), 'Associations of location and perceived environmental attributes with walking in neighborhoods', *Am. J. Health Promot.*, **18**, 239–42.

IOFT (2004), The report, 'Obesity in children and young people: a crisis in public health', has been issued by the International Obesity Task Force (IOTF) of the WHO in co-operation with the International Association for the Study of Obesity (IASO) in May 2004.

JEFFERY, R. W. (2004), 'How can health behavior theory be made more useful for intervention research?' *Int. J. Behav. Nutr. Phys. Act*, **1**: 10 (23 July 2004).

JEFFERY, R. W. and UTTER, J. (2003), 'The changing environment and population obesity in the United States', *Obes. Res.*, **11** (Oct; suppl), 12S–22S.

KELLY, M. P. (2004), Briefing paper on the Evidence of effectiveness of public health interventions – and their implications. NHS: Health Development Agency, based on Mulvihill and Quigley (2003).

KERR, N. A., YORE, M. M., HAM, S. A. and DIETZ, W. H. (2004), 'Increasing stair use in a worksite through environmental changes', *Am. J. Health Promot.*, **18** (4), 312–5.

KREUTER, M., FARRELL, D., OLEVITCH, L. and BRENNAN, L. (2000), *Tailoring Health Messages: Customizing Communication with Computer Technology*, Mahway (NJ): Lawrence Elbaum.

KUMANYIKA, S., JEFFERY, R. W., MORABIA, A., RITENBAUGH, C. and ANTIPATIS, V. J. (2002), 'Obesity prevention: the case for action', *Int. J. Obes.*, **26**, 425–36.

LANCET EDITORIAL (2004), 'Who pays in the obesity war?', *Lancet*, **363** (Jan 31), 339.

LECHNER, L., BRUG, J. and DE VRIES, H. (1997), 'Misconception of fruit and vegetable consumption: differences between objective and subjective estimation of intake', *J. Nutr. Educ.*, **29**, 313–20.

LECHNER, L., BRUG, J., DE VRIES, H., VAN ASSEMA, P. and MUDDE, A. (1998), 'Stages of change for fruit, vegetable and fat intake: consequences of misconception', *Health Educ. Res.*, **13**, 1–11.

LEFEBVRE, R. C., LURIE, D., SAUNDERS GOODMAN, L., WEINBERG, L. and LOUGHREY, K. (1995), 'Social marketing and nutrition education: inappropriate or misunderstood?', *J. Nutr. Educ.*, **27**, 1146–50.

MACINNIS, D. J., MOORMAN, C. and JAWORSKI, B. J. (1991), 'Enhancing and measuring consumers' motivation, opportunity and ability to process brand information from ads', *J. Marketing*, **55** (Oct), 32–53.

MATTHIESSEN, J., FAGT, S., BILTOFT-JENSEN, A., BECK, A. M. and OVESEN, L. (2003), 'Size makes a difference', *Public. Health Nutr.*, **6**, 65–72.

MELA, D. J. (2001), 'Determinants of food choice: relationships with obesity and weight control', *Obes. Res.*, **9** (Nov. Suppl 4), 249S–55S.

MULVIHILL, C. and QUIGLEY, R. (2003), 'The management of obesity and overweight. An analysis of reviews of diet, physical activity and behavioural approaches', *Evidence Briefing*, 1st edn (October). www.hda.nhs.uk/evidence

NESTLE, M. and JACOBSON, M. F. (1999), 'Halting the obesity epidemic: a public health policy approach', *Public Health Rep.*, **115**, 12–24.

NEW ZEALAND HEALTH STRATEGY (2001), DHB Toolkit: Obesity; edition 1 (October 2001).

NICKLAS, T. A., BARANOWSKI, T., CULLEN, K. W. and BERENSON, G. (2001), 'Eating patterns, dietary quality and obesity', *J. Am. Coll. Nutr.*, **20** (6), 599–608.

NIELSEN, S. J. and POPKIN, B. M. (2003), 'Patterns and trends in food portion sizes 1977–1998', *JAMA*, **289**, 450–3.

OBESITY (2004), London: House of Commons – Health Committee.

OENEMA, A. and BRUG, J. (2003), 'Exploring the occurrence and nature of interpersonal comparisons of one's own dietary fat intake to that of self-selected others', *Appetite*, **41** (3), 259–64.

PATTERSON, R. E., KRISTAL, A. R. and WHITE, E. (1996), 'Do beliefs, knowledge, and perceived norms about diet and cancer predict dietary change?', *Am. J. Public Health*, **86**, 1394–400.

PEETERS, A., BARENDREGT, J. J., WILLEKENS, F., MACKENBACH, J. P., MAMUN, A. A. and BONNEUX, L. (2003), 'Obesity in adulthood and its consequences for life expectancy: a life-table analysis', *Ann. Intern. Med.*, **138**, 24–32.

PETERS, J. C. (2003), 'Combating obesity: challenges and choices', *Obes. Res.*, **11** (Oct; suppl), 7S–11S.

POSTON, W. S. C. and FOREYT, J. P. (1999), 'Obesity is an environmental issue', *Atherosclerosis*, **146** (2), 201–9.

POVEY, R., CONNER, M., SPARKS, P., JAMES, R. and SHEPHERD, R. (2000), 'The theory of planned behaviour and healthy eating: examining additive and moderating effects of social influence variables', *Psychol. Health*, **14**, 991–1006.

RONDA, G., VAN ASSEMA, P. and BRUG, J. (2001), 'Stages of change, psychological factors and awareness of physical activity levels', *Health Promot. Int.*, **16**, 305–14.

ROOTMAN, I., GOODSTADT, M., HYNDMAN, B. *et al.* (2001), *Evaluation in Health Promotion: Principles and Perspectives*, Copenhagen: WHO Regional Office for Europe.

ROSENSTOCK, I. M. (1990), 'The health belief model: explaining health behavior through expectancies', in Glanz K, Lewis F M and Rimer B K, *Health Behavior and Health Education: Theory, Research, and Practice*, San Francisco CA, US: Jossey-Bass Inc, Publishers.

ROTHSCHILD, M. L. (1999), 'Carrots, sticks and promises: a conceptual framework for the management of public health and social issue behaviors', *J. Marketing*, **63** (October), 24–37.

SATIA, J. A., KRISTAL, A. R., CURRY, S. and TRUDEAU, E. (2001), 'Motivations for healthful dietary change', *Public Health Nutr.*, **4** (5), 953–9.

SHARPE, P. A., GRANNER, M. L., HUTTO, B. and AINSWORTH, B. E. (2004), 'Association of environmental factors to meeting physical activity recommendations in two South Carolina counties', *Am. J. Health Promot.*, **18**, 251–7.

SHEERAN, P. (2002), 'Intention-behavior relations: a conceptual and empirical review', in Hewstone M and Stroebe W, *European Review of Social Psychology, 12*, Chichester, John Wiley & Son, 1–36.

STORY, M. and FRENCH, S. (2004), 'Food advertising and marketing directed at children and adolescents in the US', *Int. J. Behav. Nutr. Phys. Act*, **1**, 3 (10 Febr 2004).

SWINBURN, B. A., EGGER, G. and RAZA, F. (1999), 'Dissecting obesogenic environments: the development and application of a framework for identifying and prioritizing environmental interventions for obesity', *Prev. Med.*, **29**, 563–70.

SWINBURN, B. A., CATERSON, I., SEIDELL, J. C. and JAMES, W. P. T. (2004), 'Diet, nutrition and the prevention of excess weight gain and obesity', *Public Health Nutr.*, **7** (1A), 123–46.

US DEPARTMENT OF HEALTH AND HUMAN SERVICES (2001), 'The Surgeon General's call to action to prevent and decrease overweight and obesity'. Rockville, MD. www.surgeongeneral.gov/library [based on priorities for action]

VAN LENTHE, F. and MACKENBACH, J. (2002), 'Neighbourhood deprivation and overweight: the GLOBE study', *Int. J. Obesity*, **26**, 234–40.

VAN LENTHE, F. J., BRUG, J. and MACKENBACH, J. P. (2005), 'Neighbourhood inequalities in physical activity: the role of neighbourhood attractiveness, proximity to local facilities and safety in the Netherlands', *Soc. Sci. Med.*, **60** (4), 763–75.

WAMMES, B., KREMERS, S., BREEDVELDT, B. and BRUG, J. (2005), 'Correlates of motivation to prevent weight gain: a cross-sectional study', *Int. J. Behav. Nutr. Phys. Act*, **2** (1), 1.

WARDLE, J. and JOHNSON, F. (2002), 'Weight and dieting: examining levels of weight concern in British adults', *Int. J. Obesity*, **26**, 1144–9.

WEINSTEIN, N. D. (1984), 'Why it won't happen to me: perceptions of risk factors and susceptibility,' *Health Psychol.*, **3**, 431–57.

WHO (1998), *Obesity: Preventing and Managing the Global Epidemic*. Geneva: WHO.

WHO (2003), *Diet, Nutrition and the Prevention of Chronic Disease*. Report of a Joint WHO/FAO expert consultation. Geneva 28 January-1 February 2002. WHO Tech Rep Series 916.

WHO (2004), *Global Strategy on Diet, Physical Activity and Health*. Resolution WHA57.17. Geneva, WHO.

YOUNG, L. R. and NESTLE, M. (2003), 'Expanding portion sizes in the US marketplace: implications for nutrition counseling', *J. Am. Diet Assoc.*, **103**, 231–4.

ZIZZA, C., SIEGA-RIZ, A. M. and POPKIN, B. M. (2001), 'Significant increase in young adults' snacking between 1977–1978 and 1994–1996 represents a cause for concern!', *Prev. Med.*, **32**, 303–10.

18

Fat oxidation, appetite and weight control

M. Leonhardt and W. Langhans, Swiss Federal Institute of Technology

18.1 Introduction

Obesity is now a global health problem of epidemic proportions. Worldwide more than 1 billion adults are overweight, and at least 300 million of them are obese (World Health Organization (WHO), 2004). Obesity is a major risk for chronic diseases including type 2 diabetes, coronary heart disease and different forms of cancer (World Health Organization (WHO), 2004; Office of the Surgeon General, 2001; Kopelman, 2000). The tremendous increase in obesity is supposedly related to a combination of genetic susceptibility, decreased physical activity, and a high level of dietary fat (Kopelman, 2000). Several studies in humans have demonstrated a positive relationship between the level of fat intake and body weight (Astrup *et al.*, 2000; Bray and Popkin, 1998; Huot *et al.*, 2004; Mosca *et al.*, 2004; Saris *et al.*, 2000; Satia-Abouta *et al.*, 2002). Although the important contribution of high fat intake to the development of obesity is widely accepted, it is also clear that fat cannot be the only culprit (for review see Willett, 1998), and recent findings even suggest that high fat low carbohydrate diets lead to weight loss (e.g. Brehm *et al.*, 2003). High fat diets may normally increase the obesity risk because of (i) the usually high energy density of such diets (Rolls, 2000; Westerterp-Plantenga, 2001), (ii) the often high palatability of fat-rich foods (Drewnowski, 1998), and (iii) the finding that fats seem to have a lower short-term satiating capacity than carbohydrates (for review see Blundell and Stubbs, 1999). In short-term studies, the macronutrients protein, carbohydrate and fat exert hierarchical effects on satiety, with protein having the greatest and fat the weakest effect (see Blundell and Stubbs, 1999). The macronutrients' satiating potency mainly reflects the rate at which they are oxidised, which, in turn, is inversely related to the body's storage capacity for fat (very high), carbohydrate (intermediate) and protein (low). Accordingly, a high protein high carbohydrate diet has a greater thermogenic effect than a high fat diet (for review see Westerterp-Plantenga, 2003). These findings suggest that the oxidation of metabolic fuels generates a satiety signal and, in consequence, if nutrients are stored rather than oxidised they are less satiating (for review see Friedman, 1990, 1998; Langhans, 1996). Yet, although fat seems to have a weaker short-term satiating effect than carbohydrate and protein, it is also clear that ingestion of fat does inhibit eating. Gastrointestinal peptides and proteins such as cholecystokinin (CCK) and apolipoprotein A-IV, which are released in response to fat digestion, presumably contribute to the satiating effect of fat (for review see Degen *et al.*, 2001; Ritter, 2004; Tso *et al.*, 2004; Tso and Liu, 2004). In addition, the finding that inhibition of fatty acid oxidation is associated with enhanced eating in animals and humans suggests that the oxidation of fatty acids affects food intake (for review see Langhans, 1996, 2003). In this chapter we will summarise the current knowledge about the role of fatty acid oxidation in control of energy intake as well as body weight and composition.

18.2 Inhibition of fatty acid oxidation and food intake

In 1986 Scharrer and Langhans (Scharrer and Langhans, 1986) showed that the acyl-CoA-dehydrogenase inhibitor mercaptoacetate (MA) inhibits fatty acid oxidation and stimulates eating in rats fed an 18% (w/w) fat diet. Since then the phenomenon of 'lipoprivic eating' (Ritter and Taylor, 1989) has been extended to other fatty acid oxidation inhibitors, such as methyl-palmoxirate and etomoxir (for review see Scharrer, 1999), and other species, including humans (Kahler *et al.*, 1999). The potency of MA to induce eating appears to be positively correlated with the fat content of the diet (SingerKoegler *et al.*, 1996), and MA specifically increased carbohydrate and protein but not fat intake in a macronutrient preference study (Singer *et al.*, 1998). In rats, the stimulation of eating in response to an intraperitoneal (IP) injection of MA was mainly due to a meal initiating effect, whereas meal size remained unaffected (Langhans and Scharrer, 1987b). In humans, on the other hand, etomoxir increased the size of a scheduled meal, whereas the post-meal interval remained unaffected (Kahler *et al.*, 1999).

18.2.1 Mechanism of the eating stimulatory effect of fatty acid oxidation inhibitors

So far, it is not clear whether the inhibition of fatty acid oxidation in a single organ is sufficient to increase food intake. Yet, it is known that the liver plays a key role in whole body fat metabolism. Major tasks of the liver comprise the conversion of carbohydrates into fatty acids (*de novo* lipogenesis), the uptake, storage and release of lipids and, hence, the control of blood lipid levels, and the oxidation of fatty acids, including the production of ketone bodies which serve as an energy source for other organs in fasting. Further, the liver has a very high metabolic rate, as reflected by the fact that it accounts for only 4% of body weight, but for 20% of the organism's total energy expenditure under basal conditions. Normally, the liver covers most of its own energy (ATP) needs by oxidizing fatty acids (Seifter and Englard, 1994). Therefore, it is reasonable to assume that the liver is sensitive to changes in fatty acid availability and/or metabolism.

The finding that hepatic branch vagotomy markedly attenuated the induction of eating by MA suggests that it stimulates eating by acting in the liver or in the small intestine (Langhans and Scharrer, 1987a). Lipoprivic eating appears to be triggered by a decrease in hepatic energy status because it was shown to critically depend on a decrease in hepatic ATP (Friedman *et al.*, 1999). Different metabolic inhibitors in fact synergistically decreased the hepatic ATP/ADP ratio and the phoshorylation potential, and increased food intake (Horn *et al.*, 2004; Ji *et al.*, 2000). The assumption that MA acts peripherally and probably in the liver to stimulate eating is also in line with findings demonstrating (i) that hepatic branch vagotomy eliminated the stimulating effect of MA on eating in rats receiving total parenteral nutrition (Beverly *et al.*, 1994) and (ii) that intraportal MA infusion increased afferent activity in the common hepatic branch of the vagus (Lutz *et al.*, 1997). In addition, capsaicin pretreatment, subdiaphragmatic vagotomy, and lesion of the vagal sensory terminal fields in the area postrema (AP) and in the nucleus of the solitary tract (NTS) abolished lipoprivic eating (Ritter and Taylor, 1989, 1990). Furthermore, injection of MA into the lateral or fourth ventricle of rats failed to increase food intake (Ritter and Taylor, 1989). All these findings indicate that peripheral rather than brain sensors are involved in lipoprivic eating, and that lipoprivic eating requires intact subdiaphragmatic vagal sensory neurons. It is not exactly known how this afferent signal is processed in the brain. Yet, MA increased the mRNA level of melanin-concentrating hormone (MCH) in the lateral hypothalamic area (Sergeyev *et al.*, 2000) and decreased galanin gene expression and peptide immunoreactivity in the anterior parvocellular region of the paraventricular nucleus (Wang *et al.*, 1998). The marked orexigenic effect of MCH might well contribute to MA-induced feeding, and the suppression of galanin activity is consistent with the fat-sparing stimulation of feeding by MA (Singer *et al.*, 1998).

To summarise, most results are consistent with the assumption that the liver is probably involved in lipoprivic eating; yet, the contribution of other peripheral organs, such as the small intestine, cannot be excluded.

18.3 Stimulation of fatty acid oxidation and food intake

In contrast to the strong case for an eating stimulatory effect of an inhibition of fatty acid oxidation (see above), the evidence for an eating suppressive effect of a stimulation of fatty acid oxidation, in particular in the liver, is inconsistent and comparatively weak.

18.3.1 Medium-chain triglycerides (MCT)

Several animal (Bray *et al.*, 1980; Denbow *et al.*, 1992; Furuse *et al.*, 1992) and human (Stubbs and Harbron, 1996; Van Wymelbeke *et al.*, 1998) studies suggest that medium-chain triglycerides (MCT, fatty acids = eight to twelve carbons) enhance satiety and decrease energy intake compared to long-chain triglycerides (LCT, fatty acids > 12 carbons). Medium-chain fatty acids (MCFA) are absorbed into the portal vein and are rapidly taken up and oxidised by the liver, whereas fatty acids from dietary LCT are packed into chylomicrons and bypass the liver via the lymphatic system, favoring uptake of fatty acids into adipose tissue and muscle (for review see St Onge and Jones, 2002). In addition, the transport of MCFA into the mitochondria does not require carnitine palmitoyltransferase-1 (CPT-1) and is therefore not a rate limiting step in MCFA oxidation, as it is for the oxidation of long-chain fatty acids (LCFA) (Williams *et al.*, 1968). Ingestion or administration of MCT increases fat oxidation more than LCT (DeLany *et al.*, 2000; Van Wymelbeke *et al.*, 2001), and the increase in plasma ketone bodies, e.g. β-hydroxybutyrate, after MCT administration indicates that hepatic fatty acid oxidation is increased (Krotkiewski, 2001; Nakamura *et al.*, 1994; Van Wymelbeke *et al.*, 2001).

Therefore, it is tempting to speculate that the greater hepatic uptake and oxidation of MCFA compared to LCFA is involved in the eating suppressive effect of MCT. In a recent experiment of ours, infusion of the medium-chain fatty acid caprylic acid (CA) into the hepatic portal vein increased the plasma level of β-hydroxybutyrate, indicating that hepatic fatty acid oxidation was increased. In addition, CA decreased the size of the first dark phase meal only when it was infused into the portal vein, whereas an equivalent infusion into the vena cava had no effect on short-term food intake (U. L. Jambor de Sousa *et al.*, unpublished data). These data are consistent with the assumption that an increase in hepatic fatty acid oxidation is involved in the eating suppressive effect of CA. Yet, CA also decreased the preference for saccharin solution and reduced the rate of gastric emptying, suggesting that other effects of CA might contribute to the suppression of food intake after hepatic portal vein infusion (Jambor de Sousa *et al.*, 2003). Another explanation for the eating suppressive effect of MCT might be its stimulating effect on CCK production. In rats MCT oil leads to a much greater and more prolonged secretion of CCK than beef tallow, fish oil or corn oil (Douglas *et al.*, 1990). Yet, in humans, ingestion of MCT oil does not induce CCK release (Hopman *et al.*, 1984) but reduces food intake (Stubbs and Harbron, 1996). Further, IP injection of the CCK-A receptor antagonist devazepide increased food intake in MCT- and LCT-treated rats equally so that the difference in food intake between the MCT and LCT group was maintained. These findings suggest that CCK is not an important mediator of the eating suppressive effect of MCT (Furuse *et al.*, 1992). In sum, the mechanism of the eating suppressive effect of circulating MCFA is still unknown and possibly neither related to an increase in hepatic fatty acid oxidation nor to an increase in CCK secretion. Finally, it should be mentioned that MCT did not reduce food intake in all studies (Hill *et al.*, 1993; Maggio and Koopmans, 1982). Maggio and Koopmans (1982) reported equivalent reductions of food intake in rats in response to equicaloric intragastric infusions of MCT and LCT. In this experiment short-chain triglycerides (SCT, two to six carbons) induced a greater eating suppressing effect during the first hour of eating than MCT or LCT (Maggio and Koopmans, 1982). The authors explained their findings with the fact that SCT are digested and absorbed more rapidly than MCT and LCT and therefore SCT could interact with so far unknown receptors in the gut (Maggio and Koopmans, 1982).

MCT also appears to increase energy expenditure (Kasai *et al.*, 2002), in part through activation of the sympathetic nervous system (Dulloo *et al.*, 1996), which may account for the decrease in body fat accumulation (Noguchi *et al.*, 2002). Another interesting finding is that LCFA but not MCFA oxidation is negatively correlated with fat mass (Binnert *et al.*, 1998). These findings suggest a disturbance of LCFA oxidation in obese people, who might therefore profit from a substitution of dietary LCT by MCT (Binnert *et al.*, 1998; Tsuji *et al.*, 2001).

All in all, when compared to LCT, MCT appears to reduce energy intake (Stubbs and Harbron, 1996; Van Wymelbeke *et al.*, 1998), increase energy expenditure (Kasai *et al.*, 2002) and reduce fat accumulation in adipose tissue (Tsuji *et al.*, 2001). Yet, most of the pertinent studies were acute and/or employed enormous amounts of MCT (Dulloo *et al.*, 1996; Kasai *et al.*, 2002; Stubbs and Harbron, 1996; Van Wymelbeke *et al.*, 1998). This questions the usefulness of MCT for the treatment of obesity, in particular because possible adverse symptoms such as nausea, vomiting, gastrointestinal and abdominal discomfort limit the amount of MCT that may be incorporated in the diet. Finally, negative metabolic effects of MCT, e.g. increased ketosis, *de novo* fatty acid synthesis, and hypertriglyceridemia might further limit the use of MCT in the treatment of obesity (for review see Bach *et al.*, 1996).

18.3.2 Conjugated linoleic acid (CLA)

In 1979 Pariza *et al.* (1979) described for the first time that beef contains a substance that has mutagenic inhibitory activity. Later on it was established that the anticarcinogen in beef is conjugated linoleic acid (CLA) (Pariza, 2004). CLA is a collective term for a class of conjugated dieonic isomers of linoleic acid. Most of the physiologic effects of CLA rest with the two isomers c9,t11-CLA and t10,c12-CLA (for review see Pariza, 2004). With the discovery that CLA also reduces white adipose tissue mass in many species including mouse (DeLany *et al.*, 1999; West *et al.*, 1998), rat (Azain *et al.*, 2000; Sisk *et al.*, 2001) and pig (Ostrowska *et al.*, 1999), CLA received much interest as a potential substance for the treatment of obesity in humans. Yet, CLA did not affect food intake in most studies (Azain *et al.*, 2000; DeLany *et al.*, 1999), suggesting that it mainly increases energy expenditure (West *et al.*, 1998). In addition, the t10,c12-CLA isomer produces body composition changes, whereas c9,t12-CLA is almost ineffective in reducing adipose tissue mass (Pariza *et al.*, 1999; Park *et al.*, 1999).

Several studies demonstrate that CLA increases fatty acid oxidation. For example, perfused livers from rats fed a 1% CLA mixture for two weeks produced significantly more ketone bodies than livers from 1% linoleic acid-fed rats (Sakono *et al.*, 1999) suggesting that hepatic fatty acid oxidation was increased by CLA. In line with this interpretation, Rahman *et al.* (2001) demonstrated that CLA enhanced the activity of CPT-1, a rate-limiting enzyme for fatty acid β-oxidation, in adipose tissue, muscle and liver. Yet, Martin *et al.* (2000) reported that CLA only increased adipose tissue and not liver CPT-1 activity (for review see also McLeod *et al.*, 2004; Wang and Jones, 2004). How exactly CLA stimulates fatty acid oxidation is not clear. Yet, CLA is a ligand for certain peroxisome proliferators-activated receptors (PPARs) (for review see Taylor and Zahradka, 2004) such as PPARα, which is predominantly expressed in liver, kidney and heart (Moya-Camarena *et al.*, 1999). As PPARα is involved in the regulation of inducible (peroximal β-oxidation) and constitutive (mitochondrial β-oxidation) lipid oxidation (Moya-Camarena and Belury, 1999), it is likely that CLA stimulates fatty acid oxidation by activating PPARα.

CLA may be able to reduce body fat gain and to increase lean body mass also in humans, but the effects are smaller than in comparable rodent studies. Kamphuis *et al.* (2003) demonstrated that CLA supplementation after body weight loss enhanced the regain of lean body mass and, hence, increased resting metabolic rate without affecting total body weight regain (Kamphuis *et al.*, 2003). CLA supplementation for 1 year also increased lean body mass and reduced body fat in healthy overweight humans (Gaullier *et al.*, 2004). As CLA reduces body fat, it was suggested that CLA might also positively influence risk factors for the development of atherosclerosis and insulin resistance. Most animal studies in fact support this assumption. Thus, CLA reduced plasma triglyceride and total plasma cholesterol concentration in hamsters (Gavino *et al.*, 2000) and improved insulin sensitivity in Zucker diabetic fatty rats (Houseknecht *et al.*, 1998; Ryder *et al.*, 2001). Some studies, however, reported negative effects of CLA: 1% CLA induced lipodystrophy accompanied by an increase in tumor necrosis factor (TNF)-α and uncoupling protein (UCP)-2 mRNA in white adipose tissue, as well as by marked hepatomegaly and insulin resistance in female mice (Tsuboyama-Kasaoka *et al.*, 2000). In male rats, 2% CLA induced lipid peroxidation and fat deposition in the liver (Yamasaki *et al.*, 2000), and in obese men CLA induced hyperproinsulinemia (Riserus *et al.*, 2004b) and insulin resistance (Riserus *et al.*, 2002), and increased oxidative stress and inflammatory biomarkers (for review see Riserus *et al.*, 2004a). The reason for these conflicting data is unclear and might be related to species differences and different study designs. Further, these negative effects were unfortunately caused by the isomer t10,c12-CLA, the same isomer that most potently reduces body fat (Riserus *et al.*, 2004b; Roche *et al.*, 2002). c9,t11-CLA did not induce insulin resistance; it rather improved lipid metabolism, which was presumably due to reduced hepatic expression of the sterol regulatory element-binding protein (SREBP) and the oxysterol liver x receptor (LXR)-α. Further, c9,t11-CLA reduced TNF-α expression in white adipose tissue in male ob/ob mice (Roche *et al.*, 2002) (for review see Aminot-Gilchrist and Anderson, 2004).

Overall, CLA appears to be effective in reducing fat mass and enhancing lean body mass in rodents and, to a lesser extent, also in humans without affecting food intake. As CLA influences many metabolic pathways, it is impossible to assess the contribution of changes in fatty acid oxidation to any effect of CLA on energy balance. Further studies are needed to clarify whether CLA might have negative effects, such as increased production of peroxides, increased inflammation and reduced insulin sensitivity, before the use of CLA as a supplement in human nutrition can be recommended.

18.3.3 *n*-3 polyunsaturated fatty acids (*n*-3 PUFA)

The effects of polyunsaturated fatty acids (PUFA), in particular of the *n*-3 family such as eicosapentaenoic (EPA) and docosahexaenoic acids (DHA), on food intake, body weight and composition as well as on insulin resistance have often been tested (for review see Clarke, 2000; Rivellese *et al.*, 2002). It is also well documented that *n*-3 fatty acids increase fatty acid oxidation. EPA in particular increased mitochondrial fatty acid oxidation by increasing the activity of CPT-1, whereas DHA increased mRNA of fatty acyl-CoA oxidase and, therefore, enhanced peroximal fatty acid oxidation (Madsen *et al.*, 1999). Dietary fish oil supplementation (18 or 24% of the diet w/w) reduces food intake and body weight gain in rats (Del Prete *et al.*, 2000; Hill *et al.*, 1993), and in diet-induced obese mice *n*-3 PUFA reversed excessive body weight gain (Huang *et al.*, 2004). In this study *n*-3 PUFA normalized hypothalamic neuropeptide expression, e.g., NPYmRNA in the arcuate nucleus was decreased, whereas pro-opiomelanocortin mRNA was increased by *n*-3 PUFA (Huang *et al.*, 2004). Further, in rats *n*-3 PUFA also increased brown adipose tissue UCP-1 mRNA level (Takahashi and Ide, 2000) and induced a marked stimulation of brown fat thermogenesis (Oudart *et al.*, 1997). In both studies *n*-3 PUFA had no major effect on food intake, but epididymal white fat mass was reduced by *n*-3 PUFA, suggesting that *n*-3 PUFA indeed increased energy expenditure (Oudart *et al.*, 1997; Takahashi and Ide, 2000). Finally, fish oil prevented insulin resistance induced by a high-fat (Alsaif and Duwaihy, 2004; Storlien *et al.*, 1987) or a high sucrose diet in rats (Aguilera *et al.*, 2004; Soria *et al.*, 2002).

Interestingly, *n*-3 PUFA and CLA share several characteristics. Both substances seem to act as fuel partitioners in that they shift fatty acids away from triglyceride synthesis and storage in adipose tissue towards fatty acid oxidation. This effect seems to be mainly related to the fact that CLA and *n*-3 PUFA both activate PPARs, induce genes encoding proteins involved in fatty acid oxidation (Clarke, 2000; Madsen *et al.*, 1999; Moya-Camarena *et al.*, 1999), and inhibit genes involved in lipogenesis, presumably by reducing SREBP-1 expression (Roche *et al.*, 2002; Sekiya *et al.*, 2003). *n*-3 PUFA and CLA also inhibit tumor growth, but the exact mechanism of this effect is unknown (for review see Field and Schley, 2004; Larsson *et al.*, 2004). Surprisingly, both substances had adverse effects on glycemic control in obese individuals (Mori *et al.*, 2000; Pariza *et al.*, 1999; Riserus *et al.*, 2004a, b; Woodman *et al.*, 2002). The mechanism of this negative effect is unknown, but an increase in hepatic gluconeogenesis caused by an increase in hepatic fatty acid oxidation might contribute (Woodman *et al.*, 2002).

To summarise, the amount of *n*-3 PUFA that reduced food intake in animal studies cannot be recommended for human nutrition. Whether moderate amounts of dietary *n*-3 PUFA can affect body composition and food intake is unclear. In addition, because *n*-3 PUFA affects different metabolic pathways, a possible contribution of an increase in fatty acid oxidation to any reduction in food intake and body weight by *n*-3 PUFA cannot be determined. As for CLA, further studies are necessary to test whether *n*-3 PUFA might have adverse effects on insulin sensitivity in obese people under certain circumstances.

18.3.4 High fat – low carbohydrate diet ('Atkins diet')

Over the last years, diets that restrict carbohydrate intake (low carbohydrate or 'Atkins' diet) have become very popular. Although the composition of these diets is not exactly defined, their common goal is to substantially limit carbohydrate intake. The hypothesis is that high protein, low carbohydrate diets promote the breakdown of adipose tissue in the absence of available dietary carbohydrate and, hence, result in rapid weight loss without significant adverse effects. Yet, opponents of such diets claim that a low carbohydrate diet might be dangerous because it causes an accumulation of ketone bodies in the blood and hyperlipidemia, and because it may result in abnormal metabolism of insulin and impaired liver and kidney function due to the high protein content (Bravata *et al.*, 2003).

Meanwhile, the results of several well-controlled human studies with low carbohydrate diets have been published. In most of these studies no major side effects were observed, body weight loss was achieved and, hence, certain risk factors for cardiovascular diseases or diabetes were improved (Dashti *et al.*, 2003; Meckling *et al.*, 2004; Samaha *et al.*, 2003; Sharman *et al.*, 2004; Westman *et al.*, 2002; Yancy *et al.*, 2004). In one study (Yancy *et al.*, 2004), in which the effect of a low-carbohydrate, ketogenic diet on obesity and hyperlipidemia was compared, participants' compliance with the dietary programme and weight loss were greater with the low carbohydrate than with the low fat diet (Yancy *et al.*, 2004). Similarly, others reported that subjects voluntarily reduced energy intake on a low carbohydrate diet (Brehm *et al.*, 2003). In this study, subjects were randomly assigned to 6 months of either a very low carbohydrate diet *ad libitum* or of a calorie-restricted diet with 30% of the calories as fat. Although the subjects consuming the very low carbohydrate diet were not asked to restrict their energy intake, they voluntarily reduced intake to a level comparable to that of the restricted diet group, and after 6 months on the very low carbohydrate diet subjects had lost more weight and body fat than low fat diet subjects (Brehm *et al.*, 2003). A meta-analysis reviewing 107 articles describing 94 different dietary interventions using low carbohydrate diets (Bravata *et al.*, 2003) revealed that, in obese people, weight loss was positively correlated with the duration of the diet and the restriction of energy intake, but not with restriction of carbohydrate content. Moreover, low carbohydrate diets seemed to have no adverse effects on metabolic parameters such as serum lipids, fasting serum glucose and insulin concentrations, and on blood pressure (Bravata *et al.*, 2003).

To summarise, low carbohydrate diets seem to increase the participants' compliance with a diet programme and might therefore be useful for achieving body weight loss. At present, it is unclear whether an enhanced hepatic fatty acid oxidation combined with increased plasma levels of ketone bodies enhances the satiating effect of such diets and, thus, contributes to the reduction in energy intake. Another, and probably more likely, interpretation is that subjects eat less because of the very limited choice of foods that this low carbohydrate diet offers. Finally, very little is currently known about the safety of long-term use of such diets and whether such a diet regime is also useful for weight maintenance.

18.4 Inhibition of fatty acid synthesis

Until recently, textbook knowledge held that neurons only metabolize glucose and ketone bodies and that fatty acid metabolism is irrelevant in the brain. Over the last few years this view has changed. In 2000 Loftus *et al.* (2000) demonstrated that the fatty acid synthase inhibitor C75 reduced food intake and body weight after systemic and intracerebroventricular administration in mice (Loftus *et al.*, 2000). Recently, it has been shown that chronic C75 treatment reduced food intake, adipose tissue mass and hepatic steatosis in diet-induced obese mice (Thupari *et al.*, 2004). C75 blocks the conversion of malonyl-CoA into fatty acids and, hence, increases tissue levels of malonyl-CoA (Loftus *et al.*, 2000). An increase in hypothalamic malonyl-CoA and subsequent changes in the expression of hypothalamic orexigenic (NPY, AgrP) and anorectic (POMC, CART) neuropeptides are presumably involved in the eating inhibitory effect of C75 (Kumar *et al.*, 2002). In addition, C75 reduced the activity of the energy sensor AMP-activated protein kinase (AMPK), as reflected by a reduced level of phosphorylated hypothalamic AMPKα (Kim *et al.*, 2004; Landree *et al.*, 2004). AMPK appears to control food intake by responding to hormonal and nutrient signals in the hypothalamus (Minokoshi *et al.*, 2004). The finding that AICAR, an activator of AMPK, reversed C75-induced anorexia and the reduced levels of pAMPK further suggests that C75 reduces food intake through a reduction of AMPK activity in the hypothalamus (Kim *et al.*, 2004).

Malonyl-CoA inhibits CPT 1 activity. Consequently an increased level of malonyl-CoA in the liver should decrease the activity of CPT-1 and therefore decrease hepatic fatty acid oxidation. Paradoxically, however, C75 turned out to be a CPT-1 agonist in primary hepatocytes. Thupari *et al.* (2002) demonstrated that IP injected C75 increased fatty acid oxidation in adipose tissue and liver despite a high level of malonyl-CoA. The increased fatty acid oxidation in response to C75 enhanced the cellular energy turnover and decreased hepatic fat content (Thupari *et al.*, 2002). Also in primary cultures of cortical neurons, C75 stimulated CPT-1 and increased intracellular ATP levels, similar to its effects in peripheral tissues (Kim *et al.*, 2004; Landree *et al.*, 2004).

Overall, C75 seems to decrease food intake and body weight in mice and rats, and the reduction of body weight persists even after chronic treatment. Yet, there are still several unanswered questions. Clegg *et al.* (2002) demonstrated that, in rats, IP but not ICV C75 had aversive properties. Also, IP injection of C75 induced severe loosening or liquefaction of stools in mice, and C75 did not only affect anorexigenic POMC and orexigenic NPY neurons of the hypothalamic arcuate nucleus. Rather, C75 also activated cerebellar Purkinje neurons that are not involved in control of food intake (Takahashi *et al.*, 2004), suggesting that C75 is a nonspecific neural activator. Yet, it should be mentioned that IP C75 did not always induce a conditioned taste aversion in mice (for negative results see Kim *et al.*, 2002), and the reasons for these discrepancies are unclear.

Finally, C75 increased CPT-1 activity and ATP production in neurons concomitant with a reduction in food intake, whereas Obici *et al.* (2003) demonstrated that inhibition of hypothalamic CPT-1 also decreases food intake and glucose production. Mice lacking acetyl-Co carboxylase-2 have an increased rate of fatty acid oxidation in different tissues, yet, their food intake is increased instead of reduced (Abu-Elheiga *et al.*, 2001). All in all, nutrient sensing in the hypothalamus seems to be important for the regulation of food intake and body weight, and this may also hold for fatty acids and/or fatty acid oxidation. But, further research is needed to understand the exact mechanisms involved (for review see Obici and Rossetti, 2003).

18.5 Effects of changes in fatty acid oxidation on glucose tolerance

Changes of fatty acid oxidation, in particular in liver and brain, are not only important with respect to food intake and body weight, but also for the control of glucose metabolism and, hence, insulin resistance.

In 1963 Randle *et al.* proposed that glucose and fatty acid oxidation are inversely related ('glucose-fatty acid cycle') (Randle *et al.*, 1963). Thus, an increased uptake and oxidation of non-esterified fatty acids (NEFA) and ketone bodies in peripheral tissues, such as muscle, will reduce the uptake and oxidation of glucose (Randle *et al.*, 1963; Randle, 1998). This hypothesis has been confirmed by the finding that NEFA impair peripheral and splanchnic glucose uptake (Saltiel and Kahn, 2001), enhance hepatic glucose production (Foley, 1992; Randle, 1998), and inhibit insulin suppression of glycogenolysis (Gupta *et al.*, 2000). Finally, approximately 50% of the insulin that is released into the portal vein is immediately degraded in the liver (Bergman, 2000), but a high portal vein concentration of NEFA decreases hepatic insulin clearance (Bergman, 2000). Consistent with the glucose–fatty acid cycle, a short-term inhibition of fatty acid oxidation reduces hepatic glucose output and improves fasting plasma glucose (Ratheiser *et al.*, 1991; Deems *et al.*, 1998). Diraison *et al.* (1998), however, could not find any evidence of an increased hepatic fatty acid oxidation or an increased gluconeogenesis in type 2 diabetes. Finally, prolonged inhibition of CPT-1α promoted triglyceride accumulation in liver cells and increased glucose production during a hyperinsulinemic-euglycemic clamp, suggesting that the insulin sensitivity of the liver was reduced (Dobbins *et al.*, 2001). Inhibition of fatty acid oxidation also increased the intramyocellular lipid content of muscle, and this was correlated with the occurrence of insulin resistance in rats (Dobbins *et al.*, 2001). The exact mechanism of insulin resistance due to lipid accumulation in muscle is unknown. It is likely, however, that increased cytosolic levels of long-chain fatty acyl CoAs lead to altered insulin signaling or enzyme activities (e.g. glycogen synthase), either directly or via chronic activation of mediators such as protein kinase C (Kraegen *et al.*, 2001). Accumulation of long-chain fatty acyl CoAs in neurons caused by oleic acid infusion into the third cerebral ventricle (Obici *et al.*, 2002) or by inhibiting CPT-1 improved glucose tolerance. This effect was related to a suppression of hepatic glucose production (Obici *et al.*, 2003) due to a reduced expression of hepatic glucose-6-phosphatase (Morgan *et al.*, 2004).

In general, short-term and long-term studies are necessary to examine the effect of an increased fatty acid oxidation in different tissues on insulin sensitivity in healthy individuals and in diabetic subjects.

18.6 Implications and recommendations

Many findings suggest that fatty acid metabolism is involved in the control of food intake and body weight. MCT are oxidised faster than LCT, and they seem to enhance satiety and to increase energy expenditure. Yet, large amounts of MCT cause side effects such as nausea, vomiting and abdominal discomfort. CLA and *n*-3 PUFA might be useful in the prevention of obesity, but it is presently unclear whether consumption of these fatty acids can be recommended in obese people with reduced glucose tolerance. A restricted intake of a high fat, low carbohydrate diet might be useful for achieving body weight loss, but it is uncertain whether chronic consumption of such a diet is safe and nutritionally balanced. A further risk of trying to maintain a very low carbohydrate diet intake is that people will slowly increase carbohydrate intake and eventually end up consuming a high fat high carbohydrate diet that cannot be recommended. The *de novo* lipogenesis inhibitor C75 has been tested so far only in rodents, and it is unknown whether C75 is effective and safe in humans. To summarise, all substances discussed (Fig. 18.1) are not 'miracle pills' and will not cure obesity. An increase in fatty acid oxidation might be involved in the effects of some of these substances on food intake and body composition. Yet, all of them influence several pathways, and a final judgement of the contribution of an increase in fatty acid oxidation, in particular in the liver, to satiety is impossible. At the moment it is also not clear whether an increase in hepatic fatty acid oxidation might further increase insulin resistance in diabetic patients or in people with reduced glucose tolerance.

18.7 Conclusions and future trends

As it is impossible to quantify the contribution of a change in fatty acid oxidation to the changes in food intake, as well as body weight and composition, caused by various substances, other approaches are needed to critically examine the contribution of fatty acid oxidation to the control of food intake and energy balance. A good target to manipulate fatty acid oxidation is the enzyme CPT-1, which catalyses the rate limiting step in the mitochondrial oxidation of LCFA (for review see Eaton, 2002). CPT-1 is located on the mitochondrial outer membrane and catalyzes the transfer of LCFA

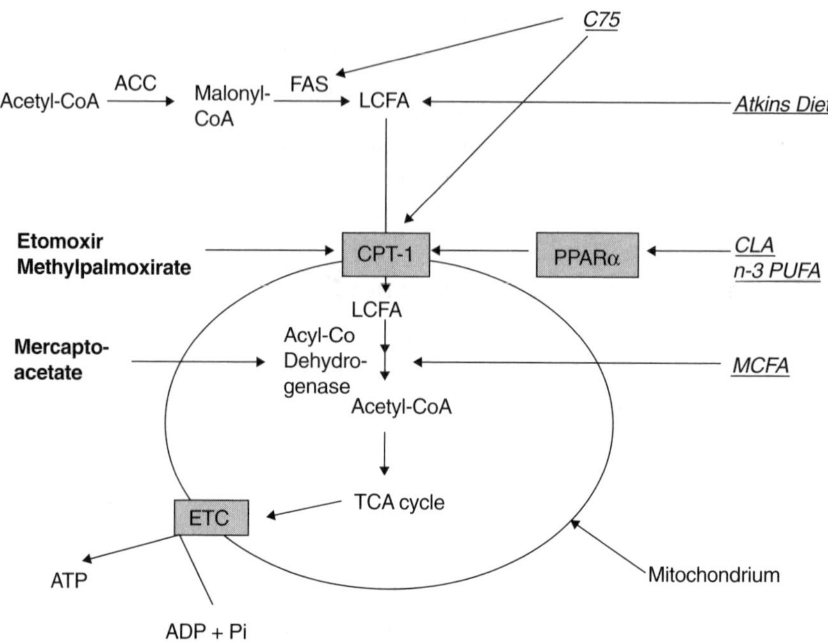

Fig. 18.1 Diagram depicting the effects of several substances on mitochondrial fatty acid oxidation; bold letters: substances that inhibit fatty acid oxidation; italic and underlined letters: substances that increase fatty acid oxidation; abbreviations: ACC: acetyl-CoA-carboxylase; FAS: fatty acid synthase; CPT-1: carnitine palmitoyltransferase-1; PPARα: peroxisome proliferator-activated receptors; TCA: tricarboxylic acid; ETC: electron transport chain; LCFA: long-chain fatty acids; MCFA: medium-chain fatty acids, CLA: conjugated linoleic acid; *n*-3 PUFA: *n*-3 polyunsaturated fatty acids.

from CoA to carnitine for translocation across the mitochondrial inner membrane. Acylcarnitine is translocated across the mitochondrial membrane in exchange for carnitine by carnitine acylcarnitine transferase and then re-esterified with CoA by the inner mitochondrial membrane CPT-2 (Park *et al.*, 1998; Steffen *et al.*, 1999). Two isoforms of CPT-1 have been identified: the liver isoform (L-CPT-1 or CPT-1α), which is expressed in most tissues, including liver, kidney, lung and heart, but not in skeletal muscle, and the muscle isoform (M-CPT or CPT-1β), which is expressed in skeletal muscle, heart and adipose tissue. The finding that adenovirus-mediated over-expression of CPT-1α in rat insulinoma INS1E cells increased fatty acid oxidation (Rubi *et al.*, 2002) confirms that transgenic over-expression of CPT-1 can be physiologically active. Therefore, transgenic animals with an increased or suppressed expression of CPT-1 should allow for a critical examination of the contribution of fatty acid oxidation to the control of food intake and body weight. Yet, it is not possible to create homozygous CPT-1 knock-out mice because this mutation is lethal (Wood *et al.*, 2003). In addition, given the complex interactions and redundancies in the physiological control of food intake and energy balance, a constitutive over-expression or suppression of CPT-1 in all organs might not allow us to identify this enzyme's role in different organs and in different metabolic situations because of developmental compensation. It is well known that transgenic animals often display phenotypical traits contrary to what might be expected: Thus, acetyl-CoA-carboxylase-2 knock-out mice showed excessive fatty acid oxidation and were resistant to obesity, whereas mice with fatty acid oxidation gene knock-outs such as the LCFA-CoA dehydrogenase knock-out mice, did not develop obesity despite reduced fatty acid oxidation (Wood, 2004).

An inducible over-expression of CPT-1α should avoid adaptive responses caused by permanent and constitutive genetic changes in classic 'knock-out' or 'knock-in' preparations. A tetra- or doxycycline (Dox)-regulated gene expression allows for such an inducible over-expression of a gene (Corbel and Rossi, 2002; Zhu *et al.*, 2002). To generate such transgenic animals it is necessary to place a Dox-dependent transcriptional activator (tTA) under the control of an organ-specific promoter and the target gene (CPT-1α) under the control of the tet operator. Both constructs have to be inserted into mice or rat genome. The resulting animal lines carrying both transgenes should show a Dox-inducible, organ-specific CPT-1α over-expression. This method allows us, for example, to generate a rat with an inducible, liver-specific over-expression of CPT-1α, and such a novel animal model could be used to examine the role of an increase in hepatic fatty acid oxidation in the control of food intake, body weight and metabolism under different conditions and without the limitation of a life-long adaptation to the change in gene expression.

Finally, most studies discussed in this chapter used male animals or subjects and did not consider sex differences related to fat metabolism. It is unknown whether the role of fatty acid oxidation in control of food intake and body weight differs between men and women. The fact that women generally have a higher amount of body fat and a higher proportion of body fat in the gluteal-femoral region, whereas men have more body fat in the abdominal (visceral) region, suggests that fat metabolism is sexually differentiated. Some other findings support this assumption: The fatty acid oxidation inhibitor MA increased food intake in male and ovariectomised female rats, but failed to stimulate eating in estradiol-treated ovariectomised rats (Geary, 2004); resting fat oxidation seems to be lower in women than in men (for review see Blaak, 2001). Although this latter observation may be related to sex differences in fat free mass and energy balance, it is clear that possible sex differences in fat metabolism and eating control deserve more attention in the future.

18.8 References

ABU-ELHEIGA, L., MATZUK, M. M., ABO-HASHEMA, K. A. and WAKIL, S. J. (2001), Continuous fatty acid oxidation and reduced fat storage in mice lacking acetyl-CoA carboxylase 2. *Science*, **291**, 2613–6.

AGUILERA, A. A., DIAZ, G. H., BARCELATA, M. L., GUERRERO, O. A. and ROS, R. M. O. (2004), Effects of fish oil on hypertension, plasma lipids, and tumor necrosis factor-alpha in rats with sucrose-induced metabolic syndrome. *Journal of Nutritional Biochemistry*, **15**, 350–7.

ALSAIF, M. A. and DUWAIHY, M. M. S. (2004), Influence of dietary fat quantity and composition on glucose tolerance and insulin sensitivity in rats. *Nutrition Research*, **24**, 417–25.

AMINOT-GILCHRIST, D. V. and ANDERSON, H. D. I. (2004), Insulin resistance-associated cardiovascular disease: potential benefits of conjugated linoleic acid. *American Journal of Clinical Nutrition*, **79**, 1159S–63S.

ASTRUP, A., GRUNWALD, G. K., MELANSON, E. L., SARIS, W. H. M. and HILL, J. O. (2000), The role of low-fat diets in body weight control: a meta-analysis of *ad libitum* dietary intervention studies. *International Journal of Obesity*, **24**, 1545–52.

AZAIN, M. J., HAUSMAN, D. B., SISK, M. B., FLATT, W. P. and JEWELL, D. E. (2000), Dietary conjugated linoleic acid reduces rat adipose tissue cell size rather than cell number. *Journal of Nutrition*, **130**, 1548–54.

BACH, A. C., INGENBLEEK, Y. and FREY, A. (1996), Usefulness of dietary medium-chain triglycerides in body weight control: Fact or fancy? *Journal of Lipid Research*, **37**, 708–26.

BERGMAN, R. N. (2000), Non-esterified fatty acids and the liver: why is insulin secreted into the portal vein? *Diabetologia*, **43**, 946–52.

BEVERLY, J. L., YANG, Z. J. and MEGUID, M. M. (1994), Hepatic vagotomy effects on metabolic challenges during parenteral-nutrition in rats. *American Journal of Physiology – Regulatory Integrative and Comparative Physiology*, **266**, R646–9.

BINNERT, C., PACHIAUDI, C., BEYLOT, M. *et al.* (1998), Influence of human obesity on the metabolic fate of dietary long- and medium-chain triacylglycerols. *American Journal of Clinical Nutrition*, **67**, 595–601.

BLAAK, E. (2001), Gender differences in fat metabolism. *Current Opinion in Clinical Nutrition and Metabolic Care*, **4**, 499–502.

BLUNDELL, J. E. and STUBBS, R. J. (1999), High and low carbohydrate and fat intakes: limits imposed by appetite and palatability and their implications for energy balance. *European Journal of Clinical Nutrition*, **53**, S148–65.

BRAVATA, D. M., SANDERS, L., HUANG, J. *et al.* (2003), Efficacy and safety of low-carbohydrate diets – a systematic review. *Journal of the American Medical Association*, **289**, 1837–50.

BRAY, G. A., LEE, M. and BRAY, T. L. (1980), Weight-gain of rats fed medium-chain triglycerides is less than rats fed long-chain triglycerides. *International Journal of Obesity*, **4**, 27–32.

BRAY, G. A. and POPKIN, B. M. (1998), Dietary fat intake does affect obesity! *American Journal of Clinical Nutrition*, **68**, 1157–73.

BREHM, B. J., SEELEY, R. J., DANIELS, S. R. and D'ALESSIO, D. A. (2003), A randomized trial comparing a very low carbohydrate diet and a calorie-restricted low fat diet on body weight and cardiovascular risk factors in healthy women. *Journal of Clinical Endocrinology and Metabolism*, **88**, 1617–23.

CLARKE, S. D. (2000), Polyunsaturated fatty acid regulation of gene transcription: a mechanism to improve energy balance and insulin resistance. *British Journal of Nutrition*, **83**, S59–66.

CLEGG, D. J., WORTMAN, M. D., BENOIT, S. C., MCOSKER, C. C. and SEELEY, R. J. (2002), Comparison of central and peripheral administration of C75 on food intake, body weight, and conditioned taste aversion. *Diabetes*, **51**, 3196–201.

CORBEL, S. Y. and ROSSI, F. M. (2002), Latest developments and in vivo use of the Tet system: *ex vivo* and *in vivo* delivery of tetracycline-regulated genes. *Current Opinion in Biotechnology*, **13**, 448–52.

DASHTI, H. M., BO-ABBAS, Y. Y., ASFAR, S. K. *et al.* (2003), Ketogenic diet modifies the risk factors of heart disease in obese patients. *Nutrition*, **19**, 901–2.

DEEMS, R. O. ANDERSON, R. C. and FOLEY, J. E. (1998), Hypoglycemic effects of a novel fatty acid oxidation inhibitor in rats and monkeys. *American Journal of Physiology – Regulatory Integrative and Comparative Physiology*, **274**, R524–8.

DEGEN, L., MATZINGER, D., DREWE, J. and BEGLINGER, C. (2001), The effect of cholecystokinin in controlling appetite and food intake in humans. *Peptides*, **22**, 1265–9.

DEL PRETE, E., LUTZ, T. A. and SCHARRER, E. (2000), Transient hypophagia in rats switched from high-fat diets with different fatty-acid pattern to a high-carbohydrate diet. *Appetite*, **34**, 137–45.

DELANY, J. P., BLOHM, F., TRUETT, A. A., SCIMECA, J. A. and WEST, D. B. (1999), Conjugated linoleic acid rapidly reduces body fat content in micc without affecting energy intake. *American Journal of Physiology – Regulatory Integrative and Comparative Physiology*, **276**, R1172–9.

DELANY, J. P., WINDHAUSER, M. M., CHAMPAGNE, C. M. and BRAY, G. A. (2000), Differential oxidation of individual dietary fatty acids in humans. *American Journal of Clinical Nutrition*, **72**, 905–11.

DENBOW, D. M., VANKREY, H. P., LACY, M. P. and WATKINS, B. A. (1992), The effect of triacylglycerol chain-length on food-intake in domestic-fowl. *Physiology and Behavior*, **51**, 1147–50.

DIRAISON, F., LARGE, V., BRUNENGRABER, H. and BEYLOT, M. (1998), Non-invasive tracing of liver intermediary metabolism in normal subjects and in moderately hyperglycaemic NIDDM subjects. Evidence against increased gluconeogenesis and hepatic fatty acid oxidation in NIDDM. *Diabetologia*, **41**, 212–20.

DOBBINS, R. L., SZCZEPANIAK, L. S., BENTLEY, B., ESSER, V., MYHILL, J. and MCGARRY, J. D. (2001), Prolonged inhibition of muscle carnitine palmitoyltransferase-1 promotes intramyocellular lipid accumulation and insulin resistance in rats. *Diabetes*, **50**, 123–30.

DOUGLAS, B. R., JANSEN, J. B. M. J., DEJONG, A. J. L. and LAMERS, C. B. H. W. (1990), Effect of various triglycerides on plasma cholecystokinin levels in rats. *Journal of Nutrition*, **120**, 686–90.

DREWNOWSKI, A. (1998), Energy density, palatability, and satiety: implications for weight control. *Nutrition Review*, **56**, 347–53.

DULLOO, A. G., FATHI, M., MENSI, N. and GIRARDIER, L. (1996), Twenty-four-hour energy expenditure and urinary catecholamines of humans consuming low-to-moderate amounts of medium-chain triglycerides: a dose–response study in a human respiratory chamber. *European Journal of Clinical Nutrition*, **50**, 152–8.

EATON, S. (2002), Control of mitochondrial beta-oxidation flux. *Progress in Lipid Research*, **41**, 197–239.

FIELD, C. J. and SCHLEY, P. D. (2004), Evidence for potential mechanisms for the effect of conjugated linoleic acid on tumor metabolism and immune function: lessons from *n*-3 fatty acids. *American Journal of Clinical Nutrition*, **79**, 1190S–8S.

FOLEY, J. E. (1992), Rationale and application of fatty-acid oxidation inhibitors in treatment of diabetes-mellitus. *Diabetes Care*, **15**, 773–84.

FRIEDMAN, M. I. (1990), Body-fat and the metabolic control of food-intake. *International Journal of Obesity*, **14**, 53–67.

FRIEDMAN, M. I. (1998), Fuel partitioning and food intake. *American Journal of Clinical Nutrition*, **67**, 513S–8S.

FRIEDMAN, M. I., HARRIS, R. B., JI, H., RAMIREZ, I. and TORDOFF, M. G. (1999), Fatty acid oxidation affects food intake by altering hepatic energy status. *American Journal of Physiology – Regulatory Integrative and Comparative Physiology*, **276**, R1046–53.

FURUSE, M., CHOI, Y. H., MABAYO, R. T. and OKUMURA, J. I. (1992), Feeding-behavior in rats fed diets containing medium chain triglyceride. *Physiology and Behavior*, **52**, 815–7.

GAULLIER, J. M., HALSE, J., HOYE, K. *et al.* (2004), Conjugated linoleic acid supplementation for 1 y reduces body fat mass in healthy overweight humans. *American Journal of Clinical Nutrition*, **79**, 1118–25.

GAVINO, V. C., GAVINO, G., LEBLANC, M. J. and TUCHWEBER, B. (2000), An isomeric mixture of conjugated linoleic acids but not pure *cis*-9, *trans*-11-octadecadienoic acid affects body weight gain and plasma lipids in hamsters. *Journal of Nutrition*, **130**, 27–9.

GEARY, N. (2004), Is the control of fat ingestion sexually differentiated? *Physiology and Behavior*, **83**, 659–71.

GUPTA, G., CASES, J. A., SHE, L. *et al.* (2000), Ability of insulin to modulate hepatic glucose production in aging rats is impaired by fat accumulation. *American Journal of Physiology – Endocrinology and Metabolism*, **278**, E985–91.

HILL, J. O., PETERS, J. C., LIN, D., YAKUBU, F., GREENE, H. and SWIFT, L. (1993), Lipid-accumulation and body-fat distribution is influenced by type of dietary-fat fed to rats. *International Journal of Obesity*, **17**, 223–36.

HOPMAN, W. P. M., JANSEN, J. B. M. J., ROSENBUSCH, G. and LAMERS, C. B. H. W. (1984), Effect of equimolar amounts of long-chain triglycerides and medium-chain triglycerides on plasma cholecystokinin and gallbladder contraction. *American Journal of Clinical Nutrition*, **39**, 356–9.

HORN, C. C., JI, H. and FRIEDMAN, M. I. (2004), Etomoxir, a fatty acid oxidation inhibitor, increases food intake and reduces hepatic energy status in rats. *Physiology and Behavior*, **81**, 157–62.

HOUSEKNECHT, K. L., VANDEN HEUVEL, J. P., MOYA-CAMARENA, S. Y. *et al.* (1998), Dietary conjugated linoleic acid normalizes impaired glucose tolerance in the Zucker diabetic fatty fa/fa rat. *Biochemical and Biophysical Research Communications*, **244**, 678–82.

HUANG, X. F., XIN, X., MCLENNAN, P. and STORLIEN, L. (2004), Role of fat amount and type in ameliorating diet-induced obesity: insights at the level of hypothalamic arcuate nucleus leptin receptor, neuropeptide Y and pro-opiomelanocortin mRNA expression. *Diabetes Obesity and Metabolism*, **6**, 35–44.

HUOT, I., PARADIS, G. and LEDOUX, M. (2004), Factors associated with overweight and obesity in Quebec adults. *International Journal of Obesity*, **28**, 766–74.

JAMBOR DE SOUSA, U. L., LEONHARDT, M. and LANGHANS, W. (2003), Effect of hepatic portal vein (HPV) caprylic acid (CA) infusion on saccharin preference and gastric emptying in male rats. *Appetite*, **40**, A338–9.

JI, H., GRACZYK-MILBRANDT, G. and FRIEDMAN, M. I. (2000), Metabolic inhibitors synergistically decrease hepatic energy status and increase food intake. *American Journal of Physiology – Regulatory Integrative and Comparative Physiology*, **278**, R1579–82.

KAHLER, A., ZIMMERMANN, M. and LANGHANS, W. (1999), Suppression of hepatic fatty acid oxidation and food intake in men. *Nutrition*, **15**, 819–28.

KAMPHUIS, M. M. J. W., LEJEUNE, M. P. G. M., SARIS, W. H. M. and WESTERTERP-PLANTENGA, M. S. (2003), The effect of conjugated linoleic acid supplementation after weight loss on body weight regain, body composition, and resting metabolic rate in overweight subjects. *International Journal of Obesity*, **27**, 840–7.

KASAI, M., NOSAKA, N., MAKI, H. *et al.* (2002), Comparison of diet-induced thermogenesis of foods containing medium-versus long-chain triacylglycerols. *Journal of Nutritional Science and Vitaminology*, **48**, 536–40.

KIM, E. K., MILLER, I., LANDREE, L. E. *et al.* (2002), Expression of FAS within hypothalamic neurons: a model for decreased food intake after C75 treatment. *American Journal of Physiology – Endocrinology and Metabolism*, **283**, E867–79.

KIM, E. K., MILLER, I., AJA, S. *et al.* (2004), C75, a fatty acid synthase inhibitor, reduces food intake via hypothalamic AMP-activated protein kinase. *Journal of Biological Chemistry*, **279**, 19970–6.

KOPELMAN, P. G. (2000), Obesity as a medical problem. *Nature*, **404**, 635–43.

KRAEGEN, E. W., COONEY, G. J., YE, J. M., THOMPSON, A. L. and FURLER, S. M. (2001), The role of lipids in the pathogenesis of muscle insulin resistance and beta cell failure in type 2 diabetes and obesity. *Experimental and Clinical Endocrinology and Diabetes*, **109**, S189–201.

KROTKIEWSKI, M. (2001), Value of VLCD supplementation with medium chain triglycerides. *International Journal of Obesity*, **25**, 1393–400.

KUMAR, M. V., SHIMOKAWA, T., NAGY, T. R. and LANE, M. D. (2002), Differential effects of a centrally acting fatty acid synthase inhibitor in lean and obese mice. *Proceedings of the National Academy of Sciences of the United States of America*, **99**, 1921–5.

LANDREE, L. E., HANLON, A. L., STRONG, D. W. *et al.* (2004), C75, a fatty acid synthase inhibitor, modulates AMP-activated protein kinase to alter neuronal energy metabolism. *Journal of Biological Chemistry*, **279**, 3817–27.

LANGHANS, W. (1996), Role of the liver in the metabolic control of eating: what we know – and what we do not know. *Neuroscience and Biobehavioral Reviews*, **20**, 145–53.

LANGHANS, W. (2003), Role of the liver in the control of glucose–lipid utilization and body weight. *Current Opinion in Clinical Nutrition and Metabolic Care*, **6**, 449–55.

LANGHANS, W. and SCHARRER, E. (1987a), Evidence for a vagally mediated satiety signal derived from hepatic fatty-acid oxidation. *Journal of the Autonomic Nervous System*, **18**, 13–8.

LANGHANS, W. and SCHARRER, E. (1987b), Role of fatty-acid oxidation in control of meal pattern. *Behavioral and Neural Biology*, **47**, 7–16.

LARSSON, S. C., KUMLIN, M., INGELMAN-SUNDBERG, M. and WOLK, A. (2004), Dietary long-chain *n*-3 fatty acids for the prevention of cancer: a review of potential mechanisms. *American Journal of Clinical Nutrition*, **79**, 935–45.

LOFTUS, T. M., JAWORSKY, D. E., FREHYWOT, G. L. *et al.* (2000), Reduced food intake and body weight in mice treated with fatty acid synthase inhibitors. *Science*, **288**, 2379–81.

LUTZ, T. A., DIENER, M. and SCHARRER, E. (1997), Intraportal mercaptoacetate infusion increases afferent activity in the common hepatic vagus branch of the rat. *American Journal of Physiology – Regulatory Integrative and Comparative Physiology*, **273**, R442–5.

MADSEN, L., RUSTAN, A. C., VAAGENES, H., BERGE, K., DYROY, E. and BERGE, R. K. (1999), Eicosapentaenoic and docosahexaenoic acid affect mitochondrial and peroxisomal fatty acid oxidation in relation to substrate preference. *Lipids*, **34**, 951–63.

MAGGIO, C. A. and KOOPMANS, H. S. (1982), Food-intake after intra-gastric meals of short-chain, medium-chain, or long-chain triglyceride. *Physiology and Behavior*, **28**, 921–6.

MARTIN, J. C., GREGOIRE, S. and SIESS, M. H. (2000), Effects of conjugated linoleic acid isomers on lipid-metabolizing enzymes in male rats. *Lipids*, **35**, 91–8.

MCLEOD, R. S., LEBLANC, A. M., LANGILLE, M. A., MITCHELL, P. L. and CURRIE, D. L. (2004), Conjugated linoleic acids, atherosclerosis, and hepatic very-low-density lipoprotein metabolism. *American Journal of Clinical Nutrition*, **79**, 1169S–74S.

MECKLING, K. A., O'SULLIVAN, C. and SAARI, D. (2004), Comparison of a low-fat diet to a low-carbohydrate diet on weight loss, body composition, and risk factors for diabetes and cardiovascular disease in free-living, overweight men and women. *Journal of Clinical Endocrinology and Metabolism*, **89**, 2717–23.

MINOKOSHI, Y., ALQUIER, T., FURUKAWA, N. *et al.* (2004), AMP-kinase regulates food intake by responding to hormonal and nutrient signals in the hypothalamus. *Nature*, **428**, 569–74.

MORGAN, K., OBICI, S. and ROSSETTI, L. (2004), Hypothalamic responses to long-chain fatty acids are nutritionally regulated. *Journal of Biological Chemistry*, **279**, 31139–48.

MORI, T. A., BURKE, V., PUDDEY, I. B. *et al.* (2000), Purified eicosapentaenoic and docosahexaenoic acids have differential effects on serum lipids and lipoproteins, LDL particle size, glucose, and insulin in mildly hyperlipidemic men. *American Journal of Clinical Nutrition*, **71**, 1085–94.

MOSCA, C. L., MARSHALL, J. A., GRUNWALD, G. K., CORNIER, M. A. and BAXTER, J. (2004), Insulin resistance as a modifier of the relationship between dietary fat intake and weight gain. *International Journal of Obesity*, **28**, 803–12.

MOYA-CAMARENA, S. Y. and BELURY, M. A. (1999), Species differences in the metabolism and regulation of gene expression by conjugated linoleic acid. *Nutrition Reviews*, **57**, 336–40.

MOYA-CAMARENA, S. Y., VANDEN HEUVEL, J. P., BLANCHARD, S. G., LEESNITZER, L. A. and BELURY, M. A. (1999), Conjugated linoleic acid is a potent naturally occurring ligand and activator of PPARalpha. *Journal of Lipid Research*, **40**, 1426–33.

NAKAMURA, T., YOSHIHARA, D., OHMORI, T., YANAI, M. and TAKESHITA, Y. (1994), Effects of diet high in medium-chain triglyceride on plasma ketone, glucose, and insulin concentrations in enterectomized and normal rats. *Journal of Nutritional Science and Vitaminology*, **40**, 147–59.

NOGUCHI, O., TAKEUCHI, H., KUBOTA, F., TSUJI, H. and AOYAMA, T. (2002), Larger diet-induced thermogenesis and less body fat accumulation in rats fed medium-chain triacylglycerols than in those fed long-chain triacylglycerols. *Journal of Nutritional Science and Vitaminology*, **48**, 524–9.

OBICI, S., FENG, Z. H., ARDUINI, A., CONTI, R. and ROSSETTI, L. (2003), Inhibition of hypothalamic carnitine palmitoyltransferase-1 decreases food intake and glucose production. *Nature Medicine*, **9**, 756–61.

OBICI, S., FENG, Z. H., MORGAN, Y., STEIN, D., KARKANIAS, G. and ROSSETTI, L. (2002), Central administration of oleic acid inhibits glucose production and food intake. *Diabetes*, **51**, 271–5.

OBICI, S. and ROSSETTI, L. (2003), Minireview: nutrient sensing and the regulation of insulin action and energy balance. *Endocrinology*, **144**, 5172–8.

OFFICE OF THE SURGEON GENERAL (2001), The surgeon general's call to action to prevent and decrease overweight and obesity. http://www.surgeongeneral.gov/library.

OSTROWSKA, E., MURALITHARAN, M., CROSS, R. F., BAUMAN, D. E. and DUNSHEA, F. R. (1999), Dietary conjugated linoleic acids increase lean tissue and decrease fat deposition in growing pigs. *Journal of Nutrition*, **129**, 2037–42.

OUDART, H., GROSCOLAS, R., CALGARI, C. *et al.* (1997), Brown fat thermogenesis in rats fed high-fat diets enriched with *n*-3 polyunsaturated fatty acids. *International Journal of Obesity*, **21**, 955–62.

PARIZA, M. W. (2004), Perspective on the safety and effectiveness of conjugated linoleic acid. *American Journal of Clinical Nutrition*, **79**, 1132S–6S.

PARIZA, M. W., ASHOOR, S. H., CHU, F. S. and LUND, D. B. (1979), Effects of temperature and time on mutagen formation in pan-fried hamburger. *Cancer Letters*, **7**, 63–9.

PARIZA, M. W., PARK, Y. and COOK, M. E. (1999), Conjugated linoleic acid and the control of cancer and obesity. *Toxicological Sciences*, **52**, 107–10.

PARK, E. A., STEFFEN, M. L., SONG, S. L., PARK, V. M. and COOK, G. A. (1998), Cloning and characterization of the promoter for the liver isoform of the rat carnitine palmitoyltransferase I (L-CPT I) gene. *Biochemical Journal*, **330**, 217–24.

PARK, Y., STORKSON, J. M., ALBRIGHT, K. J., LIU, W. and PARIZA, M. W. (1999), Evidence that the *trans*-10,*cis*-12 isomer of conjugated linoleic acid induces body composition changes in mice. *Lipids*, **34**, 235–41.

RAHMAN, S. M., WANG, Y., YOTSUMOTO, H. *et al.* (2001), Effects of conjugated linoleic acid on serum leptin concentration, body-fat accumulation, and beta-oxidation of fatty acid in OLETF rats. *Nutrition*, **17**, 385–90.

RANDLE, P. J. (1998), Regulatory interactions between lipids and carbohydrates: The glucose fatty acid cycle after 35 years. *Diabetes – Metabolism Reviews*, **14**, 263–83.

RANDLE, P. J., GARLAND, P. B., NEWSHOLME, E. A. and HALES, C. N. (1963), Glucose fatty-acid cycle – its role in insulin sensitivity and metabolic disturbances of diabetes mellitus. *Lancet*, **1**, 785–9.

RATHEISER, K., SCHNEEWEISS, B., WALDHAUSL, W. *et al.* (1991), Inhibition by etomoxir of carnitine palmitoyltransferase-I reduces hepatic glucose-production and plasma-lipids in noninsulin-dependent diabetes-mellitus. *Metabolism – Clinical and Experimental*, **40**, 1185–90.

RISERUS, U., BASU, S., JOVINGE, S., FREDRIKSON, G. N., ARNLOV, J. and VESSBY, B. (2002), Supplementation with conjugated linoleic acid causes isomer-dependent oxidative stress and elevated C-reactive protein – a potential link to fatty acid-induced insulin resistance. *Circulation*, **106**, 1925–9.

RISERUS, U., SMEDMAN, A., BASU, S. and VESSBY, B. (2004a), Metabolic effects of conjugated linoleic acid in humans: the Swedish experience. *American Journal of Clinical Nutrition*, **79**, 1146S–8S.

RISERUS, U., VESSBY, B., ARNER, P. and ZETHELIUS, B. (2004b), Supplementation with *trans*10*cis*12-conjugated linoleic acid induces hyperproinsulinaemia in obese men: close association with impaired insulin sensitivity. *Diabetologia*, **47**, 1016–9.

RITTER, R. C. (2004), Gastrointestinal mechanisms of satiation for food. *Physiology and Behavior*, **81**, 249–73.

RITTER, S. and TAYLOR, J. S. (1989), Capsaicin abolishes lipoprivic but not glucoprivic feeding in rats. *American Journal of Physiology – Regulatory Integrative and Comparative Physiology*, **256**, R1232–9.

RITTER, S. and TAYLOR, J. S. (1990), Vagal sensory neurons are required for lipoprivic but not glucoprivic feeding in rats. *American Journal of Physiology – Regulatory Integrative and Comparative Physiology*, **258**, R1395–401.

RIVELLESE, A. A., DE NATALE, C. and LILLI, S. (2002), Type of dietary fat and insulin resistance. *Lipids and Insulin Resistance: the Role of Fatty Acid Metabolism and Fuel Partitioning*, **967**, 329–35.

ROCHE, H. M., NOONE, E., SEWTER, C. *et al.* (2002), Isomer-dependent metabolic effects of conjugated linoleic acid – insights from molecular markers sterol regulatory element-binding protein-1c and LXR alpha. *Diabetes*, **51**, 2037–44.

ROLLS, B. J. (2000), The role of energy density in the overconsumption of fat. *Journal of Nutrition*, **130**, 268S–71S.

RUBI, B., ANTINOZZI, P. A., HERRERO, L. *et al.* (2002), Adenovirus-mediated overexpression of liver carnitine palmitoyltransferase I in INS1E cells: effects on cell metabolism and insulin secretion. *Biochemical Journal*, **364**, 219–26.

RYDER, J. W., PORTOCARRERO, C. P., SONG, X. M. *et al.* (2001), Isomer-specific antidiabetic properties of conjugated linoleic acid. Improved glucose tolerance, skeletal muscle insulin action, and UCP-2 gene expression. *Diabetes*, **50**, 1149–57.

SAKONO, M., MIYANAGA, F., KAWAHARA, S. *et al.* (1999), Dietary conjugated linoleic acid reciprocally modifies ketogenesis and lipid secretion by the rat liver. *Lipids*, **34**, 997–1000.

SALTIEL, A. R. and KAHN, C. R. (2001), Insulin signalling and the regulation of glucose and lipid metabolism. *Nature*, **414**, 799–806.

SAMAHA, F. F., IQBAL, N., SESHADRI, P. *et al.* (2003), A low-carbohydrate as compared with a low-fat diet in severe obesity. *New England Journal of Medicine*, **348**, 2074–81.

SARIS, W. H. M., ASTRUP, A., PRENTICE, A. M. *et al.* (2000), Randomized controlled trial of changes in dietary carbohydrate/fat ratio and simple vs complex carbohydrates on body weight and blood lipids: the CARMEN study. *International Journal of Obesity*, **24**, 1310–18.

SATIA-ABOUTA, J., PATTERSON, R. E., SCHILLER, R. N. and KRISTAL, A. R. (2002), Energy from fat is associated with obesity in US men: Results from the prostate cancer prevention trial. *Preventive Medicine*, **34**, 493–501.

SCHARRER, E. (1999), Control of food intake by fatty acid oxidation and ketogenesis. *Nutrition*, **15**, 704–14.

SCHARRER, E. and LANGHANS, W. (1986), Control of food-intake by fatty-acid oxidation. *American Journal of Physiology – Regulatory Integrative and Comparative Physiology*, **250**, R1003–6.

SEIFTER, S. and ENGLARD, S. (1994), Energy metabolism. In: Arias, I. M., Boyer, J. L., Fausto, N., Jakoby, W. B., Schachter, D. A. and Shafritz, D. A., eds. *The Liver: Biology and Pathobiology*. 3rd edn. New York: Raven Press, Ltd., pp. 323–64.

SEKIYA, M., YAHAGI, N., MATSUZAKA, T. *et al.* (2003), Polyunsaturated fatty acids ameliorate hepatic steatosis in obese mice by SREBP-1 suppression. *Hepatology*, **38**, 1529–39.

SERGEYEV, V., BROBERGER, C., GORBATYUK, O. and HOKFELT, T. (2000), Effect of 2-mercaptoacetate and 2-deoxy-D-glucose administration on the expression of NPY, AGRP, POMC, MCH and hypocretin/orexin in the rat hypothalamus. *Neuroreport*, **11**, 117–21.

SHARMAN, M. J., GOMEZ, A. L., KRAEMER, W. J. and VOLEK, J. S. (2004), Very low-carbohydrate and low-fat diets affect fasting lipids and postprandial lipernia differently in overweight men. *Journal of Nutrition*, **134**, 880–5.

SINGER, L. K., YORK, D. A. and BRAY, G. A. (1998), Macronutrient selection following 2-deoxy-D-glucose and mercaptoacetate administration in rats. *Physiology and Behavior*, **65**, 115–21.

SINGERKOEGLER, L. K., MAGLUYAN, P. and RITTER, S. (1996), The effects of low-, medium-, and high-fat diets on 2-deoxy-D-glucose- and mercaptoacetate-induced feeding. *Physiology and Behavior*, **60**, 321–3.

SISK, M. B., HAUSMAN, D. B., MARTIN, R. J. and AZAIN, M. J. (2001), Dietary conjugated linoleic acid reduces adiposity in lean but not obese Zucker rats. *Journal of Nutrition*, **131**, 1668–74.

SORIA, A., CHICCO, A., D'ALESSANDRO, M. E., ROSSI, A. and LOMBARDO, Y. B. (2002), Dietary fish oil reverse epididymal tissue adiposity, cell hypertrophy and insulin resistance in dyslipemic sucrose fed rat model. *Journal of Nutritional Biochemistry*, **13**, 209–18.

ST ONGE, M. P. and JONES, P. J. (2002), Physiological effects of medium-chain triglycerides: potential agents in the prevention of obesity. *Journal of Nutrition*, **132**, 329–32.

STEFFEN, M. L., HARRISON, W. R., ELDER, F. F. B., COOK, G. A. and PARK, E. A. (1999), Expression of the rat liver carnitine palmitoyltransferase I (CPT-I alpha) gene is regulated by Sp1 and nuclear factor Y: chromosomal localization and promoter characterization. *Biochemical Journal*, **340**, 425–32.

STORLIEN, L. H., KRAEGEN, E. W., CHISHOLM, D. J., FORD, G. L., BRUCE, D. G. and PASCOE, W. S. (1987), Fish oil prevents insulin resistance induced by high-fat feeding in rats. *Science*, **237**, 885–8.

STUBBS, R. J. and HARBRON, C. G. (1996), Covert manipulation of the ratio of medium- to long-chain triglycerides in isoenergetically dense diets: effect on food intake in *ad libitum* feeding men. *International Journal of Obesity*, **20**, 435–44.

TAKAHASHI, K. A., SMART, J. L., LIU, H. Y. and CONE, R. D. (2004), The anorexigenic fatty acid synthase inhibitor, C75, is a nonspecific neuronal activator. *Endocrinology*, **145**, 184–93.

TAKAHASHI, Y. and IDE, T. (2000), Dietary *n*-3 fatty acids affect mRNA level of brown adipose tissue uncoupling protein 1, and white adipose tissue leptin and glucose transporter 4 in the rat. *British Journal of Nutrition*, **84**, 175–84.

TAYLOR, C. G. and ZAHRADKA, P. (2004), Dietary conjugated linoleic acid and insulin sensitivity and resistance in rodent models. *American Journal of Clinical Nutrition*, **79**, 1164S–8S.

THUPARI, J. N., KIM, E. K., MORAN, T. H., RONNETT, G. V. and KUHAJDA, F. P. (2004), Chronic C75 treatment of diet-induced obese mice increases fat oxidation and reduces food intake to reduce adipose mass. *American Journal of Physiology – Endocrinology and Metabolism*, **287**, E97–104.

THUPARI, J. N., LANDREE, L. E., RONNETT, G. V. and KUHAJDA, F. P. (2002), C75 increases peripheral energy utilization and fatty acid oxidation in diet-induced obesity. *Proceedings of the National Academy of Sciences of the United States of America*, **99**, 9498–502.

TSO, P. and LIU, M. (2004), Ingested fat and satiety. *Physiology and Behavior*, **81**, 275–87.

TSO, P., SUN, W. and LIU, M. (2004), Gastrointestinal satiety signals – IV. Apolipoprotein A-IV. *American Journal of Physiology – Gastrointestinal and Liver Physiology*, **286**, G885–90.

TSUBOYAMA-KASAOKA, N., TAKAHASHI, M., TANEMURA, K. *et al.* (2000), Conjugated linoleic acid supplementation reduces adipose tissue by apoptosis and develops lipodystrophy in mice. *Diabetes*, **49**, 1534–42.

TSUJI, H., KASAI, M., TAKEUCHI, H., NAKAMURA, M., OKAZAKI, M. and KONDO, K. (2001), Dietary medium-chain triacylglycerols suppress accumulation of body fat in a double-blind, controlled trial in healthy men and women. *Journal of Nutrition*, **131**, 2853–9.

VAN WYMELBEKE, V., HIMAYA, A., LOUIS-SYLVESTRE, J. and FANTINO, M. (1998), Influence of medium-chain and long-chain triacylglycerols on the control of food intake in men. *American Journal of Clinical Nutrition*, **68**, 226–34.

VAN WYMELBEKE, V., LOUIS-SYLVESTRE, J. and FANTINO, M. (2001), Substrate oxidation and control of food intake in men after a fat-substitute meal compared with meals supplemented with an isoenergetic load of carbohydrate, long-chain triacylglycerols, or medium-chain triacylglycerols. *American Journal of Clinical Nutrition*, **74**, 620–30.

WANG, J., AKABAYASHI, A., YU, H. J. *et al.* (1998), Hypothalamic galanin: control by signals of fat metabolism. *Brain Research*, **804**, 7–20.

WANG, Y. W. and JONES, P. J. H. (2004), Dietary conjugated linoleic acid and body composition. *American Journal of Clinical Nutrition*, **79**, 1153S–8S.

WEST, D. B., DELANY, J. P., CAMET, P. M., BLOHM, F., TRUETT, A. A. and SCIMECA, J. (1998), Effects of conjugated linoleic acid on body fat and energy metabolism in the mouse. *American Journal of Physiology – Regulatory Integrative and Comparative Physiology*, **275**, R667–72.

WESTERTERP-PLANTENGA, M. S. (2001), Analysis of energy density of food in relation to energy intake regulation in human subjects. *British Journal of Nutrition*, **85**, 351–61.

WESTERTERP-PLANTENGA, M. S. (2003), The significance of protein in food intake and body weight regulation. *Current Opinion in Clinical Nutrition and Metabolic Care*, **6**, 635–8.

WESTMAN, E. C., YANCY, W. S., EDMAN, J. S., TOMLIN, K. F. and PERKINS, C. E. (2002), Effect of 6-month adherence to a very low carbohydrate diet programme. *American Journal of Medicine*, **113**, 30–6.

WILLETT, W. C. (1998), Is dietary fat a major determinant of body fat? *American Journal of Clinical Nutrition*, **67**, 556S–62S.

WILLIAMS, J. R., BROWNING, E. T., SCHOLZ, R., KREISBER, R. A. and FRITZ, I. B. (1968), Inhibition of fatty acid stimulation of gluconeogenesis by (+)-decanoylcarnitine in perfused rat liver. *Diabetes*, **17**, 194–208.

WOOD, P. A., KURTZ, D. M., COX, K. B. *et al.* (2003), Role of genetic deficiency of fatty acid oxidation in metabolic syndrome/obesity. In Medeiros-Neto, G., Halpern, A., Bouchard, C., eds. *Progress in Obesity Research*. 9th edn. Esher, UK: John Libbey Eurotext Ltd., pp. 293–6.

WOOD, P. A. (2004), Genetically modified mouse models for disorders of fatty acid metabolism: Pursuing the nutrigenomics of insulin resistance and type 2 diabetes. *Nutrition*, **20**, 121–6.

WOODMAN, R. J., MORI, T. A., BURKE, V., PUDDEY, I. B., WATTS, G. F. and BEILIN, L. J. (2002), Effects of purified eicosapentaenoic and docosahexaenoic acids on glycemic control, blood pressure, and serum lipids in type 2 diabetic patients with treated hypertension. *American Journal of Clinical Nutrition*, **76**, 1007–15.

WORLD HEALTH ORGANIZATION (WHO). (2004), Obesity and overweight (WHO global strategy on diet, physical activity and health). http://www.who.int/topics/obesity/en/

YAMASAKI, M., MANSHO, K., MISHIMA, H. *et al.* (2000), Effect of dietary conjugated linoleic acid on lipid peroxidation and histological change in rat liver tissues. *Journal of Agricultural and Food Chemistry*, **48**, 6367–71.

YANCY, W. S., OLSEN, M. K., GUYTON, J. R., BAKST, R. P. and WESTMAN, E. C. (2004), A low-carbohydrate, ketogenic diet versus a low-fat diet to treat obesity and hyperlipidemia – a randomized, controlled trial. *Annals of Internal Medicine*, **140**, 769–77.

ZHU, Z., ZHENG, T., LEE, C. G., HOMER, R. J. and ELIAS, J. A. (2002), Tetracycline-controlled transcriptional regulation systems: advances and application in transgenic animal modeling. *Seminars in Cell and Developmental Biology*, **13**, 121–8.

19

The use of very-low-calorie diets (VLCDs) and meal replacements for weight control

J. W. Anderson and E. C. Konz, University of Kentucky, USA

19.1 Introduction

The prevalence of obesity is increasing at epidemic rates in the United States and around the world (Flegal *et al.*, 2002; James *et al.*, 2001). The World Health Organization estimates that 1.3 billion people globally are overweight or obese with the UK, USA, Australia and France leading the way (International Obesity Taskforce, 2004). Almost two-thirds of adults in the United States are overweight (Flegal *et al.*, 2002) and the prevalence of extreme or Class 3 obesity has almost tripled in the last 10 years (Freedman *et al.*, 2002). According to the Behavioral Risk Factor Surveillance System conducted by state health departments in the United States in 1996, the percentage of individuals attempting to lose weight and to maintain weight was 28.8% and 35.1% among men and 43.6% and 34.4% among women, respectively (Serdula *et al.*, 1999). Unfortunately, many obese individuals are not successful at losing weight and have even more difficulty maintaining a lower body weight long term (Anderson *et al.*, 2001). Very-low-calorie diets (VLCD) have enabled many individuals to lose substantial amounts of weight and to maintain these losses long term (Anderson *et al.*, 1992, 1999, 2001; Anderson *et al.*, 1992). More recently, less intensive interventions with meal replacements (MR) using liquid meals (shakes) have emerged as an effective strategy for weight loss and weight maintenance for some individuals (Anderson *et al.*, 2004; Heymsfield *et al.*, 2003).

Over the past 20 years nutrition, physical activity and behavior modification have been combined to substantially improve weight loss and maintenance of weight loss outcomes (Anderson *et al.*, 1992, 2004). As a result, less emphasis is placed on radical restriction of energy intake and more attention is focused on successful lifestyle changes with moderation in energy intake (Rossner and Flaten, 1997). In this chapter, different dietary strategies for weight loss will be reviewed and compared. Very-low-calorie diets (VLCD) also referred to as very-low-energy diets (VLED) will receive the major focus because these diets are the most effective for fostering substantial weight loss and long-term maintenance of weight loss. Use of meal replacements will also be emphasized because these appear to be the most cost-effective approach to weight loss and maintenance. We will not review other diet approaches, pharmacotherapy or bariatric surgery.

19.2 Tailoring nutritional advice for weight control

19.2.1 Patient assessment

Nutrition recommendations are tailored to the individual's needs, capabilities and resources. The height and weight of individuals should be routinely measured and the body mass index (BMI) calculated. Most individuals with BMI values >25 kg/m^2 should be counseled about the health benefits of maintaining a BMI of <25 kg/m^2. The lifestyle approaches to management of overweight and obesity are summarized in Table 19.1 and will be discussed later. Guidance for management of overweight and obese individuals are summarized in Table 19.2. As patients are evaluated, blood pressure measurements and physical examination including inspection for *Acanthosis nigricans*, a harbinger of diabetes mellitus (Stuart *et al.*, 1998), and evidence of Cushing's syndrome, are done. The BMI is usually the starting place for decision making about nutrition recommendations. Endocrine causes of overweight, such as hypothyroidism or Cushing's syndrome, are usually excluded by examination and laboratory assessment.

Laboratory measurements of fasting plasma glucose and lipid values help in risk assessment. Having features of the metabolic syndrome indicates a higher risk for coronary heart disease (Lakka *et al.*, 2002). Presence of three of these characteristics of the metabolic syndrome indicates that this syndrome is present: waist circumference >102 cm in men and >88 cm in women; hypertriglyceridemia with fasting serum triglycerides >150 mg/dl (1.69 mmol/l); low high-density lipoprotein (HDL) cholesterol values of <40 mg/dl (1.04 mmol/l) for men and <50 mg/dl (1.29 mmol/l) for women; hypertension with values of >130/85 mm Hg; or high fasting plasma glucose of >100 mg/dl (Ford *et al.*, 2002; Grundy *et al.*, 2004). Other risk factors that affect recommendations are itemized below.

19.2.2 Special considerations

Risk factors

Overweight and obesity are independent risk factors for coronary heart disease (CHD) and premature death (Anderson and Konz, 2001). Overweight or obese women who have gained weight after 18 years of age have

Table 19.1 Lifestyle approaches to the management of overweight and obesity

Description	Components	Example	Ref.
Self-help	Encouraged to lose weight		(Heshka *et al.*, 2003)
Meal replacements (MR)	Use two MR daily	Slim-Fast®	(Heymsfield *et al.*, 2003)
Physician counseling	Mutual goal setting Physical activity Specific plan to reduce energy intake May include MR		(Bowerman *et al.*, 2001)
Community programme	Education programme Weekly group meetings Calorie-counting system Packaged food available	Weight Watchers®	(Heshka *et al.*, 2003)
Dietetic counseling	Tailored to individual		(Bowerman *et al.*, 2001)
Behavioral programme	Behavioral programme Weekly group meetings Exercise expected Record keeping		(Wadden & Foster, 2001)
Low-energy diet programme (LCD)	Behavioral programme Weekly group meetings Weekly phone calls Meal replacement use required Exercise expected Calorie-counting system Record keeping	Health Management Resources®	(Anderson *et al.*, 1992; Serdula *et al.*, 1999)

a six-fold higher risk of CHD than non-overweight women who have not gained weight since age 18 (Anderson *et al.*, 2001). Weight gain and obesity can increase risk by 90-fold compared to persons who are non-overweight and have not gained weight since adolescence (Anderson *et al.*, 2003). Major risk factors for CHD are these: family history of premature CHD; cigarette smoking; hypertension; diabetes mellitus; elevated low-density lipoprotein (LDL)–cholesterol values; low HDL–cholesterol values; age of >45 years for men and >55 years for women (Expert Panel on Detection, 2001). Other CHD risk factors to consider include these: hypertriglyceridemia (Ginsberg, 1997); elevated serum homocysteine levels (Boushey *et al.*, 1995); and elevated serum C-reactive protein levels (Ridker *et al.*, 2000). Other risk factors that contribute to disability and premature death are these: obstructive sleep apnea; excessive dyspnea with exertion; musculoskeletal problems and degenerative joint disease; varicose vein disease; gastroesophageal reflux disease; and lymphedema or elephantiasis of the lower extremities.

Table 19.2 Guidance for the management of overweight or obese individuals[a]

Weight/risk assessment	Preferred treatment	More intensive treatment	Less intensive treatment
BMI 25–30 kg/m^2 No risk factors	Meal replacements	Physician counseling	Self-help
BMI 25–30 kg/m^2 Risk factors	Physician counseling	Community programme	Meal replacements
BMI 30–35 kg/m^2	LCD programme (Behavioral programme)	LCD programme (Behavioral programme)	Dietetic counseling
BMI 35–40 kg/m^2	LCD programme	LCD programme	Dietetic counseling
BMI 40–50 kg/m^2	LCD programme	Bariatric surgery	Not recommended
BMI >50 kg/m^2	Bariatric surgery	Bariatric surgery	LCD programme

[a] This conceptual scheme follows some of the suggestions outlined by Anderson and Wadden (1999). Because effective behavioral programmes are not widely available, they are not recommended as primary choices in this outline. Pharmacotherapy may be used as adjunctive therapy in all groups except the top group with no risk factors.

Diabetes

Weight management is the most important aspect of diabetes treatment for the person with overweight or obesity (Anderson *et al.*, 2003). Virtually every overweight or obese diabetic individual should be instructed in lifestyle interventions to promote weight loss. Ongoing counseling and support is essential for these patients because most therapeutic agents for diabetes promote weight gain. Individuals of all ages and physical capabilities can be educated about ways to increase their physical activity. Reducing energy intake usually dramatically decreases blood glucose values and allows use of meal replacements and fruits with generous amounts of simple carbohydrate (Anderson *et al.*, 2003; Reynolds *et al.*, 2002; Reynolds and Anderson, 2004).

Adolescents

Overweight and obese adolescents can be effectively managed with meal replacements or low-energy diets. We have found use of two meal replacements daily, pedometers and lifestyle diaries to be effective adjuncts for management of obese adolescents (Anderson *et al.*, 2002b; Anderson, 2003b). We have modified the HMR® Healthy Solutions Programme for teenagers and use three meal replacement shakes, two meal replacement entrées, and five fruits or vegetables daily in this programme. Weight loss at 16 weeks with this approach exceeds 10% of initial body weight (Major and Anderson, 2004). Overweight adolescents have BMI >85th percentile for sex and age reflecting an adult BMI >25 kg/m^2. Obese adolescents have BMI >95th percentile for sex and age reflecting an adult BMI >30 kg/m^2. In recommending a nutrition intervention for adolescents we use these selection criteria: age >13 years; adequate sexual maturity with Tanner score of >3 and presence of menstrual periods for girls; the teenager is eager to lose weight and committed to intervention (rather than having a parent or parents who are eager with ambivalence on part of the teen); the adolescent has average intelligence (since mentally challenged individuals have difficulty grasping the complexities of the education programme); and absence of a significant psychiatric disease (such as a bipolar affective disorder). The management of overweight children is discussed elsewhere and will not be reviewed here (Yanovski and Yanovski, 2003).

Serious illnesses
After appropriate medical assessment and consultation with the appropriate medical sub-specialist and dietitian, virtually all obese adults with serious illnesses can be managed in a medically supervised LCD programme. Recently we have treated octogenarians with severe congestive heart failure, patients under treatment for life-threatening attacks of ventricular tachycardia, kidney-transplant candidates on hemodialysis or peritoneal dialysis, and liver-transplant candidates with severe liver failure.

19.3 Physical activity approaches

Increased physical activity provides many health benefits, protects from a number of chronic diseases and decreases premature mortality (Blair *et al.*, 2004; Rippe and Hess, 1998). Specifically, higher levels of physical activity compared to lower levels are associated with reduced risk for CHD, diabetes, hypertension, osteoporosis, and certain forms of cancer (e.g. breast cancer) (Rippe and Hess, 1998). In addition, increased physical activity may improve psychological health by decreasing prevalence of anxiety and depression and otherwise improving quality of life (Kiernan *et al.*, 2001; Rippe and Hess, 1998). Limited counseling, for 3–5 minutes, by primary care clinicians with one optional follow-up visit did not significantly affect levels of physical activity (Eden *et al.*, 2002). While not carefully assessed, multiple interventions – such as counseling, giving education material, clinician and patients mutually setting exercise goals, and written prescriptions – may enhance the increase in physical activity (Eden *et al.*, 2002). Current public health recommendations for physical activity are for 30 minutes of moderate intensity activity/day (Blair *et al.*, 2004). For persons with weight concerns, if 30 minutes/day does not enable them to maintain their weight, a gradual increase to 60 minutes/day is recommended (Blair *et al.*, 2004).

19.3.1 Physical activity and weight loss

Increasing physical activity without dietary changes does not appear to have a significant effect on body weight for overweight or obese subjects. However, increasing physical activity appears to be associated with slightly more weight loss than diet alone (Grilo, 1995; Miller *et al.*, 1997; Votruba *et al.*, 2000). Subjects assigned to an aerobic exercise LCD weight loss group appeared to have better dietary compliance than the LCD control group without exercise (Racette *et al.*, 2001). Increased physical activity may preserve lean body mass better than weight loss without exercise (Votruba *et al.*, 2000). The psychological benefits of adding exercise to a weight-loss programme include greater restraint in eating and less hunger (Kiernan *et al.*, 2001). Miller and colleagues (Miller *et al.*, 1997) performed a meta-analysis of 493 weight loss trials over a 25-year period. Weight loss and duration of treatment (number of studies) for different interventions were: diet alone, 10.7 kg in 15 weeks ($n = 269$); exercise alone, 2.9 kg in 21 weeks ($n = 90$); and diet plus exercise, 11.0 kg in 13 weeks ($n = 134$). Thus, the available data indicates that encouraging individuals to increase physical activity slightly enhances the weight loss associated with an energy-restricted diet and has other health and psychological benefits.

19.3.2 Physical activity and weight maintenance

Increased physical activity contributes significantly to long-term maintenance of weight loss. At an average of 2.7 years of follow-up, study subjects who had been instructed to include exercise in their LCD were maintaining a weight loss of 12.5 kg compared to 6.7 kg for control subjects instructed in the LCD without an emphasis on exercise (Anderson *et al.*, 2001). Many other reviews and meta-analyses confirm these observations (Fogelhorn and Kukkonen-Harjula, 2000; Grilo, 1995; Jeffery *et al.*, 2003; Miller *et al.*, 1997; Tremblay *et al.*, 1999). Various investigators have calculated the increase in physical activity required to enhance maintenance of weight loss but these are only estimates (Fogelhorn and Kukkonen-Harjula, 2000; Jeffery *et al.*, 2003; Schoeller, 2003). Our clinical experience is consistent with the estimate that an increase in physical activity of 1500–2000 kcal/week is minimal for successful maintenance of weight loss.

19.3.3 Practical considerations

Encouraging regular physical activity is an essential element in the weight loss plan (Rippe and Hess, 1998). Everyone can find ways to increase their level of physical activity. While commitment to physical activity enhances other elements of the lifestyle change, exercise alone is not an effective tool for promoting weight loss (Votruba *et al.*, 2000). We find pedometers to be useful adjuncts to weight loss (Anderson *et al.*, 2002a). Usually we encourage patients to obtain baseline assessments of daily steps or miles and increase this by approximately 50% initially. For people who do not wish to use pedometers, we encourage walking a specific number of minutes daily. In our HMR® Programme we encourage everyone to achieve and maintain a physical activity goal of expending 2000 kcal/week physical activity above their usual activity level. To help patients with these calculations we provide tables giving energy (kcal) expenditure per minute for different levels of physical activity for different body weights.

In the office we use multiple methods to enhance education and motivation to increase physical activity. First, we estimate the patient's current level of physical activity per day. We discuss the specific health benefits of increasing physical activity and jointly estimate how much the daily physical activity can be increased. We review a handout summarizing the health benefits of physical activity. If indicated, we give guidance for purchase of a pedometer. Then on a prescription pad we usually list three goals that with the patient we have mutually developed. The first goal relates to physical activity and indicates a specific physical activity goal such as walking 20 minutes daily (or increasing baseline pedometer steps by 50%) or doing four sets of upper body exercises with weights twice daily. The other two goals in this office visit are specific nutrition goals (e.g. use two MR daily or use diet soda instead of regular soda) and to use a specific number of fruits and vegetables daily. These physical activity and nutrition goals are usually reinforced by a dietitian and reinforced at monthly office visits. In a recent clinical study using pedometers, subjects were able to double their physical activity – increasing weekly kcal expenditure from 1500 to 3000 kcal – and sustain this increase for 6 months (Anderson *et al.*, 2002a).

19.4 Behavior modification

Several behavioral factors contribute to an individual's ability to change their lifestyle practices including societal pressures, discrimination and expectations of the individual. Behavioral treatment of obesity consists of principles and techniques to modify eating and activity habits. The focus of the treatment is for the individual to obtain skills toward a positive lifestyle change. Instructing patients in diets and physical activity regimens has little impact unless they are empowered to make these important lifestyle changes. Behavior therapy for weight management teaches individuals the process of changing their eating, physical activity, and thinking habits (Wadden *et al.*, 1999). This section will discuss behavior modification techniques to enable individuals to make these changes.

19.4.1 Dietary intake

Some behavioral strategies to modify dietary intake are to teach and incorporate tools for controlling portion size and healthier food choices (e.g. low fat food choices). Patients can be instructed on portion sizes by a registered dietitian or nutritionist and given visual examples of what an appropriate portion size is. Keeping daily food records is also an extremely useful tool in reducing food intake. The daily records should consist of the type of foods consumed, portion sizes, the amount of calories consumed, times, places and activities done when eating. Some individuals consume foods for comfort or to alleviate stress. When an individual presents who consumes food for psychological reasons, their thoughts and emotions while eating should also be discussed and recorded. Daily records allow the individual to recognize the current habits and then to focus on needed dietary changes.

Another effective method in modifying dietary intake is the use of meal replacements. Eating patterns are often altered by the use of meal replacements and the removal of their usual favorite and comfort foods. As patients decondition to intake of their usual foods, they can incorporate healthier, lower energy foods as substitutes. This process of environmental control first is 'subtractive' in that usual foods are removed and later is 'additive' in that healthier choices are brought into the environment (Reynolds and Anderson, 2004).

19.4.2 Physical activity

Often patients increase their physical activity because this is expected by their health care team, they learn new strategies for 'doable' physical activity under their specific circumstances, and they keep daily records of physical activity (Reynolds and Anderson, 2004). However, many overweight or obese individuals are reluctant to begin any physical activity due to embarrassment and/or the difficulty in including physical activity into their lifestyle because of their excess weight. Counseling individuals to incorporate physical activity slowly into their daily schedules and discussing their individual interests, preferences, and readiness for change, may ease the transition of incorporating physical activity into their daily lives.

A review of individually adapted health behavior change programmes found these programmes to be beneficial and effective for integrating physical activity. These programmes teach participants the behavioral skills needed to incorporate moderate-intensity physical activity into daily routines. Behaviors may be planned (e.g. a daily walk) or unplanned (e.g. using the stairs when the opportunity arises). All programmes reviewed incorporated the following set of skills: (1) setting goals for physical activity and self-monitoring of progress toward goals, (2) building social support for new behavioral patterns, (3) behavioral reinforcement through self-reward and positive self-talk, (4) structured problem-solving geared to maintaining the behavior change, and (5) prevention of relapse into sedentary behaviors (Preventive Health Services, 2002).

19.4.3 Changing lifestyle habits

Concentration on lifestyle changes vs. weight loss *per se* has been a major focus of behavior modification. One of the most widely used and practiced behavioral modification programmes is the LEARN® Programme for Weight Management (Brownell, 2000) developed by Kelly Brownell. The LEARN acronym was created from the first letter of the five essential components of the programme: lifestyle, exercise, attitudes, relationships and nutrition. Brownell's programme is based on the concept that individuals should change their lifestyle to better their health through practice and to incorporate healthier food choices and physical activity into their daily routines without concentrating on weight loss. People who learn new habits and practice them for at least 6 months have an excellent chance to maintain these new behaviors for long-term periods of time. It is believed that changes in lifestyle including eating habits and physical activity should promote improvements in health benefits even if weight loss is minimal.

As a clinician it is important that the patient know the rationale for changing their behavior and to target the behavior specifically. Planning a strategy for success in changing a behavior is extremely important, along with preparing for any barriers the patient may encounter while incorporating the new behavior into their lifestyle. This planning should be done in conjunction with the patient. In planning a strategy the following should be included: (1) establish a specific time and place when and where the new behavior will be incorporated; (2) have the patient keep a record of whether the behavior was accomplished or not; (3) follow-up with the individual and discuss what happened and what can be done to enhance success or problem-solve barriers in the future; and (4) reinforce success to the patient incorporating a new behavior into their lifestyle without criticizing failure or failures in their efforts.

19.4.4 Behavioral approach of the HMR® Programme for Weight Management

The philosophy of the HMR® Programme for Weight Management is that 'the real challenge in obesity treatment is in the how-tos: How does one change old, overpracticed behaviors and learn new, successful weight management behaviors in a culture and environment that is totally unsupportive of those efforts?' (Health Management Resources, 1999) The HMR® Programme focuses on Five Success Variables™ for weight and health management. The Five Success Variables™ are composed of the Programme Commitments and the Triple Imperative™. The Programme Commitments consist of mandatory weekly attendance and midweek phone call with a health educator and also daily record keeping of meal replacement use, fruit and vegetable intake and physical activity. These commitments provide the structure and the accountability that the patients need in order to learn and practice the behaviors that are imperative to successful weight management. The Triple Imperative™ consists of the following three components: (1) minimum of 2000 calories of physical activity per week; (2) minimum of 35 servings of vegetables and fruits per week (if the current weight loss programme the individual is participating in allows); and (3) use of meal replacements (for individuals in a weight loss phase this is a minimum of 35 meal replacements per week and for individuals in a weight maintenance programme, a minimum of 14 meal replacements). The Triple Imperative™ provides the patient with the skills that control the greatest degree of variability in an individual's weight management efforts (Health Management Resources, 1999).

19.5 Comparative weight loss with different nutrition approaches

Many nutrition approaches utilize meal replacements (MR) or partial meal replacements. These MR consist of liquid nutrition supplements (herein termed 'shakes'), portion-controlled meals (herein termed 'entrées'), and bars. Supplemental vitamins and minerals are also recommended.

Very-low-calorie diets (VLCD) usually provide 450–800 kcal/day (Anderson *et al.*, 1992). Usually, packets of product are mixed in water to provide ~ five shakes per day. We will review the use of these diets and our own experience (Anderson *et al.*, 2004). Low-calorie diets (LCD) usually provide 800–1500 kcal/day. These diets often include shakes, entrées and, sometimes, bars. We will review the use of these diets and our own experience (Anderson *et al.*, 2004). Energy-restricted diets (ERD): emphasize a reduction in energy intake, usually by 500–600 kcal/day; often a specific energy intake is not specified. These approaches are reviewed elsewhere and will not be discussed in this chapter (Anderson *et al.*, 2004). Portion control or food provision provides prepackaged entrées to decrease energy intake at meals. These approaches are reviewed elsewhere and will not be discussed in this chapter (Anderson *et al.*, 2004; Flechtner-Mors *et al.*, 2000). Meal replacements (MR) usually recommend the use of two MR daily; these can be shakes, entrees, or bars. We will review the use of these diets and our own experience.

Assessing weight loss with different interventions is difficult because the most important variable, the individual's commitment and desire to lose weight, cannot be accurately assessed. Extensive research indicates that persons who present to research programmes comparing drug vs. placebo lose about 3 kg or 3% of initial body weight over a 6-month period with a low-intensity intervention (Haddock, 2003). We calculated the weighted weight loss of 1499 placebo-treated subjects participating in 38 clinical trials analyzed by Haddock and colleagues (Haddock, 2003). Over an average of 26.5 weeks, these subjects lost an average of 2.9 kg or approximately 3% of their initial body weight. This may serve as a surrogate measure of the weight that subjects may lose if they visit a dietitian on a regularly scheduled basis.

Some individuals lose large amounts of weight with self-help programmes (Klem *et al.*, 1997) but they appear to be exceptions to the rule. In Table 19.3 we have summarized weight losses over 6 months reported from research studies. Most of these results have been reported previously and are summarized here to give an approximation of weight loss that might be expected with the different interventions. The rate of weight loss from representative studies is summarized in Fig. 19.1. With most weight-loss interventions the rate of weight loss is most rapid during the first 8 weeks, and is almost linear. Weight loss decelerates between 8 and 16 weeks and reaches the nadir around 16–20 weeks. Although not shown in the figure, average weight begins to increase after about 20 weeks of treatment (Anderson *et al.*, 2002a, 2004).

Although approximately one-third of the adult US population is actively attempting to lose weight (Serdula *et al.*, 1999), the natural history is for adults to gain weight (Rothacker, 2000). Our colleagues (Heshka *et al.*, 2003) attempted to estimate weight changes in a self-help group compared to subjects engaged in a community programme over a 2-year period. While the self-help group lost significant amounts of weight in the first 24 weeks (Table 19.3), by 2 years their weight had returned essentially to baseline. Information on results of dietetic counseling are limited, but in one study (Ashley *et al.*, 2001) subjects lost 4.1% of initial body weight in 24 weeks. This is in the range reported for subjects receiving placebo as part of a pharmacotherapy clinical trial (2.9%) (Haddock, 2003). As we reported (Heshka *et al.*, 2003), subjects who were given coupons to participate in a community programme without charge lost an average of 6.1% of initial body weight in 24 weeks. Providing access to two MR daily is a very cost-effective way of promoting weight loss. Our meta-analysis of four studies noted a weight loss of 9.1% at 24 weeks. These observations are supported by other analyses (Heymsfield *et al.*, 2003) and longer term studies (Blackburn and Rothacker, 2003).

Behavioral programmes require a considerably greater time commitment – weekly classes for an average of 22 weeks – than dietetic counselling or education about meal replacements. We estimated that MR use required <4 hours of education over 6 months while behavioral LED interventions required >32 hours in 6 months (Anderson *et al.*, 2004). Despite more intense intervention, ERD were associated with less average weight loss (8.5%) than were MR (9.1%) at 24 weeks (Anderson *et al.*, 2004). Behavioral LED programmes were associated with greater weight loss (11.4%) than MR at 24 weeks but these differences were not significant. While behavioral LED programmes, usually emphasizing food selection and not using MR, enable the average person to lose >10% of initial body weight, effective programmes are not widely available. Only a few US

Table 19.3 Weight loss comparisons with different diets

Group	No. of Studies	No. of Subjects	Energy intake (kcal/d)	Initial BMI (kg/m²)	Initial weight (kg)	Weight loss, 24 weeks (% initial)	95% CI (%)	Reference
Self-help	1	172	Variable	33.6	93.1	1.7	0.9–2.6	(Heshka *et al.*, 2003)
Community programme	1	175	Variable	33.8	94.2	6.1	5.0–7.1	(Heshka *et al.*, 2003)
Dietetic counseling	1	23	Variable	29.9	82.9	4.1	2.4–5.8	(Ashley *et al.*, 2001)
Meal replacement	4	579	1250	31.3	87.3	9.1	5.7–12.5	(Anderson *et al.*, 2004)
ERD	6	200	Variable	31.1	88.4	8.5	4.9–12.1	(Anderson *et al.*, 2004)
LCD	10	365	1148	36.3	101.5	11.4	8.9–13.9	(Anderson *et al.*, 2004)
Soy VLCD	8	333	468	36.2	102.7	16.5	13.9–19.1	(Anderson *et al.*, 2004)
LCD- HMR (2004)	1	265	~1000	43.7	124.7	20.1	19.1–21.1	(Anderson, 2004)
US VLCD	19	1968	434	39.6	109.9	21.3	20.1–22.5	(Anderson *et al.*, 2004)

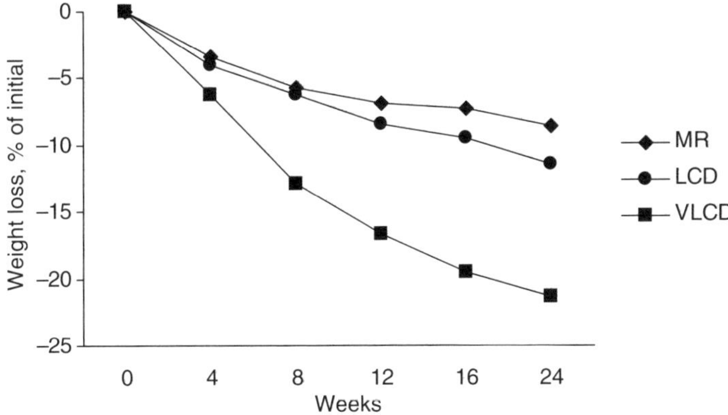

Fig. 19.1 Weight loss over time with different diets.

academic centers have reported weight losses of >10% with behavioral intervention.

VLED are associated with substantially greater weight loss than less intensive interventions. The Nutrilett® soy VLED intervention is widely used in Europe, as previously summarized (Anderson *et al.*, 2004). The clinic visits, classes and physician visits required, in aggregate, about one-third the hourly commitment that did US VLED programmes and less than half the time commitment of behavioral LED programmes. Weight loss, with this lower intensity, averaged 16.5% of initial body weight at 24 weeks (Anderson *et al.*, 2004). In our analysis of 19 reports including 1968 patients, weight loss averaged 21.3% of initial body weight with US VLED (Anderson *et al.*, 2004). Of note, we are now achieving similar weight losses with the HMR® medically supervised behavioral LED programme with better patient satisfaction and fewer side effects. As indicated in Table 19.3, our recent weight loss averages are 20.1% of initial body weight at 24 weeks.

19.5.1 Comparison of VLED and LED

Like many other clinical centers for obesity management in the 1980s, we used VLCD providing 500 kcal/day as five shakes daily (Anderson *et al.*, 1992; Wadden and Stunkard, 1986). However, as the behavioral management improved, clinical research indicated that most obese individuals could be treated as effectively with LCD of 800–1000 kcal/day in the form of shakes (Foster *et al.*, 1992; Rossner and Flaten, 1997). As the specific behavioral management improved, entrées and, later, bars were incorporated. Our early experience indicated that diabetic subjects enrolled in the intensive behavioral programme lost weight essentially as well using an evening meal of self-prepared food to substitute for two shakes as diabetic subjects randomized to use of only 5 shakes per day (Anderson *et al.*,

1994a). As indicated in Table 19.3, current patients completing our HMR® Programme using LED with shakes, entrées and bars are losing essentially the same percentage body weight as subjects previously treated with VLCD in our HMR® Programme (Anderson *et al.*, 1992) and other programmes such as Optifast® and Medifast® (Anderson *et al.*, 2004). Currently, patients enrolled in our programme select whether they want to use five shakes daily (800 kcal/day) or three shakes plus two entrées daily (820–1000 kcal/day).

19.5.2 Weight maintenance considerations

The maintenance of weight loss after various weight loss interventions is summarized in Table 19.4. In studies using MR, the use of MR is often continued for a long-term period after the weight-loss phase is completed (Blackburn and Rothacker, 2003; Flechtner-Mors *et al.*, 2000; Rothacker, 2000). Thus, it is difficult to compare results of long-term MR studies with other research reports. Nevertheless, long-term use of MR is associated with rather remarkable long-term maintenance of weight loss (Blackburn and Rothacker, 2003; Flechtner-Mors *et al.*, 2000; Rothacker, 2000). As indicated in Table 19.4, individuals who lose weight using two SlimFast® daily and then continue to use one MR daily for the next 45 months maintain ~90% of the weight lost. Further long-term controlled studies are required to confirm these preliminary observations. As previously reported in a meta-analysis (Anderson *et al.*, 2004), obese subjects treated with LED regain >80% of the weight lost over the next 54 months if there is no further intervention. Persons who lose an average of 24 kg with VLCD maintain a weight loss of ~30% at 54 months of follow-up. Our previous experience with the HMR® Programme at our institution indicates that 25% of patients are maintaining a weight loss of >10% of initial weight loss (~11 kg) at 7 years (Anderson *et al.*, 1999). Recently we obtained follow-up data for 73 morbidly obese patients who had lost >100 pounds (45.5 kg) in the HMR® programme at our institution. Follow-up weights were available for 75% of

Table 19.4 Long-term maintenance of weight loss

Diet Intervention	No. of studies (No. of subjects)	Weight loss, 6 months (kg)	Weight maintenance (kg)	Percentage weight loss maintained
MR[a]	1 (32)	8.7	7.8[c]	89.7
LCD[b]	8 (448)	8.8	2.1[d]	17.8
VLCD[b]	4 (578)	24.1	6.6[d]	29.4

[a] Data from Flechtner-Mors *et al.*, 2000.
[b] Data from Anderson *et al.*, 2004.
[c] Follow-up for 45 months.
[d] Follow-up for 54 months.

patients from 52–520 weeks. These patients lost an average of 63.3 kg and at an average of 233 weeks (4.5 years) were maintaining a weight loss of 45.5 kg (72% of weight loss). We estimated the maintenance of weight loss for the 19 patients for whom no follow-up weights were available, based on previous data (Anderson *et al.*, 1999). For the entire group of 73 patients, the estimated weight maintenance at an average of 180 weeks (3.5 years) was 59% of the weight lost.

These data support our clinical observations indicating that patients completing our behavioral LCD programme are maintaining long-term weight loss significantly better than the results reported previously (Anderson *et al.*, 1999, 2001).

19.6 Very-low-calorie diets

VLCD in the US are medically supervised diet programmes recommended for individuals with a BMI >30 kg/m^2 or for individuals with BMI >27 kg/m^2 with comorbidities such as hypertension or type 2 diabetes. VLCD are total diet replacements providing 50–70 grams of protein and 400–800 kcal/day (Anderson *et al.*, 1992).

19.6.1 Weight loss

The average rate of weight loss with VLCD is illustrated in Fig. 19.1. With an average degree of dietary compliance, men and women lose approximately 2% of initial body weight per week during the first 8 weeks of the VLCD. Patients with initial BMI values >35 kg/m^2 who have excellent compliance to the dietary regimen lose an average of approximately 30% of their initial body weight or about 35 kg (Anderson *et al.*, 1992). Morbidly obese individuals with average dietary compliance lose an average of 27% of their initial body weight or about 36 kg (Anderson *et al.*, 1992). Men, with higher initial body weights, lose more weight than women but the percentage reduction in weight does not differ significantly between sexes (Anderson *et al.*, 2001, 2004). These weight loss data relate to treatments initiated in the late 1980s and early 1990s with traditional VLCD using five shakes/day and providing ~500 kcal/day (Anderson *et al.*, 1992; Wadden *et al.*, 1992). Average weight loss in our current HMR® Programme for medically supervised patients is >20% of initial body weight for patients who complete the 12-week core programme (Gotthelf *et al.*, 2004).

19.6.2 Reduction in risk factors

Obese individuals have substantially higher risks for CHD than matched controls (Anderson and Konz, 2001; McGill *et al.*, 2002). Some of these risks are related to traditional risk factors but others appear related to inflammatory cytokines, pro-coagulant and oxidation factors associated with the obesity state (Davi *et al.*, 2002; Morrow, 2003; Sowers, 2003). Patients who present for treatment have these cardiovascular risk factors and other co-morbidities: hypertension, 68%; hypercholesterolemia, 38%; hypertriglyceridemia, 14%; diabetes, 6%; impaired fasting blood glucose, 8%; hyperuricemia or gout, 4%; degenerative joint disease, 18%; or sleep apnea, 1% (Anderson *et al.*, 1992).

Changes in major CHD risk factors for patients who had excellent adherence to the VLCD and lost ~30% of their initial body weight are summarized in Table 19.6. Serum cholesterol and LDL-cholesterol values decrease rapidly and reach a nadir after 6 weeks of weight loss. Values often increase after this time, probably related to decreased LDL-receptor activity in the liver and to continued mobilization of cholesterol from adipose tissue stores (Anderson *et al.*, 1992). Serum HDL-cholesterol values usually increase slightly in men while values in women often decrease slightly in response to VLCD (Anderson *et al.*, 1992). Fasting serum triglycerides decrease dramatically in virtually all patients with decreases ranging from 15–50% (Anderson *et al.*, 1992). Fasting serum glucose values decrease 5–10% for non-diabetic subjects and decrease dramatically by ~35% for diabetic subjects with VLCD (Anderson *et al.*, 2003). Reductions in systolic and diastolic blood pressure average about 10% and are similar in men and women (Anderson *et al.*, 1992).

19.6.3 Side effects

Obese individuals, especially women, have a high risk for gallbladder disease (Grundy, 2004). Asymptomatic or symptomatic cholelithiasis is the major side effect associated with VLCD (Schiffman *et al.*, 1995). In our clinical experience with VLCD, about 2–3% of patients develop symptoms of cholelithiasis during the weight loss phase of treatment and up to 6% require cholecystectomy during the weight loss or within 3 months of resuming their usual diet (Anderson *et al.*, 1992). Ursodeoxycholic acid can be used to reduce the frequency of cholecystitis during weight loss with VLCD but we have not used this prophylactically unless patients had symptomatic disease before starting the diet. While some clinicians provide 1–2 tablespoons of vegetable oil daily to reduce risk of gallbladder complications with VLCD, we have not seen documentation that this is effective.

Minor side effects seen in >5% of patients with VLCD are as follows: fatigue or weakness, 52%; orthostatic dizziness, 41%; constipation, 31%; diarrhea, 23%; nausea, 19%; headaches, 21%; hair loss after >20 kg weight loss, 10%; and dry skin, 6%. The fatigue or weakness is usually most marked over the first few weeks of diet and diminishes after that; sometimes patients are instructed to increase use of shakes to obtain more energy intake to alleviate fatigue. Orthostatic dizziness can often be alleviated by increased fluid intake although reductions in antihypertensive medications is required if the blood pressure is too low. Symptomatic management usually relieves the initial gastrointestinal symptoms. Weight loss can occasionally precipitate gouty arthritis or tendonitis in persons who have a diagnosis of gout; these attacks can be treated in the usual manner without interrupting the VLCD (Anderson *et al.*, 1992).

Changes in laboratory values are commonly seen with significant weight loss in VLCD programmes (Anderson *et al.*, 1992). When intakes of minerals are decreased, the body has excellent mechanisms for conserving sodium but only fair mechanisms for preserving potassium (Anderson *et al.*, 1969). Thus, VLCD should provide adequate potassium, thiazide diuretics are usually discontinued with starting the diet, and serum potassium should be monitored. Serum uric acid values usually decrease significantly but may increase for persons with hyperuricemia or gout; increases can usually be corrected by encouraging increased fluid intake or increasing the level of energy intake by about 200 kcal/day. Serum iron values usually decrease during weight loss diets representing, perhaps, an acute phase response. We often initiate iron supplements if serum iron levels drop below 30 μg/dl on two occasions or if low serum iron values are associated with development of iron-deficiency anemia.

Non-alcoholic fatty liver disease affects >67% of obese individuals and >90% of morbidly obese individuals and is the predominant cause of abnormal liver tests in obese patients (Angulo, 2002). As patients lose weight with VLCD and fat is mobilized from the liver, serum transaminase values commonly increase by two to three-fold higher than baseline values. These increases are usually transient and values return to baseline after 6–8 weeks. Patients with mild liver-test abnormalities at baseline are more likely to show significant increases than persons with normal values. If unexpected increases occur, it is important to insure that the patient is meeting the minimum nutrition prescription. Increases in serum bilirubin levels by two to three-fold with changes in serum transaminase values may be seen in patients with Gilbert's syndrome (Anderson *et al.*, 1992). As patients increase their physical activity, increases in serum creatine phosphokinase and lactic dehydrogenase may increase from baseline.

19.6.4 Long-term weight maintenance

After the safety of VLCD was accepted (Wadden *et al.*, 1983), the nutrition community raised concerns about long-term maintenance of weight loss after completing VLCD programmes. As behavioral education improved, patients began learning and practicing weight maintenance behaviors while losing weight on the VLCD programme. Results from patients treated with Optifast® (Wadden *et al.*, 1992) and HMR® (Anderson *et al.*, 1999) showed acceptable long-term maintenance of weight loss. When we did a critical meta-analysis of reports from the United States, we noted that individuals were maintaining a significantly greater percentage of their weight loss at an average 4.5 years after completing a VLCD programme than after completing LCD (Anderson *et al.*, 2001). Specifically, after VLCD, maintenance of weight loss was three-fold greater than after LCD. Studies from Europe also indicate that individuals who lose the greatest amount of weight maintain the greatest amount of weight loss long term (Astrup *et al.*, 2000; Saris, 2001; Westerterp-Plantenga *et al.*, 1998).

19.6.5 Comments

LCD use has replaced VLCD use in most medical centers because, as noted above, most individuals lose as much weight with LCD as with VLCD. Furthermore, side effects are much lower with LCD and less intensive medical monitoring is required. We rarely use diets providing <800 kcal at our medical center.

19.7 Low-calorie diet use

LCDs provide 800–1500 kcal/day from food or from MR (Anderson *et al.*, 2004). LCDs are difficult for individuals to sustain unless they have nutrition counseling and ongoing follow-up and reinforcement. Some individuals are able to maintain an energy intake of ≤1500 kcal/day using two MR shakes daily (Anderson *et al.*, 2004). Behavioral programmes with weekly classes encourage participants to maintain their energy intake at ≤1500 kcal/day (Andersen *et al.*, 1995). Intensive behavioral treatment with LCD using MR are proving to be the most efficacious intervention for moderate and severe obesity. The HMR® Programme at the University of Kentucky uses a LCD intervention with five shakes (800 kcal/day) or three shakes plus two MR entrées (800–1000 kcal/day) as the primary intervention for most patients. We have learned to encourage patients to use 'more is better' because our data indicate that patients who use additional shakes, MR entrées, or bars are less likely to eat food that is 'out of the product box'. Consequently, most of our patients successfully lose weight consuming their minimum 'prescription' intake of MR (800–1000 kcal/day) and additional products averaging about 400–600 kcal/day.

19.7.1 Weight loss

Average weight loss from LCD, as summarized in Table 19.3, is 11.4 kg. Most of the 10 studies analyzed were behavioral programmes at academic centers (Anderson *et al.*, 2004). At the HMR® Programme at the University of Kentucky we have used LCD, composed of MR, as part of an intense behavioral programme and have weight losses that average 20.1 kg (Table 19.3).

Currently, our HMR® Programmes offer treatment for overweight and obese individual with a selection of options. For persons with BMI

>35 kg/m^2, we recommend the medically supervised LCD option that includes weekly nursing visits and weekly physician visits for 8 weeks and subsequently biweekly physician visits. For persons with BMI <35 kg/m^2 we offer an intermediate option with weekly nursing visits and biweekly physician visits. For persons with BMI <30 kg/m^2 we offer the moderate option with LCD without medical supervision. Individuals enrolling in one of these three options select use of five shakes daily or three shakes plus two MR entrées daily. They are encouraged to use additional shakes, MR entrées, or bars instead of using non-product food items. In addition to these three options, patients may choose the non-medically supervised Healthy Solutions® LCD option. This option provides a minimum of three shakes, two MR entrées, and five servings of fruits or vegetables daily.

Weight losses with the four HMR® LCD options are summarized in Table 19.5. We include results for all patients who enrolled and attended one class (intention-to-treat (ITT) or last-observation-carried-forward analysis) and for patients who completed the 12-week core education programme (completers analysis). These results are obtained from three HMR® training centers, including the University of Kentucky programme, that submitted data for all patients enrolled in their programme over a 3-year period. Because these programmes are training centers, the options provided and the outcome data are essentially the same from the three centers. Medically supervised patients were those with BMI >35 kg/m^2 or having medical conditions such as diabetes that required close medical supervision. Three hundred and ninety patients enrolled in the medically supervised option. Their initial weight averaged 124.7 kg and the BMI 42.8 kg/m^2. This group of patients completed 18 weeks of treatment and lost

Table 19.5 Reduction in risk factors with weight loss for men (M) and women (W) with excellent adherence to VLCD (Modified from Anderson *et al*, 1992.)

Measurement	Sex	Initial	% change
Weight, kg	M	125.1	–28.9
	F	106.8	–29.9
Cholesterol, mmol/l	M	5.8	–23.6
	F	5.6	–16.4
LDL–cholesterol, mmol/l	M	3.9	–25.4
	F	3.6	–15.0
HDL–cholesterol, mmol/l	M	1.0	+6.1
	F	1.2	–12.2
Triglycerides, mmol/l	M	2.0	–47.3
	F	1.7	–28.9
Systolic blood pressure, mm Hg	M	143	–11.9
	F	132	–12.1
Diastolic blood pressure, mm Hg	M	92	–10.9
	F	89	–13.5

an average of 16.2% of initial body weight (ITT analysis). Of this group, 265 patients completed the 12-week core programme. These individuals had initial BMI values of 43.7 kg/m^2 and remained in treatment for an average of 24 weeks with weight losses averaging 20.1% of initial body weight (completers analysis).

For intermediate participants with BMIs of 30–35 kg/m^2, 213 patients enrolled in this option with initial weights averaging 91.9 kg and BMIs of 32.7 kg/m^2. For all patients the average weight loss was 13.3% of initial body weight in an average of 15 weeks in the programme. For patients who completed the 12-week core programme, average weight losses were 19.2% of initial body weight in an average of 21 weeks. Patients in the intermediate programme lost significantly less weight than those in the medically supervised programme.

For moderate participants with BMIs of 25–30 kg/m^2, 152 patients enrolled in this option with initial weights averaging 77.1 kg and BMIs of 28.0 kg/m^2. For all patients the average weight loss was 11.5% of initial body weight in an average of 13 weeks in the programme. For patients who completed the 12-week core programme, average weight losses were 15.5% of initial body weight in an average of 18 weeks. Average weight loss for moderate patients, as percentage of initial weight, did not differ significantly from that of patients in the intermediate option.

For Healthy Solutions® participants who did not have medical supervision and consumed vegetables and fruits in addition to five MR daily, 224 patients enrolled in this option with initial weights averaging 101.3 kg and BMIs of 35.2 kg/m^2. For all patients the average weight loss was 11.2% of initial body weight in an average of 14 weeks in the programme. For patients who completed the 12-week core programme, average weight losses were 15.4% of initial body weight in an average of 20 weeks. Weight losses for patients in the Healthy Solutions option, as a percentage of initial body weight, did not differ significantly from that for patients in the intermediate or moderate options.

19.7.2 Reduction in risk factors

Patients losing 15–20% of initial body weight have significant reductions in CHD risk factors and other co-morbid conditions such as sleep apnea and gastroesophageal reflux disease. Currently, we are analyzing outcome data for patients who have recently completed the various HMR® options. Previous analyses indicate that the percentage reduction in risk factors, such as blood pressure, parallel the percentage reduction in body weight (Anderson *et al.*, 1994b). There is a significant ($P < 0.005$) positive linear relationship between changes in these risk factors and weight: serum cholesterol, LDL-cholesterol, triglycerides, systolic and diastolic blood pressure. However, there is a significant ($P = 0.021$) negative relationship between weight loss and serum HDL-cholesterol levels (Anderson *et al.*,

1994b). Recently, we estimated the reduction in risk factors associated with weight loss from the best available meta-analyses in the literature (Anderson and Konz, 2001). These results are consistent with our own data as presented in Table 19.5. These results indicate that every 10% reduction in body weight is associated with these changes in risk factors: serum cholesterol, –9.9%; LDL–cholesterol, 6.8%; triglycerides, –19.3%; HDL–cholesterol, +1.5%; systolic blood pressure, –4.9%; and diastolic blood pressure, –3.8% (Anderson and Konz, 2001).

19.7.3 Side effects

The incidence of side effects from LCD is lower than with VLCD but the clinical symptoms and laboratory changes described above can be seen. Our experience with treating persons with weights >150 kg leads us to increase initial product prescription by ≥200 kcal and to recommend even more product use as necessary to decrease symptoms of weakness and fatigue. Symptomatic gallbladder disease is less common with LCD than VLCD but we do not have prevalence data. We do not perform ultrasound screening for gallbladder disease unless the individual has had prior symptoms clearly related to gallbladder disease. We rarely prescribe ursodeoxycholic acid prophylactically. Minor side effects are less common and less severe with LCD than with VLCD and can be managed symptomatically (Anderson *et al.*, 1992).

19.7.4 Long-term maintenance of weight loss

Data on the long-term maintenance of weight loss from behavioral LCD programmes underestimates current outcomes with more intense interventions. When individuals lose 8.8 kg in 6 months, maintenance of weight loss at 54 months averages 2.1 kg or 17.8% of weight loss (Table 19.4). Currently, patients are losing 20.1 kg in our intensive LCD (Table 19.6) but we do not have long-term maintenance data on these patients. After completing our HMR® weight loss programme patients participate in the maintenance programme for an average of 8 months, during which time their use of MR, vegetables and fruits, and physical activity are reinforced and usually become habits. Long-term experience with use of MR clearly indicate their benefits in maintenance of weight loss (Blackburn and Rothacker, 2003; Rothacker, 2000). The long-term data available for morbidly obese patients who lost ≥100 pounds using our intensive LCD programme is probably representative of long-term maintenance for all patients treated in this manner. For 54 patients who have clinic weights at ≥52 weeks, initial weight loss averaged 140 pounds and average maintenance of weight loss at 161 weeks was 100 pounds or maintenance of 71% of weight loss. We conservatively estimated maintenance of weight loss for 19 patients for whom clinic weights were not available based on our previous experience (Anderson *et al.*,

Table 19.6 Weight loss with various HMR interventions

Group	Medically supervised	Intermediate	Moderate	Healthy solutions
All enrolled patients				
Number	390	213	152	224
Initial weight (kg)	124.7	91.9	77.1	101.3
Initial BMI	42.8	32.7	28	35.2
Weeks of treatment	18	15	13	14
Weight loss (% initial)	16.2	13.3	11.5	11.2
Patients completing core				
Number	265	130	82	116
Initial BMI	43.7	33	28.2	36
Weeks of treatment	24	21	18	20
Weight loss (% initial)	20.1	17.8	15.5	15.4
SD	8.2	8.2	8.2	7.3
SE	0.50	0.72	0.91	0.68
LCI	19.1	16.4	13.7	14.1
UCI	21.1	19.2	17.3	16.7

1999). Thus, for the entire group of 74 morbidly obese patients who lost ≥100 pounds in our intense LCD programme, maintenance of weight loss at an average of 180 weeks (3.5 years) was 59% of weight lost (Anderson, 2004).

19.7.5 Comments

Intensive behavioral LCD interventions are the treatment of choice for most obese individuals. Achieving a non-obese weight requiring a weight loss of >20 kg is the goal for most obese individuals. Intensive behavioral LCD programmes are the only non-surgical approaches that meet this requirement. Currently, there are less than one effective programme per million people in the USA and probably the availability is even less in other countries. Furthermore, these programmes are expensive and are not covered by health insurance. For medically supervised programmes in the USA, the MR costs are about US$240/month and the other costs (medical visits, classes and laboratory costs) are about US$180. These costs are offset by the savings in food, snacks, restaurants and medication costs. Savings in medication costs begin immediately and can average US$100/month for persons in the medically supervised programme (Collins and Anderson, 1995; Nicholas and Anderson, 2004). Thus, weight loss of >20 kg and maintenance of weight loss of >10 kg for 5 years clearly reduces medical costs but accurate estimates are not available for the long-term.

For cost comparisons, the cost of pharmacotherapy with sibutramine or orlistat approximates US$1500/year for the medication and US$1000 for medical and laboratory monitoring. Bariatric surgery is very expensive in the USA, costing US$20000–50000 (Steinbrook, 2004). Furthermore, bariatric surgery may not reduce long-term medical costs because of the costs of medical follow-up and complications (Agren *et al.*, 2002).

19.8 Meal replacement use

Widely available MR include shakes, entrées, and bars. The nutrition profiles of some representative MR are presented in Table 19.7. Nutritionally fortified shakes are sold in cans or as powders that are mixed in water or skim milk. Shakes usually provide 100–220 kcal/serving with 10–20 grams of protein. Popular shakes are SlimFast®, HMR®, Optifast®, Revival® Soy, ScanDiet™, Nutrilett® and others. MR entrées come in shelf-stable packages or as frozen entrées. These portion-controlled meals usually provide 160–360 kcal/serving with 12–20 grams of protein. Popular entrées are HMR®, Weight Watchers®, Lean Cuisine®, Healthy Choice® and others. Many 'nutrition' bars are available. These can provide 160–250 kcal/bar with 8–15 grams of protein. Most of these do not provide the nutrition content

Table 19.7 Nutrition values for representative meal replacements

Nutrient	kcal	Protein (g)	Fat (g)	Carbohydrate (g)	Fiber (g)
HMR 70® plus shake	110	14	0.1	13	0.2
HMR® 120 shake	120	11	1.5	16	<1
HMR® 500 shake	100	10	0.5	16	1
HMR® 800 shake	170	16	2	22	<1
Optifast® 800 shake	160	14	20	3	0
Optitrim® shake	230	17	29	5	0
SlimFast® shake	220	10	2.5	40	5
SlimFast® powder shake with 8 oz fat-free milk	200	13	1	37	4
Scan-Diet™ shake	160	18	3	22	7
Nutrilett® shakes	86	12.3	1.2	6.1	3.5
Medifast 55® powder shake	90	11	0.5	13	3
Medifast 70® powder shake	100	14	1	15	3
Revival® soy shake with Splenda	125	20	2.25	6.5	1
HMR® entrée[a]	200	15	4	30	6.7
Lean Cuisine® entrée[a]	234	12.6	5.4	34	3.2
Healthy Choice entrée[a]	265	21.5	5	32	3.5
Weight Watchers® Smart Ones entrée[a]	250	14	5	36.5	3.5

[a] These are representative average nutrient compositions.

available from shakes and entrées but can provide special requirements such as soy protein (Anderson, 2003a). Bars can be used to replace meals but probably are best used as snacks to avoid consumption of higher energy and less nutritious snacks.

19.8.1 Weight loss

For 579 non-diabetic subjects completing 24-week weight loss intervention in four studies using two SlimFast® MR shakes daily, weight loss averaged 9.1% of initial body weight (Table 19.3) (Anderson *et al.*, 2004). When diabetic subjects are included in a meta-analysis of 403 completing subjects, weight loss at 3 months was 7.4% of initial body weight and at one year was 8.0% of initial body weight (Heymsfield *et al.*, 2003). These reports are consistent with our clinical research experience using three different MR shakes and observing weight losses of 7.5–9.5% of initial body weight at 24-weeks for subjects using two shakes daily and completing the intervention. Thus, instructing patients to use two MR shakes daily, giving limited advice about intake of vegetables and fruits, and providing physical activity guidance is a very cost-effective weight-reduction intervention.

19.8.2 Reduction in risk factors

Based on our previous analysis (Anderson and Konz, 2001), a weight loss of 8.5% would be expected to reduce cardiovascular risk factors as follows: fasting serum cholesterol, –7.9%; LDL–cholesterol, –5.4%; triglycerides, –15.4%; HDL–cholesterol, +1.2%; systolic blood pressures, –3.9%; and diastolic blood pressure, –2.7%. These predicted changes are similar to those noted recently in a clinical trial using a milk-based MR shake (Anderson and Hoie, 2003). When soy-based MR shakes are used, serum cholesterol and LDL–cholesterol reductions are significantly greater than with animal protein (Allison *et al.*, 2003; Anderson and Hoie, 2003; Anderson *et al.*, 1995).

19.8.3 Side effects

Side effects from MR use are uncommon. Some individuals are lactose-intolerant; most can either use a lactose-free product or use the enzyme lactase to digest the lactose. Mild gastrointestinal symptoms are usually self-limited and of short duration.

19.8.4 Long-term maintenance of weight loss

Comparable long-term information on maintenance of weight loss for MR vs. LCD or VLCD is not available. The available information indicates that daily use of one or two MR or intermittent use of MR is a very important adjunct to successful weight maintenance (Blackburn and Rothacker, 2003; Rothacker, 2000; Wadden and Stunkard, 1986). One follow-up study of 45 months for 32 subjects reports maintenance of weight loss of 7.8 kg (89.7% of the initial weight loss) (Flechtner-Mors *et al.*, 2000 Rothacker, 2000). Because most interventions with MR alone do not include a behavioral education component, it seems unlikely that use of MR alone, without increased physical activity or other modifications, will result in long-term maintenance of >50% of weight lost or >4 kg.

19.8.5 Comments

Use of MR is clearly one of the most cost-effective weight-loss interventions. Furthermore, use of two MR daily is moderately effective for weight loss with average losses exceeding those expected with clinician or dietitian counseling, community programmes, and pharmacotherapy. When most individuals modify their behavior to incorporate two MR daily, they consciously or unconsciously modify other behaviors such as physical activity and food choices. Because of the extremely favorable effects of MR use on long-term weight maintenance (Blackburn and Rothacker, 2003; Flechtner-Mors *et al.*, 2000; Rothacker, 2000) overweight and obese individuals should be strongly encouraged with ongoing reinforcement to use MR with regularity. MR are inexpensive with shakes costing <US$1 each and frozen MR entrées available for <US$1.50. When MR use, increased vegetable and fruit consumption, and increase physical activity are combined, substantial weight loss and maintenance of weight loss can be achieved.

19.9 Implications and recommendations

Obesity is a major contributor to chronic disability and premature death (Pi-Sunyer, 1993). Intentional weight loss decreases risk for CHD, diabetes and premature death (Anderson *et al.*, 2003; Anderson and Konz, 2001; Gregg *et al.*, 2003). Health care providers, psychological counselors, and other advisors should offer positive and empathetic encouragement for weight loss to overweight or obese individuals. With appropriate treatment or guidance, most obese individuals can successfully lose weight and maintain substantial and health-promoting weight losses for long-term periods. For many obese people, successful weight management requires giving behavioral strategies a very high priority and committing time and resources to these endeavors. Unfortunately, a small percentage of obese persons who were extremely obese as preschool children may require bariatric surgery to achieve health-promoting body weights. Additionally, some mentally challenged individuals and persons with significant psychiatric problems may not have the capacity to cope with the rigorous discipline required for successful weight management.

Many overweight individuals can successfully lose weight and maintain a non-obese body weight over the long-term using low-intensity interventions. Strong encouragement from the primary health care provider will stimulate certain individuals to achieve and maintain desirable body weights. Persons recently told that they have hypertension, diabetes or dyslipidemia may be motivated to lose weight to reverse these conditions and avoid medication. Meal replacements or community programmes are appropriate adjuncts to physician counseling.

Most obese individuals should be encouraged to lose >20 kg to achieve a non-obese body weight. Most individuals have difficulty losing >20 kg or >20% of their current weight without an intensive behavioral intervention. Previous intensive behavioral VLCD programmes or current intensive behavioral LCD programmes are the only effective nutritional or medical therapy with proven effectiveness in fostering weight losses of >20 kg. Unfortunately, these intensive programmes require weekly clinic visits for long-term periods, are expensive, and are not covered by health insurance plans. Innovations such as the internet (Tate *et al.*, 2003) and telephone interventions (Grant and Gotthelf, 2004) can be modestly to moderately effective with more convenience and lower expense but sustained weight losses of >10 kg probably should not be expected.

Pharmacotherapy offers promise as an adjunct to nutrition, physical activity and behavioral changes. Current agents, compared to placebo, promise weight losses averaging <4 kg (Bray and Greenway, 1999; Haddock, 2003; Halpern and Mancini, 2003; McTigue *et al.*, 2003). However, our research network is currently aware of 187 different compounds under preclinical and clinical testing by 96 companies. Currently, about 70 clinical trials are being conducted worldwide with agents having clinical promise for treatment of obesity. Preliminary data suggests that certain agents or combinations may enable obese individuals to lose 8–10 kg compared to placebo controls (Halpern and Mancini, 2003). If effective agents with an acceptable side effect profile become available, weight losses of >20 kg may be achievable with less intensive interventions than are currently required.

Bariatric surgery is gaining popularity, especially the minimally-invasive procedures (Davis, 2004). In 2004, an estimated 98 000–145 000 persons will have bariatric surgery procedures in the USA, up from 43 000 procedures performed in 2001 (Davis, 2004; Mitka, 2004). For persons with morbid obesity that has its onset before adolescence, this is the current treatment of choice (Mitka, 2004). Persons who have non-obese weights in adolescent years and become morbidly obese as adults should, in our assessment, have intensive behavioral LCD interventions before surgery. Because health insurance often provides coverage for bariatric surgery, surgery is less expensive and more convenient than an intensive behavioral LCD intervention (Brownell and Horgen, 2004). While LCD interventions carry very little risk for serious complications, bariatric surgery has a mortality risk approaching 1% and a complication rate approaching 10% (Steinbrook,

2004). Two major problems related to the popularity of bariatric surgery are, first, that many procedures are performed by surgeons with suboptimal experience and, second, that easier procedures such as gastric banding with uncertain long-term effectiveness and safety are being performed (Davis, 2004; Mitka, 2004; Steinbrook, 2004). We recommend that bariatric surgery should only be performed for morbidly obese persons who have clear indications for surgery and by experienced surgeons with documented low rates of complications and mortality.

19.10 Conclusions and future trends

The obesity epidemic must be attacked by an intensive, collaborative, focused effort involving all stakeholders. Involved groups must include these: governments at all levels; research sponsors from government, industry, and foundations; food industry; educational institutions; media; entertainment industry; high visibility spokespersons and other groups (Brownell and Horgen, 2004). Until some of these groups can collaboratively mount educational campaigns and make broad-ranging changes in many arenas, we will not make significant progress (Brownell and Horgen, 2004).

Treatment advances must continue because prevention efforts will not affect the currently obese and will only reduce the prevalence of obesity in coming generations. Genetic research is still in its infancy. Over 200 genes are identified in animals and humans that have possible links to obesity and diabetes (Snyder *et al.*, 2004). The impact of genetic polymorphism on obesity patterns in individuals must be determined and the interaction of several genetic patterns must be discerned. Lifestyle and pharmacotherapy will need to be tailored to the genetic profile of the individual.

New gut orexins are still being discovered (Kirchgessner, 2002). Over a dozen gut hormones affect eating behavior (Woods, 2004). Agonist or antagonists for these important hormones may work in concert with centrally acting, adipose-tissue active, or other agents to significantly enhance weight loss with fewer side effects. Combinations of drugs, like the fenfluramine–phentermine combination, may be substantially more effective than single agents. Pharmacogenomic information is likely to guide choices of obesity agents in the near future.

19.11 Sources of further information and advice

Health Management Resources (HMR®)	www.yourbetterhealth.com
American Dietetic Association	www.eatright.org
American Diabetes Association	www.diabetes.org
Optifast®	www.optifast.com
Slim Fast®	www.slimfast.com

Revival® Soy	www.revivalsoy.com
Scan Diet™	www.scandiet.com
eDiets®	www.ediets.com
Weight-Control Information Network (WIN) www.niddk.nih.gov/health/nutrit/win.htm	
Other websites:	www.weight.com
	www.obesity.org
	www.hcf-nutrition.org

19.12 References

AGREN, G., NARBRO, K., JONNSON, E., NASLUND, I., SJOSTROM, L. and PELTONEN, M. (2002), 'Cost of in-patient care over 7 years among surgically and conventionally treated obese patients', *Obesity Research*, **10**, 1276–83.

ALLISON, D. B., GADBURY, G., SCHWARTZ, L. G. *et al.*, (2003), 'A novel soy-based meal replacement formula for weight loss among obese individuals: a randomized controlled clinical trial', *European Journal of Nutrition*, **57**, 514–22.

ANDERSEN, R. E., WADDEN, T. A., BARLETT, S. J., VOGT, R. A. and WEINSTOCK, R. S. (1995), 'Relation of weight loss to changes in serum lipids and lipoproteins in obese women', *American Journal of Clinical Nutrition*, **62**, 350–7.

ANDERSON, D. A. and WADDEN, T. A. (1999), 'Treating the obese patient: Suggestions for primary care practice', *Archives of Family Medicine*, **8**, 156–67.

ANDERSON, J. W. (2003a), 'Diet first, then medication for hypercholesterolemia', *Journal of the American Medical Association*, **290**, 531–3.

ANDERSON, J. W. (2003b), 'Low-energy diets for intensive management of obesity in teenagers'. *Journal of the American College of Nutrition* **23**, ax. 2003b.

ANDERSON, J. W. (2004), 'Improved long-term maintenance of weight loss with ongoing involvement in weight management programme', *Obesity Research*, **12**, abstract, 156-P.

ANDERSON, J. W., BRINKMAN, V. L. and HAMILTON, C. C. (1992), 'Weight loss and 2-y follow-up for 80 morbidly obese patients treated with intensive very-low-calorie diet and an education program', *American Journal of Clinical Nutrition*, **56**, 244S–6S.

ANDERSON, J. W., BRINKMAN-KAPLAN, V. L., HAMILTON, C. C., LOGAN, J. B. and COLLINS, R. W. (1994a), 'Food-containing hypocaloric diets are as effective as liquid-supplement diets for obese individuals with NIDDM', *Diabetes Care*, **17**, 602–4.

ANDERSON, J. W., BRINKMAN-KAPLAN, V. L., LEE, H. and WOOD, C. L. (1994b), 'Relationship of weight loss to cardiovascular risk factors in morbidly obese individuals', *Journal of the American College of Nutrition*, **14**, 256–61.

ANDERSON, J. W., GREENWAY, F. L., FUJIOKA, K., GADDE, K. M., MCKINNEY, J. and O'NEIL, P. M. (2002a), 'Bupropion SR significantly enhances weight loss: a 24-week double-blind, placebo-controlled trial with placebo group randomized to bupropion SR during 24-week extension', *Obesity Research*, **10**, 633–41.

ANDERSON, J. W., HAMILTON, C. C. and BRINKMAN-KAPLAN, V. L. (1992), 'Benefits and risks of an intensive very-low-calorie diet programme for severe obesity', *American Journal of Gastroenterology*, **87**, 6–15.

ANDERSON, J. W., HERMAN, R. H. and NEWCOMER, K. L. (1969), 'Improvement of glucose tolerance of fasting obese patients given oral potassium', *American Journal of Clinical Nutrition*, **22**, 1589–96.

ANDERSON, J. W. and HOIE, L. H. (2003), Comparison of weight and lipid responses to soy and milk meal replacements. *Fifth International Symposium on the Role of Soy in Preventing and Treating Chronic Disease*, **77**, 9–21.

ANDERSON, J. W., JOHNSTONE, B. M. and COOK-NEWELL, M. E. (1995), 'Meta-analysis of effects of soy protein intake on serum lipids in humans', *New England Journal of Medicine*, **333**, 276–82.

ANDERSON, J. W., KENDALL, C. W. C. and JENKINS, D. J. A. (2003), 'Importance of weight management in type 2 diabetes: review with meta-analysis of clinical studies', *Journal of the American College of Nutrition*, **22**, 331–9.

ANDERSON, J. W. and KONZ, E. C. (2001), 'Obesity and disease management: Effects of weight loss on co-morbid conditions', *Obesity Research*, **9**, Suppl 4, 326S–34S.

ANDERSON, J. W., KONZ, E. C., FREDERICH, R. C. and WOOD, C. L. (2001), 'Long-term weight-loss maintenance: a meta-analysis of US studies', *American Journal of Clinical Nutrition*, **74**, 579–84.

ANDERSON, J. W., LUAN, J. and HOIE, L. H. (2004), 'Structured weight-loss programs: A meta-analysis of weight loss at 24 weeks and assessment of effects of intensity of intervention', *Advances in Therapy*, **21**, 61–75.

ANDERSON, J. W., VICHITBANDRA, S., QIAN, W. and KRYSICO, R. J. (1999), 'Long-term weight maintenance after an intensive weight-loss program', *Journal of the American College of Nutrition*, **18**, 620–7.

ANDERSON, J. W., WARD, A. K., GOTTHELF, L. and EARLY, J. (2002b), Response of obese adolescents to an intensive weight loss program. *Proceeding Nutrition Week* 2002, San Diego. 2-10.

ANGULO, P. (2002), 'Nonalcoholic fatty liver disease', *N Engl J Med*, **346**, 1221–31.

ASHLEY, J. M., ST JEAR, S. T., SCHRAGE, J. P. *et al.*, (2001), 'Weight control in the physician's office', *Archives of Internal Medicine*, **161**, 1599–604.

ASTRUP, A., RYAN, L., GRUNWALD, G. K., STORGAARD, M., SARIS, W., MELANSON, E. and HILL, J. O. (2000), 'The role of dietary fat in body fatness: evidence from a preliminary meta-analysis of *ad libitum* low-fat dietary intervention studies', *European Journal of Clinical Nutrition*, **83**, (Suppl 1), S25–32.

BLACKBURN, G. L. and ROTHACKER, D. (2003), Ten-year self-management of weight using a meal replacement diet plan: comparison with matched controls. *Obesity Research*, **11**, A103.

BLAIR, S. N., LAMONTE, M. J. and NICHAMAN, M. Z. (2004), 'The evolution of physical activity recommendations: how much is enough?', *American Journal of Clinical Nutrition*, **79**, (suppl), 913S–20S.

BOUSHEY, C. J., BERESFORD, S. A., OMENN, G. S. and MOTULSKY, A. G. (1995), 'A quantitative assessment of plasma homocysteine as a risk factor for vascular disease', *Journal of the American Medical Association*, **274**, 1049–57.

BOWERMAN, S., BELLMAN, M., SALTSMAN, P. *et al.* (2001), 'Implementation of a primary care physician network obesity management programme', *Obesity Research*, **9**, (Suppl 4), 321S–5S.

BRAY, G. A. and GREENWAY, F. L. (1999), 'Current and potential drugs for treatment of obesity', *Endocrine Reviews*, **20**, 805–75.

BROWNELL, K. D. (2000), *The LEARN Programme for Weight Management 2000* American Health Publishing Company, Dallas, TX.

BROWNELL, K. D. and HORGEN, K. B. (2004), *Food Fight* Contemporary Books, Chicago.

COLLINS, R. W. and ANDERSON, J. W. (1995), 'Medication cost savings associated with weight loss for obese non-insulin-dependent diabetic men and women', *Preventive Medicine*, **24**, (4), 369–74.

CONNOLLY, H. M., CRARY, J. L., MCGOON, M. D. *et al.* (1997), 'Valvular heart disease associated with fenfluramine-phentermine', *N Engl J Med*, **337**, 581–8.

DAVI, G., GUAGNANO, M. T., CIABATTONI, G. *et al.* (2002), 'Platelet activation in obese women: role of inflammation and oxidant stress', *JAMA*, **288**, 2008–14.

DAVIS, R. (2004), 'Proliferation of obesity surgeries raises alarm: Inexpert doctors, quick-fix seekers can be disastrous mix'. *USA Today*, 7D. 5-5.

EDEN, K. B., ORLEANS, T., MULROW, C. D., PENDER, N. J. and TEUTSCH, S. M. (2002), 'Does counseling by clinicians improve physical activity? a summary of the evidence for the U.S. Preventive Services Task Force', *Annals of Internal Medicine*, **137**, 208–15.

EXPERT PANEL ON DETECTION, E. A. T. O. H. B. C. I. A. (2001), 'Executive Summary of the Third Report of the National Cholesterol Education Programme (NCEP) Expert Panel on Detection, Evaluation, and treatment of high blood cholesterol in adults (Adult Treatment Panel III) ', *Journal of the American Medical Association*, **285**, 2486–97.

FLECHTNER-MORS, M., DITSCHUNEIT, H. H., JOHNSON, T. D. and SUCHARD, M. A. (2000), 'Metabolic and weight loss effects of long-term dietary intervention in obese patients: four-year results', *Obesity Research*, **8**, 399–402.

FLEGAL, K. M., CARROLL, M. D., OGDEN, C. L. and JOHNSON, C. L. (2002), 'Prevalence and trends in obesity among US adults, 1999–2000', *Journal of the American Medical Association*, **288**, 1723–7.

FOGELHORN, M. and KUKKONEN-HARJULA, K. (2000), 'Does physical activity prevent weight gain – a systematic review', *Obesity Reviews*, **1**, 95–111.

FORD, E. S., GILES, W. H. and DIETZ, W. H. (2002), 'Prevalence of the metabolic syndrome among US adults', *Journal of the American Medical Association*, **287**, 356–9.

FOSTER, G. D., WADDEN, T. A., PETERSON, F. J., LETIZIA, K. A., BARLETT, S. J. and CONILL, A. M. (1992), 'A controlled comparison of three very-low-calorie diets: effects on weight, body composition, and symptoms', *American Journal of Clinical Nutrition*, **55**, 811–7.

FREEDMAN, D. S., KHAN, L. K., SERDULA, M. K., GALUSKA, D. A. and DIETZ, W. H. (2002), 'Trends and correlates of class 3 obesity in the United States from 1990 through 2000', *Journal of the American Medical Association*, **288**, 1758–61.

GINSBERG, H. N. (1997), 'Is hypertriglyceridemia a risk factor for atherosclerotic cardiovascular disease: a simple question with a complicated answer', *Annals of Internal Medicine*, **126**, 912–4.

GOTTHELF, L., ANDERSON, J. W. and O'BRIEN, B. (2004), 'Weight loss in overweight or obese individuals with different structured intenventions in an intense behavioral programme'. *Obesity Research* **12**[abstract].

GRANT, L. and GOTTHELF, L. (2004), 'Successful weight maintenance in a telephone-based treatment programme', *Obesity Research*, **12**, abstract.

GREGG, E. W., GERZOFF, R. B., THOMPSON, T. J. and WILLIAMSON, D. F. (2003), 'Intentional weight loss and death in overweight and obese U.S. adults 35 years of age and older', *Annals of Internal Medicine*, **138**, 383–9.

GRILO, C. M. (1995), 'The role of physical activity in weight loss and weight loss management', *Med Exerc Nutr Health*, **4**, 60–76.

GRUNDY, S. M. (2004), 'Cholesterol gallstones: a fellow traveler with metabolic syndrome?', *American Journal of Clinical Nutrition*, **80**, 1–2.

GRUNDY, S. M., BREWER, B., CLEEMAN, J. I., SMITH, S. C. and LENFANT, C. (2004), 'Definition of the metabolic syndrome', *Circulation*, **109**, 433–8.

HADDOCK, C. K. (2003), 'Pharmacotherapy for obesity: a quantitative analysis of four decades of published randomized clinical trials', *International Journal of Obesity*, **26**, 262–73.

HALPERN, A. and MANCINI, M. C. (2003), 'Treatment of obesity: an update of anti-obesity medications', *Obesity Reviews*, **4**, 25–42.

HEALTH MANAGEMENT RESOURCES (1999), *HMR Programme for Weight Management Weight Loss Core Curriculum*, 1st edn, Health Management Resources, Boston, MA.

HESHKA, S., ANDERSON, J. W., ATKINSON, R. L. *et al.*, (2003), 'Weight loss with self-help compared with a structured commercial programme: a randomized trial', *Journal of the American Medical Association*, **289**, 1799–805.

HEYMSFIELD, S. B., VAN MIERLO, C., VAN DER KNAAP, H. C. M., HEO, M. and FRIER, H. I. (2003), 'Weight management using a meal replacement strategy: meta and pooling analysis from six studies', *International Journal of Obesity*, **27**, 537–49.

INTERNATIONAL OBESITY TASKFORCE. 'Global obesity'. *USA Today*. 2-5-2004.

JAMES, P. T., LEACH, R., KALAMARA, E. and SHAYEGHI, M. (2001), 'The worldwide obesity epidemic', *Obesity Research*, **9**, (Suppl. 4), 228S–33S.

JEFFERY, R. W., WING, R. R., SHERWOOD, N. E. and TATE, D. F. (2003), 'Physical activity and weight loss: does prescribing higher physical activity goals improve outcome?', *American Journal of Clinical Nutrition*, **78**, 684–9.

KIERNAN, M., KING, A. C., STEFANICK, M. L. and KILLEN, J. D. (2001), 'Men gain additional psychological benefits by adding exercise to a weight-loss program', *Obesity Research*, **9**, 770–7.

KIRCHGESSNER, A. L. (2002), 'Orexins in the brain–gut axis', *Endocrine Reviews*, **23**, 1–15.

KLEM, M. L., WING, R. R., MCGUIRE, M. T., SEAGLE, H. M. and HILL, J. O. (1997), 'A descriptive study of individuals successful at long-term maintenance of substantial weight loss', *American Journal of Clinical Nutrition*, **66**, 239–46.

LAKKA, H.-M., LAAKSONEN, D. E., LAKKA, T. A. *et al.* (2002), 'The metabolic syndrome and total and cardiovascular disease mortality in middle-aged men', *Journal of the American Medical Association*, **288**, 2709–16.

MAJOR, A. W. and ANDERSON, J. W. (2004), 'An adolescent weight reduction programme including meal replacements and parental involvement decreases body weight and fat mass of obese adolescents', *Obesity Research*, **12**, no. abstract.

MCGILL, H. C., MCMAHAN, C. A., HERDERICH, E. E. *et al.* (2002), 'Obesity accelerates the progression of coronary atherosclerosis in young men', *Circulation*, **105**, 2712–8.

MCTIGUE, K. M., HARRIS, R., HEMPHILL, B. *et al.* (2003), 'Screening and interventions for obesity in adults: summary of the evidence for the U.S. Preventive Services Task Force', *Annals of Internal Medicine*, **139**, 933–49.

MILLER, W. C., KOCEJA, D. M. and HAMILTON, E. J. (1997), 'A meta-analysis of the past 25 years of weight loss research using diet, exercise or diet plus exercise intervention', *International Journal of Obesity*, **21**, 941–7.

MITKA, M. (2004), 'Surgery for obesity. Demand soars amid scientific, ethical questions', *JAMA*, **289**, 1761–2.

MORROW, J. D. (2003), 'Is oxidative stress a connection between obesity and atherosclerosis?', *Arteriosclerosis, Thrombosis and Vascular Biology*, **23**, 368–70.

NICHOLAS, A. S. and ANDERSON, J. W. (2004), 'Reductions in blood pressure and medication costs with 100 pound weight loss', *Obesity Research*, **12**, abstract, 146-P.

PI-SUNYER, F. X. (1993), 'Medical hazards of obesity', *Annals of Internal Medicine*, **119**, 655–60.

PREVENTIVE HEALTH SERVICES (2002). 'Recommendations to increase physical activity in communities', *American Journal of Preventive Medicine,* **22**, 67–72.

RACETTE, S. B., SCHOELLER, D. A., KUSHNER, R. F. and NEIL, K. M. (2001), 'Exercise enhances dietary compliance during moderate energy restriction in obese women', *American Journal of Clinical Nutrition*, **62**, 345–9.

REYNOLDS, L. R. and ANDERSON, J. W. (2004), 'Practical office strategies for weight management of the obese diabetic individual', *Endocr. Practice*, **10**, 153–9.

REYNOLDS, L. R., KONZ, E. C., FREDERICH, R. C. and ANDERSON, J. W. (2002), 'Rosiglitazone amplifies the benefits of lifestyle intervention measures in long-standing type 2 diabetes mellitus', *Diabetes, Obesity and Metabolism*, **4**, 270–5.

RIDKER, P. M., HENNEKENS, C. H., BURING, J. E. and RIFAI, N. (2000), 'C-reactive protein and other markers of inflammation in the prediction of cardiovascular disease in women', *New England Journal of Medicine*, **342**, 836–43.

RIPPE, J. M. AND HESS, S. (1998), 'The role of physical activity in the prevention and management of obesity', *Journal of the American Dietetic Association*, **98**, (Suppl 2), S31–8.

ROSSNER, S. and FLATEN, H. (1997), 'VLCD versus LCD in long-term treatment of obesity', *International Journal of Obesity*, **21**, 22–6.

ROTHACKER, D. Q. (2000), 'Five-year self-management of weight using meal replacements: comparison with matched controls in rural Wisconsin', *Nutrition*, **16**(344), 348.

SARIS, W. H. (2001), 'Very-low-calorie diets and sustained weight loss', *Obesity Research*, **9**, (Suppl 4), 295S–301S.

SCHIFFMAN, M. L., KAPLAN, G. D., BRINKMAN-KAPLAN, V. L. and VICKERS, F. F. (1995), 'Prophylaxis against gallstone formation with ursodeooycholic acid in patients participating in a very-low-calorie diet programme', *Annals of Internal Medicine*, **122**, 899–905.

SCHOELLER, D. A. (2003), 'But how much physical activity?', *American Journal of Clinical Nutrition*, **78**, 669–70.

SERDULA, M. K., MOKDAD, A. H., WILLIAMSON, D. F., GALUSKA, D. A., MENDLEIN, J. M. and HEATH, G. W. (1999), 'Prevalence of attempting weight loss and strategies for controlling weight', *Journal of the American Medical Association*, **282**, 1353–8.

SNYDER, E. E., WALTS, B., PERUSSE, L. *et al.* (2004), 'The human obesity gene map: the 2003 update', *Obesity Research*, **12**(3), 369–439.

SOWERS, J. R. (2003), 'Obesity as a cardiovascular risk factor', *American Journal of Medicine*, **115**(8A), 37S–41S.

STEINBROOK, R. (2004), 'Surgery for severe obesity', *New England Journal of Medicine*, **350**, 1075–9.

STUART, C. H., GIKINSON, C. H., SMITH, M., BOSMA, A., BRUCE, K. and NAGAMANI, M. (1998), '*Acanthosis nigricans* as a risk factor for non insulin dependent diabetes mellitus', *Clinical Pediatrics*, **37**, 73–80.

TATE, D. F., JACKVONY, E. H. and WING, R. R. (2003), 'Effects of internet behavioral counseling on weight loss in adults at risk for type 2 diabetes: a randomized trial', *JAMA*, **289**, 1833–6.

TREMBLAY, A., DOUCET, E. and IMBEAULT, P. (1999), 'Physical activity and weight maintenance', *International Journal of Obesity*, **23**, (Suppl 3), 50S–4S.

VOTRUBA, S. B., HORVITZ, M. A. and SCHOELLER, D. A. (2000), 'The role of exercise in the treatment of obesity', *Nutrition*, **16**, 179–88.

WADDEN, T. A. and FOSTER, G. D. (2001), 'Behavioral treatment of obesity', *Medical Clinics in North America*, **84**, 441–61.

WADDEN, T. A., FOSTER, G. D., LETIZIA, K. A. and STUNKARD, A. J. (1992), 'A multicenter evaluation of a proprietary weight reduction program for the treatment of marked obesity', *Archives of Internal Medicine*, **152**, 961–6.

WADDEN, T. A., SARWER, D. B. and BERKOWITZ, R. I. (1999), 'Behavioural treatment of the overweight patient', *Bailliere's Clinical Endocrinology and Metabolism*, **13**, 93–107.

WADDEN, T. A. and STUNKARD, A. J. (1986), 'Controlled trial of very low calorie diet, behavior therapy, and their combination in the treatment of obesity', *Journal of Consulting and Clinical Psychology*, **54**, 482–8.

WADDEN, T. A., STUNKARD, A. J. and BROWNELL, K. D. (1983), 'Very low calorie diets: their efficacy, safety, and future', *Annals of Internal Medicine*, **99**(5), 675–84.

WESTERTERP-PLANTENGA, M. S., KEMPEN, K. P. G. and SARIS, W. H. M. (1998), 'Determinants of weight maintenance in women after diet-induced weight reduction', *International Journal of Obesity*, **22**, 1–6.

WOODS, S. C. (2004), 'Gastrointestinal satiety signals: I. an overview of gastrointestinal signals that influence food intake', *American Journal of Physiology, Gastrointestinal Liver Physiology*, **286**, G7–13.

YANOVSKI, J. A. and YANOVSKI, S. Z. (2003), 'Treatment of pediatric and adolescent obesity', *Journal of the American Medical Association*, **289**, 1851–3.

20

The effectiveness of popular diets: an overview

H. Raynor and R. Wing, Brown Medical School, USA

20.1 Introduction

With the prevalence of overweight and obesity increasing over the past 30 years (Flegal *et al.*, 2002), weight loss continues to be a prominent concern (Freedman *et al.*, 2001). Since there are many different commercial programmes for weight loss, the objective of this chapter is to review the research on the effectiveness of various popular adult diet programmes. This chapter begins by reporting the prevalence of weight control practices used by adults in the USA, followed by the criteria suggested by Freedman and colleagues (2001) and the Institute of Medicine (IOM) (1995) for evaluating weight loss diets and weight maintenance programmes. Then using these criteria, different dietary prescriptions for weight loss (e.g. low-fat, low-carbohydrate, and amount of dietary structure), and delivery methods used in weight loss programmes (e.g. face-to-face and Internet) are evaluated.

20.2 Weight control practices among consumers

Obesity is a major health problem and, at any given time, a large number of individuals are attempting to lose weight. Using data from the Behavioral Risk Factor Surveillance System (BRFSS) (Serdula *et al.*, 1999), a random-digit telephone survey of over 100 000 US adults, 29% of men and 44% of women reported that they were currently trying to lose weight. Body mass index (BMI) was the strongest factor related to trying to lose weight; among women, 60% of those who were overweight and 70% of those who were obese were trying to lose weight; however, interestingly, 29% of women with normal BMI (<25) also reported currently trying to lose weight. In men, 9% of normal weight, 36% of overweight, and 60% of obese respondents reported trying to lose weight. The odds of trying to lose weight were also higher in whites than blacks and increased with years of education. In women, trying to lose weight was greatest in those aged 18–29 and decreased with age, whereas in men the odds of trying to lose weight were greatest in those aged 40–49 and decreased in those over age 70.

The BRFSS also asked those who were trying to lose weight how much they would like to weigh. The median difference between current and goal weight was 8.6 kg for men and 8.9 kg for women. Approximately 37% of men and 45% of women reported a goal weight ≥10 kg below their current weight.

Those who were trying to lose weight were also asked whether they were trying to eat fewer calories or less fat to lose weight and whether they were using physical activity to lose weight. Approximately 90% reported trying to modify their diet; about half reported consuming fewer calories (with or without changing dietary fat) and 35% of men and 40% of women reported only consuming less fat. About two-thirds of men and women reported trying to increase physical activity. However, only 42% of men and 37% of women reported activity levels that satisfied the goals of engaging in 150 or more minutes per week of leisure time activity. The combination of exercising ≥150 minutes/week and any diet strategy was reported by 37% of men and 34% of women; yet, meeting the activity goal and eating fewer calories was reported by only 21.5% of men and 19.4% of women trying to lose weight. Thus, while many Americans report that they are trying to lose weight, far fewer are actually making the recommended changes of eating fewer calories and exercising more. Moreover, the duration that people engage in healthy weight loss behaviors may be very brief. While the BRFSS does not ask about the length of time weight control practices are used, French and colleagues (1999) found that, in a community sample of US adults, those who engaged in healthy weight loss behaviors only did so for about 20% of the time over a 4-year period.

20.3 Criteria for evaluating weight loss programmes

Freedman and colleagues (2001) proposed five areas in which the diet component of weight loss programmes should be evaluated. These areas include amount of weight loss and weight loss maintenance, changes in body composition, nutritional adequacy, improvements in metabolic parameters, and dietary compliance. The IOM, in their book entitled '*Weighing the Options: Criteria for Evaluating Weight Management Programmes*' (1995), expanded beyond evaluating the diet component in weight loss programmes to evaluating the whole weight loss programme. The IOM identified three criteria to consider: the match between programme and consumer; the soundness and safety of the programme; and the outcomes of the programme. We have synthesized these two approaches to develop a set of criteria to consider in discussing the variety of commercial weight loss options available to consumers.

20.3.1 Match between programme and consumer

The type of weight management programme that is most appropriate for an individual depends in large part on the degree of obesity and whether or not there are obesity-related comorbidies. For those who are overweight, but not obese, or obese without comorbidities, self-help approaches, commercial programmes, and behavioral approaches may be most appropriate. For heavier individuals and those with comorbidities, hospital-based programmes, very-low-calorie diets (VLCDs), or weight loss medications are often added. Finally, in the severely obese, surgery is a further option.

20.3.2 Weight loss and weight loss maintenance

In evaluating weight loss programmes, the emphasis should be on long-term weight loss, defined as weight loss at 1 year, and clinically significant weight losses, defined as weight losses of ≥5% of initial body weight or 1 BMI unit. Ideally, the weight management programme should also minimize loss of lean muscle and maximize loss of body fat.

20.3.3 Healthy habits for diet and physical activity

Weight loss programmes should also be evaluated in terms of the nutritional quality of the diet that is recommended. Diets which contain foods from all of the main food groups in the Food Guide Pyramid (FGP) (United States Department of Agriculture (USDA), 1996), are more likely to be nutritionally adequate and not deficient in the dietary reference intakes for the macro- and micronutrients (Institute of Medicine, 1999, 2000, 2001, 2002). Programmes should also encourage participants to achieve at least 30 minutes of moderate-intense physical activity on four or more days a week, since physical activity, independent of body weight, has been related to morbidity and mortality.

20.3.4 Metabolic parameters/safety

Weight loss diets can also affect blood lipid levels (e.g. total cholesterol, low-density lipoproteins (LDLs), high-density lipoproteins (HDLs), and triglycerides), glycemic control, blood pressure, and renal functioning. Ideally, a weight loss diet should improve most of these parameters, and minimally have no detrimental effect.

20.3.5 Compliance

In order to produce long-term weight loss, it is necessary to change eating and exercise habits long-term. Therefore, it is important to consider what types of approaches are likely to promote long-term adherence. Many factors influence adherence to a diet, including satiating quality of the diet, ease of adherence to the dietary prescription, and feelings of dietary restrictiveness and deprivation. A weight loss programme that is perceived to be easy to follow, not overly restrictive, and fits with an individual's lifestyle and eating and activity preferences should have greater long-term adherence, producing better weight loss maintenance.

20.4 Evaluating the main types of weight management programmes

There are a tremendous variety of weight loss programmes available to consumers and certainly we cannot evaluate all possible choices. In general, however, these programmes can be distinguished by the type of diet they recommend (typically a low-calorie, low-fat diet; a low-carbohydrate diet; or a diet using meal replacement products), by whether or not they include a physical activity component, and by the type of delivery format they involve (face-to-face or internet). These three components are discussed below and evaluated in terms of the criteria we have set forth.

20.4.1 Low-fat diets

Low-fat diets usually contain 20–30% energy from fat. These diets thus correspond to the government recommendations, described in the Dietary Guidelines for Americans (USDA, 2000) and The Food Guide Pyramid (USDA, 1996), and the recommendations of the American Heart Association (2000) and the American Diabetes Association (1999), which are to consume a low-fat diet (<30% energy from fat). The National Cholesterol Education Programme Step I and Step II diets (Expert Panel, 1993) and the Dietary Approaches to Stop Hypertension (DASH) from the National Heart, Lung, and Blood Institute (2003) also recommend an intake of <30% energy from fat. All of these diets also recommend weight control, by focusing on reducing caloric intake through portion control.

There are several reasons why low-fat diets have been recommended for weight loss. Cross-sectional studies examining the relationship between diet composition, energy intake, and weight status, have found a stronger relationship between dietary fat and body weight, than between energy intake and body weight (Kushi *et al.*, 1985; Dreon *et al.*, 1988; Romieu *et al.*, 1988). Longitudinal studies examining dietary predictors of weight change have also found that changes in consumption of high-fat foods and in consumption of calories from fat predict changes in weight in the general population (Klesges *et al.*, 1992) and in those trying to lose weight (Jeffery *et al.*, 1984).

Experimental studies have also found that, when the amount of fat in the diet is altered, weight change occurs. For example, investigations examining the effect of a low-fat diet on disease prevention have found that a modest amount of weight loss often occurs on a low-fat diet without specific instructions to restrict calories (Sheppard *et al.*, 1991; Chlebowski *et al.*, 1993). Four recent meta-analyses of controlled trials comparing low-fat diets with normal-fat diets under *ad libitum* conditions consistently demonstrate that a decrease in dietary fat without restriction of energy intake causes a spontaneous reduction in energy intake and a consequential modest weight loss (Bray and Popkin, 1998; Yu-Poth *et al.*, 1999; Astrup, 2000; Astrup *et al.*, 2000). Moreover, studies investigating the effect of high-fat diets on energy intake show that high-fat diets promote passive overconsumption, which increases the risk of weight gain (Stubbs *et al.*, 1995a, b).

Two hypotheses have developed as to why the amount of fat in the diet is related to energy intake and weight status. The first hypothesis focuses on the poor satiating quality of dietary fat (Gerstein *et al.*, 2004). Of the three macronutrients, protein has the strongest effect on satiation, followed by carbohydrate, and then fat (Gerstein *et al.*, 2004). The less satiating the macronutrient, the greater amount that is consumed in an eating bout (Jequier and Bray, 2002). Thus greater caloric intake occurs in a meal or snack containing high levels of fat, due to fat's less potent satiating ability. The second hypothesis for overconsumption with a high-fat diet is the effect of fat on the energy density of foods (Gerstein *et al.*, 2004). Fat increases the energy density of food. Energy density is usually expressed in kcal/g, so foods with greater energy density have more calories for a given quantity of food. Since research has shown that individuals tend to consume a similar volume or bulk of food, regardless of the food's composition (Rolls *et al.*, 2000), foods that contain a greater amount of energy per weight or volume (e.g. higher in energy density) will produce greater intake through passive ingestion (Jequier and Bray, 2002).

Dietary prescription

Low-fat diets used in weight loss programmes generally recommend a caloric intake of 1000–1500 kcal/day, with 20–30 percent calories from fat. This diet allows a wide range of food choices, with no food group or type of food completely eliminated from the diet. The emphasis in this diet is on moderation and portion control. The flexibility of these regimens should promote good long-term adherence.

Evaluation of low-fat, hypocaloric diets

A low-fat diet is the diet that has predominantly been used in standard behavioral weight loss interventions (Jeffery *et al.*, 2000); consequently there is a large amount of research that has evaluated the outcomes from a low-fat, hypocaloric diet. When used as part of a 6-month standard behavioral intervention, the average amount of weight loss achieved with a low-fat, low calorie weight loss diet is about 10.4 kg, and at 18-month follow-up (1 year after treatment), approximately 82% (8.1 kg) of that weight loss is maintained (Wing, 2004). These diets also produce decreases in percent body fat, and waist and hip circumference (Freedman *et al.*, 2001).

Participants prescribed low-fat, calorie-restricted diets as part of behavioral interventions typically report caloric intake at the end of 6 months of treatment of approximately 1300 to 1500 kcal/day, with 28 to 32% of calories from fat (Raynor *et al.*, 2004; Jakicic *et al.*, 1999). When appropriate food choices are made, a low-fat weight loss diet is nutritionally adequate (USDA, 1996). However, if proper food choices are not made, low-fat diets tend to be deficient in calcium, zinc, magnesium, iron, vitamin B12, and dietary fiber, with calcium consistently shown to be the most problematic micronutrient (Buzzard *et al.*, 1990; Insull *et al.*, 1990; Swinburn *et al.*, 1999). However, with the variety of calcium-enriched food products (i.e. orange juice, waffles, etc.) and low-fat, reduced-energy dairy products that are currently available, calcium intake on a low-fat, calorie-restricted diet may be less problematic today than previous studies have reported.

In regards to metabolic parameters, the changes in blood lipid levels that occur with a low-fat, hypocaloric diet are believed to be more of a consequence of the amount of weight loss achieved, rather than from the changes in the diet (Astrup *et al.*, 2002). A systematic review and meta-analysis of the effects of the American National Cholesterol Education Programme's dietary interventions have found that a low-fat diet with consequential weight loss is associated with a decrease in LDLs, and a normalization of triglycerides levels and the ratio of HDLs to total cholesterol (Yu-Poth *et al.*, 1999). A low-fat weight loss diet has also been found to reduce fasting insulin levels (Brinkworth *et al.*, 2004) and reduce blood pressure (Yancy *et al.*, 2004).

Adherence to low-fat, low-calorie regimens appears quite good initially, but typically declines after 6 months. Several studies have shown that weight regain after 6 months is related to increased consumption of foods with high dietary fat content and to decreased vigilance about the diet (Jeffery *et al.*, 2000). The fact that all foods can be incorporated into this diet should improve adherence. However, since the diet is based on portion-control, all foods should be weighed and measured, making adherence more difficult than a diet that requires less emphasis on portion control. In addition, since high fat foods are often preferred, reducing these types of foods in the diet may prove difficult long term.

20.4.2 Low-carbohydrate diets

The low-carbohydrate, high-protein diet, which has been promoted by Atkins and others, has recently become one of the most popular weight loss alternatives to the low-fat diet. The Atkins diet was initially published in

1972, and was updated 20 years later (1992). The premise of low-carbohydrate diets is that dietary carbohydrate should be restricted enough so that serum and urinary ketones, a byproduct of lipid oxidation, occur. As carbohydrate intake is reduced and ketosis occurs, blood glucose and insulin levels should decrease, and appetite should be suppressed. Atkins and others (1992) propose that the state of ketosis changes the metabolic state, such that increased energy expenditure occurs, making it easier to achieve a negative energy balance state, regardless of the amount of calories that are consumed. Moreover, it is proposed that since appetite is suppressed by ketosis, it is also easier to eat less, helping with rapid weight loss. However, these responses to a low-carbohydrate diet have not been established (Brehm *et al.*, 2003).

Numerous professional organizations have raised questions about the use of low-carbohydrate diets (Bravata *et al.*, 2003). These concerns include metabolic outcomes of this diet that may create negative medical consequences for individuals with cardiovascular disease, type 2 diabetes, dyslipidemia, and hypertension. Specifically, there are concerns that a low-carbohydrate diet may create a large enough accumulation of ketones to cause abnormal metabolism of insulin and impaired kidney and liver function; sodium and water depletion causing postural hypotension, constipation, and nephrolithiasis; large intakes of animal protein that may impair renal functioning; and increased consumption of saturated fats that may produce hyperlipidemia, insulin resistance and glucose intolerance.

Dietary prescription

Many of the low-carbohydrate diets that have recently been tested in randomized trials are based upon the Atkins diet (1992), in which carbohydrate intake is limited to 20 g/day for at least 2 weeks, and then carbohydrate is either increased to around 60–70 g/day, or individuals are instructed to gradually increase carbohydrate intake until a desired weight is achieved (Brehm *et al.*, 2003; Foster *et al.*, 2003; Yancy *et al.*, 2004). Other investigations have started with a dietary prescription that allows for a greater amount of carbohydrate intake, 30 g/day (Stern *et al.*, 2004), but do not allow an increase in carbohydrate intake over time. None of these prescriptions includes a calorie limit; thus, this diet allows individuals to eat as much as desired, but only from allowed (e.g. low-carbohydrate) foods.

Evaluation of low-carbohydrate diets

Several studies have compared low-carbohydrate diets to hypocaloric, low-fat diets (as described above) (Brehm *et al.*, 2003; Foster *et al.*, 2003; Samaha *et al.*, 2003; Stern *et al.*, 2004; Yancy *et al.*, 2004), with both the low-carbohydrate and low-fat diet conditions receiving education and minimal professional contact. At 6 months, all studies found greater weight loss in the low-carbohydrate diet conditions (range: –9.7 to –12.9 per cent body weight), than the low-fat diet conditions (range: –5.3 to –6.7 per cent body weight). However, few of these studies have included 12-month follow-up and those that did found no difference in weight loss between the two diets (Foster *et al.*, 2003; Stern *et al.*, 2004). In terms of body composition changes, two investigations found that there was a greater loss of fat mass than fat-free mass in both diet conditions (Brehm *et al.*, 2003; Yancy *et al.*, 2004), but only one of these investigations found that the low-carbohydrate diet produced a greater loss of both fat and fat-free mass than the low-fat diet (Brehm *et al.*, 2003). Yancy and colleagues (2004) found a greater loss of total body water in the first two weeks with the low-carbohydrate diet, but by 6 months there was no significant difference in total body water loss between the two diets.

Self-reported carbohydrate intake decreases on the low-carbohydrate diet, and with the decrease in carbohydrate intake, there is a decrease in caloric intake to the level at or slightly below what is reported in the low-fat diet condition (Brehm *et al.*, 2003; Samaha *et al.*, 2003; Stern *et al.*, 2004; Yancy *et al.*, 2004). This change in caloric intake is responsible for the weight losses seen on these regimens. Concern is raised, however, about the high amounts of saturated fat that participants consume on these diets. Brehm *et al.* (2003) found that, at 3 months, saturated fat intake had increased from 12.4% kcal to 20.7% kcal. Dietary cholesterol also increased from baseline, 215 mg/day, to 3 months, 461 mg/day. Participants on the low-carbohydrate diet report consuming more total fat, saturated fat, and dietary cholesterol; and less Vitamin C and fiber than the low-calorie, low-fat condition. At 6 months, the dietary outcomes were similar as what was reported at 3 months (Brehm *et al.*, 2003).

Several investigations have found more favorable changes in blood lipids when weight loss was achieved using a low-carbohydrate diet than a low-calorie, low-fat diet (Brehm *et al.*, 2003; Foster *et al.*, 2003; Samaha *et al.*, 2003; Stern *et al.*, 2004; Yancy *et al.*, 2004). The low-carbohydrate diet was associated with greater decreases in triglycerides (Samaha *et al.*, 2003; Yancy *et al.*, 2004) and greater increases in HDL cholesterol in some (Foster *et al.*, 2003; Yancy *et al.*, 2004), but not all investigations (Brehm *et al.*, 2003; Samaha *et al.*, 2003). No study found significant increases in total cholesterol or LDLs on low-carbohydrate diets, probably due to the weight losses produced by these regimens (Brehm *et al.*, 2003; Foster *et al.*, 2003; Sahara *et al.*, 2003; Stern *et al.*, 2004; Yancy *et al.*, 2004). Although one study found that the low-carbohydrate diet produced greater improvements in insulin sensitivity than the low-fat diet (Samaha *et al.*, 2003), others found no differences in improvements in insulin sensitivity between the two diets (Foster *et al.*, 2003; Stern *et al.*, 2004).

Since many of the low-carbohydrate diets should induce ketosis, urinary ketones provide an objective measure of dietary adherence. Adherence within the first weeks of initiating a low-carbohydrate diet appear to be good; Yancy and colleagues (2004) reported that 86% of participants on a low-carbohydrate diet tested positive for urinary ketones at 2 weeks, while Foster and colleagues (2003) reported a greater percentage of participants on the low-carbohydrate diet as compared to the low-fat diet testing positive for urinary ketones at 3 months. However, adherence appears to decrease over time. By 4 months there was no significant difference between the two diets in the percentage of participants testing positive for urinary ketones (Foster *et al.*, 2003). No relationship was found between ketosis and weight loss (Foster *et al.*, 2003).

It is important to recognize that low-carbohydrate diets eliminate many foods. This strategy, due to the decrease in variety of foods, may help to reduce intake, without having to control portion size of foods consumed (Raynor and Epstein, 2001). With the large initial weight loss on this diet, occurring without counting calories and measuring foods, adherence to this diet may be initially fairly easy. However, since many foods are eliminated from the diet, long-term adherence may be difficult.

20.4.3 Meal replacements

Dietary compliance is essential for maximizing weight loss during obesity interventions. It is believed that, over time, compliance to a weight loss diet becomes more difficult, especially with multiple dietary modifications that require many behaviors, such as measuring portions, calculating intake of several nutrients, and planning meals and snacks to meet dietary goals (Metz *et al.*, 1997).

One approach to improving dietary adherence is to simplify the diet by either providing participants with the foods they should eat in appropriate portion sizes or using meal replacement products (MRs) (Wing and Jeffery, 2001; Hannum *et al.*, 2004). MRs were initially developed for medically supervised weight loss programmes using VLCD regimens. VLCDs were diets of 400 kcal/day, in which all caloric intake was from a nutritionally balanced liquid formula. VLCDs were very effective for initial weight loss but the weight was rapidly regained when regular foods were re-introduced into the diet. This finding, coupled with evidence that liquid formula diets of 400 600, and 800 kcal/day all produced similar weight loss, led to the use of higher-calorie formula diets and the use of MRs in combination with conventional foods.

In their current form, MRs are nutritionally balanced drinks, bars, or frozen meals (or other portion controlled entrees) that are typically eaten for two meals a day in place of self-selected, conventional foods. MRs require no measurement, which increases the accuracy of self-monitoring for those meals. Moreover, meal and snack planning and making appropriate food choices requires little effort, increasing the likelihood of achieving a low-calorie, low-fat dietary intake.

Another way in which MRs may help with dietary compliance is by reducing variety in the diet (Wing and Jeffery, 2001). Previous research has documented that greater dietary variety is associated with increased intake and body weight (Raynor and Epstein, 2001). While MRs come in a variety of flavors and forms, there is still much less variety within these products than within conventional foods. Consequently, using MRs most likely decreases variety in the diet, which may assist in improving adherence to a hypocaloric diet.

Dietary prescription

Diets using MRs prescribe a hypocaloric (1200–1500 kcal/day), low-fat (<30% kcals from fat) diet, incorporating two-to-three MRs, taking the place of two meals and one snack per day (Ditschuneit *et al.*, 1999; Ashley *et al.*, 2001; Yip *et al.*, 2001; Hannum *et al.*, 2004). The third meal of the day is composed of self-selected, conventional foods and participants are encouraged to measure foods and to consume fruits and vegetables in this meal. This diet allows a wide range of food choices within the conventional meal, with no food group or type of food completely eliminated from the diet.

Evaluation of meal replacements

Most investigations examining the effectiveness of MRs on weight loss have used brief interventions of 8–12 weeks (Ditschuneit *et al.*, 1999; Yip *et al.*, 2001; Hannum *et al.*, 2004) and compared the weight losses to those achieved with a self-selected diet of the same calorie and fat level. (Ditschuneit *et al.*, 1999; Ashley *et al.*, 2001; Yip *et al.*, 2001; Hannum *et al.*, 2004). These studies consistently report better percent weight losses with the MRs than with the self-selected diet (–6.4% to –11.3% vs. –4.2% to –5.9%) (Ditschuneit *et al.*, 1999; Ashley *et al.*, 2001; Yip *et al.*, 2001; Hannum *et al.*, 2004). Ashley and colleagues (2001) found that the weight loss benefits of the MR diet compared to the conventional diet was maintained at both 12-month (–9.1% vs. –4.1%) and at 2-year follow-up (–8.5% vs. –1.5%). There was also a greater decrease in percent body fat at 1- and 2-year follow-up on the MR diet (–5.9% and –5.1%, respectively) as compared to a conventional diet (–2.6% and –2.2%, respectively) (Ashley *et al.*, 2001).

Nutrient analyses from food diaries indicate that intake on the MR diet decrease from baseline, to about 1300 to 1400 kcal per day (Ditschuneit and Flechtner-Mors, 2001; Hannum *et al.*, 2004), with one investigation showing a greater reduction in caloric intake with the MR diet than the conventional diet (Ditschuneit and Flechtner-Mors, 2001). Percentage calories from fat also decreased with MRs to <30% energy from fat, with this decrease being greater for the MR diet than the conventional diet (Ditschuneit and Flechtner-Mors, 2001; Hannum *et al.*, 2004). However, at 1-year follow-up, no differences were found in caloric and percentage dietary fat intake between the two diets (Ashley *et al.*, 2001).

Studies indicate that the nutritional adequacy of a hypocaloric, low-fat diet using MRs is very similar to that of a hypocaloric, low-fat diet using self-selected conventional foods (Ashley *et al.*, 2001; Ditschuneit and Flechtner-Mors, 2001; Hannum *et al.*, 2004). Daily servings of fruits and vegetables have been shown to increase from baseline (2.7) to 1-year (4.7) and 2-year follow-up (5.1) with the MR diet (Ashley *et al.*, 2001).

MRs have been shown to produce significant improvements in lipids, blood pressure, glucose and insulin, but it is unclear whether these changes are greater than those seen with self-selected diets. When MRs produce greater benefits, it is most likely the result of the greater weight losses they engender.

Thus, the structure and simplification provided by MR products may be helpful in the initial stages (i.e. first 3 months) of weight loss. MRs may help participants reduce caloric and fat intake, creating a greater weight loss than what is achieved with self-selected, conventional food diets.

20.5 Physical activity and weight loss programmes

Physical activity is believed to be a key component of weight loss programmes because it is the single best predictor of the long-term maintenance of weight loss (Wing, 2004). Standard behavioral weight loss interventions provide an activity prescription of expending 1000 kcal/week in moderate-intense physical activity. This activity prescription is considered to be a necessary and essential component of a successful weight loss intervention. The current focus regarding physical activity in behavioral weight loss interventions is on two areas: (1) does the physical activity prescription need to be higher than 1000 kcals/week for weight loss maintenance (Jeffery *et al.*, 2003); and (2) how should physical activity be prescribed to improve long-term adherence (Wing, 2004)? Recent research has indicated that higher levels of physical activity (2500 kcals/week) improve weight loss maintenance at 12- and 18-month follow-up as compared to the standard prescription of 1000 kcals/week (8.5 kg vs. 6.1 kg at 12 months and 6.7 kg vs. 4.1 kg at 18 months) (Jeffery *et al.*, 2004). To improve adherence to the physical activity prescription, previous research has found that prescribing short bouts (≥10 minutes) of activity (Jakicic *et al.*, 1999), having exercise equipment available at home (Jakicic *et al.*, 1999), and encouraging lifestyle activity (e.g. parking further away to encourage walking) may be helpful.

Since physical activity has been found to be so important for weight loss maintenance, it might be expected that all weight loss interventions target increasing physical activity. However, some commercial weight loss programmes do not include an activity prescription. Weight loss programmes that lack a physical activity component most likely will produce poorer weight loss maintenance than those programmes that include physical activity.

20.6 Delivery methods used in weight loss programmes

Decisions about which type of weight loss programme to select depend not only on the type of diet that is prescribed and the degree of emphasis on physical activity, but also on the treatment format. The two most common formats – face-to-face and internet programmes – are discussed below.

20.6.1 Face-to-face contact

Research programmes
There is a large body of research on the efficacy of face-to-face programmes that combine diet, physical activity, and behavior modification. These behavioral obesity interventions typically provide weekly group meetings for 6 months, followed by bimonthly and monthly group meetings for 18 months of follow-up (Wing, 2004). These interventions recommend a hypocaloric diet (1000–1500 kcal/day) and an activity prescription of 1000 kcal/wk, and teach participants behavioral skills (e.g. self-monitoring, stimulus control, positive reinforcement, pre-planning, problem-solving) for weight loss. These programmes are very effective at weight loss; on average partici-pants lose approximately 10.4 kg (or approximately a 10% weight loss) at 6 months. These programmes are also gradually becoming more successful at producing weight loss maintenance; currently, over 80% of the initial weight loss is maintained at 18-month follow-up (Wing, 2004).

Commercial programmes
Some of the elements of research weight loss programmes are included in commercial programmes. Commercial programmes recommended a hypocaloric diet and often some level of physical activity for participants. Some commercial programmes will also provide instruction on behavioral tools (e.g. self-monitoring), and provide the opportunity for regular meetings. However, most commercial programmes do not provide all of the elements that are commonly used in research programmes at the same level of intensity; thus, the commercial programmes appear to be less effective for weight loss and weight loss maintenance than the research programmes.

Most reports of the efficacy of commercial weight loss programmes are clinical series, rather than controlled trials, and often provide information only on those who remained in the treatment programme. Such studies may markedly overestimate the success of the programme. Given this concern, this chapter focuses primarily on randomized controlled trials evaluating these approaches.

Weight Watchers® (www.weightwatchers.com) is one of the few commercial programmes to evaluate its results. The Weight Watchers® programme uses a balanced deficit diet and provides lessons on behavior change and suggestions for increasing physical activity. The programme is conducted in an open-group format, with successful Weight Watchers® members serving as group leaders. Recently, a multi-center trial was conducted to evaluate the 2-year results of participation in Weight Watchers® (Heshka *et al.*, 2000). The 423 research study participants had a BMI of 27–40 kg/m^2 and were randomly assigned to a self-help programme or to Weight Watchers®. Those in the self-help condition attended a 20-minute consultation with a dietician at baseline and at week 12 and were given written materials related to weight loss. Those assigned to the Weight Watchers® condition were given vouchers to attend the commercial programme at a location convenient to them; they were instructed not to disclose the fact that they were participating in a research study.

Eighty-two percent completed the 6-month study and 70% completed 2 years. Analysis of completers showed that the Weight Watchers® group had significantly better weight losses at all time points (6 months = 5.6 vs. 1.8 kg; 12 months = 4.9 vs. 1.3 kg; 24 months = 3.0 vs. 0.0 kg). At 2 years, 52% of the Weight Watchers® group and 29% of the self-help group had decreased their BMI by 1 unit or more. Blood pressure, lipids, glucose and insulin all improved with weight loss in both conditions, but the improvement in glucose and blood pressure, per unit weight loss, was greater in the Weight Watchers® condition.

A follow-up survey of Weight Watchers® members who reached their goal weight during the treatment programme has also been reported (Lowe *et al.*, 2001). These authors weighed a sub-group of the participants and used these objective data to develop a correction factor for self-report biases. Based on corrected weights, these authors concluded that at 5-year follow-up, 42.6% of the successful Weight Watchers® members had maintained a loss of 5% or more and 18.8% maintained a loss of 10% or more. Thus, these data suggest that individuals who reach goal weight on Weight Watchers® are able to maintain significant weight losses long term.

Unfortunately, there are no empirical studies of programmes such as Jenny Craig® (www.jennycraig.com) or L.A. Weight Loss Centers®. Such studies are needed to provide an empirical basis for treatment recommendations and referrals.

20.6.2 Internet

Research programmes

Recently, several programmes have been developed using the internet for treatment delivery. Internet approaches may be particularly well suited for individuals who live far from treatment sites or have limited time to attend treatment meetings. Because they involve no face-to-face contact with a professional, internet approaches may be most appropriate for individuals with moderate degrees of obesity and no medical comorbidities.

Two research studies have been conducted by Tate and colleagues evaluating the efficacy of the internet for weight loss (Tate *et al.*, 2001, 2003). In the first of the studies, Tate compared an internet education programme with an internet behavioral treatment programme over a 6-month period (Tate *et al.*, 2001). All 91 participants were given one face-to-face group session teaching the basics of weight loss and access to a website with organized links to internet resources for weight loss. In addition, participants in the behavior therapy condition received a 24-week sequence of behavioral lessons via email and were instructed to submit weekly self-monitoring records. These records were reviewed by a behavior therapist who emailed individualized feedback to the participant. The internet behavior therapy group lost 4.1 kg at 6 months, compared to 1.6 kg in the internet education group.

Building on this, a second randomized trial was implemented to tease apart the effect of the behavioral lessons compared to the counseling (Tate *et al.*, 2003). Ninety-two participants were randomly assigned to a year-long basic internet programme or to internet plus behavioral e-counseling programme. Both groups received an initial face-to-face meeting, weekly weight loss information, and reminders to submit weekly weight data. The internet behavioral e-counseling group submitted diaries daily for 1 month and then weekly and received email communication from a therapist. Analysis of the 77 completers showed that the internet plus e-counseling group lost more weight at 6 months (–5.2 vs. –2.5 kg) and at 12 months (–5.3 vs. –2.3 kg) than basic internet. Intent-to-treat analyses confirmed this finding. These data suggest that the individualized email counseling is an important component of an effective internet weight loss programme.

The internet has also been shown to help maintain weight loss. Following a 6-month interactive TV weight loss programme, participants were randomly assigned to a frequent face-to-face programme, a minimal face-to-face programme, or internet support (Harvey-Berino *et al.*, 2004). Weight losses over the 18-month study, averaged 7.6, 5.5, and 5.1 kg for the three programmes respectively, with no significant differences among them.

Commercial programmes

Several commercial programmes are now offering internet programmes as a means of increasing their audience. To date, only one of these – ediets.com® (www.ediets.com) – has been evaluated in a randomized controlled design (Womble *et al.*, 2004). Ediets.com® allows participants to select the type of diet that they prefer (including choices of low-calorie, low-fat, or low-carbohydrate diets). Customized grocery lists are provided; there is access to on-line meetings moderated by a professional and on-line bulletin board support groups; further support is available through a 'find a buddy' programme. Participants self-report their level of cardiovascular endurance and strength, and physical activity recommendations are provided accordingly.

Womble and colleagues (2004) evaluated the efficacy of this programme in a randomized trial with 47 women (mean age = 43.7; BMI = 33.5). Participants were randomly assigned to either ediets.com® or to a weight loss manual (Learn Programme for Weight Control 2000). Both groups were seen briefly by an interventionist at baseline and at weeks 8, 16, 26, and 52. Outcome visits were held at weeks 2, 4, 8, 12, 16, 20, 26, 34, 42, and 52.

At week 16, 66% of the women were still participating. Those in the e-diets programme lost 0.7 kg on average at week 16 compared to 3.0 kg for the Learn Manual. At week 52, the e-diet group again had poorer weight loss results (0.8 kg vs. 3.3 kg).

As with the comparison between research and commercial programmes in a face-to-face format, the internet research programmes provide better weight loss outcomes than the internet commercial programme. This appears to again be a consequence of the commercial programme providing less of the structure and frequency of contact that was found to be effective in the research programmes.

20.7 Implications and recommendations

There are large numbers of individuals who are trying to lose weight. It is important to help them identify effective approaches to long-term weight control. The most successful programmes appear to be ones that include recommendations for changing both dietary intake and physical activity and provide on-going contact through either face-to-face meetings or e-mail counseling. Low-fat, low-calorie diets have been most carefully studied to date and appear to be safe and effective in producing weight losses of approximately 10% of body weight. Long-term weight loss maintenance appears to be less influenced by the specific type of diet that is prescribed than by whether or not the programme includes the combination of diet plus physical activity.

What is most striking is the discrepancy between the results achieved when these weight loss strategies are implemented in research settings compared to commercial settings. There is a tremendous need for research evaluating the success of currently available commercial weight loss programmes in order to permit consumers to select those approaches that are most effective. Moreover, it is important to determine how to better translate the approaches that are working in research settings into the commercial environment. In order to reverse the current trends in obesity, it is important to develop effective weight loss programmes that can be made available to the large number of overweight and obese individuals seeking to lose weight.

20.8 References

AMERICAN DIABETES ASSOCIATION. (1999), Clinical practice recommendations. *Diabetes Care*, **22**.

AMERICAN HEART ASSOCIATION. (2000), *Heart and Stroke Statistical Update*. Dallas: American Heart Association.

ASHLEY, J. M., ST JEOR, S. T., PERUMEAN-CHANEY, S., SCHRAGE, J. and BOVEE, V. (2001), Meal replacements in weight intervention. *Obesity Research*, **9**, 312S–20S.

ASTRUP, A. (2000), Healthy lifestyles in Europe: prevention of obesity and type 2 diabetes by diet and physical activity. *Public Health Nutrition*, **4**, 499–515.

ASTRUP, A., GRUNWALD, G. K., MELANSON, E. L., SARIS, W. H. M. and HILL, J. O. (2000), The role of low-fat diets in body weight control: a meta-analysis of *ad libitum* intervention studies. *International Journal of Obesity and Related Metabolic Disorders*, **24**, 1545–52.

ASTRUP, A., BUEMANN, B., FLINT, A. and RABEN, A. (2002), Low-fat diets and energy balance: how does the evidence stand in 2002? *Proceedings of the Nutrition Society*, **61**, 299–309.

ATKINS, R. (1992), *Dr. Atkins New Diet Revolution*. New York: Avon Books.

BRAVATA, D. M., SANDERS, L., HUANG, J., KRUMHOLZ, H. M., OLKIN, I, GARDNER, C. D. and BRAVATA, D. M. (2003), Efficacy and safety of low-carbohydrate diets: a systematic review. *Journal of the American Medical Association*, **289**, 1837–50.

BRAY, G. A. and POPKIN, B. M. (1998), Dietary fat intake does affect obesity. *American Journal of Clinical Nutrition*, **68**, 1157–73.

BREHM, B. J., SEELEY, R. J., DANIELS, S. R. and D'ALESSIO, D. A. (2003), A randomized trial comparing a very low carbohydrate diet and a calorie-restricted low fat diet on body weight and cardiovascular risk factors in healthy women. *Journal of Clinical Endocrinology and Metabolism*, **88**, 1617–23.

BRINKWORTH, G. D., NOAKES, M., KEOGH, J. B., LUSCOMBE, N. D., WITTERT, G. A. and CLIFTON, M. (2004), Long-term effects of a high-protein, low-carbohydrate diet on weight control and cardiovascular risk markers in obese hyperinsulinemic subjects. *International Journal of Obesity*, **28**, 661–70.

BUZZARD, I. M., ASP, E. H., CHLEBOWSKI, R. T. *et al.* (1990), Diet intervention methods to reduce fat intake: nutrient and food group composition of self-selected low-fat diets. *Journal of the American Dietetic Association*, **90**, 42–50, 53.

CHLEBOWSKI, R. T., BLACKBURN, G. L., BUZZARD, I. M. *et al.* (1993), Adherence to a dietary fat intake reduction programme in postmenopausal women receiving therapy for early breast cancer. *Journal of Clinical Oncology*, **11**, 2072–80.

DITSCHUNEIT, H. H., FLECHTNER-MORS, M., JOHNSON, T. D. and ADLER, G. (1999), Metabolic and weight-loss effects of a long-term dietary intervention in obese patients. *American Journal of Clinical Nutrition*, **69**, 198–204.

DITSCHUNEIT, H. H. and FLECHTNER-MORS, M. (2001), Value of structured meals for weight management: risk factors and long-term weight maintenance. *Obesity Research*, **9**, 284S–9S.

DREON, D. M., FREY-HEWITT, B., ELLSWORTH, N., WILLIAMS, P. T., TERRY, R. B. and WOOD, D. (1988), Dietary fat: carbohydrate ratio and obesity in middle-aged men. *American Journal of Clinical Nutrition*, **47**, 995–1000.

EXPERT PANEL (1993), Summary of the second report of the National Cholesterol Education Programme (NCEP) expert panel on detection, evaluation, and treatment of high blood cholesterol in adults (adult treatment panel II). *Journal of the American Medical Association*, **269**, 3015–23.

FLEGAL, K. M., CARROL, M. D., OGDEN, C. L. and JOHNSON, C. L. (2002), Prevalences and trends in obesity among US adults, 1999–2000. *Journal of the American Medical Association*, **288**, 1723–7.

FOSTER, G. D., WYATT, H. R., HILL, J. O. *et al.* (2003), A randomized trial of a low-carbohydrate diet for obesity. *New England Journal of Medicine*, **348**, 2082–90.

FREEDMAN, M. R., KING, J. and KENNEDY, E. (2001), Popular diets: a scientific review. *Obesity Research*, **9**, 1S–40S.

FRENCH, S. A., JEFFERY, R. W. and MURRAY, D. (1999), Is dieting good for you?: prevalence, duration and associated weight and behaviour changes for specific weight loss strategies over four years in US adults. *International Journal of Obesity*, **23**, 320–7.

GERSTEIN, D. E., WOODWARD-LOPEZ, G., EVANS, A. E., KELSEY, K. and DREWNOWSKI, A. (2004), Clarifying concepts about macronutrients' effects on satiation and satiety. *Journal of the American Dietetic Association*, **104**, 1151–3.

HANNUM, S. M., CARSON, L., EVANS, E. M. *et al.* (2004), Use of portion-controlled entrees enhances weight loss in women. *Obesity Research*, **12**, 538–46.

HARVEY-BERINO, J., PINTAURO, S., BUZZELL, P. and GOLD, E. C. (2004), Effect of internet support on the long-term maintenance of weight loss. *Obesity Research*, **12**, 320–9.

HESHKA, S., GREENWAY, F., ANDERSON, J. W. *et al.* (2000), Self-help weight loss versus a structured commercial programme after 26 weeks: a randomized controlled study. *American Journal of Medicine*, **109**, 282–7.

INSTITUTE OF MEDICINE (1995), *Weighing the Options: Criteria for Evaluating Weight Management Programmes*. Washington, DC: National Academy Press.

INSTITUTE OF MEDICINE (1999), *Dietary Reference Intake for Calcium, Phosphorous, Magnesium, Vitamin D, and Fluoride*. Washington, DC: National Academy Press.

INSTITUTE OF MEDICINE (1999), *Dietary Reference Intake for Thiamin, Riboflavin, Niacin, Vitamin B6, Folate, Vitamin B12, Pantothenic Acid, Biotin, and Choline*. Washington, DC: National Academy Press.

INSTITUTE OF MEDICINE (2000), *Dietary Reference Intake for Vitamin C, Vitamin E, Selenium, and Carotenoids*. Washington, DC: National Academy Press.

INSTITUTE OF MEDICINE (2001), *Dietary Reference Intake for Vitamin A, Vitamin K, Arsenic, Boron, Chromium, Copper, Iodine, Iron, Manganese, Molybdenum, Nickel, Silicon, Vanadium, and Zinc*. Washington, DC: National Academy Press.

INSTITUTE OF MEDICINE (2002), *Dietary Reference Intake for Energy, Carbohydrates, Fiber, Fat, Protein and Amino Acids (Macronutrients)*. Washington, DC: National Academy Press.

INSULL, W., HENDERSON, M. M., PRENTICE, R. L. *et al.* (1990), Results of a randomized feasibility study of a low-fat diet. *Archives of Internal Medicine*, **150**, 421–7.

JAKICIC, J. M., WINTERS, C., LANG, W. and WING, R. R. (1999), Effects of intermittent exercise and use of home exercise equipment on adherence, weight loss, and fitness in overweight women. *Journal of the American Medical Association*, **282**, 1554–60.

JEFFERY, R. W., BJORNSON-BENSON, W. M., ROSENTHAL, B. S., LINDQUIST, R. A., KURTH, C. L. and JOHNSON, S. L. (1984), Correlates of weight loss and its maintenance over two years of follow-up among middle-aged men. *Preventive Medicine*, **13**, 155–68.

JEFFERY, R. W., DRENOWSKI, A., EPSTEIN, L. H. *et al.* (2000), Long-term maintenance of weight loss: current status. *Health Psychology*, **19**, 5–16.

JEFFERY, R. W., WING, R. R., SHERWOOD, N. E. and TATE D. F. (2003), Physical activity and weight loss: does prescribing higher physical activity goals improve outcome? *American Journal of Clinical Nutrition*, **78**, 684–9.

JEQUIER, E. and BRAY, G. A. (2002), Low-fat diets are preferred. *American Journal of Medicine*, **113**, 41S–6S.

KLESGES, R. C., KLESGES, L. M., HADDOCK, C. K. and ECK, L. H. (1992), A longitudinal analysis of the impact of dietary intake and physical activity on weight change in adults. *American Journal of Clinical Nutrition*, **55**, 818–22.

KUSHI, L. H., LEW, R. A., STARE, F. J. *et al.* (1985), Diet and 20-year mortality from coronary heart disease. *The New England Journal of Medicine*, **312**, 811–8.

LOWE, M. R., MILLER-KOVACH, K. and PHELAN, S. (2001), Weight-loss maintenance in overweight individuals one to five years following successful completion of a commercial weight loss program. *International Journal of Obesity*, **25**, 325–31.

METZ, J. A., KRIS-ETHERTON, P. M., MORRIS, C. D. *et al.* (1997), Dietary compliance and cardiovascular risk reduction with a prepared meal plan compared with a self-selected diet. *American Journal of Clinical Nutrition*, **66**, 373–85.

NATIONAL HEART, LUNG and BLOOD INSTITUTE (2003), *Facts about the DASH Eating Plan*. Washington, DC: United States Department of Health and Human Services.

RAYNOR, H. A. and EPSTEIN, L. H. (2001), Dietary variety, energy regulation, and obesity. *Psychological Bulletin*, **127**, 1–17.

RAYNOR, H. A., JEFFERY, R. W., TATE, D. F. and WING, R. R. (2004), Relationship between changes in food group variety, dietary intake, and weight during obesity treatment. *International Journal of Obesity*, **28**, 813–20.

ROLLS, B. J., BELL, E. A. and WAUGH, B. A. (2000), Increasing the volume of a food by incorporating air affects satiety in men. *American Journal of Clinical Nutrition*, **72**, 361–8.

ROMIEU, I., WILLETT, W. C., STAMPFER, M. J. *et al.* (1988), Energy intake and other determinants of relative weight. *American Journal of Clinical Nutrition*, **47**, 406–12.

SAMAHA, F. F., IQBAL, N., SESHADRI, P. *et al.* (2003), A low-carbohydrate as compared with a low-fat diet in severe obesity. *New England Journal of Medicine*, **348**, 2074–81.

SERDULA, M. K., MOKDAD, A. H., WILLIAMSON, D. F., GALUSKA, D. A., MENDLEIN, J. M. and HEATH, G. W. (1999), Prevalence of attempting weight loss and strategies for controlling weight. *Journal of the American Medical Association*, **282**, 1353–8.

SHEPPARD, L., KRISTAL, A. R. and KUSHI, L. H. (1991), Weight loss in women participating in a randomized trial of low-fat diets. *American Journal of Clinical Nutrition*, **54**, 821–8.

STERN, L., IQBAL, N., SESHADRI, P. *et al.* (2004), The effects of low-carbohydrate versus conventional weight loss diets in severely obese adults: one-year follow-up of a randomized trial. *Annals of Internal Medicine*, **140**, 778–85.

STUBBS, R. J., NARBRON, C. G., MURGATROYD, R. and PRENTICE, A. M. (1995a), Covert manipulation of dietary fat and energy density: effect on substrate flux and food intake in men eating *ad libitum*. *American Journal of Clinical Nutrition*, **62**, 316–29.

STUBBS, R. J., RITZ, P., COWARD, W. A. and PRENTICE, A. M. (1995b), Covert manipulation of the ratio of dietary fat to carbohydrate and energy density: effect on food intake and energy balance in free-living men eating *ad libitum*. *American Journal of Clinical Nutrition*, **62**, 330–7.

SWINBURN, B. A., WOOLARD, G. A., CHANG, E. C. and WILSON, M. R. (1999), Effects of reduced fat diets consumed *ad libitum* on intake of nutrients, particularly antioxidant vitamins. *Journal of the American Dietetic Association*, **99**, 1400–5.

TATE, D. F., WING, R. R. and WINETT, R. A. (2001), Using internet technology to deliver a behavioral weight loss program. *Journal of the American Medical Association*, **285**, 1172–7.

TATE, D. F., JACKVONY, E. H. and WING, R. R. (2003), Effects of internet behavioral counseling on weight loss in adults at risk for type 2 diabetes: a randomized trial. *Journal of the American Medical Association*, **289**, 1833–6.

UNITED STATES DEPARTMENT OF AGRICULTURE (1996), *The Food Guide Pyramid*. Home and Garden Bulletin 252. Washington, DC: United States Department of Agriculture.

UNITED STATES DEPARTMENT OF AGRICULTURE (2000), *The Dietary Guidelines for Americans*. Home and Garden Bulletin 232. Washington, DC: United States Department of Agriculture.

WING, R. R. and JEFFERY, R. W. (2001), Food provision as a strategy to promote weight loss. *Obesity Research*, **9**, 271S–5S.

WING, R. R. (2004), Behavioral approaches to the treatment of obesity. In Bray, G., Bouchard, C. and James, T. (eds.) *Handbook of Obesity*. 2nd edn. New York: Marcel Dekker, inc.

WOMBLE, L. G., WADDEN, T. A., MCGUCKIN, B. G., SARGENT, S. L., ROTHMAN, R. A. and KRAUTHAMER-EWING, E. S. (2004), A randomized controlled trial of a commercial internet weight loss program. *Obesity Research*, **12**, 1011–8.

YANCY, W. S., OLSEN, M. K., GUYTON, J. R., BAKST, R. P. and WESTMAN, E. C. (2004), A low-carbohydrate, ketogenic diet versus a low-fat diet to treat obesity and hyperlipidemia. *Annals of Internal Medicine*, **140**, 769–77.

YIP, I., GO, V. L. W., DESHIELDS, S. *et al.* (2001), Liquid meal replacements and glycemic control in obese type 2 diabetes patients. *Obesity Research*, **9**, 341S–7S.

YU-POTH, S., ZHAO, G. ETHERTON, T., NAGLAK, M., JONNALAGADDA, S. and KRIS-ETHERTON, M. (1999), Effects of the National Cholesterol Education Programmes step I and step II dietary intervention programmes on cardiovascular disease risk factors: a meta-analysis. *American Journal of Clinical Nutrition*, **69**, 632–46.

21

Calcium and obesity

S. I. Barr, University of British Columbia, Canada

21.1 Introduction

During the past decade, both academic researchers and the general public have become increasingly interested in the possible link between low intakes of calcium (and/or dairy products) and obesity. In this chapter, I first describe the mechanisms which have been suggested to underlie this association. Next, epidemiological studies that demonstrate – or, in some cases, fail to demonstrate – associations between low calcium intake and obesity are presented. This is followed by the description of randomized human trials designed to test the hypothesis that a low-energy, calcium/dairy-rich diet leads to greater weight or fat loss than a diet with similar low energy content, but low in calcium/dairy. Also described are the results of randomized intervention trials designed to assess effects of calcium or dairy product supplementation on bone or other outcomes, but that include data on changes in body weight or composition. This section is followed by a discussion of the limited evidence from human metabolic studies. Next, gaps in the literature and future research questions are identified. The chapter concludes by addressing potential implications of this body of research for the prevention or management of obesity from the perspective of consumers, the food industry and public health strategies, and by providing sources of further information and advice.

21.2 Possible mechanisms linking calcium/dairy intake and body weight regulation

From the thermodynamic perspective, calcium or dairy products could theoretically affect energy balance by influencing energy intake, energy absorption, or energy expenditure. Evidence for each of these is examined below.

21.2.1 Energy intake

Energy intake in humans can be influenced by feelings of hunger and satiety. Although our understanding of mechanisms that may regulate hunger and satiety is expanding rapidly, to date, little work has been done to directly assess the effects of calcium or dairy products. In one randomized crossover study, 19 young adults were fed isocaloric low- and high-dairy diets (providing 500 mg and 1400 mg calcium) for 7 days each (E. Melanson, personal communication, May 2004). On the seventh day of each study period, participants rated their hunger, satiety, and fullness before and after each meal, and no differences were observed between the low- and high-dairy diets. Another randomized cross-over study in 44 young women assessed whether consumption of various beverages (one of which was milk) with a meal affected total *ad libitum* energy intake at that meal (Della Valle *et al.*, 2004). Results indicated that consumption of a caloric beverage (1% milk, orange juice with pulp, or cola, each providing 150 kcal) increased total energy intake at the meal by 104 ± 16 kcal when compared to consumption of a non-caloric beverage (water, diet cola) or no beverage. There were no differences in energy intake among the three caloric beverages, nor did perceived fullness differ, suggesting that milk did not have specific effects on satiety or energy intake. Thus, although additional research may be warranted to further explore the effects of calcium and dairy products on energy intake, hunger and satiety, the limited available data do not suggest a major effect.

21.2.2 Energy absorption

It has been known for many years that calcium can reduce fat absorption through an interaction between calcium and saturated fatty acids that results in the formation of insoluble (and therefore poorly absorbed) calcium-fatty acid soaps (Drenick, 1961). This mechanism underlies the poorer fat absorption of infants fed cow's milk compared to those fed human milk. In human milk, palmitate is primarily esterified at position two of triacylglycerol, and following lipase activity, the resulting two-monoglyceride is readily solubilized into biliary micelles and absorbed. In contrast, a greater proportion of palmitate in cow's milk is esterified at the one and three positions, so is released as the free fatty acid following lipase action. Saturated fatty acids are more slowly absorbed from the intestine, and can form poorly soluble calcium-fatty acid soaps that are excreted in the feces.

The possible contribution of this mechanism to weight loss in human adults appears modest, but possibly meaningful. In men fed relatively high-fat diets (134 g/d, 57 g as saturated fat), doubling calcium intake from 950 to 1855 mg/d increased fecal fat excretion by 4.04 g/d, representing approximately 36 kcal/d (Shahkhalili *et al.*, 2001). In another study, to date reported only in abstract form (Kunchel *et al.*, 2004), ten subjects participated in a randomized crossover study of diets with 15% protein and 500 mg or 1800 mg calcium. The percentage energy from fat and the type of fat were not specified. On the high calcium diet, fecal fat excretion increased 2.5-fold (14.2 vs. 6.0 g/d) and fecal energy excretion was 90 kcal/d higher. In other studies (Welberg *et al.*, 1994; Denke *et al.*, 1993), adding elemental calcium in amounts up to 4 g/d increased fat excretion by approximately 1% of energy intake (e.g. 30 kcal/d in a 3000 kcal diet). Collectively, these studies suggest that fecal energy excretion may increase by between 30 and 90 kcal/d on high calcium diets. Using these values to estimate the potential long-term impact of high calcium intakes, individuals on diets high in calcium and relatively high in saturated fat (compared to diets low in these components) could be predicted to lose approximately 1–4 kg of body fat in a year. Presumably, smaller losses would occur on diets lower in energy/saturated fat and with smaller increments in calcium intake.

21.2.3 Energy expenditure and substrate partitioning

Zemel and colleagues have proposed a mechanism to explain how calcium could reduce fat storage and lead to negative energy balance (Zemel, 2004). It is based on the well-established regulatory system for serum calcium: when extracellular (serum) calcium levels are low (as seen with inadequate calcium intakes), parathyroid hormone (PTH) is released and increases synthesis of $1,25(OH)_2$ vitamin D, leading to increased calcium absorption and mobilization, and restoration of serum levels. The proposed mechanism, however, relates to the actions of $1,25(OH)_2$ vitamin D in human adipocytes. In cultured human adipocytes, addition of $1,25(OH)_2$ vitamin D to the culture medium leads to a prompt increase in intracellular calcium levels (Zemel *et al.*, 2000). Intracellular calcium appears to play a regulatory role in the activity of key enzymes involved in fat synthesis, fat breakdown, and the degree of coupling of oxidative phosphorylation (and thus energy metabolism). Specifically, high intracellular calcium levels activate fatty acid synthase, inhibit fat breakdown, and maintain tightly coupled oxidative phosphorylation (Xue *et al.*, 2001; Shi *et al.*, 2002), all of which would be predicted to lead to an increase in body fat and body energy stores.

Results consistent with this proposed mechanism have been obtained using the *agouti* obese mouse model (Zemel *et al.*, 2000). These animals overexpress agouti protein, a protein that plays a role in regulation of food intake. When they are fed a highly palatable diet, they overeat and become obese. However, in a study in which the calcium content of such a palatable diet was manipulated (1.2% vs. 0.4% calcium by weight), less body weight and fat were gained on the high calcium diet, and the expected changes in enzyme activities were observed (Zemel *et al.*, 2000). Furthermore, the animals receiving a high calcium diet had significantly elevated body core temperature, which would indicate increased energy dissipation as heat (Zemel *et al.*, 2000). Additional support for the proposed mechanism was provided in another study from the same group. When *agouti* obese mice were placed on energy-restricted diets after having gained weight, greater weight loss and fat loss were seen in animals on the high calcium diets (Shi *et al.*, 2001). These studies also included treatment arms in which calcium was provided as either skim milk powder or elemental calcium (e.g. calcium carbonate, $CaCO_3$). In animals fed restricted diets, dairy calcium had greater effects on enhancing weight and fat loss as compared to elemental calcium (Shi *et al.*, 2001).

Other studies conducted with rodents, however, have not detected consistent effects of calcium on body weight or composition of lean and obese mice and rats. Zhang and Tordoff (2004) conducted a series of experiments that varied energy density of diets as well as their elemental calcium content (0.2%, 0.6% or 1.8%). Studies in female C57BL/6J mice revealed no effect of calcium on body weight or carcass fat. Female Sprague–Dawley rats fed diets with 1.8% calcium gained significantly less weight than those fed 0.2% or 0.6% calcium on the normal-energy-density diet, but this was associated with a reduced body protein content rather than a reduction in percentage body fat. In a study conducted by Papakonstantinou and colleagues (2003), male Wistar rats fed diets with 2.4% calcium (provided from non-fat dry milk) gained less weight and carcass fat than those fed diets with 0.4% calcium. However, the difference in body composition could be accounted for by increased fecal excretion of dietary lipid in the high calcium group. Furthermore, no difference in body core temperature was observed between animals on the high- and low-dairy diets (Papakonstantinou *et al.*, 2003). Thus, it appears that not all rodents respond to alterations of dietary calcium in a manner similar to the *agouti* obese mouse.

Another consideration regarding the proposed calcium mechanism is related to differences in lipogenesis between rodents and humans. As described above, $1,25(OH)_2$ vitamin D-mediated increases in adipocyte intracellular calcium concentrations cause increased expression and activity of fatty acid synthase in the *agouti* mouse model and in human adipocytes *in vitro*. However, this mechanism has not yet been demonstrated in humans *in vivo*. In this regard, it is important to note that it is generally accepted that *de novo* lipogenesis (DNL; synthesis of fatty acids *de novo* by fatty acid synthase) does not make a substantive contribution to whole body lipogenesis in humans, under most conditions (Strawford *et al.*, 2004; Hellerstein, 1999; Guo *et al.*, 2000). Although DNL can be induced by massive carbohydrate overfeeding (Pasquet *et al.*, 1992), unless carbohydrate intake exceeds total daily energy expenditure, its contribution to fat storage appears minimal. Humans thus appear to differ in this respect from rodents, in which up to 70% of palmitate is derived from DNL (Turner *et al.*, 2003). Furthermore, to the extent that DNL does occur in humans, the relative contributions of hepatic versus adipose tissue DNL are difficult to assess, and the proposed mechanism has not been assessed in human hepatocytes.

Thus, while cell culture studies and animal models can provide important insights into possible mechanisms, by themselves they do not establish that a mechanism operates or is important in humans. Given the differences in rodent and human lipid metabolism, there is reason to question whether the mechanism that could account for effects observed in the *agouti* mouse model is relevant for people. Accordingly, human studies are required to determine whether or not calcium or dairy products have important roles in body weight regulation. In the sections that follow, the human evidence currently available (from epidemiological studies, clinical trials, and metabolic studies) is examined.

21.3 Epidemiological studies

Although epidemiological studies cannot demonstrate cause and effect, they can be used to explore associations, and thus warrant discussion in terms of whether they support the link between calcium and body weight regulation.

21.3.1 Cross-sectional analyses

An early report from Zemel's group examined data from the Third National Health and Nutrition Examination Survey (NHANES-III; a representative sample of individuals living in the United States). A striking inverse association between calcium intake (estimated using a 24-hr recall) and the risk of being in the highest quartile for body fat was reported for adult women (Zemel *et al.*, 2000). Using the lowest quartile of calcium intake as the reference, women in the second, third and highest quartiles of calcium intake had a progressively lower relative risk of being in the highest body fat quartile (1.0, 0.75, 0.44 and 0.16, respectively). A limitation of this analysis was that it included only 380 of the more than 7000 women in the NHANES-III sample. Subsequently, Barr and colleagues (2004) repeated the analysis using 6878 women (selected using the same inclusion/exclusion criteria specified by Zemel). Contrary to the previous report, they did not detect a significant association between quartile of calcium intake or dairy intake and risk of being in the highest quartile for body fat: The relative risks of being in the highest body fat quartile were 1.0, 1.01, 1.01 and 0.75 as quartile of calcium intake increased (Barr *et al.*, 2004). Similar to Zemel's findings, no associations were observed in men. Reports based on the NHANES data must be interpreted cautiously, as the usual calcium intake of an individual is known to be poorly estimated by a singe 24-hr recall, and considerable misclassification can occur. Thus, the inconsistent findings and the lack of evidence for an association in men do not prove that a relationship between calcium intake and body fat does not exist.

Several smaller studies have detected cross-sectional associations between calcium and body weight or fatness, particularly in women (Jacqmain *et al.*, 2003, Davies *et al.*, 2000, Skinner *et al.*, 2003). For example, in the Quebec Family Study, 235 men and 235 women were divided into three groups based on their calcium intake, as assessed by a 3-day food record (Jacqmain *et al.*, 2003). Women who consumed less than 600 mg calcium per day weighed more and had higher percentage body fat than women with calcium intakes of 600–1000 mg/d or over 1000 mg/d. However, a possible limitation of this study is that physical activity was not included as a covariate in the analysis, and this could potentially confound an association between calcium and body fatness. As was the case in both analyses of the NHANES-III data, no associations between calcium intake and body fatness or weight were observed in men in the Quebec Family Study. Davies and colleagues (2000) reported on two cross-sectional studies in 344 young adult women, among whom calcium intake (expressed relative to protein intake) was negatively associated with body mass index (BMI; kg/m^2), and accounted for about 3% of the variance in BMI. Skinner, Carruth and colleagues assessed calcium intake in a sample of 52 children between the ages of 2 months and 6 years (Carruth and Skinner, 2001), and between 2 months and 8 years (Skinner *et al.*, 2003), and found that average calcium intake over 6 or 8 years was a significant negative predictor of percentage body fat at age 6 or 8.

21.3.2 Longitudinal analyses

In the CARDIA study, diets and health risk factors of 3157 black and white adults (initially aged 18–30) were assessed at baseline and participants were followed for 10 years (Pereira *et al.*, 2002). An inverse association was observed between the number of dairy product servings (assessed using a food frequency questionnaire) and the risk of developing components of the insulin resistance syndrome (glucose intolerance, hyperlipidemia and obesity). However, the beneficial associations with dairy product intake were restricted to those whose initial BMI was over 25 kg/m^2: in this overweight group, 64.8% of those consuming <10 dairy servings weekly became obese during the 10-yr follow-up, compared to 45.1% of those consuming ≥35 servings weekly (P for trend <0.001). In contrast, no associations were detected in those with initial BMI <25 kg/m^2.

Associations between calcium intake and change in body weight were also reported by Davies and colleagues (2000) and Lin and colleagues (2000). Davies (2000) reported associations between calcium intake (expressed relative to protein intake) and change in body weight in two longitudinal studies conducted in women aged 35–58 at baseline. In one, participants were followed every 6 months for 8 years; however, only calcium intake at baseline was used to assess the relationship with weight change. In the other, which had a 21-year follow-up, diets were assessed every 5 years and average calcium intake throughout the study was used in the analysis. The pooled data from the two studies showed an inverse association between calcium (mg/g protein) and change in body weight, which accounted for about 3% of the variance in body weight change (Davies *et al.*, 2000). Lin followed a group of 54 young adult women (aged 18–30) for 2 years, and assessed dietary calcium intake every 6 months using 3-day diet records. Average calcium intake expressed relative to energy was associated with body weight and body fat change. Additional analyses revealed that this association was confined to women who reported energy intakes below the median intake of 1876 kcal/d. In this group, total calcium intake predicted 22% of the variance in weight change ($P = 0.01$) and 17% of the variance in fat change ($P = 0.03$). However, in the women with energy intakes above 1876 kcal/d, calcium intake was not associated with weight change (4% of explained variance, $P = 0.32$) or fat change (0.2% of explained variance, $P = 0.85$) (Lin *et al.*, 2000).

Conversely, other observational studies have not detected an association between calcium and body fatness. For example, in the MIT Growth and Development Study, Phillips and colleagues (2003) followed non-obese premenarcheal girls until they were 4 years post-menarche. At annual visits, percentage body fat was assessed using bioelectrical impedance analysis, BMI z-scores were calculated, calcium intake was assessed using a food frequency questionnaire, and physical activity was assessed. An analysis of 178 girls with at least three annual visits and who had valid anthropometric and food frequency data indicated no relationship between BMI z-score or percentage body fat and measures of dairy food or calcium consumption.

Thus, although some epidemiological studies have revealed associations between calcium intake and body weight or fatness, the findings are not consistent. Randomized controlled clinical trials provide the highest level of evidence, and are discussed below.

21.4 Randomized trials in humans

In the past several years, Zemel and colleagues have reported on four randomized trials conducted to assess the effects of calcium and/or dairy product intake on weight and fat loss in overweight and obese adults. At the time of writing, all but one were available in abstract form. The published report (Zemel *et al.*, 2004a) describes the results of a 24-week study of 41 obese adults (34 women, seven men; baseline BMI = 35.0 ± 4.1 kg/m^2) who were randomly assigned to one of three diets, each with a 500 kcal/d energy deficit. Two of the diets were low in dairy products (no more than one serving per day) and included either a placebo supplement or an 800 mg calcium supplement, while the third diet was high in dairy products (three servings daily) and included a placebo supplement. Participants were counselled individually by a dietitian, and body weight, waist circumference and fat mass were measured at baseline, 12 weeks and 24 weeks. Thirty-two individuals (27 women, five men) completed the study. For each of weight loss, fat loss, trunk fat loss and waist circumference, the calcium-supplemented low-dairy group had significantly greater losses than the placebo low-dairy group, and losses among the high-dairy group were significantly greater than the calcium-supplemented low-dairy group. For example, total fat losses were 4.8 ± 1.22 kg (mean ± SE) for the low-dairy/placebo group, 5.6 ± 0.98 kg for the low-dairy/supplement group, and 7.16 ± 1.22 kg for the high-dairy group, and each group differed significantly from the two other groups. Two other studies available in abstract form also report greater fat loss in obese adults consuming high- versus low-dairy diets (Zemel *et al.*, 2002, 2003).

A different pattern of results was observed in a larger study recently reported in abstract form (Zemel *et al.*, 2004b). In this study, a similar protocol to that described above was used, except the study duration was 12 weeks instead of 24. One hundred and five overweight and obese adults began the study, 93 completed it, and 68 who complied with the protocol were included in the analysis. In contrast to the step-wise differences among the low-dairy/placebo, low-dairy/supplement and high-dairy groups reported earlier (Zemel *et al.*, 2004a), in this study there were no differences in any outcome variables between the low-dairy groups who received a placebo or an 800 mg calcium supplement. For example, fat loss averaged 2.69 ± 0.53 kg (mean ± SE) and 2.32 ± 0.87 kg in the low-dairy placebo and supplemented groups, respectively. However, the high dairy group had significantly greater fat loss than the other two groups (4.43 ± 0.53 kg), as well as significantly greater losses in weight, trunk fat and waist circumference. Possible reasons for the different pattern of results in this study, compared to the previous study, are difficult to discern, but the absence of a difference between the low-dairy groups receiving a placebo or an 800 mg calcium supplement raises questions about the hypothesis based on adipocyte intracellular calcium levels. Specifically, it is difficult to advance a mechanism based on calcium when calcium as placebo did not have any effects. Potentially, substances in dairy products other than calcium (e.g. vitamin D, bioactive peptides, amino acids) may play a role through other mechanisms (Zemel, 2004).

Insights can also be gained from large randomized trials that were conducted to assess the effects of increased calcium or dairy product intake on other outcomes, most frequently bone density or bone mass. The majority of these studies were conducted in women, but they have spanned an age range from childhood to old age. Although bone was the primary endpoint in many of these studies, most also obtained data on changes in weight (such data are needed to interpret the bone data). Some also included data on whole body fat and lean tissue as assessed by dual-energy X-ray absorptiometry (DEXA). A review of these studies was published by Barr (2003), and was updated for this chapter. To conduct the review, a MEDLINE search between the years 1966 and April 2004 was completed, in which articles containing the exploded search terms 'calcium', 'calcium citrate', 'calcium, dietary', 'calcium carbonate' or 'dairy products' were combined with those in which the search terms 'bone density', 'body weight' or 'body composition' were a focus of the article. The combined sets were limited to studies published in the English language and conducted with humans. Titles of the resulting articles were reviewed manually, and 39 randomized controlled trials of increased dairy product or calcium intake in generally healthy individuals were identified (in addition to the study by Zemel and colleagues (2004a) described above). Twenty-eight articles provided information on relative changes in body weight or composition, and an attempt was made to contact the authors of the remaining papers to obtain the relevant data.

Fourteen studies were available with data on body weight or composition in which the study protocol included increased dairy product intake for some (or all) of the study participants (nine cited in Barr, 2003; Chee *et al.*, 2003; Volek *et al.*, 2003; Farnsworth *et al.*, 2003; Bowen *et al.*, 2004; Lappe *et al.*, 2004). In ten studies, participants were randomly assigned to increased dairy product intake or to maintain their 'usual' diets; one study reported the results of a randomized crossover trial of high- and low-calcium diets; one compared supplementation with milk or a low-calcium juice; and two compared isocaloric high- and low-dairy diets during weight loss. These studies were conducted in adolescent girls, adolescent boys, premenopausal women, overweight and obese adults, women within 5 years of menopause and postmenopausal women (one of which also included men). Most studies did not detect group differences in the changes in weight, height, fat mass or lean mass, although two studies conducted in older adults observed significantly greater weight gains in the dairy supplemented groups. These dairy interventions, however, are difficult to interpret from the perspective of whether they support the concept that calcium or dairy products increase energy utilization, because in most cases diets were not tightly controlled. Any effect on weight or fat mass would depend on the extent to which compensation occurred for the additional energy contained in the dairy products.

The two studies that included high- and low-dairy diets during weight loss interventions warrant additional discussion, as attempts were made to control energy intake by providing participants with foods consistent with their allocated diets (Farnsworth *et al.*, 2003; Bowen *et al.*, 2004). Both studies consisted of 12-week periods of energy restriction in overweight and obese adults, followed by 4 weeks of energy balance. In one study (Farnsworth *et al.*, 2003), participants were randomly assigned to isoenergetic high protein (27%) or standard protein (16%) diets. The additional protein was provided primarily from dairy products, so the high protein diet contained 1600 mg calcium compared to 600 mg in the standard protein diet. Neither weight loss nor fat loss differed between diet groups. In the other study (Bowen *et al.*, 2004), all participants received high protein diets (34% energy), but protein was provided either primarily from dairy sources (2400 mg calcium) or other sources (500 mg calcium). Again, weight loss did not differ between groups, and averaged 9.0 ± 0.6 kg on the dairy protein diet and 9.3 ± 0.7 kg on the mixed protein diet. In this study, fat loss was not reported.

Randomized trials of calcium supplementation are more straightforward to interpret than are dairy interventions, as energy intake presumably does not change. Twenty relevant randomized trials were located (17 cited in Barr 2003; Rozen *et al.*, 2003; Specker and Binkley, 2003; Shapses *et al.*, 2004); these studies were conducted in children or adolescents, women during lactation, perimenopausal women, postmenopausal women (one of which included men), and during weight loss in pre- and post-menopausal women. The studies varied in length from three months to four years, and included subjects that varied in ethnicity and baseline calcium intake. In the large majority of studies, no differences in the changes in body weight or body composition were detected between the calcium and placebo/untreated groups. Only one study detected a difference in body weight change: postmenopausal women receiving 1.2 g calcium/d lost 0.35 kg/yr more than the control group during the 4-year study (Recker *et al.*, 1996). In the only study to detect a change in body composition (Riggs *et al.*, 1998), women supplemented with 1.6 g calcium/d lost more lean mass than controls during the 4-year study, although group differences in weight and fat mass were not observed. Taken together, the data from randomized trials of calcium supplementation provide little evidence to suggest that supplemental calcium affects body weight or composition over time. They are thus consistent with the recent preliminary results of Zemel *et al.* (2004b), in which no effect of calcium supplementation on body weight or composition was observed during energy restriction, but fail to support a hypothesis based on the effects of increased calcium intake.

21.5 Human metabolic studies

Few human studies have directly assessed the potential impact of calcium or dairy products on substrate oxidation or energy expenditure. However, Melanson and colleagues recently assessed these relationships using data from 35 healthy, normal-weight (BMI = 23.7 ± 2.9 kg/m^2) young adults who had previously completed a 24-h stay in a room calorimeter (Melanson *et al.*, 2003). Habitual calcium intake, assessed using a 4-d food record completed prior to the calorimetry study, was 1222 ± 116 mg/d (mean ± SE; range 485–4109 mg/d) while acute calcium intake during the 24-h study period was 1046 ± 55 mg/d (range 477–1768 mg/d). Acute calcium intake, expressed as mg/kcal, was positively correlated with fat oxidation during the 24-hr study period ($r = 0.38$, $P = 0.03$), but habitual calcium intake was not ($r = -0.06$, $P = 0.73$). Neither acute nor habitual calcium intake was significantly associated with 24-h energy expenditure, although the correlation with acute calcium intake was positive ($r = 0.26$). Thus, the data suggested that higher calcium intakes were acutely associated with increased fat oxidation, although the retrospective and cross-sectional nature of the analysis precluded strong conclusions.

These investigators subsequently conducted another study to address this question prospectively, and have reported preliminary results on resting metabolic rate (RMR) and resting respiratory quotient (RQ) (Melanson *et al.*, 2004). Eighteen overweight young adults (BMI = 27.6 ± 3.2 kg/m^2) consumed either a low-dairy diet (500 mg calcium/d) or an isocaloric high-dairy diet (1400 mg calcium/d) for 7 days. Meals were prepared in the research kitchen, and were matched for macronutrients, fibre, and saturated, monounsaturated and polyunsaturated fat. Each participant completed the low- and high-dairy dietary condition twice, with washout periods of one to three weeks between each trial (i.e. four 7-day trials were completed by each subject). The order of dietary periods was randomized across subjects, and RMR and RQ were measured on the fifth or sixth day of each dietary period. RMR was 1676 ± 214 kcal/d (mean ± SD) on the low-dairy diet and 1650 ± 212 kcal/d on the high-dairy diet ($P = 0.75$) while RQ on the low- and high-dairy diets was 0.78 ± 0.05 and 0.78 ± 0.03, respectively ($P = 0.96$). Thus, using dairy products to vary calcium intake between 500 mg/d and 1400 mg/d had no effect on resting energy expenditure or substrate oxidation. The seventh day of each dietary period was spent in the room calorimeter to provide data on 24-h energy expenditure and substrate oxidation (E. L. Melanson, personal communication, May 2004). For both the low- and high-dairy diets, one 24-h period was conducted in a state of energy balance and the second was conducted with an energy deficit induced by exercise. Twenty-four hour energy expenditure was not increased on the high- vs. the low-dairy diets, and analysis of substrate oxidation indicated no differences in 24-h respiratory quotient. During the energy balance condition, no difference in 24-h fat oxidation was observed between high- and low-dairy diets (92 ± 10 g/d vs. 100 ± 10 g/d, respectively). However, there was a significant increase in 24-h fat oxidation on the high-dairy energy deficit diet (136 ± 13 g/d) vs. the low-dairy deficit diet (106 ± 7 g/d), which appeared to occur as a result of greater fat oxidation during exercise. Thus, these results suggest that a high-dairy diet increases fat oxidation during exercise conducted on an energy-deficient diet, but do not indicate that total energy expenditure is affected. Additional studies could establish whether similar changes would be seen with an energy deficit resulting from a hypocaloric diet, rather than from increased energy expenditure as exercise.

Kunchel and colleagues (2004) have also assessed the effect of high- and low-dairy diets on 24-h energy expenditure and fat oxidation. In their study, ten subjects participated in a randomized crossover study of isocaloric diets that differed in calcium content (1800 mg vs. 500 mg). Each diet period lasted one week. No differences were observed in 24-h energy expenditure or fat oxidation, consistent with the results of Melanson and colleagues with regard to their energy balance condition.

21.6 Gaps in the literature and directions for future research

Consideration of the data presented in this review suggests that the role of calcium in body weight regulation may be complex, as results are not consistent across studies. Additional research is needed with regard to the proposed mechanism(s), and additional human clinical trials are also needed. In terms of one of the proposed mechanisms (i.e. that intracellular calcium acts as a regulator of adipocyte lipogenesis and lipolysis, and thereby affects body fatness and energy stores), more work is required to confirm its relevance in humans, and to demonstrate effects on overall energy balance. It may also be important to ascertain the relative roles of calcium intake vs. vitamin D status. Both calcium and vitamin D can affect vitamin D activity, and because the increase in intracellular calcium is mediated by $1,25(OH)_2$ vitamin D, it is possible that these two nutrients may interact. It is also possible that there may be a genetically susceptible subset of the population among whom this mechanism is important (e.g., analogous to the obesity associated with defects in the melanocortin-4 receptor) (Farooqi *et al.*, 2003). Furthermore, additional exploration of mechanisms that could explain the apparently greater effects on weight/fat loss of dairy calcium than elemental calcium is required. It has been proposed that leucine-rich whey proteins or bioactive compounds found in whey may affect adiposity and energy partitioning (Zemel, 2004), but further studies are required to demonstrate whether these apply in humans. Additional human clinical trials are essential to confirm a number of issues, including (a) whether the effects of calcium and dairy products differ; (b) whether a 'threshold' exists, such that additional calcium/dairy product intake is only effective in those with initially low intakes; (c) whether differential responses occur in men and women, or in individuals who are initially at normal weight versus those who are overweight or obese; and d) whether responses are seen only in energy-deficit conditions (vs. energy-balance conditions), and if so, what mechanism might underlie this observation. Ideally, these studies should be conducted in metabolic-ward settings in which all food and beverages are provided to participants to avoid the uncertainty associated with intakes of free-living individuals.

21.7 Implications and recommendations

Based primarily on the results of randomized controlled human trials, there is not yet consistent evidence that increasing calcium or dairy product intake will prevent weight gain or will increase weight loss on a low-energy diet. Thus, in this author's opinion, it seems premature to broadly promote increased consumer use of dairy products or calcium supplements as a public health strategy for weight management purposes, or for the food industry to develop additional calcium-fortified food products for the same purpose. In the event that additional research yields consistent findings, or clarifies subsets of the population among whom the hypothesized effects are consistently observed, such promotional efforts (if necessary, appropriately targeted) could be warranted.

However, this does not mean that it is inappropriate to encourage adequate calcium intake (primarily through food sources) as one component of a larger weight management strategy. In addition to preliminary evidence suggesting that fat loss may be enhanced, there are a number of reasons why this should occur: (a) dairy products are nutrient dense foods (e.g. Weinberg *et al.*, 2004), and as such, are particularly important in meeting nutrient needs when energy intake is limited; and (b) a generous calcium intake may reduce bone loss that can occur in association with weight loss (Ricci *et al.*, 1998; Jensen *et al.*, 2001). Furthermore, as stated by the United States Dietary Guidelines Advisory Committee (Dietary Guidelines Advisory Committee, 2005), 'There is no evidence that milk products should be avoided because of concerns that these foods are fattening'. The Committee, however, also noted that 'Because of the lack of large-scale, randomized trials or controlled feeding studies designed explicitly to test the effect of milk group intake or calcium consumption on body weight and the limitations of the studies reported above, at this time there is insufficient evidence on which to base a more definitive statement regarding the intake of milk products and management of body weight'.

Finally, although the scope of this article was intentionally limited to focus only on the role of calcium and dairy products in weight regulation, substantial evidence supports their role in maintaining health and preventing chronic conditions such as osteoporosis and fractures (Heaney, 2000), hypertension (Atallah *et al.*, 2002; Massey, 2001), and possibly colon cancer (Lipkin, 2002; Lamprecht and Lipkin, 2003). Accordingly, efforts to increase population calcium intakes may be warranted on grounds other than the potential for body weight regulation.

21.8 Sources of further information and advice

There are few sources (e.g. books, research or interest groups, professional or trade organizations) that focus specifically on the role of calcium and dairy products in prevention and management of obesity, probably because this is a relatively recent area of investigation. However, the National Dairy Council in the United States maintains a website that provides references for studies that support a link between dairy intake and body weight regulation (http://www.nationaldairycouncil.org/healthyweight/science.asp). Studies are described in one or two sentences, and a link is provided to the study abstract. The site does not, however, include references for studies that fail to detect an association. It also provides a link to an issue of the *Dairy Council Digest* titled 'Dairy foods' role in achieving a healthy weight'.

21.9 References

ATALLAH, A. N., HOFMEYR, G. J. and DULEY, L. (2002), 'Calcium supplementation during pregnancy for preventing hypertensive disorders and related problems', *Cochrane Database of Systematic Reviews*, (1), CD001059.

BARR, S. I. (2003), 'Increased calcium or dairy product intake: is body weight or composition affected in humans?', *J. Nutr.*, **133** (1), 245S–8S.

BARR, S. I., FULGONI, V. L. and PEREIRA, M. A. (2004), 'Relationship of calcium or dairy product intakes on percent body fat, BMI, and anthropometric measures in NHANES-III', *FASEB J.*, **18** (5 Part II), A873 (Abstract #583.8).

BOWEN, J., NOAKES, M. and CLIFTON, P. M. (2004), 'A high dairy protein, high-calcium diet minimizes bone turnover in overweight adults during weight loss', *J. Nutr.*, **134** (3), 568–73.

CARRUTH, B. R. and SKINNER, J. D. (2001), 'The role of dietary calcium and other nutrients in moderating body fat in preschool children', *Int. J. Obes. Relat. Metab. Disord.*, **25** (4), 559–66.

CHEE, W. S. S., SURIAH, A. R., CHAN, S. P., ZAITUN, Y. and CHAN, Y. M. (2003), 'The effect of milk supplementation on bone mineral density in postmenopausal Chinese women in Malaysia', *Osteoporos. Int.*, **14** (10), 828–34.

DAVIES, K. M., HEANEY, R. P., RECKER, R. R., LAPPE, J. M., BARGER-LUX, J., RAFFERTY, K. and HINDERS, S. (2000), 'Calcium intake and body weight', *J. Clin. Endocrinol. Metab.*, **85** (12), 4635–8.

DELLA VALLE, D. M., ROE, L. S. and ROLLS, B. J. (2004), 'Does the consumption of different beverages with a meal affect intake?', *FASEB J.*, **18** (5 Part II), A1109–10, (Abstract #727.4).

DENKE, M. A., FOX, M. M. and SCHULTE, M. C. (1993), 'Short-term dietary calcium fortification increases fecal saturated fat content and reduced serum lipids in men', *J. Nutr.*, **123** (6), 1047–53.

DIETARY GUIDELINES ADVISORY COMMITTEE (2005), '*Report of the Dietary Guidelines Advisory Committee on the Dietary Guidelines for Americans, 2005*', United States Department of Health and Human Services and United States Department of Agriculture, Washington, DC. Available at: http://www.health.gov/dietaryguidelines/dga2005/report/.

DRENICK, E. J. (1961), 'The influence of ingestion of calcium and other soap-forming substances on fecal fat', *Gastroenterology*, **41** (3), 242–4.

FARNSWORTH, E., LUSCOMBE, N. D., NOAKES, M., WITTERT, G., ARGYIOU, E. and CLIFTON, P. M. (2003), 'Effect of a high-protein, energy-restricted diet on body composition, glycemic control, and lipid concentrations in overweight and obese hyperinsulinemic men and women', *Am. J. Clin. Nutr.*, **78** (1), 31–9.

FAROOQI, I. S., KEOGH, J. M., YEO, G. S., LANK, E. J., CHEETHAM, T. and O'RAHILLY, S. (2003), 'Clinical spectrum of obesity and mutations in the melanocortin 4 receptor gene', *N. Engl. J. Med.*, **348** (12), 1085–95.

GUO, Z. K., CELLA, L. K., BAUM, C., RAVUSSIN, E. and SCHOELLER, D. A. (2000), '*De novo* lipogenesis in adipose tissue of lean and obese women: application of deuterated water and istotope ratio mass spectrometry', *Int. J. Obes.*, **24** (7), 932–7.

HEANEY, R. P. (2000), 'Calcium, dairy products and osteoporosis', *J. Am. Coll. Nutr.*, **19** (2 Suppl), 83S–99S.

HELLERSTEIN, M. K. (1999), '*De novo* lipogenesis in humans: metabolic and regulatory aspects', *Eur. J. Clin. Nutr.*, **53** (Suppl 1), S53–65.

JACQMAIN, M., DOUCET, E., DESPRES, J.-P., BOUCHARD, C. and TREMBLAY, A. (2003), 'Calcium intake, body composition, and lipoprotein–lipid concentrations in adults', *Am. J. Clin. Nutr.*, **77** (6), 1448–52.

JENSEN, L. B., KOLLERUP, G., QUAADE, F. and SORENSEN, O. H. (2001), 'Bone minerals changes in obese women during a moderate weight loss with and without calcium supplementation', *J. Bone Miner. Res.*, **16** (1), 141–7.

KUNCHEL, L. J., RIKKE, J. and ASTRUP, A. (2004), 'Effect of short-term high dietary calcium intake on 24-h energy expenditure, fat oxidation, and fecal fat excretion', *Int. J. Obes.*, **28** (Suppl 1), S34 (Abstract T6:O2-002).

LAMPRECHT, S. A. and LIPKIN, M. (2003), 'Chemoprevention of colon cancer by calcium, vitamin D and folate: molecular mechanisms', *Nature Reviews Cancer*, **3** (8), 601–14.

LAPPE, J. M., RAFFERTY, K. A., DAVIES, K. M. and LYPACZEWSKI, G. (2004), 'Girls on a high-calcium diet gain weight at the same rate as girls on a normal diet: a pilot study', *J. Am. Diet Assoc.*, **104** (9), 1361–7.

LIN, Y.-C., LYLE, R. M., MCCABE, L. D., MCCABE, G. P., WEAVER, C. M. and TEEGARDEN, D. (2000), 'Dairy calcium is related to changes in body composition during a two-year exercise intervention in young women', *J. Am. Coll. Nutr.*, **19** (6), 754–60.

LIPKIN, M. (2002), 'Early development of cancer chemoprevention clinical trials: studies of dietary calcium as a chemopreventive agent for human subjects', *Eur. J. Canc. Prev.*, **11** (Suppl 2), S65–70.

MASSEY, L. K. (2001), 'Dairy food consumption, blood pressure and stroke', *J. Nutr.*, **131** (7), 1875–8.

MELANSON, E. L., IDA, T., DONAHOO, W. T., ZEMEL, M. B. and HILL, J. O. (2004), 'The effects of low- and high-dairy calcium diets on resting energy expenditure and substrate oxidation', *FASEB J.*, **18** (5 Part II), A846 (Abstract #566.6).

MELANSON, E. L., SHARP, T. A., SCHNEIDER, J., DONAHOO, W. T., GRUNWALD, G. K. and HILL, J. O. (2003), 'Relation between calcium intake and fat oxidation in adult humans', *Int. J. Obes. Relat. Metab. Disord.*, **27** (2), 196–203.

PAPAKONSTANTINOU, E., FLATT, W. P., HUTH, P. J. and HARRIS, R. B. S. (2003), 'High dietary calcium reduces body fat content, digestibility of fat, and serum vitamin D in rats', *Obes. Res.*, **11** (3), 387–94.

PASQUET, P., BRIGANT, L., FROMENT, A., *et al.* (1992), 'Massive overfeeding and energy balance in men: the Guru Walla model', *Am. J. Clin. Nutr.*, **56** (3), 483–90.

PEREIRA, M. A., JACOBS, D. R., VAN HORN, L., SLATTERY, M. L., KARTASHOV, A. I. and LUDWIG, D. S. (2002), 'Dairy consumption, obesity, and the insulin resistance syndrome', *JAMA*, **287** (16), 2081–9.

PHILLIPS, S. M., BANDINI, L. G., CYR, H., COLCLOUGH-DOUGLAS, S., NAUMOVA, E. and MUST, A. (2003), 'Dairy food consumption and body weight and fatness studied longitudinally over the adolescent period', *Int. J. Obes. Rel. Metab. Disord.*, **27** (9), 1106–13.

RECKER, R., HINDERS, S., DAVIES, K. M. *et al.* (1996), 'Correcting calcium nutritional deficiency prevents spine fractures in elderly women', *J. Bone Miner. Res.*, **11** (12), 1961–6.

RICCI, T. A., CHOWDHURY, H. A., HEYMSFIELD, S. B., STAHL, T., PIERSON, R. N. JR. and SHAPSES, S. A. (1998), 'Calcium supplementation suppresses bone turnover during weight reduction in postmenopausal women', *J. Bone Miner. Res.*, **13** (6), 1045–50.

RIGGS, B. L., O'FALLON, W. M., MUHS, J., O'CONNOR, M. K., KUMAR, R. and MELTON, L. J. III (1998), 'Long-term effects of calcium supplementation on serum parathyroid level, bone turnover, and bone loss in elderly women', *J. Bone Miner. Res.*, **13** (2), 168–74.

ROZEN, G. S., RENNERT, G., DODIUK-GAD, R. P. *et al.* (2003), 'Calcium supplementation provides an extended window of opportunity for bone mass accretion after menarche', *Am. J. Clin. Nutr.*, **78** (5), 993–8.

SHAHKHALALILI, Y., MURSET, C., MEIRIM, I. *et al.* (2001), 'Calcium supplementation of chocolate: effect on cocoa butter digestibility and blood lipids in humans', *Am. J. Clin. Nutr.*, **73** (2), 246–52.

SHAPSES, S. A., HESHKA, S. and HEYMSFIELD, S. B. (2004), 'Effect of calcium supplementation on weight and fat loss in women', *J. Clin. Endocrinol. Metab.*, **89** (2), 632–7.

SHI, H., DIRIENZO, D. and ZEMEL, M. B. (2001), 'Effects of dietary calcium on adipocyte lipid metabolism and body weight regulation in energy-restricted aP2-agouti transgenic mice', *FASEB J.*, **15** (2), 291–3.

SHI, H., NORMAN, A. W., OKAMURA, W. H., SEN, A. and ZEMEL, M. B. (2002), '1α-25-dihydroxyvitamin D_3 inhibits uncoupling protein 2 expression in human adipocytes', *FASEB J.*, **16** (13), 1808–10.

SKINNER, J. D., BOUNDS, W., CARRUTH, B. R. and ZIEGLER, P. (2003), 'Longitudinal calcium intake is negatively related to children's body fat indexes', *J. Am. Diet Assoc.*, **103** (12), 1626–31.

SPECKER, B. and BINKLEY, T. (2003), 'Randomized trial of physical activity and calcium supplementation on bone mineral content in 3- to 5-year-old children', *J. Bone Miner. Res.*, **18** (5), 885–92.

STRAWFORD, A., ANTELO, F., CHRISTIANSEN, M. and HELLERSTEIN, M. K. (2004), 'Adipose tissue triglyceride turnover, *de novo* lipogenesis, and cell proliferation in humans measured with ^2H_2O', *Am. J. Physiol. Endocrinol. Metab.*, **286** (4), E577–88.

TURNER, S. M., MURPHY, E. J., NEESE, R. A. *et al.* (2003), 'Measurement of TG synthesis and turnover *in vivo* by $2H_2O$ incorporation into the glycerol moiety and application of MIDA', *Am. J. Physiol. Endocrinol. Metab.*, **285** (4), E790–803.

VOLEK, J. S., GOMEZ, A. L., SCHEET, T. P. *et al.* (2003), 'Increasing fluid milk favourably affects bone mineral density responses to resistance training in adolescent boys', *J. Am. Diet Assoc.*, **103** (10), 1353–6.

WEINBERG, L. G., BERNER, L. A. and GROVES, J. E. (2004), 'Nutrient contributions of dairy foods in the United States, Continuing Survey of Food Intakes by Individuals, 1994–1996, 1998', *J. Am. Diet Assoc.*, **104** (6), 895–902.

WELBERG, J. W., MONKELBAAN, J. F., DE VRIES, E. G. *et al.* (1994), 'Effects of supplemental dietary calcium on quantitative and qualitative fecal fat excretion in man', *Ann. Nutr. Metab.*, **38** (4), 185–91.

XUE, B., GREENBERG, A. G., KRAEMER, F. B. and ZEMEL, M. B. (2001), 'Mechanism of intracellular Ca_2^+ ($[Ca_2^+]_i$) inhibition of lipolysis in human adipocytes', *FASEB J.*, **15** (13), 2527–9.

ZEMEL, M. B. (2004), 'Role of calcium and dairy products in energy partitioning and weight management', *Am. J. Clin. Nutr.*, **79** (5 Suppl), 907S–12S.

ZEMEL, M. B., SHI, H., GREER, B., DIRIENZO, D. and ZEMEL, P. C. (2000), 'Regulation of adiposity by dietary calcium', *FASEB J.*, **14** (9), 1132–8.

ZEMEL, M. B., THOMPSON, W., MILSTEAD, A., MORRIS, K. and CAMPBELL, P. (2004a), 'Calcium and dairy acceleration of weight and fat loss during energy restriction in obese adults', *Obes. Res.*, **12** (4), 582–90.

ZEMEL, M. B., TEEGARDEN, D. T., VAN LOAN, M. *et al.* (2004b), 'Role of dairy products in modulating weight and fat loss: a multi-center trial', *FASEB J.*, **18** (5 Part II), A845–6 (Abstract #566.5).

ZEMEL, M. B., NOCTON, A. M., RICHARDS, J. D., *et al.* (2002), 'Increasing dairy calcium intake reduces adiposity in obese African-American adults', *Circulation*, **106** (suppl), II-610 (abstract).

ZEMEL, M. B., NOCTON, A. M., RICHARDS, J. D. *et al.* (2003), 'Dairy (yogurt) augments fat loss and reduces central adiposity during energy restriction in obese subjects', *FASEB J.*, **17** (5 Part II), A1088 (abstr).

ZHANG, Q. and TORDOFF, M. G. (2004), 'No effect of dietary calcium on body weight of lean and obese mice and rats', *Am. J. Physiol. Regul. Integr. Comp. Physiol.*, **286** (4), R669–77.

22

Community-based approaches to prevent obesity

C. Bell, Deakin University, Australia

22.1 Introduction

The obesity epidemic continues unabated. The reasons for this are neither a lack of knowledge as to the underlying causes or a lack of knowledge about how to prevent or treat the disease. Putting knowledge into practice is where the difficulty lies. Experience from other public health epidemics has shown that putting knowledge into practice at the population level is easier when behaviours are encouraged and supported by changes to the environment. Quitting smoking, for example, became easier as the price of cigarettes went up and as the number of places where you could smoke went down. Similar environmental changes are needed to prevent obesity. To date the impact of efforts to change the environment in support of changes in eating and physical activity behaviour has been patchy. This chapter will draw on learnings from other public health epidemics and evidence from community- and settings-based interventions to explain why multi-setting, multi-strategy community-based action should be the foundation of obesity prevention efforts. It will outline the core elements necessary to set up and sustain a community-based obesity prevention (CBOP) programme using the example of the Be Active Eat Well project in Australia. The chapter will also provide insight into the central role that community-based demonstration programmes should play in national and international strategies as governments gear up to control the epidemic.

22.2 What has worked in other public health epidemics?

The key lesson from efforts to control epidemics of infectious and non-infectious causes of death in many high-income countries has been to develop strategies that address both behavioural and environmental determinants (Swinburn *et al.*, 1999). The epidemiological triad, originally used as a model for controlling infectious disease, has been particularly useful in helping to identify these determinants. The triad divides them into a connected 'triangle' of host (h), vector (v) and environment (e), with the agent (a) being the final common pathway that leads to disease, injury or death. The triad is applicable not only to infectious diseases such as malaria, but also to injuries and non-communicable disease (Haddon, 1980). In the case of road traffic injuries (RTIs) the 'agent' is speed. The 'vectors' are the motor vehicles that bring the 'host' (driver/passenger) in contact with the agent and 'environment' encompasses the road conditions, terrain, weather, road rules and other factors that influence the speed at which the vehicle can travel safely. By combining strategies that influence vectors, hosts and environments, countries such as Australia have seen dramatic and continuing reductions in RTIs (Ozane-Smith, 2004). Reductions have occurred via ad campaigns and driver education (h), regulations and laws (e) on drink driving (h), seat belts (e), driver licenses (h), median barriers and improved roads (e), improved car safety (v), vehicle inspection certificates (v) and changes in public attitudes (e). Success in controlling this epidemic has been achieved in the face of substantial barriers including the proliferation of motor vehicles and social norms such as drinking and driving, and speeding. It is worth noting that new barriers to safe driving continue to arise, demanding new solutions. Mobile phone use, for example, is common among Melbourne metropolitan drivers (Timperio *et al.*,2002), and the risks of collision and fatality from driving while using a mobile phone are similar to those for drunken driving (Redelmeier and Tibshirani, 1997). Tighter legislation (e) and ad campaigns (h) are currently being put in place to reduce RTIs from mobile phone use while driving.

The epidemiological triad is also applicable to obesity (Swinburn and Egger, 2002). For obesity, the agent is chronic positive energy imbalance. The 'vectors' that deliver excess energy to the host, leading to passive overconsumption (Blundell and King, 1996) are largely energy dense foods (mainly high fat foods), energy dense beverages (high sugar, fat or alcohol), and large portion sizes (Rolls *et al.*, 2000, 2002). The vectors of low energy expenditure are two types of machines – those that reduce the energy cost of work or transport (e.g. electric appliances, cars) and those that promote passive recreation (e.g. television, videos). The 'host' factors include age, gender, genetic make-up, physiological factors (e.g. hormonal status, metabolic rate), behaviours, and personal attitudes and beliefs. The 'environmental' factors can be considered in four different categories – the physical environment (what is available?), the economic environment (what are the financial factors, both income and costs?), the policy environment (what are the rules?), and the socio-cultural environment (what are society's attitudes, beliefs, perceptions and values?) (Swinburn *et al.*, 1999). Because they are of a manageable size, communities are the level of society where action in each of these areas can best be achieved.

22.2.1 Lack of impact of single strategy or single setting interventions

Evidence from the literature suggests that single strategy approaches such public education about healthy choices (Jeffery and French, 1999) or single setting approaches such as a school-based programmes (Sahota *et al.*, 2001a, b) or workplace programmes (Jeffery and French, 1999) are going to be insufficient to achieve the intervention dose required to reverse the current trends in obesity.

School-based approaches are attractive for preventing childhood obesity because they provide access to a large number of children, the programmes are generally well received by stakeholders, and they have proven successful in influencing dietary and physical activity knowledge and behaviour, as well as health behaviours beyond those that were originally planned (Edmunds and Ziebland, 2002). Few, however, have demonstrated any long-term impact on weight, including those that have gone beyond using single strategies. Short- to medium-term studies have produced decreases in childhood obesity of up to 25% and over 1.1 BMI units (Flores, 1995; Robinson, 1999; Manios and Kafatos, 1999). Longer-term trials have shown around 5% reduction in obesity rates.

One might expect a home-based approach to obesity prevention to be beneficial. Indeed, many scholars consider the home and family environment crucial for shaping children's physical activity and eating patterns (Davison and Birch, 2001). Food availability and accessibility, parental role modelling, television viewing and child-parent interactions in the home are important (Campbell and Crawford, 2001), and parent participation in physical activity has been positively related to activity in children, particularly girls (Sallis *et al.*, 1988). Children in Australia watch an average of 23 hours of television per week at home (Zuppa *et al.*, 2003), and other studies have shown children's television viewing to be associated with both parental viewing practices and their monitoring of their children's viewing hours (Davison and Birch, 2001). Opportunities for influencing the home are limited however, because it is difficult to access. There is also a danger that interventions directed only at the home may encourage the prevailing but counterproductive attitude that parents and, to a lesser degree, children be held responsible for their own weight. Mass media is probably the easiest way to access parents and families and to deliver action messages in relation to making the home environment less obesogenic.

Studies in other settings, such as churches, have shown an impact on weight, at least in the short term (Bell *et al.*, 2001), but the best evidence of what works for children comes from studies that link settings.

The school-based programmes that have shown the largest impact on obesity have been those that included efforts to reduce television viewing; an activity that occurs at home. Two major US school-based studies have successfully implemented such programmes (Gortmaker *et al.*, 1999, Robinson, 1999). These studies suggest that interventions, at least for children, need to occur in at least two settings to be effective. This makes sense given that children do not spend all their time in school. In Australia for example, 37% of children's daily energy intake is consumed in the school environment on a school day, but only 16% of energy is consumed in the school environment over the period of a year when holidays and weekends are taken into account (Bell and Swinburn, 2004). A significant proportion of their energy intake and energy expenditure occurs in settings other than school. The value of a multi-setting approach can also be seen with breastfeeding. Increased rates of breastfeeding (both initiation and duration) have been demonstrated through programmes that include antenatal education for parents, the adoption and promotion of Baby Friendly environments; increased support for existing professional and trained volunteers to support breastfeeding in the 6-month postnatal period (Fairbank *et al.*, 2000). Several large-scale, longitudinal studies have demonstrated a strong protective effect of exclusive breastfeeding against the development of obesity in later childhood (Armstrong and Reilly, 2002; Dietz, 2001).

The above-mentioned lack of impact using single setting or single strategy interventions and the rapid increase in obesity has led to a welcome shift in our approach to the epidemic. Governments and public health professionals are being urged to take a broader view of what constitutes evidence for taking action (Swinburn *et al.*, 2005) and researchers are being urged to look for outcomes that inform interventions rather than identify problems (Robinson and Sirard, 2005). The best place for this action and research to come together is the community and the approach with the greatest likelihood of effect is one that encompasses multiple strategies (social marketing, policy change, environmental change, management of current overweight and obesity), in multiple settings and sectors, across both sides of the energy balance equation. A comprehensive approach to obesity prevention is one that simultaneously addresses as many of the underlying behavioural and environmental causes of obesity as possible.

22.3 Elements in a community-based approach to obesity prevention

The race began in 1903 as a publicity stunt for *L'Auto*, a French newspaper. Now it is an annual event that draws together 21 teams of 189 competitors and millions of spectators from around the world. *Le Tour de France* is amazing not only for the incredible endurance and athleticism of the participants, but also for the teamwork involved in winning the yellow jersey worn by the overall race leader. The elements that make up a successful *Tour de France* team also provide insight into the design and implementation of a successful community-based obesity prevention programme. These elements can be summarised as follows: a well-defined goal and a plan to get there; identity and social marketing; training; empowering partnerships; inspiring leadership; sponsorship and; responsive and relevant evaluation. Each of these headings is elaborated below using examples from 'Be Active Eat Well'. Be Active Eat Well (BAEW) is a 3-year obesity prevention programme in Colac, a small (population 11 000) rural town in the Barwon South Western region of Victoria, Australia. The programme began in mid-2002 with baseline measurements being taken in early 2003. Follow-up measures are planned for early 2006.

22.3.1 An achievable aim and a plan to get there

For teams in the *Tour de France* there is a single aim: to have their team leader in the yellow jersey when the race finishes on the Champs Elysees in Paris. The aim is well defined and is simple enough that it is recognised, not only by members of the team, but also by those looking on. The aim remains unchanged during the race and teams wouldn't compete unless they thought the goal was achievable. Exactly the same type of aim is required for community-based obesity prevention programmes: clear, well recognised, unchanging and achievable. The aim defines the reason a programme exists and it should be easily described. The aim of BAEW is to improve the health and well-being of children aged 2 to 12 years and to strengthen the local community through healthy eating and physical activity promotion. This aim is clear to the extent that people understand what 'health and well-being' and 'strengthen the local community' mean. In this programme, 'health and well-being' refers to the physical activity patterns, healthy eating and weight status of children, and 'strengthen the local community' means building capacity within the community to promote physical activity and healthy eating.

Once the aim has been decided, a good plan is required. In the build-up phase to the *Tour de France*, each team puts a series of strategies in place that are designed to help them win. Lance Armstrong and his 'US Postal Service' (now Discovery Channel) team are known for their meticulous planning in preparation for the race. No other team spends as much time going over the routes that will be ridden during the race and preparing strategies that will help them avoid losing time or riders on dangerous parts of the ride and that will give them an advantage over other teams. This planning extends to the selection of those who will ride in the team. Similarly, community-based obesity prevention programmes require an outline of the strategic direction that will be taken to achieve the overall aim. There are various theoretical frameworks available to help draw up a plan (Sanderson *et al.*, 1996). In BAEW we used a process developed by

Swinburn and Egger (Swinburn *et al.*, 1999) dubbed the ANGELO process based on the use of an Analysis Grid for Environments Linked to Obesity. Using this process, a group of informed stakeholders 'scan' the local environment and identify specific prevention strategies. The exact combination of strategies is determined by local relevance, probably impact, changeability, and resource constraints. In this first phase of the planning process, the programme itself has not yet begun and therefore planning is driven by a combination of past experience, theoretical best practice, and the experience of others. In BAEW, this was achieved by bringing together the physical activity and nutrition skills of the local community with knowledge of best practice based on published literature. A shortened version of the resulting action plan is shown in Table 22.1.

The second phase of the planning process occurs during the implementation of the action plan and it involves making changes to the plan in response to progress made and changes in circumstances. In the *Tour de*

Table 22.1 Action plan strategies for the BAEW project and the settings/sectors in which they are applied

Strategy	Setting/Sector
To achieve a high awareness of the 'Be Active, Eat Well' messages among parents and children	Home, school, community using print and other media
To build Colac community capacity to promote physical activity and healthy eating	Home, school, community
To evaluate the process, impact and outcomes of the 'Be Active Eat Well' project	
To significantly decrease the time spent watching TV and playing on computers or electronic games	Home
To significantly decrease the consumption of high sugar drinks and to promote the consumption of water	Home, school
To significantly decrease the consumption of energy dense snacks and significantly increase consumption of fruit	Home, school
To significantly increase the proportion of primary school children living within 1.5 km who walk/cycle to and from school	Transportation sector (local government)
To significantly increase the amount of active play after school and on weekends	Home, school, parks and recreation areas, sport clubs
To improve the quality of deep-fried takeaway chips (French fries)	Fast food outlets
To pilot a healthy lifestyle programme for parents and carers of children aged 2–12 years, focusing on healthy eating, physical activity and parenting skills	Community

France, this second phase is equivalent to the strategies that teams employ during the race. Each team has a team manager (*Directeur Sportif*) who follows the race and provides strategies and tactics for the riders as the race progresses. A strategy that the US Postal Team (2004) employed to great effect was to lead from the front. In the 2004 tour the US Postal team dominated at the front of the *peleton* (French for 'herd' and refers to the main field of riders). They set the pace and effectively tired out the other teams so that Armstrong's lead could be established and protected. Flexibility in strategic direction needs to be encouraged in CBOP programmes and for evaluation purposes, records should be kept of the changes that occur. In BAEW the action plan is considered a 'living' document because changes in strategic direction are recorded as the project progresses. The objective focused on fast food outlets, for example (see Table 22.1), was originally 'to investigate the potential for improving the quality (fat content and type) of deep-fried foods'. This investigation was carried out in the first year of the project and it was decided that there was in fact potential for improving the quality (lowering total fat and saturated fat) of hot chips (French fries) sold in local Fast Food outlets (excluding franchises). A survey of the fat content of the chips revealed that the percentage of fat in hot chips sold at local outlets ranged from 10.4% to 18.5% and the National Heart Foundation of Australia recommend 8.4%. Also, through discussion with the outlet operators and using community surveys, it was discovered that both operators and customers were willing to support a 'healthier chips' initiative. With this new information, the objective was updated and became 'to improve the quality of deep-fried takeaway chips'. Importantly, the original objective was retained in the action plan for process evaluation purposes.

CBOP programmes should also have the equivalent of a *Directeur Sportif* to guide the project. In most cases, this takes the form of a reference or 'expert' committee. Discussed further below, members of a reference committee bring a helicopter view to the project, helping to maximise opportunities and minimise risk. A good example of the importance of having a reference committee arose in the BAEW project when reporters from a television show with a reputation for sensation and controversy came looking for a 'before and after' story on overweight children. The reference committee was able to meet, provide strategic advice and call on media experts who were in turn able to contact the shows producers. Ultimately, a sensational enough story could not be found and it did not run.

22.3.2 Identity and social marketing

It is essential that CBOP programmes establish a strong identity early on. In most cases this means developing a project name, logo, catch-phrase or slogan in line with the project's aim. In the *Tour de France*, teams are identified by their sponsors. Sponsors include a range of businesses such as cellular phone companies (T Mobile Team), food companies (*Brioches la*

Boulangère), and banks (*Credit Agricole*). Most have little to do with cycling, but their names have become synonymous with a team of riders and their performance in the race. This model highlights the importance of developing a strong identity (or name) even if it is not closely related to the project goal. A name brings tangibility to a project when it is still being developed and when it may be difficult to articulate what the aims or the benefits of the project are. BAEW inherited its name from the original project proposal as it was passed on to the community by the funding body, and a decision was made to keep it because it was simple, it described the purpose of the project well and people latched on to it quickly. An alternative way of building project identity is to engage the target population in developing a name. This helps the target population understand what the project is about while also bringing a target population 'flavour' to the project which should help with uptake of the project activities and their sustainability. In BAEW, this process was used to develop the 'making it easy' strap line linked to the project name. This catch phrase helped reflect the overall goal of the project and it also summarised the key social marketing message of making it easier for the target population and the broader community to make healthy eating choices, to reduce sedentary behaviour and to be physically active. A marketing company was then invited to develop the project logo (Fig. 22.1).

Unlike teams in the *Tour de France*, CBOP programmes generally don't have a high degree of recognition, at least at the start. Thus there is a need to market the project identity. There is also a need to market health messages via social marketing to support the target population in their efforts to make behavioural changes. At a community level, the experience or capacity to do social marketing well is often not available and this is an area where training is needed or where outside expertise should be sought. In BAEW, an academic expert was invited to come and run a two day workshop (at the beginning of the intervention period) on social marketing (Donovan and Henley, 2003). Using skills from the workshop, a social marketing plan was developed and it was decided that, while the project team would come up with the messages to go out into the community, a professional marketing company would be contracted to market these messages. Figure 22.2 summarizes the overall messages promoted by BAEW, and Fig. 22.3 shows how a message about walking was marketed to children via the school newsletter.

The link between social marketing and intervention activities is important. There is little point in marketing a *Tour de France* team that does not ride in the race. Similarly in community-based interventions, there is little value in a marketing campaign that is not underpinned by action on the ground. For this reason, BAEW messages are closely linked to action plan objectives and, importantly, their release is timed to either promote the uptake of an activity or behaviour or to sustain it. For example, considerable social marketing occurred around the launch of Choice Chips (see

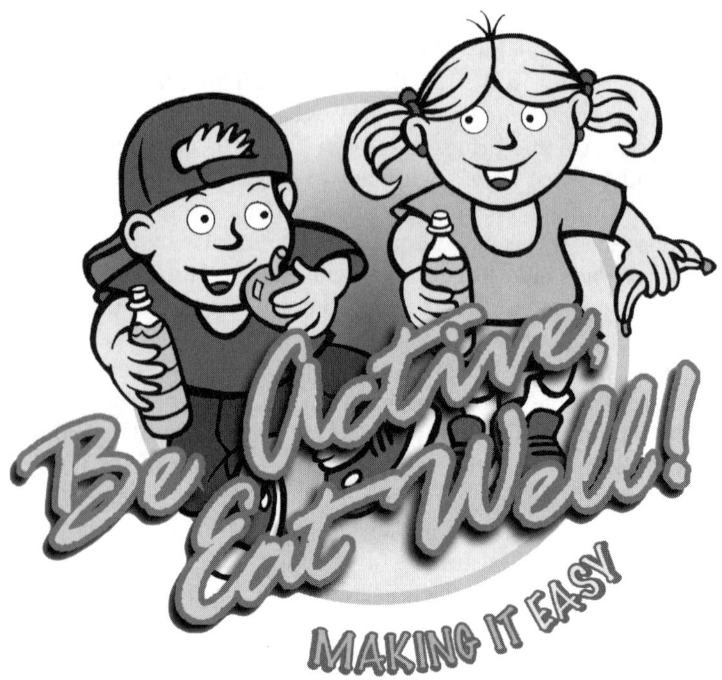

Fig. 22.1 'Be Active Eat Well' logos (supplied courtesy of Thirteenth Beach Marketing Services Pty Ltd).

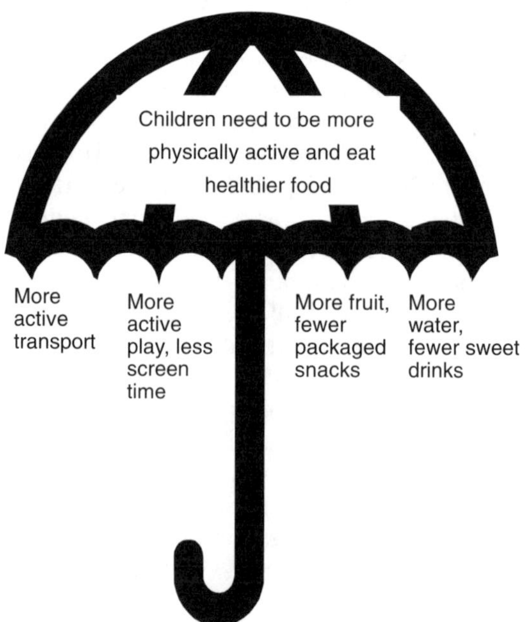

Fig. 22.2 Overall and specific communication messages in the BAEW project.

objective 9 in Table 22.1). A vast amount of work went into establishing a system for measuring the fat content of the chips, sourcing frying fats that contained less saturated fat, developing an award system that offered recognition to outlets meeting certain criteria and in talking to outlet managers about the feasibility of changing current practices. This behind the scenes work culminated in a Choice Chips launch by the Mayor who presented bronze awards to participating Outlets. The launch was designed to bring recognition to participating Outlets, to encourage non-participating stores to join Choice Chips and to send a message to consumers that quality matters as much as quantity when it comes to improving eating patterns.

At least two of these goals were achieved. In the lead-up to the launch, two outlets that had been reluctant to join the programme joined, presumably to take advantage of the marketing. On-going social marketing has served to encourage outlets to achieve higher awards through improved deep-frying practices and to inform consumers of which stores are participating and what level of fat quality they have achieved. This has taken the form of in-store posters and publication of information about participating stores in local newspapers. In 2005 all seven participating outlets have achieved a gold award (see Fig. 22.4).

A final point in relation to developing an identity and marketing project messages is that the messages need to be consistent. The project needs to

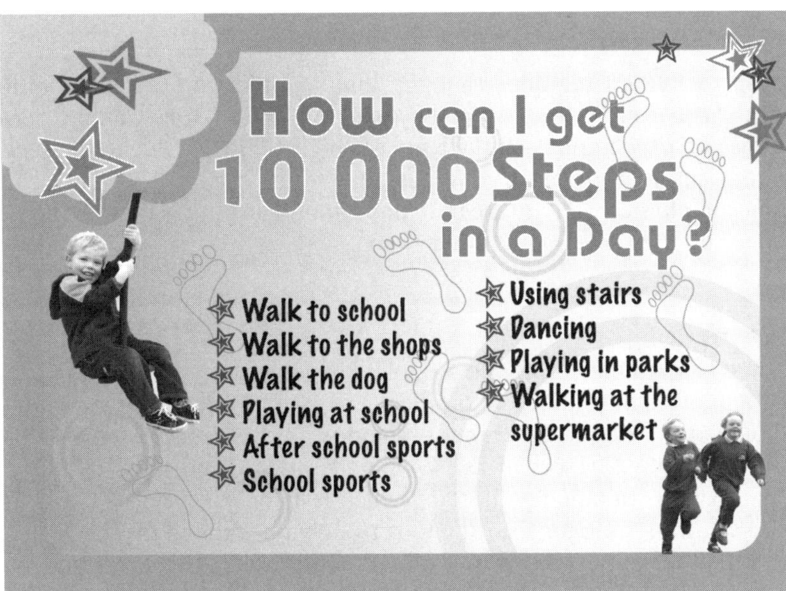

Fig. 22.3 Excerpt from one of the BAEW newsletters promoting walking (supplied courtesy of Thirteenth Beach Marketing Services Pty Ltd).

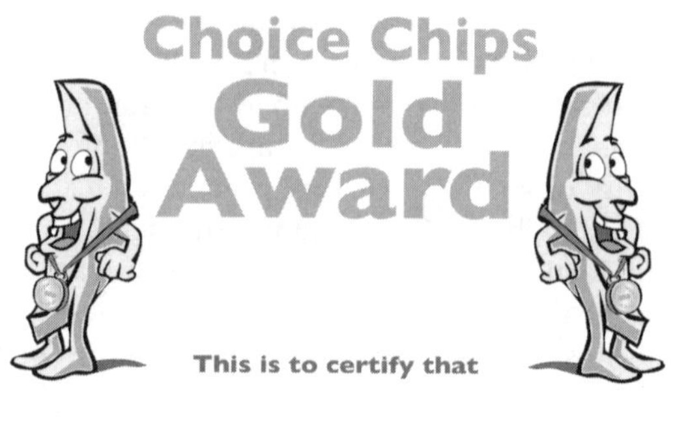

has applied to meet the Gold Award criteria

- Chips that have less than 10% fat
- Oil that has a saturated fat content less than 20%
- Chips used are greater than 12 mm in diameter
- Choice Chips guidelines of cooking followed

Project Dietician

Mayor of Colac Otway Shire

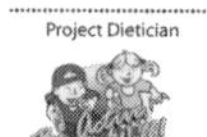

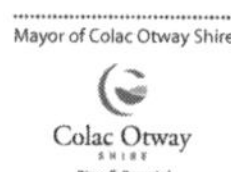

Fig. 22.4 Poster showing the gold 'Choice Chips' award (supplied courtesy of Thirteenth Beach Marketing Services Pty Ltd).

live up to the expectations that the target population associate with it. Lance Armstrong's team have become recognised for winning performances and expectations on the team are high. Similarly, due to the success of the social marketing, BAEW has got the message across that healthy eating and physical activity are both important. The onus is now on the team to translate these messages into action.

22.3.3 Training

The need for training is often overlooked in community-based intervention programmes. Great intervention ideas are often initiated in communities without considering whether the community has the capacity to make them work. In contrast, riders in the *Tour de France* spend most of the year preparing and training for the race which lasts only 3 weeks. People have criticised Armstrong for focusing too strongly on training for the *Tour* and ignoring other important races on the cycling circuit. This focus and training, however, has led to him becoming the first ever cyclist to win seven consecutive tour titles.

22.3.4 Build-up phase

Training begins with an audit of existing knowledge, skill, talent and experience. Cyclists are selected for the *Tour de France* based on these factors and similarly, the selection of staff and stakeholders for community-based interventions should be based, at least partly, on existing capacity, experience and talent. There needs to be a core group of people who understands what it will take for the project to succeed (experience), and who have the necessary skills to achieve success. This group also needs to have the skills to learn and adapt. Existing capacity in the BAEW project took the form of staff from four organisations representing skills in health promotion, local governance, evaluation and knowledge of the community. The role these organisations play and how they are structured in relation to BAEW is discussed further in the section on empowering partnerships. In the case of obesity prevention, there may be very few people in a community with experience in promoting physical activity and healthy eating at a population level. However, there will be people with a strong interest in these areas, with a willingness to learn, and with skills that could be transferred. Sports coaches are one example. In BAEW, local sports clubs were challenged to think beyond traditional competitive structures and skill acquisition to the broader role they could play in promoting physical activity. By shifting their emphasis, local Soccer, Tennis, Field Hockey and Tai Kwon Do clubs have succeeded in increasing the numbers of children who are active after school as well as boosting their own memberships by around 15%.

Once existing capacity has been identified, the continuation of the build-up phase involves identifying gaps in knowledge or skills and supplying the education or expertise necessary to fill them. In BAEW, this occurred in close proximity to the development of the action plan. An informal needs assessment process was conducted by local University staff, and key stakeholders were asked what their training requirements were. Subsequently, staff from the University with particularly skills in community-based obesity prevention, conducted a training workshop with ~30 people from the community including people from local government, schools, day care facilities and the local health service. This training workshop served to inform people about the size of the obesity epidemic, up-skill them in promoting physical activity and healthy eating and also to provide evidence from the literature on what interventions are most likely to work. This information was then fed into the action plan. Once the action plan had been developed, training in social marketing was identified as a further need and expertise was brought in (see section on Identity and Social Marketing).

22.3.5 Maintenance phase

The maintenance phase involves continuing education and the transfer of skills to others in the community. In BAEW, regular updates in nutrition (and physical activity) occur as part of a region-wide nutrition network.

Twenty to thirty members of the network meet four times a year to discuss the progress of nutrition-related projects in the region and to hear invited speakers present on project relevant topics, such as healthy school canteens. The network also produces a newsletter that is distributed to over 70 people throughout Victoria. BAEW project staff have also participated in and presented at a range of relevant conferences, which builds up their presentation skills and transfers information about BAEW beyond the boundaries of the community. As the project has progressed and more people have become involved, various tasks and skills have also been transferred. The walking school bus is a good example. Project staff saw starting a walking school bus (a group of children who are walked to school under the supervision of two adult volunteers) as one strategy for achieving the objective of increasing the proportion of primary school children living within 1.5 km who walk/cycle to and from school. A team from local government was identified as the most suited group to apply for funding and to implement a walking bus programme. The application to the Victorian Health Promotion Foundation was successful and one bus began at one of the schools under the responsibility of the local government's Transportation Officer. Ideally, the walking school bus should also be an opportunity to engage parents in the task of walking children to school. Unfortunately, this has been difficult to achieve, in large part because the local government has not communicated well with the community, but also because parents find it hard to find the time to walk their children to school. Grandparents, police-officers or retirees may make better volunteers. For the sustainability of CBOP programmes, continuing education and skill transfer is vital. In the case of the walking school bus, training in communication skills may have given the bus a better chance of survival. It appears that walking and cycling to school may have increased however, even without the formal walking school bus programme.

22.3.6 Empowering partnerships

In 2005, 21 teams of nine riders took part in the *Tour de France* and of those nine riders, only one rider from one team can win. The others ride on his behalf. So strongly is this notion of selflessness expressed in these teams that the term for those who ride on behalf of their leader is 'domestiques' or servants. The value of bringing this kind of attitude to the partnerships between stakeholders that support community-based interventions cannot be understated. Partnerships are necessary to ensure the right strings are pulled to achieve action, that existing capacity is used to full extent, that additional expertise is provided, that opinion leaders in the community are engaged throughout the project and that risks associated with the intervention can be managed. In essence, partners form a support crew whose combined expertise and efforts are used to empower staff to achieve the projects stated goal. In BAEW, the original partners were people from the local area health service (with skills in health promotion and dietetics), local government (skills in health and recreation planning), the local University (skills in project implementation and evaluation) and the State-wide health service (skills in health promotion and public health and also sponsors of the project). This group formed an implementation committee whose primary responsibility, as the name suggests, was to implement the project during the initial stages. This included project planning, identifying target groups and key settings, conducting an informal needs assessment, and building the foundations of an action plan. The committee also identified gaps in the community's ability to run the project and created opportunities for increasing capacity (e.g. workshop in social marketing).

Like members of a *Tour de France* team, the partners supporting community-based interventions should have specialised skills that can be called on at various stages during the project. Specialists in community-based obesity prevention include those with skills in nutrition, physical activity, health promotion, community development, programme management and communications. Other key specialists are local champions (people known to the community who are passionate about the cause) and people with influence at a local level but also at a State or National level who can link the project with broader strategies and policies. Also, like a *Tour de France* team, not all these skills are required at once. Often it is a matter of letting a specialist 'do their thing' while others simply ride in the same direction. In BAEW, this process of partner engagement is managed in two ways. Firstly, the partners involved with the day-to-day running of the project have been split into two groups: a local steering committee – the engine room where decisions about the project are made by project staff, parents, representatives from schools and sports clubs and other interested members of the community; and a reference committee that meets less frequently with skills in health promotion, evaluation, local government and representation from the funding organisation who provide advice, support and leadership. Secondly, working groups have been set up that focus on individual project objectives (Fig. 22.5).

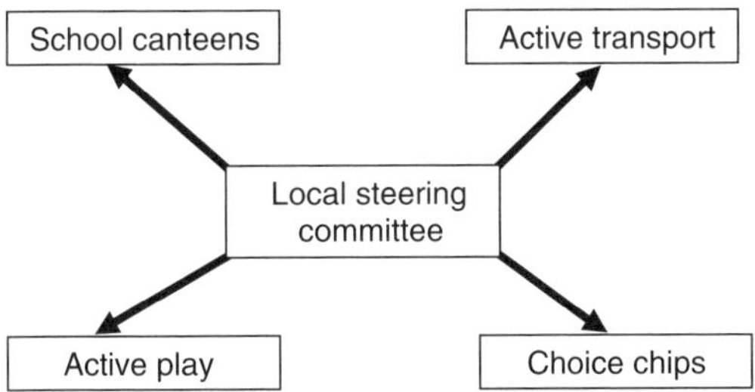

Fig. 22.5 Examples of working groups that have stemmed from the local steering committee.

These working groups allow members of the community to engage with the project in areas of interest without being overwhelmed by the project as a whole. They also allow the project to achieve considerably more than would otherwise be possible. An example is the Choice Chips working group. Led by a local dietitian, this working group have successfully engaged 7 of the 13 Fast Food Outlets. Working with the Outlet managers the impact of this group can be readily seen in the lower average fat content of chips from 12.4% to 9.5%, a reduction of 46 kg of total fat per week. It can also be seen in the reduced proportion of saturated fat in chips (5.2% to 1.7%), a reduction of 55 kg per week.

22.3.7 Inspiring leadership

When health promotion projects such as Be Active Eat Well are set up, more often than not, the first task is employing someone to implement the action plan. This position often bears the title 'Project Worker' and the person filling the position is thought of as the one who does the work. This is appropriate to the extent that they are the person primarily responsible for the implementation of the action plan. But considering them solely as a worker is too narrow a view and one that leads to unmet expectations. More than one health promotion project has fallen over because the project worker was expected to run things single-handedly. Also, due to the nature of the work and the funding available, project worker positions are often filled by young, enthusiastic, intelligent and creative people who, by virtue of their youth, lack the status required within a community to get things done. A more accurate title for this vital role is 'Project Coordinator' and a more complete role definition includes leadership, coordination and implementation. To refer once again to the *Tour de France* analogy, a project coordinator should be the one who wears the yellow jersey, who leads the project and becomes the person that people identify the project with. They are the one who has the most to gain if the project is successful and the most to lose if it is not. As a leader they need to be the catalyst for change by developing the projects direction, aligning people (and particularly the partners) with that direction and helping people to keep moving in the right direction by motivating and inspiring them. Their next role is that of coordination. Rather that asking 'how can I implement this objective?' the project coordinator needs to ask 'who can I get to help me implement this objective?' In this way, the coordinator will succeed not only in expanding their capacity to achieve the objectives set out in the action plan, but they will also increase the buy-in from the project stakeholders and they will have more time to attend to achieving objectives that are best suited to the coordinator's role. These include taking the lead on building community capacity for obesity prevention, social marketing and process evaluation. With their knowledge of the action plan and links with stakeholders, the project coordinator is the best person to identify training needs within the community and to ensure that the training is provided. Also, as the person with their finger on the pulse, they are well placed to market the projects key messages and to ensure that community awareness of the project is high. The third critical role for the project coordinator is documenting the projects progress and updating or revising implementation strategies.

When BAEW began, we had too narrow view of what the project workers role entailed. However, with some valuable input from the local health promotion officer and with the realisation that the action plan was too big for one person, the role has gradually become one of coordinator and leader. Progress has been significantly enhanced as a result.

22.3.8 Sponsorship (flexible resources)

Because obesity prevention does not happen quickly and because a comprehensive approach requires multiple strategies in multiple settings, we need to rethink the way community-based obesity prevention projects are funded. Currently, the systems governing the funding process do not encourage sustainability, flexibility or accountability and rarely do they encourage good evaluation. What is needed is a shift in how funding is provided, an expansion of potential funding sources, and a change in our view of the overall process from one of funding to one of sponsorship.

The CBOPs' funding is required for three distinct purposes: initiation, implementation and evaluation. The initiation or pump-priming funding covers the costs of preparing an action plan, developing a project identity and, most importantly, bringing in capacity in the form of additional staff and/or training. Traditionally, government and non-government organisations (NGOs) have funded community based programmes and these organisations are well suited to providing pump priming funding for CBOPs because they have a responsibility to the community and a mandate to take the lead on public health initiatives. They will also benefit from the publicity that comes from launching new initiatives.

Implementation funding generally covers the cost of social marketing, equipment, purchasing 'off-the-shelf' programmes, intervention activities and ongoing support for the project coordinator. There are advantages in terms of sustainability, flexibility and security in getting this funding from multiple sources. Thus an array of funding bodies, including businesses, community funding agencies, trusts and foundations, as well as government agencies and NGOs, should be approached to provide implementation funding. The task of selling the project to these other agencies is made easier because the project has already been initiated and, with an action plan in place, the funding can be linked to tangible objectives. Take the example of the walking school bus in the Be Active Eat Well project. Not only did the local council's successful application bring additional resources to the project but, as mentioned earlier, it brought skills to the local community in terms of making funding applications.

The third purpose for funding in CBOP programmes is evaluation. Because of their vested interest in the outcome, the primary funding agency (i.e. the agency who provided pump-priming funding) should be the main source of evaluation funding. However, to maximise the funding available for this vital part of the project other sources should also be considered. Universities are an obvious choice. The project may be able to access evaluation funding through University research funding streams and also benefit from their evaluation expertise. The strong link the Be Active, Eat Well project has with Deakin University has led to both these benefits.

The process described above fits better with the notion of sponsorship than it does with funding. A sponsor is a person or an organisation that pays for, or plans and carries out, a project or activity. The dictionary adds 'one that pays the cost of a radio or television programme in return for advertising time during its course'. Asking the question, 'who will get the most return?' for sponsoring a certain aspect of the project is a helpful way to identify who potential sponsors could be and it helps project staff recognise that sponsors need to get a return on their investment.

It is difficult to make a direct comparison between sponsorship of a *Tour de France* team and sponsorship of a community-based obesity prevention project as the roles of the sponsors are quite different. However, it is interesting to note that the recognition businesses gain from sponsoring *Tour de France* teams is sufficient to warrant huge investment.

22.4 Evaluating community-based projects for obesity prevention

The *Tour de France* is awash with statistics. The total distance in 2004 was 3395 km. There were 20 stages and 1 prologue – 6 of which were mountain stages, 11 were flat and 3 were time trials. Each of the 189 riders is timed over each stage and riding speed is also recorded. And the value of these statistics? To know how a rider or team is progressing during a race and to determine the eventual winner. Similarly, evaluation data are essential for community-based obesity prevention programmes to assess progress on stated objectives and determine the overall project impact. The evaluation component of the Be Active Eat Well project is described here as one example of a responsive and relevant evaluation plan.

There are a number of useful frameworks and guides to evaluating health promotion programmes that can be applied to CBOP programmes (Services, 2002, Nutbeam, 1998, Glasgow *et al.*, 1999). All highlight the importance of writing smart goals and objectives: specific, measurable, achievable, relevant and time-bound. BAEW has built these features into each of the objectives contained in the action plan and the stakeholders have agreed to an evaluation outcome for each. Moreover, each underlying strategy has process evaluation measures. After the action plan and associated evaluation plans were developed, baseline data were collected capturing information about the target population and their environment as it influences eating patterns and physical activity. We measured children's weight, height, waist and lunchbox contents and asked those aged 8 years and over to complete an additional questionnaire on food, physical activity and self esteem. We also asked parents questions about their child's eating and physical activity patterns, aspects of the home environment (e.g. family television viewing patterns), and aspects of the local neighbourhood (e.g. perceived safety for children riding bikes and walking). This was done by telephone interview. Key informant interviews were conducted with staff at schools to determine what barriers exist to healthy eating and physical activity in those settings. At the whole-of-community level we assessed the capacity of key stakeholders to promote healthy eating and physical activity and other relevant factors, such as the fat content of hot chips and the availability of playgrounds. Several of the instruments used are available on our website (www.deakin.edu.au/hbs/who-obesity). A unique feature of the BAEW evaluation is that data are not collected for research purposes only. It is also used to inform intervention activities and social marketing. For example, our data on walking to school indicate that over 50% of children who live within walking distance of their school are in fact driven. This information helps us target the intervention activities and it can be used in social marketing. Part way through the intervention we conducted a mid-intervention survey to get a sense of people's awareness of the project and what changes they may have made in response to the project. At the end of the intervention we will follow-up each of the baseline surveys to assess overall impact.

Comparison data for the BAEW intervention was collected from a group of similar schools randomly selected from the rest of the Barwon-South Western region. These schools were comparison schools, but we also intend to use their data as a baseline for ongoing monitoring. The State of Victoria does not currently have a monitoring programme and we are hopeful that BAEW can stimulate interest in establishing such a programme. For example, knowledge that 28% of a region's children aged 4 to 12 years were overweight or obese and that prevalence was increasing at a rate of 1 percentage point per year, would provide an ideal backdrop for assessing if a community-based prevention programme was successful in attenuating or reversing this trend. It is also potent information for advocacy.

Good communication is the second important aspect of evaluation. Results of the evaluation need to be distributed wisely and widely. Process evaluation data needs to be distributed in a useful format to stakeholders throughout the implementation of the project so that it can be used to inform intervention activities. Impact data is useful to a much wider audience from project participants, to advocacy groups, State policy makers, City Councils and those running similar projects. Outcomes and recommendations from the data need to be targeted to each of these audiences. Writing newspaper articles is a very useful way of learning how to write interesting, relevant and succinct project summaries.

22.4.1 Results of the mid-intervention survey

The impact of the BAEW intervention on overweight and obesity prevalence remains to be determined. However, results of our mid-intervention survey conducted with a random selection of participating families ($n = 30$) and with several key stakeholders ($n = 19$) have been very encouraging. After approximately 2 years of intervention activities, both families and stakeholders were aware of key project messages and awareness related closely to 'intervention dose'. Both parents and stakeholders could see the benefits of the programme for themselves and the wider community and the BAEW team, project coordinators in particular, received high praise for their work. In response to BAEW, most families reported limiting the consumption of sweet drinks (68.2%), participating in the after-school activity programme (67.9%) and providing healthier lunch box foods (57.1%). Changing the choice of takeaway foods (3.6%) was the change that the BAEW project had least impact on and, interestingly, 32% of respondents said they had made no changes because they considered their family to be healthy already. Schools reported increased availability of healthy foods at the school canteen, the introduction of fruit breaks during class where only fruit or vegetable sticks can be consumed and increased physical activity through increased class physical activity time. Sporting clubs reiterated that the after-school activity programme (ASAP) had increased their memberships. Good partnerships have been established between the target population, stakeholders and the project team and the capacity of the Colac community to promote healthy eating and physical activity has increased through training and reorientation of existing services.

22.5 Conclusions

Like the racers on day one of the *Tour de France*, we cannot see the 'obesity prevention' finish line. While we know where we are heading, the timeframe is uncertain and we are still working out the best way to get there. Because of this uncertainty, community-based prevention programmes like BAEW need to be established nationally and internationally so that we can learn from each other. If the programmes are coordinated appropriately and they run alongside a comprehensive monitoring system, they will improve our understanding of how to intervene effectively, serve as models for the implementation of intervention strategies in other communities, increase capacity for sustained action and enhance community ownership. They can also be used as the building blocks for policy implementation at a national and international level. In Australia a national action agenda has been put in place with the aim of assisting Australians to enjoy high levels of good health by promoting healthy weight (National Obesity TaskForce, 2003). Setting up community demonstration areas is one of four national strategies designed to achieve this goal. As other governments gear up to control the obesity epidemic worldwide, they will be looking for guidance on the way ahead. A linked network of comprehensive community-based prevention programmes is a good place to start.

22.6 Acknowledgements

I thank all those involved in implementing the Be Active Eat Well project in Colac and the Colac community for the enthusiastic way they have embraced the project. Also, Professor Boyd Swinburn, Annie Simmons, Peter Kremer, Andrea Sanigorksi and other members of the Sentinel Site team at Deakin University. Be Active Eat Well is funded by the Department of Human Services, Victoria and support and evaluation of the project is funded by the Commonwealth Department of Health and Aging. Colin Bell is supported by a Victorian Health Promotion Foundation Public Health Fellowship.

22.7 References

ARMSTRONG, J. and REILLY, J. J. (2002), *Lancet*, **359**, 2003–4.

BELL, A. C., and SWINBURN, B. (2004), *Eur. J. Clin. Nutr.*, **58**, 258–63.

BELL, A. C., SWINBURN, B. A., AMOSA, H. and SCRAGG, R. K. (2001), *Int. J. Obes. Relat. Metab. Disord.*, **25**, 920–7.

BLUNDELL, J. E. and KING, N. A. (1996), *Ciba. Found. Symp.*, **201**, 138–54; discussion 154–8, 188–93.

CAMPBELL, K. and CRAWFORD, D. (2001), *Aust. J. Nutr. Diet.*, **58**, 19–25.

DAVISON, K. K. and BIRCH, L. L. (2001), *Obes. Rev.*, **2**, 159–71.

DIETZ, W. H. (2001), *JAMA.*, **285**, 2506–7.

DONOVAN, R. and HENLEY, N. (2003), *Social Marketing. Principles and Practice*, IP Communications, Melbourne.

EDMUNDS, L. D. and ZIEBLAND, S. (2002), *Health Educ. Res.*, **17**, 211–20.

FAIRBANK, L., O'MEARA, S., RENFREW, M. J. *et al.* (2000), *Health Technol. Assess*, **4**, 1–171.

FLORES, R. (1995), *Public Health Rep.*, **110**, 189–93.

GLASGOW, R. E., VOGT, T. M. and BOLES, S. M. (1999), *Am. J. Public Health*, **89**, 1322–7.

GORTMAKER, S. L., PETERSON, K., WIECHA, J. *et al.* (1999), *Arch. Pediatr. Adolesc. Med.*, **153**, 409–18.

HADDON, W., JR. (1980), *Public Health Rep.*, **95**, 411–21.

JEFFERY, R. W. and FRENCH, S. A. (1999), *Am. J. Public Health*, **89**, 747–51.

MANIOS, Y. and KAFATOS, A. (1999), *Public Health Nutr.*, **2**, 445–8.

NATIONAL OBESITY TASKFORCE (2003), Department of Health & Ageing, Canberra.

NUTBEAM, D. (1998), *Health Promo. Int.*, **13**, 27–44.

OZANE-SMITH, J. (2004), *Aust. N. Z. J. Public Health*, **28**, 109–12.

REDELMEIER, D. A. and TIBSHIRANI, R. J. (1997), *N. Engl. J. Med.*, **336**, 453–8.

ROBINSON, T. N. (1999), *JAMA*, **282**, 1561–7.

ROBINSON, T. N. and SIRARD, J. R. (2005), *Am. J. Prev. Med.*, **28**, 194–201.
ROLLS, B. J., ENGELL, D. and BIRCH, L. L. (2000), *J. Am. Diet. Assoc.*, **100**, 232–4.
ROLLS, B. J., MORRIS, E. L. and ROE, L. S. (2002), *Am. J. Clin. Nutr.*, **76**, 1207–13.
SAHOTA, P., RUDOLF, M. C., DIXEY, R., HILL, A. J., BARTH, J. H. and CADE, J. (2001a), *BMJ*, **323**, 1027.
SAHOTA, P., RUDOLF, M. C., DIXEY, R., HILL, A. J., BARTH, J. H. and CADE, J. (2001b), *BMJ*, **323**, 1029–32.
SALLIS, J. F., PATTERSON, T. L., MCKENZIE, T. L. and NADER, P. R. (1988), *J. Dev. Behav. Pediatr.*, **9**, 57–61.
SANDERSON, C., HAGLUND, B., TILLGREN, P. *et al.* (1996), *Health Prom. Int.*, **11**, 143–6.
SWINBURN, B. and EGGER, G. (2002), *Obes. Rev.*, **3**, 289–301.
SWINBURN, B., EGGER, G. and RAZA, F. (1999), *Prev. Med.*, **29**, 563–70.
SWINBURN, B., GILL, T. and KUMANYIKA, S. (2005), *Obesity Reviews*, **6**, 23–33.
TIMPERIO, A., CRAWFORD, D., BURNS, C. and CAMERON-SMITH, D. (2002), *J. Am. Diet. Assoc.*, **102**, 88–91.
UNITED STATES DEPARTMENT OF HEALTH AND HUMAN SERVICES (2002), *Physical Activity Evaluation Handbook*, US. Department of Health and Human Services, Centers for Disease Control and Prevention, Atlanta, GA.
ZUPPA, J. A., MORTON, H. and METHA, K. P. (2003), *Nutr. Diet.*, **60**, 78–84.

23

Behavioural and metabolic targets for the prevention and control of obesity

M. S. Westerterp-Plantenga, Maastricht University, The Netherlands

23.1 Introduction

Body-weight management is the control of body weight through promoting a stable balance between energy intake and energy expenditure. Energy intake must be balanced against energy requirements to ensure that storing energy as fat is avoided. The key behavioural target for preventing and treating overweight and obesity is dietary restraint, or inhibition of eating. The key body-weight management targets for metabolic intermediates are satiety, thermogenesis, oxidation of fat, storage of fat, body composition and energy efficiency. These targets include sustaining satiety even when energy intake is lower than the energy requirement; preventing a decrease in thermogenesis during e.g. weight loss; increasing fat oxidation, thus limiting fat storage; increasing energy expenditure by increasing relative fat-free mass; and promoting energy inefficiency during body-weight gain or regain.

The metabolic roles of ingredients in body-weight control encompass satiety, with respect to energy intake, thermogenesis and body composition, with respect to energy expenditure, and fat-oxidation and energy efficiency in relation to energy storage.

23.2 Controlling energy intake through eating behaviour

Preventing and treating overweight and obesity through dietary restraint, or inhibition of eating, is a key target, and both people who are overweight and researchers seek strategies to support restrained eating behaviour. These strategies include the effects of meal frequency, energy density and portion size, and often appear to have a strong relationship with macronutrient composition. The evidence for the effects of these strategies is described below.

23.2.1 Meal frequency

Managing diet by controlling meal frequency is equivalent to using or influencing macronutrient composition. For instance, this strategy could operate by limiting fat intake. Fat has a high energy density and a high palatability, and over-consumption, corresponding to excess energy intake, is often a problem. A relatively high meal frequency implies a high carbohydrate and low fat ingestion, and promotes control of food intake. However, reducing fat intake must allow for the fact that some fats have beneficial effects, such as conjugated linoleic acid and diacylglycerol, as discussed below.

Daily energy intake appears to be regulated more accurately in nibblers than in meal-feeders.[1] Moreover, Drummond *et al.*[2] showed an inverse relationship between eating frequency and body weight in male, but not female, non-obese adults who reported valid dietary intakes. An even greater appetite control was associated with a manipulated increased frequency of eating in lean males,[3] and acute appetite reduction was associated with a manipulated increased frequency of eating in obese males.[4]

The combination of these data suggests that improvements in appetite control appear when energy intake is spread evenly over the course of a day. The mechanism behind this may be that the macronutrient composition modulates meal frequency by modulating blood glucose patterns. It was observed that variations in habitual subject-specific meal frequency were primarily explained by the macronutrient composition of the food, i.e. the percentage energy from CHO or from fat. Secondary effects were the frequency of the total of transient and dynamic blood glucose declines, and sweetness perception and hunger suppression. Habitual meal frequency is supposed to be the result of a partly genetically determined sweetness perception,[5] which is inversely related to hunger suppression during standard consumption, and positively related to CHO intake.[6] A relatively high proportion of CHO in energy intake leads to relatively higher than average blood glucose levels during baselines, and to shorter inter-meal intervals.[6] The proportion of CHO in the diet is inversely related to the energy density of food intake, and therefore inversely related to energy intake.[6–8] High intake of simple carbohydrates may drive meal frequency through blood glucose dynamics, inducing a vicious circle of blood glucose dynamics driving carbohydrate (and/or energy) intake.

23.2.2 Energy density

Energy density is an important characteristic of macronutrient composition.

Energy density is defined as follows:

$$\begin{aligned} ED = (&\text{kJ carbohydrate} + \text{kJ protein} + \text{kJ fat} \\ &+ \text{kJ alcohol})/(\text{g carbohydrate} + \text{g protein} + \text{g fat} \\ &+ \text{g alcohol} + \text{g water and undigestible parts}) \end{aligned}$$

Energy density represents metabolisable energy/gross weight, or kJ/g since the Atwater factors are defined like this, and does not represent energy/volume.

Energy density has different short-term and long-term effects. In the short term, food intake and not energy intake is monitored, and, as a consequence, energy density affects energy intake.[7–12] However, observations during the inter-meal interval indicate that possible long-term effects may be different.

Having observed that, during meals, the body monitors the weight of food and not the energy, and given that energy balance is achieved over a week, the body might somehow correct for passive over- or under-consumption following high or low energy-dense meals over longer periods of time. Average daily energy intake (ADEI) is related to the energy density (ED) of the food, including water in the food, if ED is determined by specific macronutrients. Conversely, if ED is only determined by the weight of water, it is not related to ADEI.[8] A closer assessment of the effects of ED from food or drinks on ADEI showed that only the energy density from food ($r = 0.97$; $P < 0.0001$), and not the energy density from drinks, contributed significantly to EI. Thus, for the average daily energy intake, the energy density from food is an important determinant, but the energy density from drinks is not.[13]

Another characteristic of ADEI is that not all food is consumed in identical portion sizes. It appears that obese women take larger portions of food with a high energy density than non-obese women do, and also larger than standard sizes. They take smaller portions of food with a low energy density in comparison with the non-obese, and also in comparison with the standard sizes. In the non-obese, portion sizes are almost standard portion sizes.[11] In healthy, non-obese males, portion size is inversely related to the energy densities of snacks of 7.6–16.5 kJ/g.[16] So, in daily life, portion sizes appear to be a learned, or culturally determined, modulating factor that may have become a habit, compensating for the straightforward effect of ED on ADEI.[8,11]

In a long-term experiment, a clear effect of dietary restraint was shown in relation to energy density and fat content of food. After 6 months, a reduced fat diet in combination with unrestrained eating behaviour (which resulted in positive energy intake compensation) resulted in weight maintenance.[7] Weight reduction was the consequence of a reduced fat diet in combination with restrained eating behaviour (which did not compensate for the reduced energy intake).[7] A full fat diet combined with unrestrained eating behaviour led to increased energy intake and body weight.[7] Restrained eating behaviour with a full fat diet prevented such an increase in energy intake and body weight.[7] Thus dietary restraint compensated for an increase in ED, whereas lack of dietary restraint compensated for a decrease in ED.[7]

This indicates that dietary restraint is a modulating factor in the effect of energy density on energy intake in the long term, and thus energy intake is not only determined by energy density. More appropriately, it is determined by the characteristics of the macronutrients, mainly fat and carbohydrate, which contribute to variations in energy intake, but are modulated by eating behaviour.

23.2.3 Dietary restraint

Eating behaviour may be one of the determinants for predicting prevention or promotion of weight regain after a weight reduction programme. Eating behaviour with respect to dieting can be characterised using questionnaires, like the Herman–Polivy[15] eating restraint questionnaire, and the Three Factor Eating Questionnaire (TFEQ) by Stunkard and Messick.[16,17] The Herman–Polivy restraint scale measures the extent to which people display concern with their weight and diet chronically to control it.[18] In the Herman–Polivy restraint construct, disinhibition of restraint is measured implicitly. Relatively high scores on the Herman–Polivy restraint questionnaire are observed in the obese, and these scores correlate positively with BMI;[17] moreover, high scores imply a relationship with failure to maintain weight.

The Three Factor Eating Questionnaire discriminates between successful energy intake restriction and disinhibition of restraint. Normal weight, restrained eaters succeed in keeping their weight at a certain level for a relatively long time by maintaining a low energy intake in relation to a relatively low energy expenditure.[19] Their relatively low scores on the Herman–Polivy restraint scale indicate that they are relatively less weight-conscious,[19] and their relatively high scores on the cognitive restraint factor (TFEQ)[16] reflect that they are mainly food concerned. In several long-term studies on weight maintenance, it appears that an increase in cognitive restraint during the diet, possibly together with a decrease in disinhibition and a decrease in general hunger, is an important determinant of subsequent weight maintenance.[7,21,22] An increase in dietary restraint often explains the success of placebo groups in longer-term experiments.

23.3 Satiety

A strong factor in controlling food intake at a certain level is satiety. Investigating the mechanisms of satiety could help us to understand how to trigger these mechanisms and, thus, allow the possibility of giving the subject the feeling of satiety without the primary drive for satiety: food intake.

23.3.1 Central and peripheral mechanisms

Energy expenditure determines energy requirements,[23–25] and, in principle, energy intake is regulated physiologically by means of hunger and satiety.[26,27] With respect to food intake control in humans, in terms of meal size and meal frequency, two features are worth considering. First is the distinction between satiation and satiety. Satiation refers to the processes that bring a period of eating to an end; these processes influence the size of meals and snacks. Satiety refers to the inhibition of hunger and further eating that arises as a consequence of food ingestion, and determines intermeal intervals, or meal frequency, by determining the next meal initiation. Second is the initiation of these overlapping physiological responses as a result of the properties of food and the act of ingesting. The quantity and quality of the food determines the intensity and duration of the biological processes generated. This situation supports the idea of the different satiating power of different types of food,[8,26–30] which can be recognised at the level of:

- psychological events (hunger, perception, cravings, and hedonic sensations) and behavioural operations (meals, snacks, energy, and macronutrient intakes);
- peripheral physiology and metabolic events; or
- neurotransmitter and metabolic interactions in the brain.

The expression of appetite reflects the synchronous operation of events and processes at all three levels. Neural events trigger and guide behaviour, but each act of behaviour involves a response in the peripheral physiological system; in turn, these physiological events are translated into neurochemical activity in the brain. This activity represents the strength of motivation and the willingness to refrain from feeding. Viewed in this way, the psychobiological system permits an understanding of the inter-relationships among behavioural events that comprise eating, peripheral physiology and metabolism, and central neurochemical processes.[27]

The autonomic nervous system and the release of a variety of hormones, such as leptin[31] from the pituitary, have to be considered as the main effector systems.[32] In humans, pathological effects, such as those demonstrated by craniopharyngioma patients showing hyperphagia, have been related to dysfunction of leptin receptors in the hypothalamus,[33] also indicating the hypothalamic function.

The central and peripheral processes that affect hunger and satiety are signals during and after ingestion of food that lead to sensory-specific satiety, sensory satiety, post-prandial and post-absorptive satiety. Hunger and satiety are also affected by external factors that affect energy expenditure, such as physical activity, hypobaric hypoxia and changes in environmental temperature.

23.3.2 Sensory-specific satiety

After feeding to satiety, humans reported that the taste of the food on which they had been satiated tasted almost as intense as when they were hungry, though much less pleasant.[34,35] Analysing the neural control of feeding in the macaque monkey (*Macaca fascicularis*), by recording the activity of single neurons during feeding, has shown that a population of neurons in the lateral hypothalamus respond to the sight and/or taste of food only when the monkey is hungry.[34,35] The modulation of reward of a motivationally relevant sensory stimulus such as the taste of food according to motivational state, for example hunger, appears to be an important way in which motivational behaviour is controlled.[34–36] The subjective correlate of this modulation is that food tastes pleasant when hungry, and tastes hedonically neutral when it has been eaten to satiety.[35] Activity in the primary taste area (frontal opercular and insular taste cortices as well as the nucleus of the solitary tract) does not reflect the pleasantness of the taste of a food, but rather its sensory qualities independently of motivational state.[34–37] On the other hand, activity in the secondary taste area (the caudolateral orbitofrontal cortex) and in the lateral hypothalamus is modulated by satiety, and may be related to whether a food tastes pleasant, and to whether the food should be eaten.[34–37]

It was also found in humans that the pleasantness of the taste of food eaten to satiety decreased more than for foods that had not been eaten. This implies that, if a variety of foods is available, the total amount consumed will be more than when only one food is offered repeatedly.[38] This effect has been termed 'sensory-specific satiety'.[38] Sensory-specific satiety occurs in relation to the sight, as well as taste and odour of the food.[34] Enhanced eating when a variety of foods is available may have had evolutionary advantages, by ensuring that different foods with important different nutrients were consumed when they became available. However, with a wide variety of foods constantly available today, this response can lead to overeating and obesity.

23.3.3 Sensory satiety

In addition to sensory-specific satiety, a relationship between sensory perception and food preference with respect to satiety has been shown in rats.[39]

Perception of polyunsaturated fatty acids (PUFAs) has been demonstrated, showing that they inhibit delayed rectifying K^+ channels (DRK channels) in mammalian taste receptor cells.[39] Interestingly, the effects were only seen for *cis*-PUFAs (arachidonic, linoleic and linolenic acid). Moreover, DRK channels in the tongue tissue of rats with a preference for high fat diets (Osborne–Mendel rats), were less sensitive to the *cis*-PUFAs, than the DRK channels of rats preferring diets high in carbohydrate (S5B).[40]

In humans, fat-specific satiety was demonstrated following two weeks of using either oil containing linoleic acid or oil containing oleic acid, but there was no change in general satiety.[41] Moreover, differences in taste perception between humans were shown to exist at a low concentration of linoleic acid. Tasters appeared to terminate eating a food containing linoleic acid due to satiety, whereas non-tasters terminated eating due to a decrease in pleasantness of taste.[42]

23.3.4 Satiety in the post-prandial phase

The integrated role of gastric distension, emptying, and contractions within the complex series of physiological and biochemical events surrounding meal patterning has recently been recognised.[26,43,44] The role of the stomach in hunger and satiety has been demonstrated by increases in hunger ratings associated with the time at which 90% of a test meal had emptied from the stomach.[26] It has been suggested that foods which empty slowly from the stomach sustain satiety and delay the onset of hunger in humans.[44] Gastric emptying may play a role in this relationship, although it is likely that gastric sensations interact with related factors such as the subsequent delayed (and thus prolonged) elevation in blood glucose.[26,45,46]

It has also been suggested that gastric stretch receptors and contractions indicate the volume of stomach contents to the organism, whereas various peptides secreted from, or induced by, the alimentary tract, indicate energy content. Such peptides include food intake inhibitors such as cholecystokinin (CCK), serotonin (5HT), corticotrophin-releasing factor (CRF), somatostatin, enterostatin, bombesin, glucagon and glucagon-like peptide (GLP-I and -II). GLP-I, for instance, is related to the control of insulin, and to satiety, but its effect is diminished in the visceral obese.[26] For some of these subjects, it has been questioned whether the experimental results of hypophagia were actually caused by satiety, or by nausea induced by non-physiological quantities of the peptides.[26] Other peptides believed to stimulate food intake include neuropeptide Y (NPY), galanin, and endogenous opiods. It may be that peptides which reduce food intake signal via the central nervous system to the ventromedial hypothalamus (VMH), and peptides which stimulate food consumption may signal through the central nervous system to the lateral hypothalamus (LH).[26]

The presence of food, particularly fat, in the upper small intestine stimulates the release of CCK, which has both peripheral and central receptors.[47,48] CCK is known to serve regulatory roles in bile secretion, gastric emptying, and the exocrine pancreas. Additionally, CCK relays signals to the brain through the vagus nerve, inhibiting eating behaviour in humans and causing meal termination.[49] Conversely, as nutrient delivery to the intestine decreases, CCK release and vagal activity are reduced, so that eating behaviour is no longer inhibited. Antagonists to CCK have been shown to increase food intake in rats, whereas CCK stimulants have been shown to decrease food intake in both rats and humans.[26]

In rats, increased serotenergic (5HT) transmission has been shown to decrease food intake, acting peripherally, and possibly via the central nervous system (CNS) as well. In humans, the hypophagic actions of serotonin have been studied extensively. Synthesis of 5HT in the brain depends on the availability of tryptophan, its amino acid precursor. Thus, dietary factors influencing blood tryptophan concentration may influence 5HT synthesis. Such dietary factors include other amino acids, which compete with 5HT uptake across the blood-brain barrier, and carbohydrate, which may have a diluting effect on tryptophan concentrations.

Some data indicate that the hypophagic actions of serotonin work preabsorptively, possibly through interactions with CCK and enterostatin.[26] Changes in serotonin metabolism have been reported in many cases of individuals with disordered eating, including anorexia, bulimia, obesity, and type 2 diabetes mellitus. Some investigators have proposed that serotonin may play a role in macronutrient preferences, including carbohydrate cravings, and fat avoidance, but this has been refuted by others.[26]

Corticotrophin-releasing factor (CRF), a 41-residue peptide located in neurons throughout the brain, particularly the paraventricular nucleus, is believed to suppress food intake, and also to stimulate thermogenesis.[50–52] These actions may occur via the sympathetic nervous system and/or via mediation of the actions of serotonin. Alterations in the responses of adrenocorticotrophin hormone (ACTH) and cortisol to CRF have also been reported in some conditions of disturbed eating behaviour, such as anorexia nervosa.[53] It has also been suggested that CRF, which is stimulated by exercise, may mediate the effects of post-exercise anorexia and elevated energy expenditure, being strongest immediately following a bout of exercise.[50–52] CRF is also released during the stress response, therefore CRF may be a factor in the down-regulation of food intake during stress, possibly along with noradrenaline.[50–52]

The most potent endogenous appetite stimulant known in humans, thus far, is neuropeptide Y (NPY), which acts through the central nervous system, possibly through noradrenergic mechanisms.[26] High levels of NPY have been found in the human hypothalamus.[54] In both rats and humans, starvation is associated with elevated levels of NPY, which are reversed by re-feeding. Some investigators have suggested that disturbed patterns or activity of NPY may occur in patients with anorexia and bulimia nervosa.[26]

Galanin, another peptide with hyperphagic activity, is secreted from the intestine and Islets of Langerhans, relaying signals to receptors in the paraventricular nucleus.[55] In both animals and humans, it is recognized that some kinds of stress can reduce food intake (possibly mediated through CRF), whereas other types of stress can stimulate food intake.[55] Endogenous opiods (beta-endorphin, dynorphin, and encephalines) are believed to induce stress-related hyperphagia, acting on several sites in the hypothalamus. Some data, but not all, suggest that these compounds may influence meal size and macronutrient preference (for fat rather than simple carbohydrate) in humans.[56]

23.3.5 Satiety in the post-absorptive phase

Once nutrients cross from the intestinal tract into the blood and become available for metabolism, they may exert post-absorptive food intake regulation. Satiety and hunger seem to be related to metabolic events surrounding nutrient processing, utilisation, and storage.[26] Thus, it logically follows that carbohydrate, with its rapid uptake and metabolism, would play an important role in short-term food intake regulation. For example, carbohydrate stores in humans range from approximately 150 to 500 grams, depending on body size, exercise and state of nutrition.[26] This is rather low in relation to the 200 to 500 grams of carbohydrate consumed in a typical daily diet. Conversely, the amount of fat and protein in the body are quite high in relation to daily dietary intake. Given each of these relative turnovers, and the complete dependence of the central nervous system (CNS) on glucose as a metabolic fuel, the role of carbohydrate, particularly blood glucose, in the regulation of food intake and energy balance has long been an intense focus of research.[26]

In the 1950s, Jean Mayer conducted an elaborate series of experiments in mice and rats leading to the formulation of the glucostatic theory.[57–59] Based on blood glucose concentration, or arterio-venous differences, he postulated that the rate of glucose utilization by privileged brain regions determined nutrient ingestion.[57–59] When blood glucose was monitored continuously in fasting, time-blinded humans, transient declines in 89% of the cases were associated with spontaneous meal requests or changes in hunger ratings.[26] This technique has been extended for longer durations, in the post-absorptive and post-prandial states, throughout inter-meal intervals, and during exercise in time-blinded humans. As would be expected, the shape of the glucose curve varied following ingestion of different macronutrients, e.g. a 1000 kJ drink of a simple carbohydrate produced a sharp rise and subsequent fall in blood glucose. These characteristic rapid drops in blood glucose following the post-absorptive rise have been termed 'dynamic declines', because they do not originate from a stable baseline, whereas transient declines do originate from a stable baseline.

During dynamic declines in blood glucose, meal requests occurred in 87% of the cases.[46] When an isovolumetric, 1000 kJ, high fat drink was consumed, the rise in blood glucose was more gradual and prolonged. The next spontaneous meal request came during the dynamic decline that followed the drink-induced rise. However, since the rise and fall in blood glucose was of longer duration, the second meal request came later after consuming the high fat drink than after the simple carbohydrate drink. These interactions were proposed as early as 1916, and by the originator of the glucostatic theory.[60–62] More recently, the term 'glucodynamic' has been proposed as a more accurate reflection of the response of the brain (and perhaps liver) to continuously changing blood glucose, metabolism in general, and the processes by which different systems within the organism are integrated in metabolic regulation.[47] Evidence thus far indicates that patterns of plasma glucose, particularly the transient and dynamic declines, play a role in determining meal initiation and inter-meal intervals. Thus, the role of glucose in food intake regulation has shifted from that of a satiety signal to that of a meal initiation signal.[26]

Maintenance of adequate carbohydrate within the body is of vital importance (particularly to the CNS), yet the amount of dietary carbohydrate consumed each day is similar to the amount stored as glycogen. Therefore, a 'glycogenostatic' theory of food intake regulation has emerged, based on the notion that the body adjusts its food intake to ensure that ample glycogen stores are maintained.[26] The original data supporting this theory came from studies in mice, but have not been confirmed in all studies in humans. Recent data have suggested that, when glycogen stores are depleted by exercise or by energy intake restriction, the relationship between blood glucose patterns and meal requests is disturbed, perhaps due to removal of the carbohydrate buffer reserve.[26] It may be that the goal of maintaining ample blood glucose for normal CNS functioning, as predicted by the glucostatic model by Mayer, could be considered as an additional daily goal. Since the glucostatic and glycogenostatic models complement each other, this may be an example whereby long-term food intake regulation is a summation of short-term regulations.

23.3.6 Role of the liver in the metabolic control of food intake

Although hepatic metabolic signals are not necessary to maintain food intake and body weight, a large body of evidence indicates that such signals play a role in the control of eating.[60] Total parenteral nutrition and peripheral administration of various metabolites (e.g. glucose, pyruvate, lactate, hydroxybutyrate) generally inhibit eating. On the other hand metabolic inhibitors such as the glucose antimetabolite 2-deoxy-D-glucose, fatty acid oxidation inhibitors,[61] the fructose analogue 2,5-anhydro-D-mannitol (2,5AM), and the sodium pump inhibitor ouabain, have been shown to stimulate eating under various conditions.[60] Many of these effects are particularly pronounced when the substances are infused into the hepatic portal vein, and are markedly attenuated when the hepatic branch of the vagus is disconnected.[60] This suggests that the observed effects on eating originate in the liver and are mediated by hepatic afferent nerves. In addressing these issues, it must be kept in mind that the hepatic afferent nerves involved are also part of a complex network that plays an important role in blood glucose regulation, electrolyte/fluid balance, and other regulatory systems, which may interact with mechanisms of food intake control.[60]

Taken together, satiety is generated by sensory, post-ingestive and post-absorptive mechanisms, which may be targets for sustaining or enhancing satiety while reducing energy intake.

23.4 The effects of conjugated linoleic acid and other ingredients on energy efficiency and body composition

Post-ingestive and post-absorptive mechanisms support the dynamic state of satiety during the inter-meal interval. These mechanisms imply effects on metabolic targets such as 'satiety hormones', thermogenesis and fat oxidation. Thus, satiety is often affected in relation to or coinciding with these metabolic targets, and therefore satiety due to post-ingestive or post-absorptive processes is referred to as metabolic satiety. In the longer term, energy efficiency and body composition can be affected by certain ingredients. The following sections include the scientific evidence for the possible body-weight control effects of conjugated linoleic acid, capsaicine, green tea, diacylglycerol and protein, and illustrate these with possible applications in body-weight management research.

23.4.1 Metabolic targets and conjugated linoleic acid

Conjugated linoleic acid (CLA) is naturally found in beef, milk and milk products, since it is an intermediate in the biohydrogenation of linoleic acid, which occurs in the rumen through the action of bacteria.[62,63] CLA refers to a group of positional and geometrical isomers of linoleic acid containing conjugated double bonds. The natural form is predominantly the *cis*-9, *trans*-11 isomer.

Numerous physiological effects in relation to body weight control have been attributed to CLA in animals. In different animal models, CLA has been shown to reduce body fat[67–74] and to increase lean body mass.[64,66–68] However, effects on body weight are controversial. Some investigators found reduced body weight after a CLA diet,[68,69,71] whereas others found no effect[64,67,70–72] or an increase in body weight.[72] Furthermore, CLA intake has been associated with increased energy expenditure.[65,70,73]

A few human studies on the effect of CLA on body weight, BMI and/or fat mass, showed that though fat mass[74,75] and sagittal abdominal diameter[76] were lowered by CLA, this did not result in body weight loss.[74–79] While subjects are in a state of weight regain, CLA reduces fat uptake into adipocytes by lowering the lipoprotein lipase activity[64,66] as well as stearoyl-CoA desaturase,[80] thus blocking body fat gain instead of reducing body fat level.

The effects of CLA are illustrated by the following example. After a very low calorie diet that significantly lowered body weight, per cent body fat,

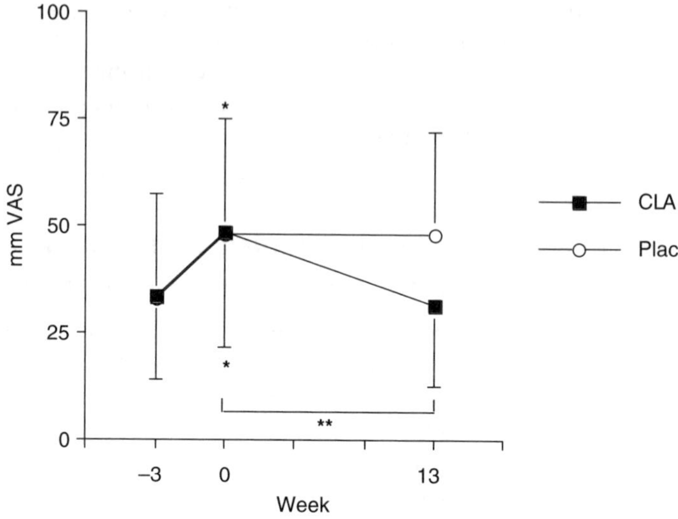

Fig. 23.1 Feelings of hunger measured with an anchored 100 mm visual analogue scale (VAS) before VLCD (–3) after VLCD and before intervention (0) and at 13 weeks of intervention with 1.8 or 3.6 g conjugated linoleic acid/d (CLA, $n = 27$) and 1.8 or 3.6 g placebo/d (oleic acid, $n = 27$). The results are presented as CLA and placebo, with the low and high dosage combined. * Repeated measures ANOVA for all subjects together showed a significant increase in feelings of hunger from week –3 to week 0 ($P < 0.001$). ** Multiple regression showed that the feelings of hunger during intervention was decreased by CLA compared to placebo (Regression coefficient 14.0 (25.0–3), ($P < 0.05$). After Kamphuis *et al.*[82]

fat mass, fat free mass, resting metabolic rate, respiratory quotient, plasma glucose, insulin, triacylglycerol, free fatty acids, glycerol and β-hydroxy butyrate concentrations, CLA (1.8 or 3.6 g/d) or placebo was administrated to subjects over 13 weeks, during which time body weight was regained. The regain of fat free mass was increased by CLA, independently of per cent body weight regain and physical activity. As a consequence of the increased regain of fat free mass, resting metabolic rate increased. Substrate oxidation and blood plasma parameters were not affected by CLA.[81] Coinciding with the increase in resting metabolic rate, post-absorptive feelings of fullness and satiety were increased and feelings of hunger were decreased after 13 weeks, independently of per cent of body weight regain[82] (see Figs. 23.1, 23.2). Thus, the increase in satiety coincided with increased thermogenesis, which was related to increased fat free mass, the main metabolic target in this respect. However, although the metabolic target was affected by CLA, this did not result in a better weight maintenance compared with the placebo, since dietary restraint tended to increase and disinhibition tended to decrease in the placebo group.[81,82]

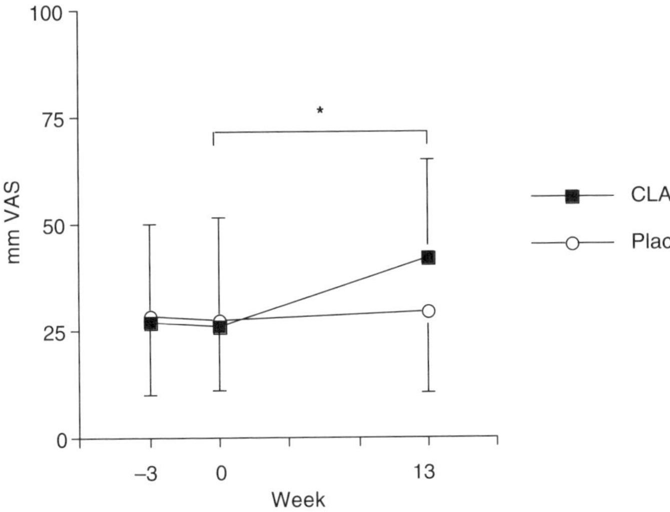

Fig. 23.2 Feelings of satiety measured with an anchored 100 mm visual analogue scale (VAS) before VLCD (–3) after VLCD and before intervention (0) and at 13 weeks of intervention with 1.8 or 3.6 g conjugated linoleic acid/d (CLA, $n = 27$) and 1.8 or 3.6 g placebo/d (oleic acid, $n = 27$). The results are presented as CLA and placebo, with the low and high dosage combined. ** Multiple regression showed that the feelings of hunger during intervention was increased by CLA compared to placebo (Regression coefficient 12.2 (0.9–23.5), ($P < 0.05$). After Kamphuis *et al.*[82]

23.4.2 Metabolic targets and capsaicin

Capsaicin has been reported to reduce adiposity in rats, which can be explained partly by the enhancement of energy and lipid metabolism via catecholamine secretion from the adrenal medulla through sympathetic activation of the central nervous system.[83,84] In a series of human studies, Yoshioka *et al.*[85–88] showed an increase in diet-induced thermogenesis and a decrease in respiratory quotient (RQ) immediately after a meal to which red pepper (capsaicin) was added, implying a shift in substrate oxidation from carbohydrate to fat. This increase in the facultative phase of diet-induced thermogenesis was probably due to beta-adrenergic stimulation.[85] They also showed a decreased appetite, decreased cumulative food intake[86] and increased energy expenditure[86,88] after consumption of red pepper.

In these studies, capsaicin was given orally as red pepper. Therefore, the reduction in energy intake could have been due to the sensory effect of capsaicin or the post-ingestive, gastro-intestinal effect. The separate sensory and gastro-intestinal contributions to satiety were assessed by offering the same dosage of capsaicin in tomato juice (sensory and gastro-intestinal exposure), or in capsules (gastro-intestinal exposure) that were swallowed with tomato juice. Average daily energy intake over two days was lower after capsaicin capsules, and also after capsaicin in tomato juice. Capsaicin in tomato juice had a stronger effect than capsaicin in capsules. Energy intake was decreased through reducing fat intake and increasing carbohydrate intake, thus decreasing the energy density of food intake. Despite the decreased food intake, satiety was still raised. Thus, in the short term, both oral and gastro-intestinal exposure to capsaicin increased satiety and reduced energy and fat-intake; the stronger reduction with oral exposure indicating an additional sensory effect. The reduction in satiety that occurred, despite the lower food intake, was related to continuously increased thermogenesis,[89,90] which may be considered as the main long-term metabolic effect of capsaicin.[89] However, long-term weight maintenance again appeared to fail with capsaicin, probably due to lack of compliance because of its pungency.[89]

23.4.3 Metabolic targets and green tea

Anti-obesity properties have been claimed for green tea (epigallocatechin gallate plus caffeine), and ascribed to increased thermogenesis and fat-oxidation.[91–96] Green tea contains caffeine, which may stimulate thermogenesis and fat oxidation through the inhibition of phosphodiesterase and through adenosine antagonism.[91] Human studies have shown that caffeine does indeed stimulate thermogenesis and fat oxidation.[92–97] In addition, green tea contains large amounts of catechins, which may stimulate thermogenesis and fat oxidation through inhibition of catechol *O*-methyl-transferase.[95]

Dulloo *et al.*[96] showed that the effect of green tea was greater than can be attributed to its caffeine content alone. In a study investigating the effects of green tea on weight maintenance, after body-weight loss in moderately obese subjects in relation to habitual caffeine intake, metabolic as well as satiety parameters were determined. It appeared that habitually high caffeine consumers reduced weight, fat-mass and waist circumference more than habitually low caffeine consumers; and resting energy expenditure (REE) was reduced less and respiratory quotient was reduced more during weight loss. In the low caffeine consumers, green tea still reduced body weight, waist, RQ and body fat during weight maintenance, while REE was increased compared to a restoration of these variables with a placebo. In the high caffeine consumers, no effects due to green tea were observed during weight maintenance.

High caffeine intake was associated with body-weight loss through thermogenesis and fat oxidation, and with suppressed leptin in women. Green tea improved weight maintenance through thermogenesis and fat oxidation only in habitual low caffeine consumers. There was no difference in satiety between subjects with a habitual low caffeine intake who received green tea or placebo, although the placebo group regained body weight and the green-tea group did not. Increased fat oxidation and thermogenesis was an important metabolic effect that contributed to sustaining satiety.[98,99] However, in the long term, this appeared to be effective with respect to weight maintenance only in subjects who did not consume high amounts of caffeine already, indicating that the pitfall here is habituation, probably due to saturation of the enzyme system.[8,99]

23.4.4 Metabolic targets and diacylglycerol

Normal fat intake in the diet occurs largely as triacylglycerides (TG), although small amounts of diacylglycerol (DG) are usually present. Recent studies suggest that modest intakes of DG might have a beneficial effect on lipid metabolism in rats as well as in humans. Compared to TG, consumption of DG seems to produce lower post-prandial elevation of plasma TG concentrations[100,101] in humans and fasting serum TG levels in rats[102,103] and humans.[104] Reduced total body fat accumulation[105] and visceral fat accumulation[106] in rats and humans[107,108] by DG have also been reported. These effects appear most likely to be attributable to differences in DG utilization, especially the promotion of enhanced (post-prandial) β-oxidation.[103,108] This is probably due to enhanced post-absorptive availability of free fatty acids in the portal circulation. Notably, DG oil has the same digestion and absorption routes as comparable TG oils, along with similar bioavailability and physiological fuel value.[109]

In a respiration chamber study by Kamphuis *et al.*,[110] the effects of partial replacement of TG by DG on substrate oxidation, energy metabolism, respiratory quotient (RQ), relevant blood parameters and measures of appetite were assessed. Fat oxidation appeared to be higher and RQ lower with DG than with TG. Feelings of hunger, appetite, estimated prospective food intake and desire to eat were all lower with DG from the second day onwards, when the mean plasma β-hydroxy-butyrate level was also higher in the DG subjects. Consumption of DG in place of TG did not appear to alter total energy expenditure, but produced metabolic effects, particularly increased fat oxidation, associated with improved appetite control and energy balance.

23.4.5 Metabolic targets and protein

Protein may play a role in the treatment of obesity and subsequent weight maintenance. Treatment of obesity is beneficial in that weight loss reduces the risk for mortality and morbidity in obese subjects. Even modest weight loss, 5 to 10% of the initial body weight, has beneficial health effects,[111–113] and such weight loss is a realistic goal for most subjects.[111,113] However long-term maintenance of weight loss can be described as unsuccessful.[20] Most studies on weight maintenance show that weight regain is usually the case,[114–118] indicating that subjects are not able to change their eating and activity behaviour adequately.[20] In this context, it has been suggested that aiming for a more favourable body composition during weight regain, i.e. consisting of a larger fat-free mass, may slow weight regain. This is based upon previous observations that weight regain is slower when the composition of the weight regained consists of a greater fat-free mass.[118] With this in mind, studies have been carried out to evaluate increased protein intake, because of its contribution to the storage of fat-free mass,[119] its low energy efficiency during overfeeding,[120,121] and its increased satiety effect, despite similar energy intake.[28,122]

The 'Stock hypothesis' states that, during overfeeding, a relatively high percentage of energy as protein might have a limiting effect on body weight gain in humans through an energy efficiency effect.[120,121] A 3-month weight maintenance study assessed whether this would apply to body-weight regain, thus promoting weight maintenance using the favourable satiety, body composition and energy efficiency effects of an elevated protein consumption. It appeared that, during weight maintenance, the group with additional protein intake (18 en % vs. 15 en% protein intake) showed a 50% lower body weight regain, which consisted only of fat-free mass, a 50% decrease in energy efficiency, and increased satiety, while energy intake did not differ and a lower increase was found in triacylglycerol and leptin. At the same time, resting metabolic rate, respiratory quotient, total energy expenditure, and increases in other blood parameters did not differ between the groups that regained weight or remained relatively weight stable. Thus, a 20% higher protein intake during weight maintenance after weight loss resulted in a 50% lower body-weight regain, with the body weight regained consisting only of fat-free mass, increased satiety and decreased energy efficiency. Here again, an increase in satiety coincided with relatively higher thermogenesis, which was due to the improvement of body composition in favour of fat-free body mass.[123] These metabolic targets sustained an increase in dietary restraint similar to the placebo group, yet were more effective due to the increased metabolism on an increased protein diet.

23.5 Energy intake, expenditure and storage: a synthesis

Energy expenditure determines energy requirement, and if energy expenditure is not met or is exceeded, energy stores are depleted or increased, respectively. Since humans are genetically programmed to survive during famine, storage of excess energy intake is a strong characteristic, based upon a redundant metabolic system that aims for high energy efficiency i.e. high weight gain with little energy intake. In many societies today, famine is rare and the effects of this energy storage response are exaggerated, resulting in overweight and obesity, with several co-morbidities.

To prevent or treat overweight/obesity, body-weight control needs to be managed in spite of the tendency of the human metabolism to store energy.

Energy intake needs to be controlled, and energy efficiency needs to be lowered. Dietary restraint is an important mechanism to reduce energy intake. Dietary restraint needs to be supported by feelings of satiety, along with lack of hunger, desire to eat or appetite. These may be achieved by 'fooling' the subject with e.g. low energy density foods which have low fat content; frequent yet small carbohydrate-rich meals so that less energy is ingested; or by adjusting portion sizes to energy density thus 'normalising' energy intake. These measures all are based upon reducing fat intake (since this is a source of over-consumption or excess energy intake, though particular fats or fatty acids may be beneficial) while keeping carbohydrate intake and protein intake constant, thus reducing energy intake. These measures may fit in a certain society and culture.[124]

Another approach, also aimed at promoting dietary restraint through sustaining satiety, assesses particular satiety mechanisms and aims to stimulate these without stimulating food intake. These mechanisms focus on special pathways that affect metabolic targets such as thermogenesis and fat oxidation, and often satiety as well. The most promising ingredients are those that continue to affect metabolic targets in the longer term, during weight maintenance, and result in a better body composition together with higher thermogenesis and fat oxidation. Examples are, as described above, green tea, red pepper, protein, CLA and diacylglycerol. In practice, these treatments may be alternated to avoid habituation. Taken together, the metabolic targets of lean body mass, thermogenesis and fat oxidation, promote total energy expenditure and metabolic satiety at the same time. Problems that could prevent success in weight management are lack of sustained dietary restraint, habituation and non-compliance.

23.6 Future trends

Overweight and obesity will continue to increase unless a famine occurs. One future trend will be to characterise subjects with a predisposition to fat storage and lack of dietary-related discipline[125,126]. This way, the possible success of different treatments may be predicted. At the same time, the actual results will also be refined e.g. by describing the metabolic pathways still more accurately and adding genetic backgrounds to these, resulting in metabolomics.

The effect of macronutrient composition still needs to be better understood. For instance, if one aims for a high protein content of food, how is the fate of carbohydrate and fat affected? Another area where understanding is poor, is how taste perception could affect energy intake in a desirable way, opposing overeating rather than promoting it.

An overall consideration for the future is the importance of assessing subject-specific sensitivity for all possible treatments, as well as the effects on metabolic parameters.

23.7 References and further reading

1 WESTERTERP-PLANTENGA, M. S., WIJCKMANS-DUYSENS, N. E. G. and TEN HOOR, F. (1994), Food intake in the daily environment after energy-reduced lunch related to habitual meal frequency. *Appetite*, **22**, 173–82.

2 DRUMMOND, S. E., CROMBIE, N. E., CURSITER, M. C. and KIRK, T. R. (1988), Evidence that eating freqency is inversely related to body weight status in male, but not female, non-obese adults reporting valid dietary intakes. *Int. J. Obes. Relat. Metab. Disord.*, **22**, 105–12.

3 SPEECHLY, D. P. and BUFFENSTEIN, R. (1999), Greater appetite control associated with an increased frequency of eating in lean males. *Appetite*, **33**, 285–97.

4 SPEECHLY, D. P., ROGERS, G. G. and BUFFENSTEIN, R. (1999), Acute appetite reduction associated with an increased frequency of eating in obese males. *Int. J. Obes. Relat. Metab. Disord.*, **23**, 1151–9.

5 DE CASTRO, J. M. (1999), Behavioral genetics of food intake regulation in free-living humans. *Nutrition*, **15**, 550–4.

6 MELANSON, K. J., WESTERTERP-PLANTENGA, M. S., CAMPFIELD, L. A. and SARIS, W. H. M. (1999), Blood glucose and meal patterns in time-blinded males, after aspartame, carbohydrate, and fat consumption, in relation to sweetness perception. *Br. J. Nutr.*, **82**, 437–46.

7 WESTERTERP-PLANTENGA, M. S., WIJCKMANS-DUIJSENS, N. E. G., VERBOEKET-VAN DE VENNE, W. P. G., DE GRAAF, K., VAN HET HOF, K. H. and WESTSTRATE, J. A. (1998), Energy intake and body weight effects of six months reduced or full fat diets, as a function of dietary restraint. *Int. J. Obes. Relat. Metab. Disord.*, **22**, 14–22.

8 WESTERTERP-PLANTENGA, M. S. (2001), Analysis of energy density of food in relation to energy intake regulation in humans. *Br. J. Nutr.*, **85**, 351–61.

9 BELL, E. A. and ROLLS, B. J. (2001), Energy density of foods affects energy intake across multiple levels of fat content in lean and obese women. *Am. J. Clin. Nutr.*, **73** (6), 999–1000.

10 ROLLS, B. J. and BELL, E. A. (1999), Intake of fat and carbohydrate: role of energy density. *Eur. J. Clin. Nutr.*, **53**, S166–73.

11 WESTERTERP-PLANTENGA, M. S., PASMAN, W. J., YEDEMA, M. J. W. and WIJCKMANS-DUIJSENS, N. E. G. (1996), Energy intake adaptation of food to extreme energy densities of food by obese and non-obese women. *Eur. J. Clin. Nutr.*, **50**, 401–7.

12 WESTERTERP-PLANTENGA, M. S. (2000), Eating behaviour in humans, characterized by cumulative food intake curves – a review. *Neurosci. Biobehav. Rev.*, **24**, 239–48.

13 WESTERTERP-PLANTENGA, M. S. (2004), Effects of energy density of daily food intake on long term energy intake. *Phys. Behav.*, **81**, 765–71.

14 GREEN, S. M., BURLEY, V. J. and BLUNDELL, J. (1994), Effect of fat- and sucrose-containing foods on the size of eating episodes and energy intake in lean males: potential for causing overconsumption. *Eur. J. Clin. Nutr.*, **48**, 547–55.

15 HERMAN, C. P. and POLIVY, J. (1980), Restrained eating. In A. Stunkard (ed) *Obesity*, W. B. Saunders, Philadelphia, pp 208–24.

16 STUNKARD, A. J. and MESSICK, S. (1985), The three factor eating questionnaire to measure dietary restraint, disinhibition, and hunger. *J. Psychosom. Res.*, **29**, 71–83.

17 WESTERTERP-PLANTENGA, M. S., WOUTERS, L. and TEN HOOR, F. (1991), Restrained eating, obesity, and cumulative food intake curves during four course meals. *Appetite*, **16**, 149–58.

18 HEATHERTON, T. F., HERMAN, C. P., POLIVY, J., KING, G. A. and MCGREE, S. T. (1988), The (mis)measurement of restraint; an analysis of conceptual and psychometric issues. *J. Abn. Psych.*, **97** (1), 19–28.

19 TUSCHL, R. J., PLATTE, P., LAESSLE, R. G., STICHLER, W. and PIRKE, K. M. (1990), Energy expenditure and every day eating behavior in healthy young women. *Am. J. Clin. Nutr.*, **52**, 81–6.

20 WESTERTERP-PLANTENGA, M. S, KEMPEN, K. P. G. and SARIS, W. H. M. (1998), Determinants of weight maintenance in women after diet-induced weight reduction. *Int. J. Obes. Relat. Metab. Dis.*, **22**, 1–6.

21 LEJEUNE, M. P. G. M., HUKSHORN, C. J., SARIS, W. H. M. and WESTERTERP-PLANTENGA, M. S. (2003), Effect of dietary restraint during and following pegylated recombinant leptin treatment (PEG-OB) of overweight men. *Int. J. Obes. Relat. Metab. Disord.*, **27**, 1494–9.

22 LEJEUNE, M. P. G. M., VAN AGGEL-LEIJSSEN, D. P. C., VAN BAAK, M. A. and WESTERTERP-PLANTENGA, M. S. (2003), Effects of dietary restraint versus exercise during weight maintenance in obese men. *Eur. J. Clin. Nutr.*, **57**, 1338–44.

23 WESTERTERP, K. R. and ELBERS, J. M. H. (1999), Gender differences, energy balance, and effects of sex steroid hormones on circulating leptin levels. In: Westerterp-Plantenga M. S., Steffens A. B. and Tremblay A. (eds). *Regulation of Food Intake and Energy Expenditure.* EDRA: Milan; pp. 305–24.

24 WESTERTERP, K. R. and GORAN, M. I. (1999), Age and energy balance. In: Westerterp-Plantenga M. S., Steffens A. B. and Tremblay A. (eds). *Regulation of Food Intake and Energy Expenditure.* EDRA: Milan; pp. 325–48.

25 WESTERTERP, K. R. (1999), Exercise and energy balance. In: Westerterp-Plantenga M. S., Steffens A. B. and Tremblay A. (eds). *Regulation of Food Intake and Energy Expenditure.* EDRA: Milan, pp. 349–61.

26 MELANSON, K. J., WESTERTERP-PLANTENGA, M. S., CAMPFIELD, L. A. and SARIS, W. H. M. (1999), Short term regulation of food intake in humans. In: Westerterp-Plantenga M. S., Steffens A. B. and Tremblay A. (eds). *Regulation of Food Intake and Energy Expenditure.* EDRA: Milan; pp. 37–58.

27 HETHERINGTON, M. and BLUNDELL, J. E. (1999), Eating disorders. In: Westerterp-Plantenga M. S., Steffens A. B. and Tremblay A. (eds). *Regulation of Food Intake and Energy Expenditure.* EDRA: Milan, pp. 98–121.

28 WESTERTERP-PLANTENGA, M. S., ROLLAND, V., WILSON, S. A. J. and WESTERTERP, K. R. (1999), Satiety related to 24h diet-induced thermogenesis during high protein/carbohydrate versus high fat diets, measured in a respiration chamber. *Eur. J. Clin. Nutr.*, **53**, 1–8.

29 WESTERTERP-PLANTENGA, M. S. and VERWEGEN, C. R. T. (1999), The appetizing effect of an alcohol aperitif in overweight and normal weight humans. *Am. J. Clin. Nutr.*, **69**, 205–12.

30 WESTERTERP-PLANTENGA, M. S., KOVACS, E. M. R. and MELANSON, K. J. (2002), Habitual meal frequency and energy intake regulation in partially temporally isolated men. *Int. J. Obes. Relat. Metab. Disord.*, **26**, 102–10.

31 CAMPFIELD, L. A. and SMITH, F. J. (1999), OB Protein pathway – a link between adipose tissue mass and central neural networks. In: Westerterp-Plantenga M. S., Steffens A. B. and Tremblay A. (eds). *Regulation of Food Intake and Energy Expenditure.* EDRA: Milan, pp. 85–98.

32 STEFFENS, A. B. and VAN DIJK, G. (1999), Central nervous control of food intake, metabolism, and body weight. In: Westerterp-Plantenga M. S., Steffens A. B. and Tremblay A. (eds). *Regulation of Food Intake and Energy Expenditure.* EDRA: Milan, pp. 121–34.

33 ROTH, C., WILKEN, B., HANEFELD, F., SCHROTER, W. and LEONHARDT, U. (1998), Hyperphagis in children with craniopharyngioma is associated with hyperleptinaemia and a failure in the downregulation of appetite. *Eur. J. Endocrinol.*, **138**, 89–91.

34 ROLLS, E. T. (1999), Taste and olfactory processing in the brain, and its relation to the regulation of food intake. In: Westerterp-Plantenga M. S., Steffens A. B. and Tremblay A. (eds). *Regulation of Food Intake and Energy Expenditure.* EDRA: Milan, pp. 19–36.

35 ROLLS, E. T., MURZI, E., YAXLEY, S., THORPE, S. J. and SIMPSON, S. J. (1986), Sensory-specific satiety: food-specific reduction in responsiveness of ventral forebrain neurons after feeding in the monkey. *Brain. Res.*, **368**, 79–86.

36 ROLLS, E. T., SIENKIEWICZ, Z. J. and YAXLEY, S. (1989), Hunger modulates the responses to gustatory stimuli of single neurons in the orbitofrontal cortex. *Eur. J. Neurosci.*, **1**, 53–60.

37 CRITCHLEY, H. D. and ROLLS, E. T. (1996), Hunger and satiety modify the responses of olfactory and visual neurons in the primate orbitofrontal cortex. *J. Neurophysiol.*, **75**, 1673–86.

38 ROLLS, B. J., ROLLS, E. T., ROWE, E. A. and SWEENEY, K. (1981), Sensory-specific satiety in man. *Physiol. Behav.*, **27**, 137–42.

39 GILBERTSON, T. A., FONTENOT, T., LIU, L., ZHANG, H. and MONROE, W. T. (1997), Fatty acid modulation of K^+ channels in taste receptor cells: gustatory cues for dietary fat. *Am. J. Physiol.*, **272**, C1203–10.

40 GILBERTSON, T. A., LIU, L., YORK, D. A. and BRAY, G. A. (1998), Dietary fat preferences are inversely correlated with peripheral gustatory fatty acid sensitivity. *Ann. N. Y. Acad. Sci.*, **855**, 165–8.

41 KAMPHUIS, M. M. J. W., WESTERTERP-PLANTENGA, M. S. and SARIS, W. H. M. (2001), Fat specific satiety in humans for fat high in linoleic acid versus fat high in oleic acid. *Eur. J. Clin. Nutr.*, **55**, 499–508.

42 KAMPHUIS, M. M. J. W. and WESTERTERP-PLANTENGA, M. S. (2001), Taste perception of free fatty acids, i.e. CLA. *Int. J. Obes. Rel. Metab. Disord.*, **25**, S51.

43 VAN ITALLIE, T. B. (1990), The glucostatic theory 1953–1988: Roots and branches. *Int. J. Obes. Rel. Metab. Disord.*, **14**, 1–10.

44 BRAY, G. A. (1996), Static theories in a dynamic world: a glucodynamic theory of food intake. *Obes. Res.*, **4**, 489–92.

45 LEATHWOOD, P. and POLLET, P. (1998), Effects of slow release carbohydrates in the form of bean flakes on the evolution of hunger and satiety in man. *Appetite*, **10**, 1–11.

46 MELANSON, K. J., WESTERTERP-PLANTENGA, M. S., SARIS, W. H. M. and CAMPFIELD, L. A. (1999), Blood glucose patterns and appetite in time-blinded humans: carbohydrate versus fat. *Am. J. Physiol.*, **77** (Regulatory Integrative Comp. Physiol. 46): R337–45.

47 FRENCH, S. J., MURRAY, B., RUMSEY, R. D. E., SEPPLE, C. P. and READ, N. W. (1993), Is cholecystokinin a satiety hormone? Correlations of plasma cholecystokinin with hunger, satiety and gastric emptying in normal volunteers. *Appetite*, **21**, 95–104.

48 SMITH, G. P. and GIBBS, J. (1985), The satiety effect of cholecystokinin: recent progress and current problems. *Ann. N. Y. Acad. Sci.*, **448**, 424–30.

49 KISSILEFF, H. R., PI-SUNYER, F. X., THORNTON, J. and SMITH, G. P. (1981), C-terminal octapeptide of cholecystokinin decreases food intake in man. *Am. J. Clin. Nutr.*, **34**, 154–60.

50 RICHARD, D. (1993), Involvement of corticotrophin-releasing factor in the control of food intake and energy expenditure. *Ann. N. Y. Acad. Sci.*, **456**, 155–72.

51 RICHARD, D. (1995), Exercise and the neurobiological control of food intake and energy expenditure. *Int. J. Obes. Rel. Metab. Disord.*, **19**, S73–9.

52 RIVEST, S. and RICHARD, D. (1990), Involvement of corticotrophin-releasing factor in the anorexia induced by exercise. *Brain Res. Bull.*, **25**, 169–72.

53 BERGH, C. and SODERSTEN, P. (1996), Anorexia nervosa, self-starvation and the reward of stress. *Nature Med.*, **2**, 21–2.

54 ADRIAN, T. E., ALLEN, J. M., BLOOM, S. R. *et al.* (1983), Neuropeptide Y distribution in the human brain. *Nature*, **306**, 584–6.

55 WOODS, S. C. (1986), Central nervous system control of nutrient homeostasis. In: Bloom F. (ed). *Handbook of Physiology, Section I: The Nervous System Volume 4, Intrinsic Regulatory Systems of the Brain.* American Physiological Society: Bethesda MD, pp. 365–411.

56 STRUBBE, J. H. (1994), Circadian rhythms of food intake. In: Westerterp-Plantenga M. S., Fredrix E. W. H. M. and Steffens A. B. (eds). *Food Intake and Energy Expenditure.* CRC Press: London., pp. 155–174.

57 MAYER, J. M. (1952), The glucostatic theory of regulation of food intake and the problem of obesity. *Bull. N. Engl. Med. Cent.*, **14**, 43–9.

58 MAYER, J. M. (1953), Glucostatic mechanisms in the regulation of food intake. *N. Engl. J. Med.*, **249**, 13–6.

59 MAYER, J. M. (1955), Regulation of energy intake and body weight, the glucostatic theory and the lipostatic hypothesis. *Ann. N. Y. Acad. Sci.*, **63**, 15–43.

60 LANGHANS, W. (1999), Metabolic control of food intake. Role of the liver. In: Westerterp-Plantenga M. S., Steffens A. B. and Tremblay A. (eds). *Regulation of Food Intake and Energy Expenditure.* EDRA: Milan, pp. 185–99.

61 HINDERLING, V. B., SCHRAUWEN, P., LANGHANS, W. and WESTERTERP-PLANTENGA, M. S. (2002), The effect of Etomoxir on 24 h substrate oxidation and satiety in humans. *Am. J. Clin. Nutr.*, **76**, 141–7.

62 KEPLER, C. R., TUCKER, W. P. and TOVE, S. B. (1970), Biohydrogenation of unsaturated fatty acids. IV. Substrate specificity and inhibition of linoleate delta-12-*cis*, delta-11-*trans*-isomerase from *Butyrivibrio fibrisolvens*. *J. Biol. Chem.*, **245** (14), 3612–20.

63 KEPLER, C. R., TUCKER, W. P. and TOVE, S. B. (1971), Biohydrogenation of unsaturated fatty acids. V. Stereospecificity of proton addition and mechanism of action of linoleic acid delta 12-*cis*, delta 11-*trans*-isomerase from *Butyrivibrio fibrisolvens*. *J. Biol. Chem.*, **246** (9), 2765–71.

64 PARK, Y., ALBRIGHT, K. J., LIU, W., STORKSON, J. M., COOK, M. E. and PARIZA, M. W. (1997), Effect of conjugated linoleic acid on body composition in mice. *Lipids*, **32** (8), 853–8.

65 WEST, D. B., DELANY, J. P., CAMET, P. M., BLOHM, F., TRUETT, A. A. and SCIMECA, J. (1998), Effects of conjugated linoleic acid on body fat and energy metabolism in the mouse. *Am. J. Physiol.*, **275**, R667–72.

66 PARK, Y., STORKSON, J. M., ALBRIGHT, K. J., LIU, W. and PARIZA, M. W. (1999), Evidence that the *trans*-10,*cis*-12 isomer of conjugated linoleic acid induces body composition changes in mice. *Lipids*, **34** (3), 235–41.

67 PARK, Y., ALBRIGHT, K. J., STORKSON, J. M., LIU, W., COOK, M. E. and PARIZA, M. W. (1999), Changes in body composition in mice during feeding and withdrawal of conjugated linoleic acid. *Lipids*, **34** (3), 243–8.

68 DELANY, J. P., BLOHM, F., TRUETT, A. A., SCIMECA, J. A. and WEST, D. B. (1999), Conjugated linoleic acid rapidly reduces body fat content in mice without affecting energy intake. *Am. J. Physiol.*, **276**, R1172–9.

69 AZAIN, M. J., HAUSMAN, D. B., SISK, M. B., FLATT, W. P. and JEWELL, D. E. (2000), Dietary conjugated linoleic acid reduces rat adipose tissue cell size rather than cell number. *J. Nutr.*, **130** (6), 1548–54.

70 WEST, D. B., BLOHM, F. Y., TRUETT, A. A. and DELANY, J. P. (2000), Conjugated linoleic acid persistently increases total energy expenditure in AKR/J mice without increasing uncoupling protein gene expression. *J. Nutr.*, **130** (10), 2471–7.

71 SISK, M. B., HAUSMAN, D. B., MARTIN, R. J. and AZAIN, M. J. (2001), Dietary conjugated linoleic acid reduces adiposity in lean but not obese Zucker rats. *J. Nutr.*, **131** (6), 1668–74.

72 MINER, J. L., CEDERBERG, C. A., NIELSEN, M. K., CHEN, X. and BAILE, C. A. (2001), Conjugated linoleic acid (CLA), body fat, and apoptosis. *Obes. Res.*, **9** (2), 129–34.

73 OHNUKI, K., HARAMIZU, S., OKI, K., ISHIHARA, K. and FUSHIKI, T. (2001), A single oral administration of conjugated linoleic acid enhanced energy metabolism in mice. *Lipids*, **36** (6), 583–7.

74 BLANKSON, H., STAKKESTAD, J. A., FAGERTUN, H., THOM, E., WADSTEIN, J. and GUDMUNDSEN, O. (2000), Conjugated linoleic acid reduces body fat mass in overweight and obese humans. *J. Nutr.*, **130** (12), 2943–8.

75 MOUGIOS, V., MATSAKAS, A., PETRIDOU, A. *et al.* (2001), Effect of supplementation with conjugated linoleic acid on human serum lipids and body fat. *J. Nutr. Biochem.*, **12**, 585–94.

76 RISERUS, U., BERGLUND, L. and VESSBY, B. (2001), Conjugated linoleic acid (CLA) reduced abdominal adipose tissue in obese middle-aged men with signs of the metabolic syndrome: a randomised controlled trial. *Int. J. Obes. Relat. Metab. Disord.*, **25** (8), 1129–35.

77 BERVEN, G., BYE, A., HALS, O. *et al.* (2000), Safety of conjugated linoleic acid (CLA) in overweight and obese human volunteers. *Eur. J. Lipid. Sci. Technol.*, **102**, 455–62.

78 ZAMBELL, K. L., KEIM, N. L., VAN LOAN, M. D. *et al.* (2000), Conjugated linoleic acid supplementation in humans: effects on body composition and energy expenditure. *Lipids.*, **35** (7), 777–82.

79 SMEDMAN, A. and VESSBY, B. (2001), Conjugated linoleic acid supplementation in humans – metabolic effects. *Lipids*, **36** (8), 773–81.

80 CHOI, Y., KIM, Y. C., HAN, Y. B., PARK, Y., PARIZA, M. W. and NTAMBI, J. M. (2000), The *trans*-10,*cis*-12 isomer of conjugated linoleic acid downregulates stearoyl-CoA desaturase 1 gene expression in 3T3-L1 adipocytes. *J. Nutr.*, **130** (8), 1920–4.

81 KAMPHUIS, M. M. J. W., LEJEUNE, M. P. G. M., SARIS, W. H. M. and WESTERTERP-PLANTENGA, M. S. (2003), The effect of conjugated linoleic acid supplementation after weight loss on body weight regain, body composition, and resting metabolic rate in overweight subjects. *Int. J. Obes. Relat. Metab. Disord.*, **27** (7), 840–7.

82 KAMPHUIS, M. M. J. W., LEJEUNE, M. P. G. M., SARIS, W. H. M. and WESTERTERP-PLANTENGA, M. S. (2003), Effect of conjugated linoleic acid supplementation after weight loss on appetite and food intake in overweight subjects. *Eur. J. Clin. Nutr.*, **57** (10), 1268–74.

83 KAWADA, T., HAGIHARA, K. and IWAI, K. (1986), Effects of capsaicin on lipid metabolism in rats fed high fat diet. *J. Nutr.*, **116**, 1272–8.

84 KAWADA, T., SAKABE, S., WATANABE, T., YAMAMOTO, M. and IWAI, K. (1988), Some pungent principles of spices cause the adrenal medulla to secrete catecholamine in anesthesized rats. *Proc. Soc. Exp. Biol. Med.*, **188**, 229–33.

85 YOSHIOKA, M., LIM, K., KIKUZATO, S. *et al.* (1995), Effects of red-pepper diet on the energy metabolism in men. *J. Nutr. Sci. Vitaminol.*, **41**, 647–56.

86 YOSHIOKA, M., ST-PIERRE, S., SUZUKI, M. and TREMBLAY, A. (1998), Effects of red pepper added to high-fat and high-carbohydrate meals on energy metabolism and substrate utilization in Japanse women. *Br. J. Nutr.*, **80**, 503–10.

87 YOSHIOKA, M., ST-PIERRE, S., DRAPEAU, V. *et al.* (1999), Effects of red pepper on appetite and energy intake. *Br. J. Nutr.*, **82**, 115–23.

88 YOSHIOKA, M., DOUCET, E., DRAPEAU, V., DIONNE, I. and TREMBLAY, A. (2001), Combined effects of red pepper and caffeine consumption on 24 h energy balance in subjects given free access to foods. *Br. J. Nutr.*, **85**, 203–11.

89 LEJEUNE, M. P. G. M., KOVACS, E. M. R. and WESTERTERP-PLANTENGA, M. S. (2003), Effect of capsaicin on substrate oxidation and weight maintenance after modest body weight loss in human subject. *Br. J. Nutr.*, **90**, 651–9.

90 WESTERTERP-PLANTENGA, M. S., SMEETS, A. and LEJEUNE, M. P. G. M. (2004), Oral and gastro-intestinal satiety effects of capsaicine on food intake. *Appetite*, **42**, 408.

91 DULLOO, A. G., SEYDOUX, J. and GIRARDIER, L. (1992), Potentiation of the thermogenic antiobesity effects of ephedrine by dietary methylxanthines: adenosine antagonism or phosphodiesterase inhibition? *Metabolism*, **41**, 1233–41.

92 DULLOO, A. G., GEISSLER, C. A., HORTON, T., COLLINS, A. and MILLER, D. S. (1989), Normal caffeine consumption: influence on thermogenesis and daily energy expenditure in lean and postobese human volunteers. *Am. J. Clin. Nutr.*, **49**, 44–50.

93 ASTRUP, A., TOUBRO, S., CANNON, S., HEIN, P., BREUM, L. and MADSEN, J. (1990), Caffeine: a double-blind, placebo-controlled study of its thermogenic, metabolic, and cardiovascular effects in healthy volunteers. *Am. J. Clin. Nutr.*, **51**, 759–67.

94 BRACCO, D., FERRARRA, J. M., ARNAUD, M. J., JEQUIER, E. and SCHUTZ, Y. (1995), Effects of caffeine on energy metabolism, heart rate, and methylxanthine metabolism in lean and obese women. *Am. J. Physiol.*, E671–8.

95 BORCHARDT, R. T. and HUBER, J. A. (1975), Catechol *O*-methyltransferase. Structure-activity relationships for inhibition by flavonoids. *J. Med. Chem.*, **18**, 120–2.

96 DULLOO, A. G., DURET, C., ROHRER, D. *et al.* (1999), Efficacy of a green tea extract rich in catechin polyphenols and caffeine in increasing 24-h energy expenditure and fat oxidation in humans. *Am. J. Clin. Nutr.*, **70**, 1040–5.

97 RUMPLER, W., SEALE, J., CLEVIDENCE, B. *et al.* (2001), Oolong tea increases metabolic rate and fat oxidation in men. *J. Nutr.*, **131**, 2848–52.

98 WESTERTERP-PLANTENGA, M. S., LEJEUNE, M. P. G. M. and KOVACS, E. M. R. (2003), Effect of green tea on body weight maintenance after body-weight loss as a function of habitual caffein intake. *Appetite*, **40**, 402.

99 KOVACS, E. M. R., LEJEUNE, M. P. G. M., NIJS, I. and WESTERTERP-PLANTENGA, M. S. (2004), Effects of green tea on weight maintenance after body-weight loss. *Br. J. Nutr.*, **91**, 431–7.

100 TAGUCHI, H., WATANABE, H., ONIZAWA, K. *et al.* (2000), Double-blind controlled study on the effects of dietary diacylglycerol on postprandial serum and chylomicron triacylglycerol responses in healthy humans. *J. Am. Coll. Nutr.*, **19**, 789–96.

101 WATANABE, H., ONIZAWA, K., TAGUCHI, H. *et al.* (1997), Effects of diacylglycerols on lipid metabolism in human. *Nippon. Yukagaku. Kaishi.*, **46**, 309–14.

102 HARA, K., ONIZAWA, K., HONDA, H., OTSUJI, K., IDE, T. and MURATA, M. (1993), Dietary diacylglycerol-dependent reduction in serum triacylglycerol concentration in rats. *Ann. Nutr. Metab.*, **37**, 185–91.

103 MURATA, M., IDE, T. and HARA, K. (1997), Reciprocal responses to dietary diacylglycerol of hepatic enzymes of fatty acid synthesis and oxidation in the rat. *Br. J. Nutr.*, **77**, 107–21.

104 YAMAMOTO, K., ASAKAWA, H., TOKUNAGA, K. *et al.* (2001), Long-term ingestion of dietary diacylglycerol lowers serum triacylglycerol in type II diabetic patients with hypertriglyceridemia. *J. Nutr.*, **131**, 3204–7.

105 WATANABE, H., ONIZAWA, K., TAGUCHI, H. *et al.* (1997), Nutritional characterization of diacylglycerols in rats. *J. Japan. Oil. Chem. Soc.*, **46**, 301–7.

106 MURASE, T., MIZUNO, T., OMACHI, T. *et al.* (2001), Dietary diacylglycerol suppresses high fat and high sucrose diet- induced body fat accumulation in C57BL/6J mice. *J. Lipid. Res.*, **42**, 372–8.

107 NAGAO, T., WATANABE, H., GOTO, N. *et al.* (2000), Dietary diacylglycerol suppresses accumulation of body fat compared to triacylglycerol in men in a double-blind controlled trial. *J. Nutr.*, **130**, 792–7.
108 WATANABE, H., NAGAO, T., GOTO, N. *et al.* (1998), Long-term effects of dietary diacylglycerols on body fat metabolism in man. *Nippon. Yukagaku. Kaishi.*, **47**, 369–76.
109 TAGUCHI, H., NAGAO, T., WATANABE, H. *et al.* (2001), Energy value and digestibility of dietary oil containing mainly 1,3-diacylglycerol are similar to those of triacylglycerol. *Lipids*, **36**, 379–82.
110 KAMPHUIS, M. M. J. W., MELA, D. M. and WESTERTERP-PLANTENGA, M. S. (2003), Diacylglycerols affect substrate oxidation and appetite in humans. *Am. J. Clin. Nutr.*, **77** (5), 1133–9.
111 GOLDSTEIN, D. J. (1992), Beneficial effects of modest weight loss. *Int. J. Obes. Relat. Metab. Disord.*, **16**, 397–415.
112 WING, R. R., JEFFERY, R. W., BURTON, L. R., THORSON, C., KULLER, L. H. and FOLSOM, A. R. (1992), Change in waist–hip ratio with weight loss and its association with change in cardiovascular risk factors. *Am. J. Clin. Nutr.*, **55**, 1086–92.
113 GAAL, L. F., VAN WAUTERS, M. A. and DE LEEUW, I. H. (1997), The beneficial effects of modest weight loss on cardiovascular risk factors. *Int. J. Obes. Relat. Metab. Disord.*, **21**, S5–9.
114 WADDEN, T. A., STUNKARD, A. J. and LIEBSCHUTZ, J. (1998), Three-year follow-up of the treatment of obesity by very low calorie diet, behavior therapy, and their combination. *J. Consult. Clin. Psychol.*, **56**, 925–8.
115 KRAMER, F. M., JEFFERY, R. W, FORSTER, J. L. and SNELL, M. K. (1989), Long-term follow-up of behavioral treatment for obesity: patterns of weight regain among men and women. *Int. J. Obes. Relat. Metab. Disord.*, **13**, 123–36.
116 PASMAN, W. J., WESTERTERP-PLANTENGA, M. S., MULS, E., VANSANT, G., VAN REE, J. and SARIS, W. H. M. (1997), The effectiveness of long-term fiber supplementation on weight maintenance in weight reduced women. *Int. J. Obes. Relat. Metab. Disord.*, **21**, 548–55.
117 PASMAN, W. J., WESTERTERP-PLANTENGA, M. S. and SARIS, W. H. M. (1997), The effectiveness of long-term supplementation of carbohydrate, chromium, fiber and caffeine on weight maintenance. *Int. J. Obes. Relat. Metab. Disord.*, **21**, 1143–51.
118 PASMAN, W. J., SARIS, W. H. M., MULS, E., VANSANT, G. and WESTERTERP-PLANTENGA, M. S. (1999), The effect of exercise training on long-term weight maintenance in weight-reduced men. *Metabolism*, **48**, 15–21.
119 JEAN, C., ROME, S., MATHE, Y., *et al.* (2001), Metabolic evidence for adaptation to a high protein diet in rats. *J. Nutr.*, **131**, 91–8.
120 STOCK, M. J. (1999), Gluttony and thermogenesis revisited. *Int. J. Obes. Relat. Metab. Disord.*, **23**, 1105–17.
121 DULLOO, A. G.and JACQUET, J. (1999), Low-protein overfeeding: a tool to unmask susceptibility to obesity in humans. *Int. J. Obes. Relat. Metab. Disord.*, **23**, 1118–21.
122 WESTERTERP-PLANTENGA, M. S. (2003), The significance of protein in food intake and body-weight regulation. *Curr. Opin. Clin. Nutr. Metab. Care.*, **6**, 635–9.
123 WESTERTERP-PLANTENGA, M. S., LEJEUNE, M. P. G. M., NIJS, I., VAN OOIJEN, M. and KOVACS, E. M. R. (2004), High protein intake sustains weight maintenance after weight loss in humans. *Int. J. Obes. Relat. Metab. Disord.*, **28**, 57–64.
124 HOFSTEDE, G. (1984), *Cultures Consequences. International Differences in Work-Related Values*. New Delhi: Sage Publications.
125 VOGELS, N. and WESTERTERP-PLANTENGA, M. S. (2005), Categorical strategies based on subject characteristics of dietary restraint and physical activity, for weight maintenance. *Int. J. Obes.*, **29**, 849–57.
126 VOGELS, N., MARIMAN, E. C. M., BOUWMAN, F. G., KESTER, A. D. M., DIEPVENS, K. and WESTERTERP-PLANTENGA, M. S. (2005), Relationship of weight maintenance and dietary restraint with PPARY 2, GRL and CNTF polymorphisms. *Am. J. Clin. Nutr.* (in press).

24

A commercial R&D perspective on weight control foods and ingredients

D. J. Mela, Unilever Food & Health Research Institute, The Netherlands

24.1 Introduction

Chapters by Popkin and by van Trijp *et al.* in this volume indicate the magnitude of the weight control problem and its implications. Other chapters, particularly by Raynor and Wing and by Anderson and Konz, indicate the very great interest in weight control amongst consumers, and the wide range of different weight management plans, programmes and products available to them and health professionals. Lastly, additional chapters highlight a very wide array of compositional options and potential 'functional' agents and targets that might be used in selecting and constructing the formulations for commercial weight control products. Many of these are evaluated mainly from a perspective of basic research, which aims to understand the systems influencing energy balance and how these may be targeted and affected by specific ingredients. This chapter will adopt a slightly different perspective, considering where the basic science has taken us, and what is required to translate that information into effective and marketable commercial food products.

24.2 Commercial approaches to weight control

The epidemic of obesity has raised interest and commercial opportunities in three major types of consumer benefit areas:

(a) everyday weight control: 'weight-friendly' products
(b) active weight loss: products and plans for dieters

(c) control of co-morbidities: products to help reduce risk of obesity-related diseases.

24.2.1 'Weight-friendly' products

'Weight-friendly' products include everyday foods which are naturally low in energy content (e.g. waters, soups, vegetables), and the so-called 'diet' or 'light' versions of more energy-rich products (e.g. soft drinks, spreads). Public health approaches to weight control are aimed towards changing consumer behaviour to increase relative intakes from the former group, especially foods which are naturally low in energy and rich in nutrients. Commercial R&D tends to be focused on technology to enhance the appeal of this group of foods, but also to deliver technology for reducing energy content of higher-energy manufactured foods. Legislation relating to claims may help protect consumers, but can unfortunately also constrain innovation and marketing of both types of products. For example, draft European regulations have proposed that a 'low energy' claim would be allowed only on products with up to 0.4 kcal/g (1.7 kJ/g) for solids or 0.2 kcal/ml (0.8 kJ/ml) for liquids (Council of the European Union, 2004). These criteria would exclude 'low energy' claims for many unprocessed and relatively low energy density products such as apples, strawberries, peas, and lean fish and meats. On the other hand, the advantage of these criteria is that they allow manufacturers to identify and make claims for existing products which presently are not recognised (by marketers or consumers) as 'low energy', and also provide clear targets for product development.

To reduce the energy content of manufactured foods, the emphasis of technology is on making significant changes while still retaining the desired sensory quality and shelf-stability. Energy reduction, usually by replacement of fat or sugars, has long been a target for new product development, with obvious success in some segments (e.g. soft drinks, dairy) and less sustained success in others (e.g. savoury snacks, baked goods, confectionery). The types of problems encountered trying to successfully develop and market reduced-energy products are described by Parr *et al.* (2001). Legislation also affects the economic incentives for companies to reduce the energy content of products. For example, a significant change in product composition and quality may be required to meet a proposed 30% reduction in energy content needed for a 'reduced-energy' claim (e.g. Council of the European Union, 2004). Smaller reductions in energy content may be feasible and of benefit to consumers (especially if these occur across a broad range of standard products); however, this may incur considerable cost to the manufacturer (ingredient cost and sourcing, re-testing for acceptability and shelf-life, labelling, production line modifications, etc.), without them being able to recoup costs through marketing using 'reduced-energy' nutrition claims. The result is pressure toward an 'all or none' approach to reducing energy content in a relatively small number of manufactured foods, in place of more widespread but modest innovation. This also contributes toward the appearance of nutritionally impressive, but poorly accepted, reduced-energy versions of products. This, in turn, generates a negative spiral where consumers are apprehensive about the quality of products with 'low' or 'reduced-energy' claims, and commercial marketers hesitate to invest further in reducing the energy content of products.

'Weight-friendly' products are generally seen as beneficial for weight control simply because of their lower energy content per unit. Product claims are, in most cases, correspondingly limited to statements relating to energy content, perhaps with some proviso that they may only help weight control as a part of an energy-controlled diet. In some cases, these products are aligned with, or form the basis of, a commercial weight loss programme (see chapter by Raynor and Wing in this volume). Although it seems self-evident that increasing the availability and use of low or reduced-energy products should help in weight control (Lowe, 2003), evidence remains largely circumstantial (Rolls *et al.*, 2004; Poppitt and Prentice, 1996; see chapters in this volume by Stubbs *et al.*; Whybrow *et al.*; Miller-Jones *et al.*). Nevertheless, there remains a significant opportunity for both industry and consumers to benefit from marketing of appealing low- and reduced-energy everyday foods, and a challenge to companies to successfully develop and market these.

24.2.2 Active weight loss products and plans

Although not necessarily intrinsically different from products described in Section 24.2.1 above, products for weight loss may be distinguished by their marketing and claims, or clear alignment with specific weight control plans. In other words, they are not just marketed on their nutritional content, but depend upon consumers' beliefs in the functionality of the products for weight loss or maintenance. Where products are intended to be used within a particular weight loss programme, consumer involvement may be much higher than for the casual use of reduced-energy products.

Chapters in this book by Raynor and Wing and by Anderson and Konz describe much of the range of different commercial food plans and products. From a product formulation perspective, these may be classified as follows:

Energy control

Specific branded ranges of portion-controlled or low- or reduced-energy products intended to support flexible individual or commercial group weight control programmes.

Macronutrient control

Products based around reduction or enrichment in a particular component or characteristic of foods (e.g. low carbohydrate, high fibre, low glycemic index, etc.), usually aligned to specific popular weight control programmes which advocate this approach (rather than an emphasis on energy content).

Meal replacement
Fortified or nutritionally complete products intended to provide a structured and limited energy intake through partial or total replacement of self-selected foods.

Because the commercial success of these products is closely related to consumer beliefs in the value of a particular diet plan or approach, manufacturers have a much greater interest in scientific credibility and substantiation of efficacy, an issue considered in a following section.

24.2.3 Control of co-morbidities

Obesity is increasingly recognised as a serious health issue by both health professionals and individual consumers. It would be unrealistic to expect that the problem of obesity will disappear, so management of co-morbidities becomes an increasingly important and attractive area for food product innovation. For many years, food products have been available with claims relating to reduction of cardiovascular disease through cholesterol lowering. The staggering increase in prevalence of diabetes and the constellation of conditions known as the 'metabolic syndrome' (Meigs, 2002) will give increasing impetus to the development and mainstream marketing of products oriented toward managing risks associated with these. For example, it is estimated that about 35% of Americans born in the year 2000 will develop diabetes (Narayan *et al.*, 2003). Food formulations and ingredients that aid in management of blood glucose responses or perhaps insulin sensitivity will be of growing interest, along with control of blood pressure and lipid levels. At the very least, products oriented toward weight control will have to ensure they do not exacerbate these associated disease risks. The potential types of products and technologies behind them will not be considered further here, but may represent a growth area associated with the weight control foods market.

24.3 Formulating weight control products

Responsible and successful development of weight control products is driven towards products that fulfil three key aspects, relating to scientific substantiation, commercial execution and consumer behaviour:

(a) efficacy: does it really work when used as recommended?
(b) feasibility: can it be made into a successful commercial product?
(c) compliance: will consumers use it as recommended, on a sustained basis?

24.3.1 Formulation: ingredients

Variations in the composition of weight loss products may directly affect energy intake or expenditure, and products or plans may offer further advantages in convenience, taste etc., which affect degree and duration of compliance with individual or group weight loss programmes.

Macronutrient and energy content

A long history of research shows that relatively wide variations in the macronutrient composition of the diet have fairly marginal effects on loss or expenditure of energy through reduced absorption, increased excretion, or metabolic efficiency during weight maintenance or loss (see Chapter 5 of Mela and Rogers, 1998). This is confirmed in studies carried out under both highly controlled conditions or within the context of relatively free-living diet interventions (Brehm *et al.*, 2005; Diaz *et al.*, 2005; Verboeket-van de Venne *et al.*, 1996; Abbott *et al.*, 1988; Hill *et al.*, 1991; Hurni *et al.*, 1981; Lean and James, 1988; Leibel *et al.*, 1992; Yang and van Itallie, 1976). The main exception to this may be protein (Westerterp, 2004; chapter by Clifton in this volume), where small added energy losses could be of value in long-term weight maintenance, though this thermogenic effect probably adds little in the context of active weight loss diets. Nevertheless, at equal energy intakes, consumer-perceivable weight loss may be much greater at the start of a hypocaloric low carbohydrate diet, largely due to much greater water losses (Yang and van Itallie, 1976). This rapid early weight loss may be highly motivating to consumers, as evidence that the diet 'works', even though this does not really reflect the loss of body fat.

Together, the literature leads clearly to the conclusion that, even if energy expenditure is marginally increased through changes in macronutrient sources, overall energy balance on diets of different compositions largely or wholly reflects changes in energy intake. In other words, 'calories count', and diets largely work via their effects on food purchase and consumption behaviour. The pattern of intake can, of course, also have varying nutritional and health implications, and some products and plans are not nutritionally balanced in line with more general 'healthy eating' guidance (Freedman *et al.*, 2001; Kennedy *et al.*, 2001). However, regardless of macronutrient composition, the key factor for weight loss is ultimately intensity and duration of compliance with a reduced energy intake (Dansinger *et al.*, 2005). Other chapters of this book focus in depth on how variations in food composition (macronutrients, fibre, energy density, sensory characteristics, portion size) and their metabolism (fat oxidation, glycemic response) may influence feelings of hunger and freely-selected energy intake, and thereby enhance weight control.

The primary goal, therefore, for selection of the macronutrient and energy content of products, is to achieve reduced energy intake through a format and pattern of consumption that ensure overall good nutritional quality and balance, with a convenience, simplicity and acceptability (including effects on hunger and mood) that supports sustained use for weight loss and maintenance. Beyond this, selection of specific types and content of macronutrients, and possible 'functional' ingredients, may be used to confer added health benefits, improved appetite control, or small additional losses of energy through excretion or metabolism.

'Functional' ingredients

Many 'functional' weight control agents have been available in the form of food supplements or pills, and also proposed or used as ingredients for mainstream food products. Main targets for these, the types of ingredients available, and evidence of efficacy (or not) are reviewed elsewhere in this book (chapters by Westerterp-Plantenga; Leonhardt and Langhans) and several recent reviews (Kovacs and Mela, in press; St Onge, 2005; Pittler and Ernst, 2004; Saper *et al.*, 2004), and will not be considered here.

Functional ingredients may affect energy balance and weight control through three possible routes.

Reduce voluntary energy intake

Enhanced satiety or food intake control via action in the gut or post-absorptive (metabolic or central) action.

Interfere with energy uptake

Reduced energy absorption, usually by inhibition of gastrointestinal lipase or amylase (or saccharidase) activity, fat 'binding', or fat or carbohydrate modification.

Alter energy metabolism

Increased energy losses through thermogenesis, or through influencing nutrient partitioning (ratio of fat: lean tissue lost or gained).

Enhancement of satiety and appetite control seems to be the most attractive of these. It is a motivating and believable claim area, large and consumer-perceivable effects are possible, and there are many food components and compositions which can already be shown to affect these processes (at least in the short term). Interference with energy uptake has generally had limited application in foods, due to potential side effects and loss of micronutrients. Enhancement of metabolism may be most beneficial for weight maintenance rather than loss, because only relatively small effects are likely to be safe for extended periods. On the other hand, prevention of reduction in resting energy expenditure occurring during negative energy balance may provide more scope for metabolic agents to improve weight loss rates.

Overall, evidence for efficacy and safety of a variety agents proposed to act on each of these routes remains somewhat mixed. While there are a number of candidate agents with reasonable evidence of plausibility and (usually modest) efficacy, there is presently no 'magic bullet' with proven functionality and safety in foods. Unfortunately, in addition to some excellent research by established centres of expertise, the research literature is also cluttered with studies of questionable validity or inappropriate design and interpretation. The poor quality and dubious results of some commercially driven studies, often carried out in collaboration with 'rent-a-scientist' contract or academic researchers, tends to undermine the credibility of the entire functional foods area. In other cases, clinical weight control trials on specific agents have been carried out before enough is really known to select the appropriate study design and power. The tendency for 'cook and look' rather than hypothesis-driven research contributes to many inconsistent and sometimes irrelevant results. Section 24.4 considers these issues in greater depth.

24.3.2 Formulation: feasibility

Evidence of efficacy should be necessary, but is by no means sufficient, to make an ingredient or technology a good candidate for use in a commercial weight control products. Some proposed functional ingredients may demonstrate efficacy under certain conditions, but few are currently used in mass market foods. This is largely due to the different criteria, particularly the technical demands and regulatory standards, that are applied to food products in comparison with food supplements. In order for a functional food ingredient to be considered and accepted for mainstream food use, and a new food product to come to market, a number of criteria need to be satisfactorily addressed. These aspects are listed and described in Table 24.1, and commercial research and development programmes need to consider these in addition to the mechanistic and clinical data which are the focus of this review.

In addition to these practical considerations for development, there are major issues around the marketing execution of finished products, which can spell the difference between success and failure. An example of this is product placement within the retail setting. Should specially formulated weight loss products be mixed in amongst standard products, or in a separate area with foods for other special dietary needs, or perhaps with the personal care or cosmetics sections of a supermarket?

24.4 Efficacy testing of weight control products

Products orientated toward active weight control are marketed toward, and depend upon, consumer beliefs in efficacy. For a responsible commercial manufacturer, efficacy is the most fundamental criterion which a candidate active ingredient, product formulation, or plan should fulfil.

Table 24.1 Feasibility: factors influencing selection and application of ingredients and technologies for weight control products (Adapted from Kovacs and Mela (in press) with permission of Blackwell Publishers).

Quality and quantity of scientific support for efficacy	Regulatory agencies, including those involved in advertising standards and consumer protection, require that scientific evidence supports the product claims in the product as used by the intended target group. In addition, a record of clinical research published in mainstream scientific journals is needed to gain desired endorsement from recognised independent experts and organisations.
Safety and toxicology	A thorough safety dossier is required as part of due diligence as well as regulatory approval, and to reassure consumers and external experts. Unlike medications and supplements, where access can be controlled or warnings and contraindications stated on the label, foods must be safe for consumption by all healthy people, including children and pregnant or lactating women.
Regulatory approval for specific food compositions	Regulations often specify what levels, purpose, and product formats are allowable for a specific ingredient. These may limit amounts to a level below what is required for health benefits, or restrict use to less favourable product formats.
Sensory quality	Functional ingredients may impart unwanted tastes, flavours, colours or textures to products, either immediately or after processing or during shelf life. A range of secondary technologies (e.g. encapsulation, antioxidants, flavour masking agents) may be required to overcome this.
Stability (including processing and shelf-life)	Active ingredients must be shown to remain active and bioavailable after relevant processing steps (e.g. high shear or temperature) and through the product shelf-life. The added ingredients must also not diminish stability of the product itself, e.g. lead to more rapid loss of quality or microbial safety.
Sourcing (defined specification, source reliability, quality control)	Ingredients need to be reliably available to the product supply chain, in required quantities, in forms with known and stable composition, bioavailability and activity. This can be a particular problem for using plant extracts or with specialised ingredients or technologies where the number of suppliers or production capacity is limited. In the latter case, significant capital investments in new facilities may be required. Although this raises business risk, limited ingredient supply or high specifications can also act as a barrier against competitors.
Proprietary opportunities	There is a major competitive advantage for ingredients or technologies protected by patents or exclusive licensing arrangements. Concepts that can be readily copied are less likely to attract the investments needed to get them to market. This can be particularly problematic for 'natural'

	compounds and extracts, though there can still be proprietary opportunities, e.g. related to specific compositions with added benefits (such as improved stability or bioavailability), or more efficient production routes (implying greater profit margins for a particular producer).
Dosing level and schedule	In order to be effective in a food format, a functional ingredient must work within a dose level and pattern of intake which is feasible through foods. For example, if efficacy required ingestion several times a day at regularly spaced intervals, then delivery through food is problematic. If it must be taken before meals, then this also limits the range of suitable food formats. Ingredients that must be used at high levels (several grams) create problems for product formulation and quality.
Cost (of development and ingredient)	Cost margins for foods are considerably lower than for medications and supplements. A proven ingredient in a popular, trusted brand may command a significant price premium, but this is the exception in a generally price-competitive market. This means that sustained high sales volumes are usually required to recoup the investments in research and development. Those costs, plus costs of safety testing and regulatory approval processes, will also be much higher for novel ingredients and technologies.
Appropriate food vehicle (technical and ethical)	Certain ingredients may not be feasible or bioavailable in particular product formats, or require significant process or recipe modifications. Examples are lipid-based ingredients for very low-fat foods, aqueous ingredients for dry foods, or insoluble ingredients in beverages. Ethical issues may also determine the appropriate food carriers for functional ingredients or added nutrients, for example, whether it is appropriate to add these to foods which otherwise have a poor nutritional value or high energy content. Sometimes these can bring conflicting nutritional goals into focus, e.g. the addition of iron to chocolate confectionery popular with children and young adult women (groups at risk of iron deficiency), or a weight control ingredient in a popular but energy dense snack food format.
Marketing strategy and claims	Functional ingredients need to be aligned with the desired image of the brand or product. For example, an agent with an apparently drug-like activity may not be suitable for a brand characterised by 'natural' values. Similarly, ingredients are preferred if they can directly support a claim which is legally allowed, readily understood, and credible, meaningful and motivational to consumers.

24.4.1 Evidence base for efficacy of weight control approaches

The quality and quantity of evidence supporting particular weight control agents or approaches is inconsistent. Although publicly funded clinical and academic centres may carry out studies of diet composition, there is a strong bias in funding and publication toward conventional approaches with generally accepted credibility. Thus, for example, the period 1960 through 2000 produced an extensive literature on use of reduced-fat diets in weight control. However, up until the beginning of 2003, there had been virtually no major research group publishing first-quality studies of low-carbohydrate diets, and there are still few well-controlled long-term studies focussed specifically on high-protein interventions (Freedman *et al.*, 2001; Kennedy *et al.*, 2001; Tapper-Gardzina *et al.*, 2002).

Commercial backing is generally required and more common for assessments of specific programmes, food categories, products, or ingredients. Tsai and Wadden (2005) have recently noted the relative lack of evidence to support efficacy of a number of major commercial internet-based and self-help programmes. It might be argued that, since many programmes are largely intended to promote, guide and sustain consumer use of widely accepted dietary strategies, the question is not really one of efficacy, but of different techniques for gaining compliance with these. At the other extreme, there is an extensive series of studies supporting the effectiveness and safety of meal replacements (Heymsfield *et al.*, 2003; chapter by Anderson and Konz in this volume).

Unfortunately, there is also a very large number of putative weight control agents – mostly in the form of over-the-counter pills and food supplements – which lack even rudimentary supporting clinical evidence for their claims (Saper *et al.*, 2004). Indeed, in a continuing review of ingredients being sold over-the-counter, by mail order and on the internet, we (unpublished) found that about 50% either lack any supporting scientific evidence or have been tested and found not to be effective. Several others had only *in vitro* evidence of a plausible mechanism, and many had modes of action or chemical characteristics which would raise questions of safety and suitability for food use. In some areas of the world (including, increasingly, the United States), this proliferation of dubious products is due to weaknesses in regulatory systems, which allow for categories of products with unproven efficacy (e.g. Office of Dietary Supplements, 2005). However, even where regulations should prohibit many of the claims which are being made (e.g. in the European Union), local enforcement may be relatively lax or the system simply overwhelmed by the number of products appearing.

24.4.2 Approaches to efficacy testing

The gold standard for substantiation of efficacy is the randomised (placebo-)controlled intervention trial. However, studies of dietary or product intervention for weight control present some particular difficulties, relative to testing of single functional agents or drugs.

First, it is almost impossible to make studies 'blind' where the intervention is a programme, specific product type or overall dietary stategy. Thus, comparison against a fair and appropriate control is critical to interpretation. In the case of testing meal replacers (chapter by Anderson and Konz), the comparison is usually against a professionally delivered 'traditional' diet plan intended to achieve a similar energy intake, which allows a fair and conservative test against a real and appropriate alternative. A blind intervention or placebo control would simply not be possible.

There are, unfortunately, many situations where foods have been tested using designs which are unbalanced in a way that leaves serious questions about interpretation. For example, Wien *et al.* (2003) compare a fixed portion of energy from almonds to a freely selected portion of carbohydrate-rich foods. This design was then used to attribute benefits for body weight to the almonds rather than the structure that the almond condition imposed on subjects. Arguably, a more appropriate design would have been to make both conditions either fixed or freely selected. A similar approach is illustrated by studies such as Zemel *et al.* (2004). In this case, results from the use of (low energy) dairy products are ascribed to the specific effects of calcium intake or dairy products. A more likely explanation is that benefits derive from the general effect of inserting a set of low-energy products into the diet, which subjects may use in place of higher energy alternatives. Although this type of design may reasonably be seen as 'proof of product', it is certainly not proof of a specific ingredient or class of foods. More appropriate controls in this case would have been nutritionally equivalent products made from non-dairy sources or varied only in calcium content. Despite the alternative explanations for results in both of the examples here, these were used as the basis for extensive publicity about the putative weight control benefits of almonds and dairy products.

Second, it is useful to recognise that testing efficacy of many diet plans is really about testing compliance. As noted previously, many or most interventions of foods or diets work by facilitating or enhancing degree and duration of compliance with a reduced energy intake. As recently shown by Dansinger *et al.* (2005), differences in 'efficacy' of different diet approaches often can be reduced to a question of compliance. Although this may seem like a trivial distinction, it implies that greater success should be achieved with a diet plan where a given reduction in intake energy is simpler, more attractive or easier to maintain. As a result, these subjective characteristics will be major sources of variance in apparent diet efficacy, often more so than the nutritional composition.

Compared to the testing of whole foods or diets, testing of 'functional' ingredients should be much more straightforward in both execution and interpretation, since single agents lend themselves to a standard placebo-controlled design. However, there is a tendency to move too quickly to

Table 24.2 Efficacy: information used to maximise cost-efficiency and sensitivity in clinical weight control (weight change) trials of ingredients and products

Parameter	Application in clinical trials
Mechanism of action (e.g. appetite suppression or energy expenditure)	Basic study design (e.g. fixed or free energy intake) and selection of primary and secondary outcome measures (potential claims)
Bioavailability of active agent	Agent source, vehicle and dosage
Dose-response and duration of activity	Quantity, frequency, timing of agent
Expected change and variability in key outcome measures	Power calculations, study design, duration and subject numbers
Dietary interactions	Dietary regimen, timing and food format
Effectiveness in catabolic vs. anabolic conditions	Basic study design (e.g. weight loss vs. weight re-gain)
Anticipated/desired product claims	Study design and primary outcome measures
Potential side effects	Secondary outcome measures (safety)
Target population and contraindications	Subject recruitment and screening

clinical weight loss trials, before researchers have sufficient information to determine how best to design an efficacy trial, or even whether such a trial is warranted.

Table 24.2 lists a number of factors which should, if at all possible, be established prior to undertaking a clinical weight loss efficacy trial. Such trials are time-consuming and extremely expensive; thus, there are considerable savings to be made from carrying out more basic research, which can enhance the sensitivity and probability of 'success' of a longer-term study. There are many examples where relatively inexpensive background research might have greatly helped to refine the sensitivity and increase the value of clinical trials. In some cases, this is as fundamental as knowing whether an agent affects intake, uptake or expenditure of energy – questions which are (compared to a long-term clinical trial) relatively simple and inexpensive to answer empirically.

For example, clinical studies of conjugated linoleic acid (CLA) in weight control have used a variety of designs and produced a large number of conflicting results (for reviews see Wang and Jones, 2004; Kovacs and Mela, in press). This may be partly attributed to the surprising gaps in knowledge of how CLA affects whole body substrate utilisation or perhaps appetite control in humans. Despite almost 10 years of cellular, animal and human clinical trials of CLA, there are, as of this writing, almost no published data on its proximate mode of action with regard to energy balance or body composition. Similarly, clinical trials with diglyceride-rich (DG) oils (e.g. Maki *et al.*, 2002) were apparently carried out in the absence of clear understanding on whether it affects human energy expenditure, appetite, or both. Data from a subsequent short-term experiment indicates that DG is more likely to affect appetite control than energy expenditure (Kamphuis *et al.*, 2003). This information could have been used to improve the sensitivity and generate support for claims in the earlier clinical trial, for example by using a freely chosen rather than prescribed energy intake, and including secondary measures (leading to potential claims) relating to feelings of hunger and satiety. As a last example, there have also been several clinical weight loss trials of chitin, a putative dietary fat 'binder', leading to mostly negative results (e.g. Ernst and Pittler, 1998; Pittler *et al.*, 1999; Schiller *et al.*, 2001; Ni Mhurchu *et al.*, 2004). Much of that cost and effort might be saved by first just assessing whether chitosan actually has a meaningful effect on fat excretion – apparently it does not (Gades and Stern, 2002; 2003; Guerciolini *et al.*, 2001).

24.5 Summary and conclusions

There are opportunities to benefit consumers through a wide range of commercial products and plans that help in weight loss and control. Key goals for R&D in responsible companies are to develop products and plans that are proven safe and effective, that can be effectively and profitably executed through commercial production and marketing, and that gain and maintain sustained use by consumers. In most cases, products for active weight loss will work by offering consumers relatively simple, acceptable, and sustainable approaches to reducing energy intake. 'Functional' ingredients may add modestly to this, especially where they help in reducing food intake and related feelings of hunger and food deprivation.

Moving from a formulation idea to a real product requires that many issues of feasibility are satisfied, from scientific substantiation, through material sourcing and manufacturing production, to brand image and marketing claims. Testing of efficacy in appropriately designed and controlled studies is critical to making honest and attractive claims. Understanding how an ingredient or product works and what claims are desired can help to design resource-efficient trials with more power to convincingly demonstrate efficacy and support product promotion.

24.6 Future trends

> 'Prediction is very difficult, especially of the future'
>
> (Niels Bohr).

There has always been an ebb and flow of fashion in commercial diet products and plans, reflecting emerging science, celebrity or diet 'guru' endorsement, media hype, and the desire of consumers to believe that the next new diet will deliver their goal of a slim body with minimal effort.

With regard to macronutrients, recent years have seen marked swings from an emphasis on low fat foods, followed by a brief but dramatic rebound in the use of low carbohydrate diets, leading at this moment of writing to a growing interest in carbohydrate quality (e.g. diets based on glycemic index) and higher protein intakes. The latter is also stimulating a renewed focus on specific amino acids and their ratios (e.g. Layman, 2003). These trends, too, may be taken briefly to extremes, before the settling down to credible claims based on an appropriate balance of safety and efficacy.

Other benefit areas are likely to begin to take on added importance in the weight control market. As noted previously, the emerging epidemic of diabetes and 'metabolic syndrome' will be a factor in selection of macronutrient profiles and potential functional agents. Formulations and ingredients that can be convincingly shown to maximise body lean:fat ratio will also be a focus of continued research. This is taking on added importance with the ageing of Western populations, where loss of lean body mass is seen as a major contributor to frailty (Bales and Ritchie, 2002), paradoxically occurring side-by-side with increasing obesity in older adults (Roubenoff, 2004).

Services to support weight control are popular, although in some cases the appropriate business model is still unclear. A number of examples are available for monitoring of diet or activity, individually-tailored (internet-based) feedback, on-line clubs and support groups etc. Current research in genetics and genomics raises the possibility of improved personalisation of individual dietary advice, although there are no well-substantiated examples of this in the weight control area (e.g. Viguerie *et al.*, 2005). Despite optimistic predictions (Marti *et al.*, 2004), there are also serious questions of how realistic and effective this would be, and significant possibilities for diagnostic services to intentionally or unintentionally mislead consumers. Although such testing by itself may be quite interesting and motivating for consumers, responsible companies and regulators will have to be convinced of the reliability, sensitivity and specificity of the tests, and the degree to which they really improve weight control success.

We can expect to see increasing segmentation of the weight control market, in terms of consumers and benefits. In particular, with the dramatic rise in child obesity, there are significant needs and opportunities for weight control solutions appropriate for use within families. The weight control food market has also been largely oriented toward women, and there remains a challenge to design products and marketing strategies to increase uptake by men. Lastly, there may be increasing differentiation between products for active weight loss vs. subsequent weight maintenance (prevention of regain).

24.7 Implications and recommendations

The key determinant of outcomes from any weight control diet, regardless of composition or putative rationale, is compliance.

Oddly, though, this rather obvious conclusion is not reflected in the world of weight control research. Weight loss trials still collect and report mountains of physiological, anthropometric, dietary and clinical chemical data. Yet it is surprisingly rare to see any corresponding quantitative data on the subjective 'experience' of dieting and its link to compliance or outcomes. How (un)pleasant, easy/difficult, (in)convenient was it? How hungry did people feel? What were the effects on their mood or perceived 'energy' levels? These data are easily and reliably collected and analyzed (certainly in comparison to the ever-dubious dietary intakc data), are likely to have important explanatory power, and can be used to underpin attractive product claims. Even where diets produce similar rates of weight loss (which often happens in trials using highly motivated subjects and regular clinical follow-up), these types of 'soft' measures may still differentiate between diets and individuals. This can tell us something about which approaches might be more readily maintained and, therefore, successful in the real world.

Increasingly, the question for nutritionists and food companies is not 'Does this (. . . low-carb, low-fat, high fibre, etc., etc.) diet/plan work?' We know diet plans *can* work, so long as energy intake is less than expenditure. The real issues are, therefore, about designing plans and products that *will* work. This means thinking about foods, rather than just nutrients. It means making the experience as pleasant, easy and convenient as possible, within a nutritional context that is proven effective, balanced and sustainable. In other words, what the science ultimately tells us is that we need to put more effort into evaluating weight control from the perspective of the consumer.

24.8 References

ABBOTT, W. G., HOWARD, B. V., CHRISTIN, L. *et al.*, (1988), 'Short-term energy balance: relationship with protein, carbohydrate, and fat balances', *Am. J. Physiol.*, **255** (3 Pt 1), E332–7.

BALES, C. W. and RITCHIE, C. S. (2002), 'Sarcopenia, weight loss, and nutritional frailty in the elderly', *Ann. Rev. Nutr.*, **22**, 309–23.

BREHM, B. J., SPANG, S. E., LATTIN, B. L., SEELEY, R. J., DANIELS, S. R. and D'ALESSIO, D. A. (2005), 'The role of energy expenditure in the differential weight loss in obese women on low-fat and low-carbohydrate diets', *J. Clin. Endocrinol Metab.*, **90** (3), 1475–82.

COUNCIL OF THE EUROPEAN UNION (2004), 'Proposal for a Regulation of the European Parliament and of the Council on nutrition and health claims made on foods'. www.ihta.org/content/CouncilClaims17Feb.pdf. Accessed 8 April 2005.

DANSINGER, M. L., GLEASON, J. A., GRIFFITH, J. L., SELKER, H. P. and SCHAEFER, E. J. (2005), 'Comparison of the Atkins, Ornish, Weight Watchers, and Zone diets for weight loss and heart disease risk reduction: a randomized trial', *JAMA*, **293** (1), 43–53.

DIAZ, E., GALGANI, J., AGUIRRE, C., ATWATER, I. J. and BURROWS, R. (2005), 'Effect of glycemic index on whole-body substrate oxidation in obese women', *Int. J. Obes. Relat. Metab. Disord.*, **29** (1), 108–14.

ERNST, E. and PITTLER, M. H. (1998), 'Chitosan as a treatment for body weight reduction? A meta-analysis', *Perfusion*, **11**, 461–5.

FREEDMAN, M. R., KING, J. and KENNEDY, E. (2001), 'Popular diets: A scientific review', *Obes. Res.*, **9** (Suppl. 1), 1S–40S.

GADES, M. D. and STERN, J. S. (2002), 'Chitosan supplementation does not affect fat absorption in healthy males fed a high-fat diet, a pilot study', *Int. J. Obes. Relat. Metab. Disord.*, **26** (1), 119–22.

GADES, M. D. and STERN, J. S. (2003), 'Chitosan supplementation and fecal fat excretion in men', *Obes. Res.*, **11**, 683–8.

GUERCIOLINI, R., RADU-RADULESCU, L., BOLDRIN, M., DALLAS, J. and MOORE, R. (2001), 'Comparative evaluation of fecal fat excretion induced by orlistat and chitosan', *Obes. Res.*, **9** (6), 364–7.

HEYMSFIELD, S. B., VAN MIERLO, C. A., VAN DER KNAAP, H. C., HEO, M. and FRIER, H. I. (2003), 'Weight management using a meal replacement strategy: meta and pooling analysis from six studies', *Int. J. Obes. Relat. Metab. Disord.*, **27** (5), 537–49.

HILL, J. O., PETERS, J. C., REED, G. W., SCHLUNDT, D. G., SHARP, T. and GREENE, H. L. (1991), 'Nutrient balance in humans: effects of diet composition', *Am. J. Clin. Nutr.*, **54**, 10–7.

HURNI, M., BURNAND, B., PITTET, P. H. and JÉQUIER, E. (1982), 'Metabolic effects of a mixed and a high-carbohydrate low-fat diet in man, measured over 24 h in a respiration chamber', *Br. J. Nutr.*, **47**, 33–43.

KAMPHUIS, M. M., MELA, D. J. and WESTERTERP-PLANTENGA, M. S. (2003), 'Diacylglycerols affect substrate oxidation and appetite in humans', **77** (5), 1133–9.

KENNEDY, E. T., BOWMAN, S. A., SPENCE, J. T., FREEDMAN, M. and KING, J. (2001), 'Popular diets: correlation to health, nutrition, and obesity', *J. Am. Diet. Assoc.*, **101** (4), 411–20.

KOVACS, E. M. R. and MELA, D. J. (in press), 'Metabolically-active functional food ingredients for weight control', *Obes. Rev.*

LAYMAN, D. K. (2003), 'The role of leucine in weight loss diets and glucose homeostasis', *J. Nutr.*, **133** (1), 261S–7S.

LEAN, M. E. J. and JAMES, W. P. T. (1988), 'Metabolic effects of isoenergetic nutrient exchange over 24 hours on relation to obesity in women', *Int. J. Obes. Relat. Metab. Disord.* **12**, 15–27.

LEIBEL, R. L., HIRSCH, J., APPEL, B. E. and CHECANI, G. C. (1992), 'Energy intake required to maintain weight is not affected by wide variation in diet composition', *Am. J. Clin. Nutr.*, **55**, 350–5.

LOWE, M. R. (2003), 'Self-regulation of energy intake in the prevention and treatment of obesity: is it feasible?', *Obes. Res.*, **11** (suppl), 44S–59S.

MAKI, K. C., DAVIDSON, M. H. and TSUSHIMA, R. *et al.* (2002), 'Consumption of diacylglycerol oil as part of a reduced-energy diet enhances loss of body weight and fat in comparison with consumption of a triacylglycerol control oil', *Am. J. Clin. Nutr.*, **76** (6), 1230–6.

MARTI, A., MORENO-ALIAGA, M. J., HEBEBRAND, J. and MARTINEZ, J. A. (2004), 'Genes, lifestyle and obesity', *Int. J. Obes.*, **28**, S29–36.

MEIGS, J. B. (2002), 'Epidemiology of the Metabolic Syndrome, 2002', *Am. J. Manag. Care*, **8**, S283–92.

MELA, D. J. and ROGERS, P. J. (1998), *Food, Eating and Obesity: The Psychobiological Basis of Appetite and Weight Control*, London, Chapman & Hall.

NARAYAN, K. M., BOYLE, J. P., THOMPSON, T. J., SORENSEN, S. W. and WILLIAMSON, D. F. (2003), 'Lifetime risk for diabetes mellitus in the United States', *JAMA*, **8**, **290** (14), 1884–90.

NI MHURCHU, C., POPPITT, S. D., MCGILL, A-T, LEAHY, F. E., BENNETT, D. A., LIN, R. B., ORMROD, D., WARD, L., STRIK, C. and RODGERS, A. (2004), 'The effect of the dietary supplement, Chitosan, on body weight: a randomised controlled trial in 250 overweight and obese adults', *Int. J. Obes. Relat. Metab. Disord.*, **28**, 1149–56.

OFFICE OF DIETARY SUPPLEMENTS, NATIONAL INSTITUTES OF HELATH (2005), 'Dietary supplements: background information', http://ods.od.nih.gov/factsheets/DietarySupplements.asp#about. Accessed 3 April 2005.

PARR, H., KNOX, B. and HAMILTON, J. (2001), 'Problems and pitfalls in the reduced fat food product development process', *Food Indust. J.*, **102** (7), 50–60.

PITTLER, M. H., ERNST, E. (2004), 'Dietary supplements for body-weight reduction: a systematic review', *Am. J. Clin. Nutr.*, **79** (4), 529–36.

PITTLER, M. H., ABBOT, N. C., HARKNESS, E. F. and ERNST, E. (1999), 'Randomized, double-blind trial of chitosan for body weight reduction,' *Eur. J. Clin. Nutr.*, **53**, 379–81.

POPPITT, S. D. and PRENTICE, A. M. (1996), 'Energy density and its role in the control of food intake: evidence from metabolic and community studies', *Appetite*, **26**, 153–74.

ROLLS, B. J., ELLO-MARTIN, J. A. and TOHILL, B. C. (2004), 'What can intervention studies tell us about the relationship between fruit and vegetable consumption and weight management?', *Nutr. Rev.*, **62**, 1–17.

ROUBENOFF, R. (2004) 'Sarcopenic obesity: the confluence of two epidemics', *Obes. Res.*, **12** (6), 887–8.

SAPER, R. B., EISENBERG, D. M. and PHILLIPS, R. S. (2004), 'Common dietary supplements for weight loss', *Am. Fam. Physician*, **70** (9), 1731–8.

SCHILLER, R. N., BARRAGER, E., SCHAUSS, A. G. and NICHOLS, E. J. (2001), 'A randomized, double-blind, placebo-controlled study examining the effects of a rapidly soluble chitosan dietary supplement on weight loss and body composition in overweight and mildly obese individuals', *J. Am. Nutraceut. Assn.*, **4**, 34–41.

ST ONGE, M. P. (2005), 'Dietary fats, teas, dairy, and nuts: potential functional foods for weight control?', *Am. J. Clin. Nutr.*, **81** (1), 7–15.

TAPPER-GARDZINA, Y., COTUGNA, N. and VICKERY, C. E. (2002), 'Should you recommend a low-carb, high-protein diet?', *Nurse Practitioner*, April, 52–59.

TSAI, A. G. and WADDEN, T. A. (2005), 'Systematic review: an evaluation of major commercial weight loss programs in the United States', *Ann. Int. Med.*, **142** (1), 56–66.

VERBOEKET-VAN DE VENNE, W. P., WESTERTERP, K. R., HERMANS-LIMPENS, T. J., DE GRAAF, C., VAN HET HOF, K. H. and WESTSTRATE, J. A. (1996), 'Long-term effects of consumption of full-fat or reduced-fat products in healthy non-obese volunteers: assessment of energy expenditure and substrate oxidation', *Metabolism*, **45** (8), 1004–10.

VIGUERIE, N., VIDAL, H. AND ARNER, P. *et al.* (2005), 'Adipose tissue gene expression in obese subjects during low-fat and high-fat hypocaloric diets,' *Diabetologia*, **48** (1), 123–31.

WANG, Y. W. and JONES, P. J. H. (2004), 'Conjugated linoleic acid and obesity control: efficacy and mechanisms', *Int. J. Obes. Relat. Metab. Disord.*, **28**, 941–55.

WESTERTERP, K. R. (2004) 'Diet induced thermogenesis', *Nutr. Metab.*, **1**, 5 (doi:10.1186/1743-7075-1-5).

WIEN, M., SABATE, J. M., IKLE, D. N., COLE, S. E. and KANDEEL, F. R. (2003), 'Almonds vs. complex carbohydrates in a weight reduction programme', *Int. J. Obes.*, **27**, 1365–72.

YANG, M. U. and VAN ITALLIE, T. B. (1976), 'Composition of weight lost during short-term weight reduction. Metabolic responses of obese subjects to starvation and low-calorie ketogenic and nonketogenic diets', *J. Clin. Invest.*, **58** (3), 722–30.

ZEMEL, M. B., THOMPSON, W., MILSTEAD, A., MORRIS, K. and CAMPBELL, P. (2004), 'Calcium and dairy acceleration of weight and fat loss during energy restriction in obese adults', *Obes. Res.*, **12** (4), 582–90.

Index

LIBRARY, UNIVERSITY OF CHESTER